DEVELOPMENTAL MOTOR DISORDERS

THE SCIENCE AND PRACTICE OF NEUROPSYCHOLOGY
A Guilford Series

Robert A. Bornstein, *Series Editor*

DEVELOPMENTAL MOTOR DISORDERS: A NEUROPSYCHOLOGICAL PERSPECTIVE
Deborah Dewey and David E. Tupper, *Editors*

COGNITIVE AND BEHAVIORAL REHABILITATION:
FROM NEUROBIOLOGY TO CLINICAL PRACTICE
Jennie Ponsford, *Editor*

APHASIA AND LANGUAGE: THEORY TO PRACTICE
Stephen E. Nadeau, Leslie J. Gonzalez Rothi, and Bruce A. Crosson, *Editors*

PEDIATRIC NEUROPSYCHOLOGY: RESEARCH, THEORY, AND PRACTICE
Keith Owen Yeates, M. Douglas Ris, and H. Gerry Taylor, *Editors*

THE HUMAN FRONTAL LOBES: FUNCTIONS AND DISORDERS
Bruce L. Miller and Jeffrey L. Cummings, *Editors*

DEVELOPMENTAL MOTOR DISORDERS

A

NEUROPSYCHOLOGICAL

PERSPECTIVE

Edited by

DEBORAH DEWEY   DAVID E. TUPPER

Series Editor's Note by Robert A. Bornstein

THE GUILFORD PRESS
New York   London

© 2004 The Guilford Press
A Division of Guilford Publications, Inc.
72 Spring Street, New York, NY 10012
www.guilford.com

Printed in the United States of America

This book is printed on acid-free paper.

Last digit is print number: 9 8 7 6 5 4 3 2 1

Library of Congress Cataloging-in-Publication Data

Developmental motor disorders : a neuropsychological perspective / edited by Deborah
Dewey, David E. Tupper.
    p. cm.—(The science and practice of neuropsychology)
  Includes bibliographical references and index.
  ISBN 1-59385-064-6 (hard)
  1. Movement disorders in children. 2. Pediatric neuropsychology. I. Dewey, Deborah.
II. Tupper, David E. III. Series.
  RJ496.M68D485 2004
  618.92′ 8—dc22

                                         2004005223

About the Editors

Deborah Dewey, PhD, is a Canadian Institutes of Health Research Investigator and an Associate Professor of Pediatrics at the University of Calgary. She is also a member of the Behavioural Research Unit at Alberta Children's Hospital. Dr. Dewey is on the editorial board of *Developmental Neuropsychology* and has served as a grant reviewer for Canadian and international funding agencies. She is actively involved in grant-funded research on the neurobehavioral outcomes associated with developmental coordination disorder, learning disabilities, autism spectrum disorders, and attention-deficit/hyperactivity disorder, as well as the developmental outcomes of infants with very low birth weight. Dr. Dewey's research interests also encompass pediatric health psychology issues such as family adjustment to chronic disease and physical activity in preschool-age children.

David E. Tupper, PhD, a board-certified neuropsychologist, is Director of the Neuropsychology Section at Hennepin County Medical Center in Minneapolis and is Associate Professor of Neurology at the University of Minnesota Medical School. He is coauthor or editor of several books, including *Soft Neurological Signs, The Neuropsychology of Everyday Life,* and *Human Developmental Neuropsychology,* and is series editor for the Plenum Series in Russian Neuropsychology. Dr. Tupper's clinical and research interests include neuropsychological aspects of motor disorders in children, cross-cultural neuropsychological assessment, and lifespan developmental neuropsychology.

Contributors

Timo Ahonen, PhD, Department of Psychology, University of Jyväskylä, Jyväskylä, Finland

Anna Barnett, PhD, Department of Experimental Psychology, Oxford University, Oxford, United Kingdom, and School of Psychology and Human Development, Institute of Education, University of London, London, United Kingdom

Virginia W. Berninger, PhD, Department of Educational Psychology, University of Washington, Seattle, Washington

Thomas A. Blondis, MD, Department of Pediatrics, University of Chicago School of Medicine, Chicago, Illinois

Shauna Bottos, BA, Behavioural Research Unit, Alberta Children's Hospital, Calgary, Alberta, Canada

Lindsay Bunn, MS, Department of Psychology, University of Waterloo, Waterloo, Ontario, Canada

Marja Cantell, PhD, Department of Pediatrics, University of Calgary, and Behavioural Research Unit, Alberta Children's Hospital, Calgary, Alberta, Canada

Lynn Chapieski, PhD, Blue Bird Clinic for Pediatric Neurology, Texas Children's Hospital, Houston, Texas

Bryant J. Cratty, EdD, Department of Physiological Sciences, University of California, Los Angeles, California

Susan G. Crawford, MSc, Behavioural Research Unit, Alberta Children's Hospital, Calgary, Alberta, Canada

Deborah Dewey, PhD, Department of Pediatrics, University of Calgary, and Behavioural Research Unit, Alberta Children's Hospital, Calgary, Alberta, Canada

Ameet Dhillon, MSc, OT, Department of Occupational Therapy, University of Toronto, Toronto, Ontario, Canada

Digby Elliott, PhD, Department of Kinesiology, McMaster University, Hamilton, Ontario, Canada

Reint H. Geuze, PhD, Department of Psychology, Developmental and Clinical Neuropsychology, University of Groningen, Groningen, The Netherlands

Farrah Hirji, BSc, OT, Department of Occupational Therapy, University of Toronto, Toronto, Ontario, Canada

Merrill Hiscock, PhD, Department of Psychology, University of Houston, Houston, Texas

Laura Ho, MSc, Department of Exercise Science, Arnold School of Public Health, University of South Carolina, Columbia, South Carolina

Megan Hodge, PhD, Department of Speech Pathology and Audiology, University of Alberta, Edmonton, Alberta, Canada

Bonnie J. Kaplan, PhD, Department of Pediatrics, University of Calgary, and Behavioural Research Unit, Alberta Children's Hospital, Calgary, Alberta, Canada

Libbe Kooistra, PhD, Department of Pediatrics, University of Calgary, and Behavioural Research Unit, Alberta Children's Hospital, Calgary, Alberta, Canada

Dawne Larkin, PhD, School of Human Movement and Exercise Science, University of Western Australia, Nedlands, Australia

Motohide Miyahara, PhD, School of Physical Education, University of Otago, Dunedin, New Zealand

Judith Peters, MSc, Department of Physiotherapy, Great Ormond Street Hospital for Children, and School of Psychology and Human Development, Institute of Education, University of London, London, United Kingdom

Jan P. Piek, PhD, School of Psychology, Curtin University of Technology, Perth, Australia

Thelma M. Pitcher, PhD, School of Psychology, Curtin University of Technology, Perth, Australia

Helene J. Polatajko, PhD, OT, Department of Occupational Therapy, University of Toronto, Toronto, Ontario, Canada

Kelly Pryde, BSc, Department of Psychology, University of Waterloo, Waterloo, Ontario, Canada

Sylvia Rodger, PhD, Department of Occupational Therapy, School of Health and Rehabilitation Sciences, University of Queensland, Brisbane, Australia

Eric A. Roy, PhD, Department of Kinesiology, University of Waterloo, Waterloo, Ontario, Canada

Isabel M. Smith, PhD, Departments of Pediatrics and Psychology, Dalhousie University, and Psychological Services, IWK Health Centre, Halifax, Nova Scotia, Canada

Sandra K. Sondell, PhD, Department of Child and Adolescent Psychiatry, Hennepin County Medical Center, Minneapolis, Minnesota

Janet Summers, MSc (deceased), School of Occupational Therapy, Curtin University of Technology, Perth, Australia

David E. Tupper, PhD, Neuropsychology Section, Hennepin County Medical Center, and Department of Neurology, University of Minnesota Medical School, Minneapolis, Minnesota

Helena Viholainen, MEd, Niilo Mäki Institute, University of Jyväskylä, Jyväskylä, Finland

Leslie Wellman, MSc, Department of Communication Disorders, Glenrose Rehabilitation Hospital, Edmonton, Alberta, Canada

Harriet G. Williams, PhD, Department of Exercise Science, Arnold School of Public Health, University of South Carolina, Columbia, South Carolina

Brenda N. Wilson, MS, OT, Behavioural Research Unit, Alberta Children's Hospital, Calgary, Alberta, Canada

Peter Wilson, PhD, Department of Psychology and Disability Studies, Royal Melbourne Institute of Technology, Melbourne, Australia

Series Editor's Note

Developmental Motor Disorders: A Neuropsychological Perspective, edited by Deborah Dewey and David E. Tupper, is the fifth volume in The Science and Practice of Neuropsychology series. Reflecting the importance and rapid expansion of knowledge in this area, this is the second volume of the series related primarily to disorders in children. The volume takes a unique focus on motor disorders and their fundamental role in human development, and complements the earlier volume on pediatric neuropsychology, edited by Yeates, Ris, and Taylor. Dewey and Tupper have assembled an all-star group of authors who represent the broad range of perspectives that are required for thorough consideration and appreciation of the complexities of this area. This volume reflects the central theme of the series, which is the vital integration of theory, research, and practice. This integration is fundamental to all disciplines working within the field of neuropsychology.

In this series, neuropsychology is defined broadly as the study of brain–behavior relationships, incorporating the perspectives of the full range of related disciplines. Although some volumes in the series will undoubtedly be of greater interest to specific subsets of readers, it is intended that the series be of interest to scientists and practitioners in all of the disciplines that address questions of brain and behavior in research and/or applied contexts. A wide range of topics is covered, and includes reviews of emerging technologies and their potential impact on the science and clinical understanding of neuropsychology.

This volume on the developmental motor disorders brings together topics that are rarely addressed from the neuropsychological perspective, but nonetheless have broad implications for effective functioning of children (and adults). Problems with motor control are commonly associated with more generalized disorders, but frequently are overlooked in favor of disorders of cognition and behavior. Similarly, the role of disorders of other neurocognitive systems (e.g., visuomotor integration) in motor development and performance is infrequently addressed from a neuropsychological perspective. Thus Dewey and Tupper bring into focus a series of issues that have profound theoretical and practical significance for all neurobehavioral disciplines. Although the volume focuses on children, it has important messages for investigators and practitioners who work primarily with adult populations.

ROBERT A. BORNSTEIN

Preface

Movement is something most of us take for granted. Our first movements take place *in utero* and over the course of our life we produce millions upon millions of movements. Movement allows us to meet our basic needs, to communicate, and to learn. For most individuals, movement develops into an automatic process that does not demand conscious effort. Do any of us contemplate how we will put one foot in front of the other as we walk down stairs, how we pronounce the *s* in the word *snow*, or even how we form letters on paper to write articles or books? It is only when movement is impaired in some manner that the extreme importance of motor competency comes to the fore.

Individuals vary in their ability to perform coordinated actions; we are all more or less clumsy or coordinated in different activities at various times in our lives. Some of these motoric differences appear because of innate or inherited personal characteristics, some because of abnormalities in the brain or body acquired after birth, and some because of faulty or incomplete physical experiences when learning more complex motor behaviors. Scientists and practitioners have noted unusual movement characteristics for many years, but it has only been in the past century that more refined efforts have been made to study the neural and mental processes that underlie motor behavior and movement disorders. Still, pediatric neuropsychology and related disciplines have yet to develop a more integrated perspective on developmental motor impairments, although many children with motor anomalies are seen clinically every day.

The origins of this volume can be traced back to an International Neuropsychological Society conference in 1996, where we discussed putting together a book on neuropsychological aspects of motor disorders in children, as there was nothing comprehensive in the literature on this topic. However, with the impending birth of twins to Deborah Dewey, the book was put on hold. A few years later, we renewed our discussions, identified an interested publisher, and began working on this book, the first to address childhood motor disabilities from a neuropsychological perspective.

The volume brings together leading experts who comprehensively examine the neural and behavioral bases of developmental motor disorders. It reviews important current applied research on developmental motor disorders and provides vital clinical knowledge for anyone working with or studying children with developmental motor disorders. The book is organized into four parts. Part I focuses on basic neuroscientific and motor development foundations and neurological and neuropsychological assessment practices. An eloquent discussion of the history of motor disorders and motor development provides the context within which our current understanding of childhood motor disorders is placed. The neuroimaging, neurological, and neuropsychological assessment methods that have been used with children with motor disorders are critically examined, and new and innovative methods of assessing motor functioning in children are presented. The relative merits of these various approaches to assessment, and the need for an assessment process that integrates information from these various sources, are also examined.

In the second part of the book, various clinical neurological disorders that show motor symptoms, such as cerebral palsy, muscular dystrophy, autism, Down syndrome, and Tourette syndrome, are presented, and the neurological and neuropsychological characteristics of these disorders are discussed. Overviews of the motor and perceptual–motor problems that are associated with acquired conditions of childhood, such as head injury, pediatric stroke, HIV, and toxin exposure, are also provided.

Part III examines the neurological and neuropsychological basis and characteristics of well-known developmental motor disorders such as developmental coordination disorder, disorders of written language, and developmental phonological disorder. Finally, Part IV focuses on clinical and research issues associated with motor problems in children, such as manual skill asymmetries, comorbidities with other developmental disorders, and socioemotional effects. In addition, intervention methods currently used with children with motor difficulties are critically reviewed.

We believe that by reviewing current research on developmental motor disorders from a neuropsychological perspective, this volume, with chapters written by recognized experts in the field, provides a unique contribution to pediatric neuropsychology. We hope that the book appeals to a wide audience of scientists and practitioners from the various disciplines who work with and investigate movement disorders in children, including neuropsychologists, child psychologists, school psychologists, pediatric neurologists, developmental pediatricians, speech–language pathologists, occupational therapists, physiotherapists, and movement scientists.

As with many projects that take time to come to fruition, some sad events can occur during the process. During the writing of this book, Janet Summers, one of the contributors, was diagnosed with a glioblastoma multiforme brain tumor. Sadly, she passed away in September 2003.

On a happier note, during the writing of this book two of the authors found the time to get married. As one of these authors stated, "Maybe that's a notable fact, if only because it reflects the [time that has] passed since we began working on the chapter. If you should want to embellish the story by claiming that the chapter led us to matrimony, I would not contradict you." Without in any way taking credit (or responsibility) for their marriage, we wish them the best.

This book could not have been completed without the assistance of a number of agencies and individuals, all of whom deserve our gratitude. We would like to thank the Alberta Children's Hospital Foundation and the Canadian Institutes of Health Research, which have provided funding to Deborah Dewey. We would especially like to thank the authors for their contributions and their willingness to respond to our editorial suggestions. We appreciate the time and energy that they devoted to the book, at times under trying circumstances. Any edited book is only as good as its contributors, and we are particularly grateful for their expert, professional chapters. We wish to acknowledge Dr. Dawne Larkin, who read and commented on the drafts of a number of chapters in this volume. We owe thanks to Rochelle Serwator, our editor at The Guilford Press, for her guidance and encouragement from the beginning of the project to the end. We would also like to thank Bob Bornstein for inviting us to include the book in his Science and Practice of Neuropsychology series; we are pleased that we can contribute to this important area in pediatric neuropsychology. Finally, we want to thank our families for their support, understanding, and patience.

Contents

DEVELOPMENTAL MOTOR DISORDERS

PART I
FOUNDATIONS

CHAPTER 1

Motor Disorders
and Neuropsychological Development

A HISTORICAL APPRECIATION

DAVID E. TUPPER
SANDRA K. SONDELL

To gain an appreciation of the neuropsychological aspects of childhood motor disorders, it is beneficial to begin by reviewing important aspects of their history. The history of such disorders is complex and can be traced in literature relating to adult movement disorders, motor development, the development and organization of the nervous system, and the study of various developmental disorders. Each of these elements adds important information to our current understanding of childhood motor disorders. Therefore, it is the purpose of this chapter to trace these themes in historical perspective and to place them into our current neuropsychological understanding.

The early history of motor disorders is characterized by the writings of many astute scientific observers and the first explorations of the relationship between brain damage and obvious dysfunctional motor behavior. Early identification of motor disorders primarily focused on observations of individual adult patients or small groups of patients. Disorders began to be differentiated and elaborated on as additional observations were compared to earlier reports. In the first part of the 20th century (1910–1960), there was increased interest in childhood motor disorders, which were primarily either classified as a type of cerebral palsy or associated with educational impairment (Cratty, 1994). Between 1940 and 1960, incoordination in children was differentiated from cerebral palsy and was posited to be correlated with learning disorders, perceptual dysfunctions, and hyperactivity in children. The motor syndromes were identified by several different terms including *minimal brain damage, delayed maturation,* and *minimal cerebral palsy.* The recent history of motor disorders, since 1960, has been characterized by more precise research methods with increasing differentiation of the various motor disorders found in children.

3

EARLY HISTORY

Involuntary Movement Descriptions from the Middle Ages

The first description of motor disorders is traced back to the middle ages (1027–1348) and to the epidemic known as the dancing manias (Barbeau, 1981). This epidemic has been known by many different names including St. John's or St. Vitus's dance in Germany, Dance de St. Guy in France, and most commonly called chorea sancti viti. This dancing mania, similar to epileptic seizures, was mainly thought to be a hysterical disease associated with vivid hallucinations, such as seeing the Virgin Mary. It has been described as compulsive dancing, in which crowds of people suddenly form circles and start dancing for hours until exhausted. People affected by this epidemic were also observed to have abdominal swelling, which they cured by wrapping cloths tightly around their waists. Temkin (1971, cited in Park & Park, 1990) provided a description of the mania, "their limbs jerked and they collapsed snorting, unconscious, and frothing" (p. 513).

The cause of the dancing manias was believed to be demonic in nature, cured by praying to the saints (St. John and St. Vitus). In the 16th century, Aurelous von Hohenheim (1493–1541), also known as Paracelsus, was the first to dispel this notion. He named the dancing manias *choreas* from the Latin "to dance." An astute observer of signs and symptoms, he divided the choreas into three types: chorea imaginitiva (arising from imagination, such as Chorea Sancti Viti), chorea lasciva (arising from sensual desire and associated with passionate excitement), and chorea naturalis (arising from physical causes). He identified chorea naturalis as a milder, more common form of the choreas that had continued into the 16th century. Paracelsus associated this milder form with anxiety and confusion and described symptoms including involuntary laughter without howling or screaming, with an urge to dance (Park & Park, 1990). Paracelsus's belief that chorea naturalis had a natural cause was confirmed in 1607 by Shenckius of Graffenberg (Barbeau, 1981).

Although Paracelsus was the first to differentiate various forms of the dancing manias, and to name them choreas, Thomas Sydenham, also known as the "English Hippocrates," is known as the father of chorea (Goetz, Chmura, & Lanska, 2001b). Sydenham was a conscientious and keen physician who was interested in epidemic illnesses. He was known as one of the early medical epidemologists, and relied more on bedside experience and observation than on book learning. Although Sydenham completed several writings describing fevers, gout, hysteria, measles, chicken pox, dysentery, and scarlet fever, he received the most recognition for his description of chorea minor, or acute chorea. In 1686, Sydenham published, a now famous book, *Schedula Monitoria de Novae Febris Ingressa*, which discussed chorea minor. It was not until much later that chorea minor became known as Sydenham's chorea, when Charcot associated it with his name. Following is the description of Sydenham's chorea taken from his book (as cited in Barbeau, 1981):

> St. Vitus Dance is a sort of convulsion which attacks boys and girls from the tenth year until they have done growing. At first it shows itself by a halting, or rather an unsteady movement of one of the legs, which the patient drags. Then it is seen in the hand of the same side. The patient cannot keep it a moment in its place, whether he lay it upon his breast or

any part of his body. Do what he may, it will be jerked elsewhere convulsively. If any vessel filled with drink be put into his hand, before it reaches his mouth, he will exhibit a thousand gesticulations like a mountebank. He holds the cup straight, as if to move it to his mouth, but has his hand carried elsewhere by sudden jerks. Then, perhaps, he contrives to bring it to his mouth. If so, he will drink the liquid off at a gulp, just as if he were trying to amuse the spectators by his antics . . . now this affection arises from some humor falling on the nerves, and such irritation causes the spasm. (p. 5)

Movement Descriptions from the 18th to Early 20th Centuries

Chorea, Athetosis, Tics, and Tremors

Chorea continued to be studied throughout the 18th and 19th centuries with increased differentiation made between types of chorea. The list of distinguished publishers on chorea includes Richard Mead in 1751, Ewart in 1798, Cullen in 1785, Bouteille, who introduced the works to France in 1810, Roger in 1866, and finally, Charcot, Romberg, and the school of Guy's Hospital in London, all of whom made chorea known as an important disease (Barbeau, 1981).

As the details of chorea were being detailed, James Parkinson (1755–1824) identified a new disease, which he termed *shaking palsy*, in which he described six subjects with tremors. While Parkinson was better known at the time as a political lobbyist and anthropologist, he is best known in the medical world for his 1817 publication, *An Essay on the Shaking Palsy*. Parkinson's essay was the first to identify this condition, and his report gives an almost complete description of the illness, including the typical tremor, festination, slow movements, and classical gait. The one thing not identified by Parkinson was the rigidity often associated with the disease. As Parkinson's essay was not widely distributed, his observations had little impact during his lifetime. However, when Charcot came across Parkinson's essay in the late 1800s, Charcot recommended that the disease be named in Parkinson's honor, calling it Parkinson's disease, rather than paralysis agitans (Barbeau, 1981; Goetz et al., 2001b).

Jean-Martin Charcot (1825–1893) is known as the father of clinical neurology. In addition to making supplementary contributions to the identification of Parkinson's disease and Sydenham's chorea, including developing diagnostic detection methods for differentiating tremors and describing the neurological foundation of chorea, Charcot impacted the field of neurology with two important themes. The first theme, which continues to influence modern movement disorder specialists, is the importance of clinical prioritization and emphasis on visual observation. The second theme is the need for careful, anatomical–clinical correlations. Charcot favored a hereditary basis for almost all primary neurological disorders, and he proposed that phenotypical expression of the disorders could be widely variable (Goetz et al., 2001b).

Charcot's student, George Gilles de la Tourette, is known for describing a form of motor disease which included multifocal tic disorders marked by explosive utterances of words or sounds. Although Gilles de la Tourette's name is now associated with the disorder, it is likely that Charcot was a primary figure in the identification of the disease. In 1885, Gilles de la Tourette made a historical *tour d'horizon*, in which he differentiated tics from choreas and compared his *maladie des tics convulsifs* to the "jumping," seen by George Beard of Maine, Latah of Malaysia, and Myriachit of Siberia; however, Tourette syndrome is now clearly differentiated from these conditions. Whereas patients with Tourette syndrome suffer from similar symptoms as those suffering from the "jumping" conditions, repeated, involuntary motor tics were not a symptom of the other conditions. The modern definition of Tourette syndrome contains all the symptoms described by Charcot and Gilles de la Tourette, including childhood onset, motor and vocal tics, natural waxing and waning, and chronicity, as well as behavioral correlates, or "mental tics," such as obsessions, compulsions, inattentiveness, and hyperactivity (Barbeau, 1981; Goetz, Chmura, & Lanska, 2001a).

Interest in movement disorders and scientific observation increased in the United States during the mid-1800s, and much attention was given to a form of chorea described as familial and chronic. The first observation of chronic, familial chorea was printed in the first edition of *The Practice of Medicine* in 1842, in a letter written by Dr. Charles Oscar Waters in 1841 to Dunglison. In that letter, Dr. Waters described the disease, known as *magrums*, which means "fidgets" in Dutch, and indicated the hereditary nature of the disease as well as a distinction from ordinary chorea. The letter stated, "First, it rarely occurs before adult age. Second, it never ceases spontaneously. Third, when fully developed, it wants the paroxysmal character" (as cited in Barbeau, 1981, p. 10). In 1948, the third edition of Dunglison's *The Practice of Medicine* described a similar report by Charles R. Gorman (Barbeau, 1981).

It was not until the work of George Huntington (1850–1916), however, that the aforementioned disorder became well known (Barbeau, 1981; Lanska, 2000; Lanska, Goetz, & Chmura, 2001). Huntington was 8 years old when he first saw "that disorder" as he accompanied his father to work. In an address to the New York Neurological Society (cited in Barbeau, 1981) in 1909, he said:

> I recall it as vividly as though it had occurred but yesterday. It made a most enduring impression, every detail of which I recall today, an impression which was the very first impulse to my choosing chorea as my virgin contribution to medical lore. . . . We suddenly came upon two women, mother and daughter, both tall, thin, almost cadeverous, both bowing, twisting, grimacing. . . . From this point on, my interest in this disease has never wholly ceased. (p. 11)

Huntington's paper, *On Chorea*, written in 1872, was the first complete description of the disease, which was accomplished through the study of his father's and grandfather's clinical notes. In his paper, Huntington gave the following description:

> The hereditary chorea, as I shall call it, is confined to certain and fortunately a few families, and has been transmitted to them, an heirloom from generations away back in the dim past. It is spoken of by those in whose veins the seed of the disease are known to exist, with a kind of horror, and not at all alluded to except through dire necessity, when it is mentioned as "that disorder." It is attended generally by all the symptoms of common chorea, only in an aggravated degree, hardly ever manifesting itself until adult or middle life, and then coming on gradually, but surely, increasing by degrees, and often occupying years in its development, until the hapless sufferer is but a quivering wreck of his former self. It is as common and is indeed, I believe, more common among men than among women, while I am not aware that season or complexion has any influence on the matter. There are marked peculiarities in this disease; (1) its hereditary nature, (2) a tendency to insanity

and suicide, (3) its manifesting itself as a grave disease only in adult life. (Barbeau, 1981, p. 12)

At the same time, William Alexander Hammond (1828–1900) described a new disease, which he termed *Athetosis*, meaning "without fixed position" in Greek. Hammond became a key figure of neurology in the United States and wrote the first American neurological text in 1871, titled *Treatise on Diseases of the Nervous System*, in which he described one of his patients with the disease. In his paper, he hypothesized the cause of the disease of athetosis to be in the corpus striatum. In 1890, Hammond's son performed an autopsy of the original patient and confirmed the localization to be in the corpus striatum. Several other physicians described similar disorders by different names and it was not until 1886 that Griedenberg gave credit to Hammond for differentiating this disease from other forms of chorea. Griedenberg termed Hammond's disease *choreo-athetosis*, which is now the term most commonly used (Barbeau, 1981; Lanska et al., 2001).

Also around this time, William Osler (1849–1919) further differentiated forms of choreic disorders. His publication in 1894, *On Chorea and Choreiform Affections*, provided a framework for chorea and identified two, new, similar disorders. Osler's paper was a report that integrated the study of 410 cases of chorea which had been studied from 1880 to 1894. In his paper, Osler distinguished between chorea minor (Sydenham's chorea), chorea major (dancing mania), choreiform affections/pseudo-choreas (including tics), and secondary/symptomatic choreas (including posthemiplegic choreoathetosis and Huntington's disease). Most of Osler's work concentrated on Sydenham's chorea, which he described as: "An acute disease of childhood . . . characterized by irregular, involuntary movements, a variable amount of physical disturbance, and associated very often with arthritis and endocarditis" (Lanska et al., 2001, p. 751).

Cerebral Palsy

Symptoms of cerebral palsy were first described as cerebral atrophy in children by Jean Croveilheir in 1829, Gilbert Breschet in 1831, Claude Francois von Lallemond in 1834, and Carl Rokitansky in 1835; however, William John Little (1810–1894) is known as the first person to associate the adult problems to a pathological event that occurred at birth. Little was drawn to this field because of his own acquired deformity of clubfoot, the result of childhood poliomyelitis. Little's 1843 lecture series, which was later published in monograph form, titled "Deformities of the Human Frame," described motor distortions and spasmodic rigidity of newborn infants. In a monograph of his lectures published in 1853, "On the Nature and Treatment of the Deformities of the Human Frame," Little described 24 patients with motor deformities associated with complications of labor and delivery—including prematurity, labor requiring forceps, severe asphyxia, and convulsions at birth. Little had carefully investigated and documented possible etiological factors and, in 1861, defended his thesis, titled "On the Influence of Abnormal Parturition, Difficult Labours, Premature Birth, and Asphyxia Neonatorum, on the Mental and Physical Condition of the Child, Especially in Relation to Deformities" (Little, 1862), which stated that these complications can cause permanent central nervous system damage (Accardo, 1989; Dunn, 1995; George, 1992; Schifrin & Longo, 2000). Following is Little's description of cerebral palsy, which came to be known as Little's disease (as cited in Dunn, 1995):

> The object of this communication is to show that the act of birth does occasionally imprint upon the nervous and muscular systems of the nascent infantile organism very serious and peculiar evils. . . . The forms of abnormal parturition which I have observed to precede certain mental and physical derangements of the infant consisted of difficult labours—i.e., unnatural presentations, tedious labours from rigidity of maternal passages or apertures, instrumental labours, labours in which turning was had recourse to, breech presentations, premature labours, and cases in which the umbilical cord had been entangled around the infant's neck or had fallen down before the head . . . asphyxia neonatorum, thorough resulting injury to nervous centers, is the cause of the commonest contractions which originate at the moment of birth, namely, more or less general spastic rigidity, and sometimes of paralytic contraction. . . . The former class of affections may be described as impairment of volition, with tonic rigidity and ultimately structural shortening, in varying degrees, of a few or many of the muscles of the body. Both lower extremities are more or less generally involved. Sometimes the affection of one limb only is observed by the parent, but examination usually shows a smaller degree of affection in the limb supposed to be sound . . . in most cases, after a time, owing to structural shortening of the muscles and of the articular ligaments, and perhaps to some change of forms of articular surfaces, the thighs cannot be completely abducted or extended, the knees cannot be straightened, nor can the heels be properly applied to the ground. . . . The muscles feel harder than natural to the age. . . . The muscles of speech are commonly involved. . . . Often during the earliest months of life deglutition is impaired. . . . The intellectual functions are sometimes quite unaffected, but in the majority of cases the intellect suffers—from the slightest impairment . . . up to entire imbecility. . . . Some cases present distinct convulsive twitchings of face or limbs during first days after birth, open or suppressed convulsions, opisthotonos, or laryngismus. In some instances the persistent rigidity of muscles commences or is observed shortly after birth, in others it escapes observation until the lapse of some weeks or months.(p. F210)

At his thesis defense, members of the audience have been noted for commenting on the novelty and originality of his subject matter. In the years following Little's thesis, increased attention was given to researching and describing the motor effects of birth defects; however, no clear distinctions were made until 1888, when William Osler gave a series of lectures at the Infirmary for Nervous Diseases in Philadelphia, titled "The Cerebral Palsies of Children." In his lectures, Osler gave credit to Little for identifying the relationship between complications of labor and delivery to bilateral spastic hemiplegia. Osler's research was the most comprehensive of its time as a result of documentation of both his own patients and those existing in the literature equaling 151 cases; emphasis on the importance of correlating pathological findings with clinical symptoms; studies of cases from birth, as well as those acquired after 1 year of life; and the study of autopsies. Osler classified the cerebral palsies into infantile hemiplegia, bilateral spastic hemiplegia, and spastic paraplegia, based on the distribution/location and neuroanatomical pathology (Longo & Ashwal, 1993).

Sigmund Freud, mostly recognized for his work in psychiatry, contributed significantly to the area of cerebral palsy in children. Before his work on psychoanalytic theory, Freud was interested in neuroanatomy and neuropathology. From 1891 to 1897, he published several monographs and papers on the topic of cerebral palsy (Freud, 1897, 1968). His primary contributions to this field included the following: (1) He described a new form of cerebral palsy (choreatiform paresis); (2) he reclassified the cerebral palsies; (3) he challenged Little's assumption that cerebral palsy was due to perinatal asphyxia, stating that no etiology could be determined but, rather, that many factors were associated with developing cerebral palsy including congenital factors, those acquired during birth, and those acquired postnatally; and (4) he was the first to observe visual field deficits in patients with hemiplegia. Freud's classification of the cerebral palsies included the following categories: general cerebral spasticity (Little's disease), paraplegic spasticity (bilateral cerebral lesions), bilateral spastic hemiplegia, and generalized congenital "chorea" and bilateral athetosis (Freud, 1968; George, 1992; Longo & Ashwal, 1993).

The contributions of Little, Osler, and Freud were notable in their time given that neurology and pediatrics were both newly emerging fields of medicine, as most researchers were uninterested in newborn diseases because they were viewed as fatal diseases. Although Freud's work was well regarded, his interest in psychiatry took him away from his work on cerebral palsy. Thus, because Freud did not pursue his research further, Little's hypothesis that cerebral palsy was caused by birth asphyxia remained the predominant belief. It has not been until recently that research has shown that perinatal asphyxia and low birth weight explain the development of cerebral palsy in only a minority of the cases. The cause of cerebral palsy in the majority of patients is still unknown.

Muscular Dystrophy

In 1861, in the second edition of his book *Paraplégie Hypertrophique de l'Enfance de Cause Cérébrale*, Guillaume B.A. Duchenne (1806–1875) of Bologne, France, described a boy with progressive muscle disease, with onset in early childhood, significant physical–motor handicap, and death in early adulthood (Beighton & Beighton, 1986). Duchenne, who is considered the founder of French neurology, had an unusual career, including never holding an academic post or a hospital appointment. Nevertheless, he produced numerous articles and monographs on electrophysiology and neurological disorders and was one of the first to use photography to illustrate disease processes. In his later 1872 book on electrical stimulation of muscle, Duchenne provided an extensive, illustrated account of the disorder that now bears his name (DeVivo, Darras, & Jones, 2003).

Little and Meryon had briefly reported this entity several years earlier (Darras, Menache, & Kunkel, 2003). In 1852, Meyron accurately described the clinical course of the disease in four brothers, and in 1853 Little reported on two brothers who were unable to walk after the age of 11 years due to abnormal increase of muscle bulk combined with contraction and adipose degeneration. Although initially described as hypertrophic paraplegia of infancy due to a cerebral disease, Duchenne later recognized that the disorder was muscular in origin and proposed criteria for its diagnosis. Subsequently, in 1879 during a series of five lectures on this topic at University College Hospital, London, Gowers reviewed the literature and described 21 personal cases as reflective of "pseudohypertrophic dystrophy." Gowers (1886) later described in more detail the way an affected child rises from the floor to reach a standing posture, now considered a classic early indicator of muscular dystrophy called Gowers's maneuver or Gowers's sign (Darras et al., 2003).

Further histopathological characterization of muscular dystrophy occurred in the second half of the 19th century by Erb, Becker, and others, and in the 20th century, blood creatine kinase elevation was identified as a marker. Although Duchenne or early-onset muscular dystrophy and more benign, later-onset Becker muscular dystrophy were noted to have similar features and familial patterns in the early clinical descriptions, it was not known until the early 1980s, due to advances in molecular genetics, that a gene on the short arm of the X chromosome (Xp21) was responsible for this disorder, and that an abnormality in the transcription of a protein product called dystrophin underlies the disorders. Thus, the clinical cases recognized a century earlier are now known as dystrophinopathies (see Darras et al., 2003).

Apraxia

Description of cortical-level motor disorders began in the late 1800s following Broca's reports of localized cerebral lesions leading to neurological disorders. Steinthal in 1871 was the first to use the term *apraxia* to refer to disorders where the common feature was the inability to perform motor activity correctly on command. Other neurologists in the late 19th century, including Hughlings Jackson and Finkelnburg, described cases with disordered movements, but it was not until the beginning of the 20th century that Hugo Liepmann, a German neurologist and student of Carl Wernicke, began to report and theorize about disorders of purposeful action (Heilman & Rothi, 1997).

Liepmann (1900/1988; see also Kimura, 1980) began the first systematic studies of limb apraxia when he studied a right-handed civil servant who suddenly developed limb apraxia as a result of apoplexy. His goal was to demonstrate that the patient displayed apraxia as a disorder of motor planning rather than as a result of a perceptual or language/symbolic disorder associated with left-hemisphere language systems. In Liepmann's view, correct execution of a gesture requires the existence of a motor program, based on a correct spatial and temporal sequence of single movements and developed as a visual representation. Based on his analysis of a number of cases, he posited that the left hemisphere of right-handers not only mediates language but also contains movement formulas that store information regarding skilled and purposive movments. Liepmann's neuroanatomical interpretation of apraxia required three components: (1) left-hemisphere programming of the gesture, (2) control of the right-hemisphere motor regions via midcallosal pathways, and (3) motor planning as the province of cortical regions and subjacent white matter (Faglioni & Basso, 1985). Any of a variety of apraxia types could be the result from lesions in various components of this network (Heilman, Watson, & Rothi, 2000). Therefore, consistent with his mentor's influence, Liepmann was one of the most influential contributors at the turn of the 20th century to an information-processing view of apraxia.

After World War I, and based on the increase in proponents of a "holistic" approach to understanding cerebral organization, there was a loss of interest in apraxia and similar connectionist approaches. In addition, Liepmann and followers investigated apraxia in adults only, with little application to studies of developmental types of apraxia.

RECENT HISTORY

Motor Development

Until the early 20th century, at which time the first documented papers on normal motor development in infancy through childhood were written, the history of motor disorders was primarily centered around the observation of abnormal motor behaviors. Some early investigators such as Wilhelm Preyer (1882, 1885, 1888) recognized the importance of motor development in the general study of child development. Preyer, in fact, noted in chick embryos that motor activity develops early during gestation; a fetus during the second trimester is capable of movement but does not directly respond to sensory stimulation; this principle is called the developmental primacy of the motor system over the sensory systems. His view was that the motor system matures in advance of the sensory systems, so that early movements result solely from discharge of motor neurons. Early precursors to reflex theories such as those proposed by Pavlov (1927) and Sherrington (1906) were also developed at this time.

The most well-known 20th-century individuals identified as being the first to study motor development are Arnold Gesell (1880–1961) and Myrtle McGraw (1899–1988), who believed that motor behavior is predetermined and that children acquire motor skills as a result of biological/neural maturation. In 1941, Gesell characterized the maturational component in behavioral development by "inevitableness and surety" (Wolff, 1982, p. 118). As a result of the belief in biological maturation, the prominent area of research became normative, age-graded descriptions of motor milestones. Gesell's normative studies began in 1919, when he created permanent longitudinal records of motor behavior using motion pictures of 107 children from neonate to 56 weeks and followed them at 18 months and 2, 3, 4, 5, and 6 years. This extensive observation of motor behavior was accompanied by notes on "language behavior." The data described four schedules of development which included motor behavior, language behavior, adaptive behavior, and personal–social behavior. Gesell disliked statistics and disapproved of the use of an exact score; thus he correlated a child's developmental stage by comparing the percentage of children at a specific age who were able to complete the behavior in question. McGraw was the first researcher in the early motor development of infants to challenge the predetermined epigenetic view. She adopted a view that emphasized reciprocal effects in the relationship between structure and function (Gottlieb, 1998). McGraw believed that exposure to movement or stimulation could modify the development of peripheral and central nervous system structures. She also provided detailed descriptions of motor development in her writings (McGraw, 1935, 1945).

A notable difference between Gesell and McGraw was that McGraw believed in a cortical inhibition hypothesis. Specifically, she believed that reflex-based movements begin to come under cortical control. In contrast, Gesell believed in self-regulating fluctuations affected by genes, neural structure, and peripheral factors, which limit motor behavior. Nonetheless, the work of Gesell and McGraw was similar in that they both assumed that structural changes in the central nervous system directly determine behavioral changes. Subsequent investigations paralleled Gesell and McGraw's normative studies and attempted to further clarify the stages of development; hence, until the 1980s, most research on motor development stemmed from the belief that motor skill acquisition was the result of the biological maturation process (Ball, 1977; Hopkins, Beek, & Kalverboer, 1993; Wolff, 1982).

Ozeretskii,[1] Bernstein, and Other Russian Work

At the same time as the ascendancy of maturational hypotheses, measurement of motor skills was also peaking interest (see Doll, 1946). Nikolai Ozeretskii developed the first assessment instrument, initially published in Russian in 1925, to measure motor behavior, or as he described, to measure "motor idiocy" (Ozeretskii, 1925, 1929). While first working at the Moscow Neurological Institute and later at the Leningrad Pedagogical Institute, Ozeretskii established tasks that spanned different motor skill categories with varying levels of difficulty. His test further differentiated the tasks based on age. This scale incorporated tests of general static coordination, dynamic coordination of the hands (see Figure 1.1), general dynamic coordination, motor speed, simultaneous voluntary movements, and synkinesia or associated involuntary movements. This scale was the first comprehensive attempt at developmental motor assessment.

Ozeretskii's scale was quickly adapted worldwide and translated into many different languages (Doll, 1946; Lassner, 1948; Oseretzky, 1925, 1931). Subsequent incarnations of the scale have maintained the focus on developmentally or age-based motor tasks. The Lincoln–Oseretsky Motor Development Scale (Sloan, 1955) and the Bruininks–Oseretsky Test of Motor Proficiency (Bruininks, 1978) are both more contemporary descendants of Ozeretskii's original scale.

Nicholai Bernstein was a Russian physiologist and influential motor skills theorist during the 1930s and 1940s, whose work will be discussed later in the chapter. He primarily approached the study of movements as a dynamic system, based on the Russian view of activity as a defining feature of living organisms. He stated that elaborations of a motor skill cannot be equated with repetition of the same neural commands but, rather, involved the development of an ability to solve or complete the motor task differently each time. Bernstein thus suggested that movement is directed by the neural equivalent of a goal, or a model of the desired completed act (Bernstein, 1967). Unfortunately, because Bernstein's theories did not follow mainstream Pavlovian reflex thinking, his work was not fully accepted for political reasons within his own country, and only in the past 30 years has his influence for motor control theories been recognized. Interestingly, due to these political factors, Bernstein's only monograph on motor development, written in the 1940s and unpublished, was thought lost and only found in the late 1980s. It was published in Russian in 1991, and published in English in 1996 (Bernstein, 1996); Bernstein's ideas on motor control and dexterity in children remain relevant today.

A more recent investigator of motor development is the Russian developmental psychologist Alexandr Zaporozhets. Much of his early work concerned the nature and development of perception and thought in children, and he worked during the 1930s in the Kharkov Institute of Education. However, during World War II, Zaporozhets worked at a rehabilitation hospital and became involved in scientific and practical aspects of restoring disrupted motor functions after injuries. From 1942 to 1960 he conducted many investigations into the development of human voluntary

---

[1]In this chapter we use the direct Russian transliteration of Ozeretskii's name. It should be noted that it has also been Anglicized into various forms such as Oseretzky or Oseretsky.

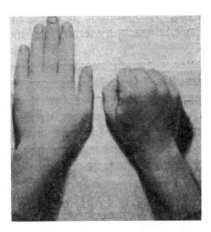

FIGURE 1.1. Ozeretskii's Test of Reciprocal Coordination. The child is required to alternately open and close each hand. From Ozeretskii (1929, p. 24).

movements and their rehabilitation after central nervous system trauma; his results were published in monograph form in Russian only (Zaporozhets, 1960). His major conclusions were that voluntary motor acts consist of two component parts, including initial orienting reactions that are genetically formed and develop early in life, and executive motor reactions, that are learned later in life based on environmental feedback.

Motor Awkwardness

At the same time as preliminary research was being conducted on normal motor development, some of the first descriptions of childhood motor dysfunction not associated with cerebral palsy were provided. The distinction between adult apraxia, a loss of acquired skilled actions, and developmental dyspraxia, the failure to acquire motor skills in a normal fashion, was generally not differentiated previously in terms of etiology (Morris, 1997). Apparently, interest was increasing regarding this type of motor disorder in children, as Collier identified a group of children as "congenitally maladroit," and Dupré and other clinicians in France during the 1910s and 1920s described children with motor awkwardness as "motorically deficient" ("debilite motrice," Dupré, 1925; see also Ford, 1966). Samuel Orton termed this abnormal clumsiness *developmental dyspraxia* in 1937. He thought that it could be due to both neurological and nonneurological factors. It was not until the 1960s that attempts were made to classify children with varying motor dysfunction (Kessler, 1980; Koupernik, MacKeith, & Francis-Williams, 1975).

In 1975, Gubbay defined the clumsy child syndrome in the following manner: "The clumsy child is to be regarded as one who is mentally normal, without bodily deformity, and whose physical strength, sensation, and co-ordination are virtually normal by the standards of routine conventional neurological assessment, but whose ability to perform skilled, purposive movement is impaired" (p. 246). Since Gubbay's description, little progress has been made in further describing and differentiating the syndrome, although it has been referred to by many names including clumsiness, developmental dyspraxia, developmental apraxia and agnosia, apractognosia, and developmental coordination disorder. This latter term is used in the fourth edition of the *Diagnostic and Statistical Manual of Mental Disorders* (American Psychiatric Association, 1994), which describes the syndrome as "performance in daily activities that require motor coordination is substantially below that expected given the person's chronological age and measured intelligence. This may be manifested by marked delays in achieving motor milestones (e.g. walking, crawling, sitting), dropping things, 'clumsiness,' poor performance in sports, or poor handwriting" (p. 54). Little is still known regarding the etiology or prognosis of developmental coordination disorder. Although it has been determined that while some children's motor impairments are observed to improve over time, this is not an absolute truth. Further, it is believed that the co-occurrence of motor problems, learning difficulties, and behavior problems persist across the lifespan. Still, many questions remain regarding motor development and motor incoordination (Henderson, 1993).

Minimal Brain Dysfunction and Soft Signs

Another theme that has evolved in recent history is minimal brain dysfunction (MBD) and "soft signs," also known as soft neurological signs, minor neurological signs, equivocal signs, and nonfocal neurological signs (Kessler, 1980; Tupper, 1987). Samuel Orton was among the first to describe the association between children with learning disabilities and mild motor incoordination in the 1930s (Orton, 1937). In 1947, Bender (1947, 1956) was the first to use the term *soft neurological signs*, which increased interest in this area.

During the 1940s, 1950s, and 1960s a number of clinicians and researchers studied a heterogeneous group of children with behavioral and learning disorders who were found to demonstrate mild abnormalities similar to children with definitive cerebral dysfunction. Most influential was the two-volume book by Strauss and colleagues titled *Psychopathology and Education of the Brain-Injured Child* (Strauss & Kephart, 1955; Strauss & Lehtinen, 1947). In this book, the authors defined what subsequent authors termed the *Strauss syndrome*: difficulty in figure–ground perception, abnormal distractibility, conceptual rigidity, hyperactivity, and motor awkwardness. The authors hypothesized a unitary syndrome of cerebral dysfunction, which led to a generalized notion of MBD in children that included motoric incoordination as a primary manifestation. Similar to Strauss's thinking, A. Jean Ayres (1972, 1985) formulated a theory of developmental disorders based on difficulty with sensory integration with motor systems. Fortunately, the limitations of such unitary thinking are more apparent now, and motor impairment is not necessarily considered a direct result of generalized cerebral damage.

By the 1970s, the association of motor dysfunction with other childhood disorders became known as "soft signs" indicating that the meaning of the sign was unclear and was not specific to a disease or etiology; however, the sign could be correlated with the disorder (Tupper, 1987). Later, during the 1980s, specific motor soft signs were found to have neurophysiological associations and, thus, are now found to be useful in the differential diagnosis of motor disorders (Deuel, 2002; Deuel & Robinson, 1987).

In summary, following the early descriptive history of clinical motor abnormalities, significant contributions have been made to the field of motor development and motor disorders of childhood in the last 50 to 100 years. These contributions include incorporation and refinement of various developmental models and testing approaches, as well as improved methods of understanding developmental motor conditions and motor skills (see Forssberg, 1998; Manoel & Connolly, 1998).

CONTEMPORARY ISSUES

A number of contemporary issues are relevant to the study of developmental motor disorders. A comprehensive neuropsychological approach to developmental motor disorders needs to consider important aspects of the approach or theory used in studying motor development, the nature of the development and acquisition of motor skills, and appropriate assessment methods (Segalowitz & Hiscock, 2002). Knowledge gained during the long history of motor disorders should guide future theoretical development and practical applications in this area. New technologies such as molecular genetics and functional neuroimaging may shape our understanding of the biological basis of childhood motor disorders.

Approaches to Motor Development

The study of the emergence of motor skills has figured prominently in the scientific study of human development (Espenschade, 1947; Thelen, 2000). Human infants are born with little control over their bodies, yet over the course of several years, they become able to sit, stand, walk, run, climb, and speak. While the emergence of motor skills is most dramatic in the first few years of life, increasing refinement of motor capabilities and acquisition of new motor milestones occurs in a fairly predictable manner for most children. Presently, the contemporary study of motor development contributes both empirically and theoretically to larger questions of development and developmental change in psychology.

As noted previously, early theories relating to motor development were often based on the maturational–biological hypotheses of Gesell and McGraw. It was not until the 1980s that improved measurement stimulated advanced research in motor skills acquisition and development (Adolph, Weise, & Marin, 2003). The neuromuscular maturation hypothesis decreased in popularity among researchers in the 1980s and emphasis was placed on the contributions of many other factors in motor development, such as peripheral factors, perceptual information, and learning during adaptive control of movements (see Williams, 1983; Zanone, 1990).

The most common of the contemporary theories included the information-processing approach, the dynamic systems approach, initially associated with the work of Bernstein in the 1960s and later expanded by Esther Thelen in the 1970s, and the ecological or perception–action approach, first associated with the work of James and Eleanor Gibson (Gibson, 1966). In 1975, Ounsted wrote, "We must know our own animal if we are to be good ethologists . . . for those interested in the brain and its development quantitative ethology is the best, and indeed the only, way in which the actual workings of the untrammelled brain can be studied properly" (as cited in Kalverboer, 1993, p. 3). Motor development theories have therefore shifted from having a sole focus on understanding of biological processes to incorporating organismic interactions with the environment.

Initially, developmental cognitive psychology was mainly interested in the information-processing approach, which assumed that motor coordination is determined by genetic, neural, cognitive, and environmental factors during development (Hopkins et al., 1993; Lockman, 1990). The information-processing approach emphasized what has to be done for motor behavior but did not answer the question of how it is done. The dynamic systems approach, associated with Bernstein (1967, 1996) and Thelen (1995, 2000), attempted to answer the question of how the brain controls the muscles to create motor behavior in the presence of external, environmental changes. This approach posits that the acquisition of motor skills is determined by the interaction of many factors, including peripheral factors, perceptual and learning factors, and muscle development. All these factors are believed to contribute equally and none of the factors can work alone. For example, the ability to walk is acquired when a child has muscle strength to carry himself, slimmed body proportions, balance control, brain maturation, and a goal of somewhere to go. The ecological or perception–action approach, associated primarily with Gibson (1966), asserts that perception and movement are linked and are inseparable. Thus, movement requires perceptual information and perceptual information requires movement. "For example, exploratory movements of the eyes, head, body, and extremities generate perceptual information in light, sound, muscles, and skin. Actions likewise generate more information for perceptual systems" (Adolph et al., 2003, p. 135). More recently, the natural–physical approach has attempted to integrate Bernstein and Thelen's dynamic systems approach with Gibson's ecological and perception–action approach, in order to identify how patterns of motor behaviors are produced (Hopkins, 2001; Hopkins et al., 1993).

One of the more enduring aspects of the early maturational theories, especially for neurology and neuropsychology, is their focus on developmental norms. The early descriptive work of Gesell and colleagues (Gesell, 1933; Gesell & Amatruda, 1947; Knobloch & Pasamanick, 1974) emphasized the orderly, sequential acquisition of motor behaviors that represent attainment of "milestones" in the normal child. Delay in the attainment of motor milestones is considered an indicator of pathology, and developmental "norms" represent the typical performances of "average" children. However, among normal children there will be variation in motor abilities; numerous factors such as genetics, practice or training, encouragement, and the child's own drive or motivation will affect performance. Many of the current neuropsychological tests use age-related normative data on motor performance and tend to be quantitatively based, thus implicitly following maturational theories. They do not take into account recent theories of motor development.

Pyramidal and Extrapyramidal Systems

The phrase *movement disorders* is a simple and handy way of describing a group of disorders that are characterized by complex and sometimes heterogeneous clinical signs (Lohr, Wisniewski, & Lohr, 1987). Two neural systems, operating semi-independently, are involved in human motor activity, and differentiation of disorders attributable to each of these has been important in the study of motor disorders. The pyramidal system is the executive system responsible for the initiation of voluntary skilled movements involving rapid and precise control of the extremities. It consists of precentral motor cortex and corticospinal tract and is connected to spinal motor neu-rons. Other motor structures, including the cerebellum, the basal ganglia, and brain stem areas such as the red nucleus and substantia nigra, form a vaguely defined extrapyramidal system. The extrapyramidal system is more concerned with alterations and adjustments in posture and with modification and coordination of movements ini-tiated by the pyramidal system.

As described previously, the early history of movement disorders was character-ized by descriptions of chorea and other involuntary movement abnormalities, which ultimately have been associated with extrapyramidal structures (see also Clarke & O'Malley, 1996; Finger, 1994). According to Albanese (1989), the pyramids were the first part of the motor system to be studied morphologically, in the 17th century. Neu-roanatomists in the early portion of the 20th century, particularly Mingazzini and Wil-son in 1912, introduced the notion of an extrapyramidal set of neural structures in-volved in motor control. Vogt in 1911 defined the syndrome of the corpus striatum, which included athetosis, associated involuntary movements, and rhythmic oscilla-tions. Subsequently, although the concepts of pyramidal and extrapyramidal systems have not been universally accepted, they remain useful to help distinguish lesions in primary motor tracts from lesions in the "motor ganglia."

With the exception of congenital motor disorders such as cerebral palsy (diplegia, paraplegia), hemiparesis and hemiplegia remain the most obvious motor symptoms as-sociated with childhood-acquired pyramidal system involvement. Extrapyramidal sys-tem disorders in childhood are also easily recognized and described and include a number of disorders that show both motor and behavioral/cognitive abnormalities. Important extrapyramidal or subcortical motor disorders discussed further in this book include tics, childhood choreas, dystonias, and Gilles de la Tourette syndrome (see Angelini, Balottin, Lanzi, & Nardocci, 1987, for clinical descriptions of additional extrapyramidal disorders in childhood).

Motor Control and Skilled Movement

Theories of motor control relevant to childhood motor disorders have been summa-rized by Shumway-Cook and Woollacott (1995). The major theories include the fol-lowing: (1) reflex theory, where reflexes have been described by Sherrington as the building blocks of complex motor behavior; (2) hierarchical theory, based on the con-cepts of Hughlings Jackson and recognizing the hierarchy of the neural organization of motor systems; (3) motor programming theories, which include a central motor pat-tern in the brain; (4) systems theory, based on Bernstein's thinking and including a dis-tributed model of mechanical muscle control; (5) dynamical action theory, which tries to find mathematical descriptions of self-organizing systems; (6) parallel distributed processing theory, suggesting simultaneous but complementary nervous system pro-cessing of motor information; (7) task-oriented theories, which involve a functional perspective to understand how a nervous system accomplishes motor tasks; and (8) ecological theory, based on Gibson's work, which considers the child an active ex-plorer of the environment. Thus, a historical perspective on motor control theories suggests a general trend from reactive sensory–motor theories to theories that involve perception–action interactions, and from the nervous system to the organism–environ-ment interface.

Rosenbaum (1991) has outlined four contemporary issues or problems in the study of motor control and skilled movements. Underlying these problems are the two main questions of how as humans we control our movements, and how we maintain stability in our movements at the same time. A complete neurophysiological understanding of the motor system must account for both movement control and stability. We include a brief review of these issues to sensitize neuropsychologists to important concerns inherent in motor control research.

The first issue outlined by Rosenbaum (1991) can be described as the *degrees-of-freedom* problem. Physical tasks can be performed in a variety of ways, in fact, an infinite variety; this capacity is called motor equivalence. For example, we can write our signature (or anything, for that matter) using any of a number of body parts: our right hand, our left hand, a pen between our teeth, a pen between our toes, and so on. In all cases, the signature would look comparable (see Figure 1.2). The problem for neuropsychological theory is to understand how particular movements are selected given that there are more degrees of freedom available in the muscles and joints than in the required task performance. A number of physiological and psychological solutions have been studied, including efficiency constraints, synergies, and biomechanical effects such as gravity. In any case, however, a simple movement can be a complex thing for a nervous system to execute in an accurate and efficient manner.

The second problem, the *serial-order* problem, has to do with how motor behaviors are sequenced. Many motor behaviors are sequenced in complex ways, and the order must be accurate for the individual to complete the task appropriately (e.g., speaking or writing). Speech errors such as spoonerisms suggest that there are distinct levels of representation in the planning and production of speech that may become affected

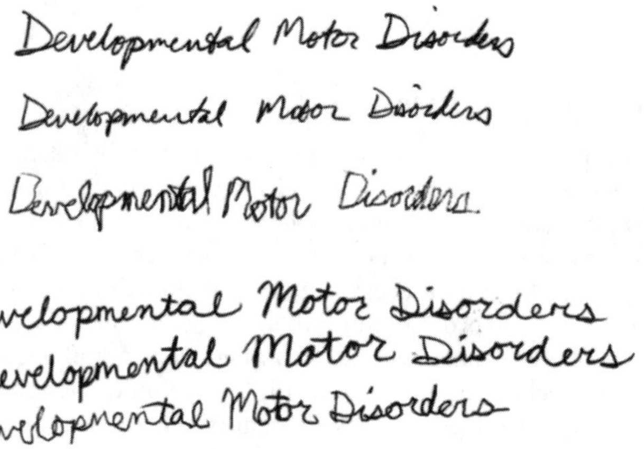

FIGURE 1.2. A demonstration of consistency and constancy with motor equivalence in graphomotor skills. The top three lines were written by the senior author of this chapter, and the bottom three lines by his 16-year-old daughter. The first two lines by each writer show the consistency of their dominant hand writing styles (both intraindividual and, to some degree, interindividual), while the bottom line for each writer demonstrates the constancy of writing form with their nondominant hand, albeit with deterioration in quality for this less practiced task.

in motor disorders. In fact, if motor behaviors were not sequenced and planned accurately (e.g., with coarticulation), then speeded activities would be executed extremely slowly. Recognizing this important feature, Luria (1973) described a "kinetic melody" as a basis for competent motor activities. Studies of motor behavior mistakes, or action slips, provide some information about the psychological foundations of complex motor activity.

How individuals coordinate motor activity and perception lies at the core of the *perceptual–motor integration* problem. Woodworth's (1899) early research on voluntary movements suggested that virtually all aiming movements proceed in a two-stage fashion, with an initial ballistic phase followed by a corrective phase. A key concept that needs to be incorporated into developmental motor theories is the importance of feedback in such movements. Movement never occurs in a behavioral vacuum; movements are both influenced by perception and also influence perception. Negative and positive feedback processing is essential for accurate movement. Movement is also organized with respect to the spatial coordinates of the body and the spatial coordinates of external space, and these forms of information need to be integrated in the motor system.

The final motor control problem can be described as the *skill-acquistion* problem—how motor skills are acquired. The problem of skill acquisition continues to be studied in many contexts and is perhaps more psychological in nature (Cox, 1934). Naturally, this is a critical core issue in motor control, and it consists of several subproblems, such as the extent to which motor skills are innate versus learned, how learned motor skills are acquired, what learner factors (e.g., age, neurological status, and motivation) influence skill acquisition, the role of feedback or practice, and others. Many contemporary theories of skill acquisition recognize the need for mental representations in the planning and execution of actions, and current cognitive neuroscience research deals with representations of object-oriented actions, mental motor imagery, and similar topics (for further examples, see Clearfield & Thelen, 2001; Connolly & Forssberg, 1997; Jeannerod, 1997).

New Technologies: Functional Neuroimaging and Molecular Genetics

Our understanding of the cerebral organization of childhood motor disorders has historically been advanced on the basis of description of clinical cases and lesion studies. In very recent history, there have been a number of new technologies developed that hold considerable promise to help us understand better the cytogenetics, neuroanatomy, and neurophysiology of these disorders, as well as the normal functioning of the developing human brain. Functional neuroimaging and molecular genetic technology will guide the future history of our understanding of childhood motor disorders.

Functional neuroimaging techniques include structural magnetic resonance imaging (MRI), positron emission tomography (PET), single photon emission computed tomography (SPECT), and functional magnetic resonance imaging (fMRI). Chapter 2 discusses each of these techniques and their application to the study of motor development in more detail; for examples of each of these technologies applied to the study of developmental disabilities, the reader can consult Durston and colleagues (2001) about structural MRI, Chugani and Chugani (2002) concerning PET and SPECT, Filipek (1997) for structural neuroimaging, Price and Friston (2003) about the blood oxygen level–dependent (BOLD) technique of fMRI, and Lyon and Rumsey (1996) for future directions in neuroimaging of developmental disorders.

Information on morphological aspects of development has been accumulating for many years, but only recently have there been significant advances in understanding the molecular basis of developmental processes. More detailed understanding of the cytogenetic and molecular genetic aspects of a number of childhood motor disorders with these new technologies has already occurred, including pathogenetic mechanisms for muscular and myotonic dystrophy, Huntington's chorea, Tourette syndrome, and many other developmental disabilities. Genetic mutations, impaired genetic transcription, specific chromosomal or gene abnormalities, programmed cell death, and abnormal expansion of trinucleotide repeat regions are all mechanisms being explored for their relationship to various developmental neurological disorders and degenerative conditions (Breg, 1996). The molecular genetics of various developmental neurological disorders are discussed in detail in relevant chapters in this book.

CONCLUSIONS

The study of childhood motor disorders has engendered a long and profitable history. A veritable survey of prominent neurological and psychological figures has provided valuable past information to guide future efforts in the exploration of the neuroscientific foundations and clinical treatment methods for children with developmental and acquired disorders of motor behavior. The study of childhood motor disorders involves an understanding of normal and abnormal motor development, the cerebral organization of the motor system, skill acquisition and movement control, and clinical conditions affecting motor skills of children. Future research will continue to be dependent on insightful clinicians and researchers who can make best use of the past research and newer technological advances.

REFERENCES

Accardo, P. (1989). William John Little and cerebral palsy in the nineteenth century. *Journal of the History of Medicine and Allied Sciences, 44,* 56–71.

Adolph, K. E., Weise, I., & Marin, L. (2003). Motor development. In L. R. Nadel (Ed.), *Encyclopedia of cognitive science* (Vol. 3, pp. 134–137). London: Nature.

Albanese, A. (1989). Extrapyramidal system and extrapyramidal disorders. In F. C. Rose (Ed.), *Neuroscience across the centuries* (pp. 97–109). London: Smith-Gordon.

American Psychiatric Association. (1994). *Diagnostic and statistical manual of mental disorders* (4th ed.). Washington, DC: Author.

Angelini, L., Balottin, U., Lanzi, G., & Nardocci, N. (Eds.). (1987). *Extrapyramidal disorders in childhood.* Amsterdam: Excerpta Medica.

Ayres, A. J. (1972). *Sensory integration and learning disorders.* Los Angeles: Western Psychological Services.

Ayres, A. J. (1985). *Developmental dyspraxia and adult-onset apraxia.* Torrance, CA: Sensory Integration International.

Ball, R. S. (1977). The Gesell developmental schedules: Arnold Gesell (1880–1961). *Journal of Abnormal Child Psychology, 5*(3), 233–239.

Barbeau, A. (1981). History of movement disorders and their treatment. In A Barbeau (Ed.), *Disorders of movement* (pp.1–28). Philadelphia: Lippincott.

Beighton, P., & Beighton, G. (1986). *The man behind the syndrome.* Berlin: Springer-Verlag.

Bender, L. (1947). Childhood schizophrenia: Clinical study of one hundred schizophrenic children. *American Journal of Orthopsychiatry, 17,* 40–46.

Bender, L. (1956). *Psychopathology of children with organic brain disorders.* Springfield, IL: Thomas.

Bernstein, N. (1967). *The co-ordination and regulation of movements.* Oxford, UK: Pergamon Press.

Bernstein, N. A. (1996). *Dexterity and its development* (M. L. Latash & M. T. Turvey, Eds.). Mahwah, NJ: Erlbaum.

Breg, W. R. (1996). The genetics of embryonic development. In A. J. Capute & P. J. Accardo (Eds.), *Developmental disabilities in infancy and childhood, Vol. I: Neurodevelopmental diagnosis and treatment* (2nd ed., pp. 91–111). Baltimore: Brookes.

Bruininks, R. H. (1978). *Bruininks–Oseretsky test of motor proficiency: Examiner's manual.* Circle Pines, MN: American Guidance Service.

Chugani, D. C., & Chugani, H. T. (2002). Positron emission tomography (PET) and single photon emission computed tomography (SPECT) in developmental disorders. In S. J. Segalowitz & I. Rapin (Eds.), *Handbook of neuropsychology: Vol. 8, Part I. Child neuropsychology* (2nd ed., pp. 195–215). Amsterdam: Elsevier.

Clarke, E., & O'Malley, C. D. (1996). *The human brain and spinal cord: A historical study illustrated by writings from antiquity to the twentieth century.* San Francisco: Norman.

Clearfield, M. W., & Thelen, E. (2001). Stability and flexibility in the acquisition of skilled movement. In C. A. Nelson, & M. Luciana (Eds.), *Handbook of developmental cognitive neuroscience* (pp. 253–266). Cambridge, MA: MIT. Press.

Connolly, K. J., & Forssberg, H. (Eds.). (1997). *Neurophysiology and neuropsychology of motor development* (Clinics in Developmental Medicine, Nos. 143/144). London: MacKeith Press.

Cox, J. W. (1934). *Manual skill: Its organization and development.* London: Cambridge University Press.

Cratty, B. J. (1994). *Clumsy child syndromes: Descriptions, evaluation and remediation.* Langhorne, PA: Harwood.

Darras, B. T., Menache, C. C., & Kunkel, L. M. (2003). Dystrophinopathies. In H. R. Jones, Jr., D. C. DeVivo, & B. T. Darras (Eds.), *Neuromuscular disorders of infancy, childhood, and adolescence: A clinician's approach* (pp. 649–699). Amsterdam: Butterworth-Heinemann.

Deuel, R. K. (2002). Motor soft signs and development. In S. J. Segalowitz & I. Rapin (Eds.), *Handbook of neuropsychology: Vol. 8, Part I. Child neuropsychology* (2nd ed., pp. 367–383). Amsterdam: Elsevier.

Deuel, R. K., & Robinson, D. J. (1987). Developmental motor signs. In D.E. Tupper (Ed.), *Soft neurological signs* (pp. 95–129). Orlando, FL: Grune & Stratton.

DeVivo, D. C., Darras, B. T., & Jones, H. R., Jr. (2003). Introduction: Historical perspectives. In H. R. Jones, Jr., D. C. DeVivo, & B. T. Darras (Eds.), *Neuromuscular disorders of infancy, childhood, and adolescence: A clinician's approach* (pp. 3–17). Amsterdam: Butterworth-Heinemann.

Doll, E. A. (Ed.). (1946). *The Oseretsky Tests of Motor Proficiency: A translation from the Portuguese adaptation.* Circle Pines, MN: American Guidance Service.

Duchenne, G. B. A. (1861). *Paraplégie hypertrophique de l'enfance de cause cérébrale* (2nd ed.). Paris: Ballière et Fils.

Dunn, P. M. (1995). Dr. William Little (1810–1894) of London and cerebral palsy. *Archives of Disease in Childhood, 72,* F209–F210.

Dupré, E. (1925). *Pathologie de L'Imagination et de L'Emotivite.* Paris: Pavot.

Durston, S., Hulshoff, H. E., Casey, B. J., Giedd, J. N., Buitelaar, J. K., & van Engeland, H. (2001). Anatomical MRI of the developing human brain: What have we learned? *Journal of the American Academy of Child and Adolescent Psychiatry, 40*(9), 1012–1020.

Espenschade, A. (1947). Motor development. *Review of Educational Research, 17,* 354–361.

Faglioni, P., & Basso, A. (1985). Historical perspectives on neuroanatomical correlates of limb apraxia. In E. A. Roy (Ed.), *Neuropsychological studies of apraxia and related disorders* (pp. 3–44). Amsterdam: North-Holland.

Filipek, P. A. (1997). Structural variations in measures in the developmental disorders. In R. W. Thatcher, G. R. Lyon, J. Rumsey, & N. Krasnegor (Eds.), *Developmental neuroimaging: Mapping the development of brain and behavior* (pp. 169–186). San Diego, CA: Academic Press.

Finger, S. (1994). *Origins of neuroscience: A history of explorations into brain function.* New York: Oxford University Press.

Ford, F. R. (1966). *Diseases of the nervous system in infancy, childhood, and adolescence* (5th ed.). Springfield, IL: Charles C. Thomas.

Forssberg, H. (1998). The neurophysiology of manual skill development. In K. J. Connolly (Ed.), *The psychobiology of the hand* (Clinics in Developmental Medicine, No. 147) (pp. 97–122). London: MacKeith Press.

Freud, S. (1897). *Die infantile Cerebrallahmung.* Vienna, Austria: Holder.

Freud, S. (1968). *Infantile cerebral paralysis.* Coral Gables, FL: University of Miami Press.

George, M. S. (1992). Changing nineteenth century views on the origins of cerebral palsy: W. J. Little and Sigmund Freud. *Journal of the History of the Neurosciences, 1,* 29–37.

Gesell, A. (1933). Maturation and the patterning of behavior. In C. Murchison (Ed.), *Manual of child psychology* (pp. 209–235). Worcester, MA: Clark University Press.

Gesell, A., & Amatruda, C. S. (1947). *Developmental diagnosis.* New York: Hoeber.

Gibson, J. J. (1966). *The senses considered as perceptual systems.* Boston: Houghton Mifflin.

Gilles de la Tourette, G. (1885). Etude sur une affection nerveuse caracterisée par de l'incoordination motrice accompagnée d'echolalie et de coprolalie. *Archives de Neurologie, 9*(19), 185.

Goetz, C. G., Chmura, T. A., & Lanska, D. J. (2001a). History of tic disorders and Gilles de la Tourette syndrome: Part 5 of the MDS-sponsored history of movement disorders exhibit, Barcelona, June 2000. *Movement Disorders, 16*(2), 346–349.

Goetz, C. G., Chmura, T. A., & Lanska, D. J. (2001b). Seminal figures in the history of movement disorders: Sydenham, Parkinson, and Charcot: Part 6 of the MDS-sponsored history of movement disorders exhibit, Barcelona, June 2000. *Movement Disorders, 16*(3), 537–540.

Gottlieb, G. (1998). Myrtle McGraw's unrecognized conceptual contribution to developmental psychology. *Developmental Review, 18,* 437–448.

Gowers, W. R. (1886). *A manual of diseases of the nervous system.* London: Churchill.

Gubbay, S. (1975). *The clumsy child: A study of developmental apraxic and agnostic ataxia.* London: Saunders.

Hammond, W. A. (1871). *A treatise on diseases of the nervous system.* New York: Appleton.

Heilman, K. M., & Rothi, L. J. G. (1997). Limb apraxia: A look back. In L. J. G. Rothi & K. M. Heilman (Eds.), *Apraxia: The neuropsychology of action* (pp. 7–18). Hove, UK: Psychology Press.

Heilman, K. M., Watson, R. T., & Rothi, L. J. G. (2000). Praxis. In C. G. Goetz & E. J. Pappert (Eds.), *Textbook of clinical neurology* (pp. 49–55). Philadelphia: Saunders.

Henderson, S. E. (1993). Motor development and minor handicap. In A. F. Kalverboer, B. Hopkins, & R. Geuze (Eds.), *Motor development in early and later childhood: Longitudinal approaches* (pp. 286–306). New York: Cambridge University Press.

Hopkins, B. (2001). Understanding motor development: Insights from dynamical systems perspectives. In A. F. Kalverboer & A. Gramsbergen (Eds.), *Handbook of brain and behaviour in human development* (pp. 591–620). Dordrecht: Kluwer Academic.

Hopkins, B., Beek, P. J., & Kalverboer, A. F. (1993). Theoretical issues in the longitudinal study of motor development. In A. F. Kalverboer, B. Hopkins, & R. Geuze (Eds.), *Motor development in early and later childhood: Longitudinal approaches* (pp. 343–371). New York: Cambridge University Press.

Huntington, G. (1872). On chorea. *Medical and Surgical Reporter, 26*, 317–321.

Jeannerod, M. (1997). *The cognitive neuroscience of action.* Cambridge, MA: Blackwell.

Kalverboer, A. F. (1993). Motor development in children at risk: Two decades of research in experimental clinical psychology. In A. F. Kalverboer, B. Hopkins, & R. Geuze (Eds.), *Motor development in early and later childhood: Longitudinal approaches* (pp. 1–14). New York: Cambridge University Press.

Kessler, J. W. (1980). History of minimal brain dysfunctions. In H. E. Rie & E. D. Rie (Eds.), *Handbook of minimal brain dysfunctions: A critical view* (pp. 18–51). New York: Wiley-Interscience.

Kimura, D. (1980). *Translations from Liepmann's essays on apraxia* (Research Bulletin #506). London, Ontario: Department of Psychology, University of Western Ontario.

Knobloch, H., & Pasamanick, B. (Eds.). (1974). *Gesell and Amatruda's developmental diagnosis: The evaluation and management of abnormal neuropsychologic development in infancy and early childhood* (3rd ed., rev. and enlarged). Hagerstown, MD: Harper & Row.

Koupernik, C., MacKeith, R., & Francis-Williams, J. (1975). Neurological correlates of motor and perceptual development. In W. M. Cruickshank & D. P. Hallahan (Eds.), *Perceptual and learning disabilities in children. Vol. 2: Research and theory* (pp. 105–135). Syracuse, NY: Syracuse University Press.

Lanska, D. J. (2000). George Huntington (1850–1916) and hereditary chorea. *Journal of the History of the Neurosciences, 9*(1), 76–89.

Lanska, D. J., Goetz, C. G., & Chmura, T. A. (2001). Seminal figures in the history of movement disorders: Hammond, Osler, and Huntington: Part 11 of the MDS-sponsored history of movement disorders exhibit, Barcelona, June 2000. *Movement Disorders, 16*(4), 749–753.

Lassner, R. (1948). Annotated bibliography on the Oseretsky tests of motor proficiency. *Journal of Consulting Psychology, 12*, 37–47.

Liepmann, H. (1988). Apraxia. In J. W. Brown (Ed.), *Agnosia and apraxia: Selected papers of Liepmann, Lange, and Pötzl* (pp. 3–39). Hillsdale, NJ: Erlbaum. (Original work published 1900)

Little, W. J. (1862). On the influence of abnormal parturition, difficult labour, premature birth, and asphyxia neonatorum on the mental and physical condition of the child, especially in relation to deformities. *Transactions of the Obstetrical Society of London, 3*, 293.

Lockman, J. J. (1990). Perceptuomotor coordination in infancy. In C. A. Hauert (Ed.), *Developmental psychology: Cognitive, perceptuo-motor, and neuropsychological perspectives* (pp. 85–111). Amsterdam: North-Holland.

Lohr, J. B., Wisniewski, A. A., & Lohr, M. A. (1987). A brief history of disorders of movement. In J. B. Lohr & A. A. Wisniewski (Eds.), *Movement disorders: A neuropsychiatric approach* (pp. 3–14). New York: Guilford Press.

Longo, L. D., & Ashwal, S. (1993). William Osler, Sigmund Freud and the evolution of ideas concerning cerebral palsy. *Journal of the History of the Neurosciences, 2*, 255–282.

Luria, A. R. (1973). *The working brain: An introduction to neuropsychology.* New York: Basic Books.

Lyon, G. R., & Rumsey, J. M. (1996). Neuroimaging and developmental disorders: Comments and future directions. In G. R. Lyon & J. M. Rumsey (Eds.), *Neuroimaging: A window to the neurological foundations of learning and behavior in children* (pp. 227–236). Baltimore: Brookes.

Manoel, E. deJ., & Connolly, K. J. (1998). The development of manual dexterity in young children. In K. J. Connolly (Ed.), *The psychobiology of the hand* (Clinics in Developmental Medicine, No. 147) (pp. 177–198). London: MacKeith Press.

McGraw, M. B. (1935). *Growth: A study of Johnny and Jimmy*. New York: Appleton-Century-Crofts.

McGraw, M. B. (1945). *The neuromuscular maturation of the human infant*. New York: Columbia University Press.

Morris, M. K. (1997). Developmental dyspraxia. In L. J. G. Rothi & K. M. Heilman (Eds.), *Apraxia: The neuropsychology of action* (pp. 245–268). Hove, UK: Psychology Press.

Orton, S. T. (1937). *Reading, writing, and speech problems in children*. New York: Norton.

Oseretzky, N. I. (1925). Eine metrische Stufenleiter zur Untersuchung der motorischen Begabung bei Kindern [A metric scale for the study of the motor ability of children]. *Zeitschrift Fuer Kinderforschung, 30*, 300–314.

Oseretzky, N. (1931). *Psychomotorik: Methoden zur Untersuchung der Motorik* [Methods of investigation of psychomotor activity]. Leipzig: Verlag von Johann Ambrosius Barth.

Osler, W. (1894). *On chorea and choreiform affections*. Philadelphia: Blakiston.

Ozeretskii, N. I. (1925). Metricheskaya skala dlya issledovaniya motornoi odarennosti y detei i podrostkov [A metric scale for investigating motor abilities in young children and youth]. In M. Gurevich (Ed.), *Voprosy Pedologii I Detskoi Psihkonevrologii* (Vypusk 2, pp. 334–346). Moskva: Izd-vo.

Ozeretskii, N. I. (1929). *Metod Massovoi Otsenki Motoriki u Detei i Podrostkov* [A group method for motor appraisal of young children and youth]. Moskva: Gosud. Meditsinskoe Izd-vo.

Park, R. H. R., & Park, M. P. (1990). Saint Vitus' dance: Vital misconceptions by Sydenham and Bruegel. *Journal of the Royal Society of Medicine, 83*, 512–515.

Parkinson, J. (1817). *Essay on the shaking palsy*. London: Whittingham and Rowland for Sherwood, Neely, and Jones.

Pavlov, I. P. (1927). *Conditioned reflexes: An investigation of the physiological activity of the cerebral cortex* (G. V. Anrep, Trans.). London: Oxford University Press.

Preyer, W. T. (1882). *Die Seele des Kindes*. Leipzig: Grieben.

Preyer, W. T. (1885). *Specielle Physiologie des Embryo*. Leipzig: Grieben.

Preyer, W. T. (1888). *The mind of the child, Part I: The senses and the will* (H.W. Brown, Trans.). New York: Appleton.

Price, C. J., & Friston, K. J. (2003). Functional neuroimaging studies of neuropsychological patients. In T. E. Feinberg & M. J. Farah (Eds.), *Behavioral neurology and neuropsychology* (2nd ed., pp. 97–104). New York: McGraw-Hill.

Rosenbaum, D. A. (1991). *Human motor control*. San Diego, CA: Academic Press.

Schifrin, B. S., & Longo, L. D. (2000). William John Little and cerebral palsy: A reappraisal. *European Journal of Obstetrics and Gynecology and Reproductive Biology, 90*, 139–144.

Segalowitz, S. J., & Hiscock, M. (2002). The neuropsychology of normal development: Developmental neuroscience and a new constructivism. In S. J. Segalowitz & I. Rapin (Eds.), *Handbook of neuropsychology. Vol. 8, Part I: Child neuropsychology, Part I* (2nd ed., pp. 7–27). Amsterdam: Elsevier.

Sherrington, C. (1906). *The integrative action of the nervous system*. New York: Charles Scribner's Sons.

Shumway-Cook, A., & Woollacott, M. H. (1995). *Motor control: Theory and practical applications*. Baltimore: Williams & Wilkins.

Sloan, W. (1955). The Lincoln–Oseretsky Motor Development Scale. *Genetic Psychology Monographs, 51*, 183–252.

Strauss, A. A., & Kephart, N. C. (1955). *Psychopathology and education of the brain-injured child, Vol. II: Progress in theory and clinic*. New York: Grune & Stratton.

Strauss, A. A., & Lehtinen, L. E. (1947). *Psychopathology and education of the brain-injured child, Vol. I*. New York: Grune & Stratton.

Sydenham, T. (1686). *Schedula Monitoria de Novae Febris Ingressu*. Londini: W. Kettilby.

Thelen, E. (1995). Motor development: a new synthesis. *American Psychologist, 50*, 79–95.

Thelen, E. (2000). Motor development as foundation and future of developmental psychology. *International Journal of Behavioral Development, 24*(4), 385–397.

Tupper, D. E. (1987). The issues with "soft signs." In D. E. Tupper (Ed.), *Soft neurological signs* (pp. 1–16). Orlando, FL: Grune & Stratton.

Williams, H. G. (1983). *Perceptual and motor development*. Englewood Cliffs, NJ: Prentice-Hall.

Wolff, P. H. (1982). Theoretical issues in the development of motor skills. In M. Lewis & L. T. Taft (Eds.), *Developmental disabilities: Theory, assessment, and intervention* (pp. 117–134). New York: SP Medical and Scientific Books.

Woodworth, R. S. (1899). The accuracy of voluntary movement. *The Psychological Review (Monograph Suppl.), III*(2) (Whole No. 13).

Zanone, P. G. (1990). Perceptuo-motor development in the child and the adolescent: Perceptuo-motor coordination. In C. A. Hauert (Ed.), *Developmental psychology: Cognitive, perceptuo-motor, and neuropsychological perspectives* (pp. 309–338). Amsterdam: North-Holland.

Zaporozhets, A. V. (1960). *Razvitie Proizvolnykh Dvizhenii* [Development of voluntary movements]. Moskva: Izd-vo.

CHAPTER 2

Neuroimaging of Developmental Motor Disorders

DEBORAH DEWEY
SHAUNA BOTTOS

A wide selection of imaging techniques has become available in the past decade that allow for the *in vivo* examination of brain structure, biochemistry, and function. These techniques serve an important role in advancing our understanding of both normal and atypical brain development and provide a means of exploring the etiological substrates implicated in motor disorders. Studies comparing children with a specific impairment to their normally developing peers have provided invaluable insights into the mechanisms involved in pathological developmental processes and the plasticity of the human brain. Research has also begun to examine the relationship between imaging findings early in childhood and long-term neurological and cognitive sequelae.

This chapter begins with a discussion of the predominant neuroimaging techniques currently in use with children, followed by a discussion of the unique methodological challenges posed when imaging children. The most common applications of imaging from infancy to adolescence are then explored, with a focus on children at risk for the development of cerebral palsy and related movement disorders. As noted in Chapter 18, children with developmental disorders such as learning disabilities attention-deficit/hyperactivity disorder, and autism frequently display motor problems. Therefore, recent imaging studies with these populations are briefly touched on. The chapter concludes with an overview of the findings of imaging studies that have investigated adult-onset motor disorders, specifically Parkinson's disease, Huntington's disease, and dystonia.

IMAGING MODALITIES

Ultrasonography

Cranial ultrasonography (US) is the most widely available and commonly used neuroimaging technique with children. In US, a transducer emits high-frequency sound waves that reflect off tissue interfaces to produce images of good clarity (Hoon,

Belsito, & Nagae-Poetscher, 2003). Because cranial US is noninvasive, can be delivered at bedside, and does not require sedation, intravenous contrast, or exposure to ionizing radiation, it is the ideal screening tool for neonatal brain imaging, especially among fragile preterm infants (Boyer, 1994). While it provides a good assessment of brain structure and brain maturation, it is of greatest utility in detecting abnormalities in periventricular white matter, although its sensitivity for detecting diffuse or subtle white matter abnormalities is poor (Debillon et al., 2003; Maalouf et al., 2001). US provides less even coverage of the brain compared with other imaging techniques such as magnetic resonance imaging (MRI). Therefore, identification of abnormalities in deeper and peripheral structures, such as the basal ganglia and cortex, is more challenging using this technique (Maalouf et al., 2001).

Computer Tomography

The computer tomography (CT) scan is a computer-enhanced X-ray of brain structure. With this technique, multiple X-rays are shot from many angles, and the computer combines the readings to create a vivid image of a horizontal slice of the brain. The entire brain can be visualized by assembling a series of images representing successive slices of the brain. Of the new imaging techniques, the CT scan is the least expensive and, hence, one of the most widely used in research. Similar to US, CT does not require sedation, and the scans can be completed relatively quickly, making it suitable for assessing high-risk newborns and cases of trauma (Boyer, 1994). Limitations include exposure to iodizing radiation, artifact from the bones of the skull, and confinement to one plane of acquisition (Hoon et al., 2003).

Positron Emission Tomography

In research on how brain and behavior are related, positron emission tomography (PET) has proven especially valuable. While CT scans can only portray brain *structure*, PET scans are able to map actual *activity* in the brain over time. In PET scans, radioactively tagged chemicals are introduced into the brain, serving as markers of blood flow or glucose metabolism, which can be monitored with X-rays. Thus, PET scans provide color-coded maps illustrating areas of high activity in the brain over time. In this way, one is able to pinpoint brain areas involved when the individual performs particular cognitive or motor activities. Because this type of scan monitors chemical processes, it can also be used to study the activity of specific neurotransmitters. A limitation of PET is its low spatial resolution. Moreover, due to radiation exposure, PET scans may have limited applications with children, although they have been frequently used to study neurological diseases in children (Hoon et al., 2003).

Single-Photon Emission Computed Tomography

Single-photon emission computed tomography (SPECT) relies on the detection of emitted photons from proton-rich unstable isotopes after captivation of an orbiting electron (Lammertsma, 2001). Similar to PET, the injection of a tracer allows one to follow cerebral blood flow, which varies as a function of metabolic rate, thereby revealing areas of higher and lower brain activity (Hoon et al., 2003). When compared to PET, however, SPECT has been reported to have lower resolution. At present, few pediatric patients undergo this procedure as it requires exposure to high levels of radiation.

Magnetic Resonance Imaging

MRI uses magnetic fields, radio waves, and computerized enhancement to map out brain structure and brain function. The mechanism of the MRI image is based on the behavior of hydrogen protons in a magnetic field. Radiofrequency pulses cause protons to absorb energy, and when these pulses terminate, the protons begin a process of relaxation (Frank & Pavlakis, 2001). These changes are detected when imaging and can be visualized on the scan. MRI scans provide much clearer and more detailed images of brain structure than do CT scans, producing three-dimensional pictures of the brain that have remarkably high resolution. Indeed, as a result of improved tissue resolution, MRI has replaced CT for most clinical indications (Hoon et al., 2003). Other advantages of MRI over other neuroimaging techniques include the lack of bone artifact and the absence of ionizing radiation (Hoon et al., 2003; Maalouf et al., 1999). The production of high-quality images on MRI scans make them ideal for observing normal and abnormal myelination processes, including the more subtle lesions evident in the white matter of the brain, which frequently go undetected by US and CT (Maalouf et al., 2001). Limitations to MRI include the equipment's sensitivity to motion, lengthy imaging time, and the need for sedation (Hoon et al., 2003).

Functional Magnetic Resonance Imaging

Functional magnetic resonance imaging (fMRI) uses conventional magnetic resonance (MR) scanners with upgraded hardware and fast imaging techniques to observe alterations in blood flow (Krasuski, Horwitz, & Rumsey, 1996). When multiple MR images are acquired rapidly, small changes in signal intensity are used to determine focal areas of activation. These changes are caused by variations in the local vascular oxygenated and deoxygenated hemoglobin concentrations. Thus, both structural and functional images are produced. Because there are no radioisotope injections (Hoon et al., 2003), fMRI may be especially applicable for children. However, in cases in which task performance cooperation is required, this technique may be limited to children capable of carrying out such tasks (e.g., older or nonimpaired children).

Diffusion-Weighted Imaging

Diffusion-weighted imaging (DWI) is a relatively recent innovation that depends on the slow random motion (diffusion) of water molecules in the central nervous system (Le Bihan, 1995). An apparent diffusion coefficient is computed, which represents differences in water diffusion in various brain tissues (Hoon et al., 2003). The limitations of DWI, such as sensitivity to movement and a relatively lengthy imaging time, are similar to MRI. DWI has recently been used with premature infants and shows great promise in the detection of periventricular white matter injury in this population (Inder, Huppi, Zientara, et al., 1999).

METHODOLOGICAL ISSUES IN PEDIATRIC NEUROIMAGING

The development of these neuroimaging techniques has made it possible to study neural development in normal children, as well as those with developmental disorders. However, with the increasing use of neuroimaging during infancy and childhood, there has been an increased recognition of the many methodological, conceptual, and practical issues that are unique to pediatric populations.

Prior to the emergence of fMRI, functional neuroimaging studies were limited to using PET and MRI. With pediatric populations, the use of both of these techniques was cause for concern. PET required the injection of radiopharmaceuticals. Because of the known risks of radiation to children, this imaging modality was limited to very sick children for whom the clinical benefit potentially outweighed the risks (Bookheimer, 2000). MRI required that children be sedated. Although the use of anesthesia for sick children for whom there would be some clinical benefit was not an issue, its use with children for research purposes was controversial. Thus, only with the recent advances in imaging techniques has it been possible to expand neuroimaging investigations to the general pediatric population.

Neuroimaging studies with adults have typically focused on how a specific operation is performed in the brain, which allowed investigators to use single-group designs. In contrast, imaging studies with children have often examined how children with a particular disorder or disability differ from typically developing children. Therefore, in studies with children, multigroup designs have been necessary. These multigroup designs are associated with unique challenges in terms of the choice of control groups, dependent measures and analysis tools (see Bookheimer, 2000).

When brain activation on imaging is used as the outcome measure, a number of variables could affect the findings of studies involving children such as the choice of the comparison group, task difficulty, performance level, and stimulus intensity. Some studies have compared the brain activation of children with and without a disability while they perform a task, whereas other studies have compared children's performance on a task with that of adults. Both of these experimental designs are problematic as any differences in task performance and, hence, activation patterns, could reflect familiarity with the task as opposed to the underlying research question (Bookheimer, 2000). Indeed, it has been demonstrated that increased practice (or experience) on several types of tasks may alter not only the intensity of activation but also the brain regions which are activated (Raichle et al., 1994). Variables such as task difficulty, performance level, and stimulus intensity have also been found to have an effect on brain activation. For example, investigations have found that increasing task difficulty, the rate of task performance, or the intensity of the stimulus presentation has resulted in increased brain activation (e.g., Fox & Raichle, 1986; Just, Carpenter, Keller, Eddy, & Thulborn, 1996). Thus, if groups of subjects are not well matched and variables such as task difficulty are not controlled for, making comparisons between groups and interpreting differences in brain activation present a major challenge for the investigators.

Distinct anatomical features during childhood may also affect brain activation patterns. It is well known that as children develop, the ratio of gray to white matter in the brain decreases, a process that continues well into adolescence (Sowell, Thompson,

Holmes, Jernigan, & Toga, 1999). Individual differences in rates of myelination may account for differences in both activation patterns and magnitude (Bookheimer, 2000) and therefore deserve careful consideration when applying neuroimaging techniques to children, particularly when making interindividual comparisons.

Another difficulty with imaging children concerns their size. The small size of neonates, particularly their shorter neck and smaller head compared to adults, is often not well suited to the geometry of MR imaging techniques (Boyer, 1994). Because magnets are shimmered to offer the highest signal in the center of the coil, an area that may be out of reach for the infant, images will offer less contrast to noise and may, as a result, yield artificially low estimates of brain activity (Bookheimer, 2000).

A practical consideration that is important when imaging children is their inability to monitor their own small movements (Bookheimer, 2000). MRI techniques are particularly sensitive to head motion, which affects the degree of contrast to background noise on the image (Bookheimer, 2000; Boyer, 1994). Furthermore, because children tend to be frightened more easily than adults, the experimenter has the added responsibility of determining a priori which children will be satisfactory participants and desensitizing them to what will be required. Ensuring that children remain awake and cooperative throughout the procedure may also pose a challenge with some children, particularly those with poorer attention spans.

Relative to their healthy peers, high-risk children, such as those born prematurely or of low birth weight, require that even more precautions be taken when they are subjected to imaging. Concerns that must be addressed include dealing with challenges related to their small size and their fragility. A significant risk may be associated with the moving of fragile infants to imaging facilities located outside the neonatal intensive care environment because many of them require ventilatory assistance, multiple indwelling catheters, vasopressor support, infusions, and warming lights (Ment et al., 2002). Moreover, depending on the severity of organ diseases, the premature neonate requires careful monitoring of blood gases, blood pressure, heart and respiratory rate, temperature, fluid balance, and electrolytes (Boyer, 1994). Recognition of the different spectrum of diseases encountered in the premature neonate compared to those found in full-term neonates, older infants, and children is also necessary (Boyer, 1994; Ment et al., 2002).

In summary, neuroimaging with children requires several considerations pertaining to the experimental design development and the interpretation of findings, which are not encountered when imaging adults. As well, practical considerations, such as determining a priori the child's suitability for imaging and ways to sustain the child's interest while participating in the procedure, are unique to the pediatric population. High-risk infants bring with them additional considerations and pose an even greater challenge to imaging research.

NEUROIMAGING IN CEREBRAL PALSY

The morphological and functional development of the human brain involves a complex temporally and spatially ordered sequence of events. As such, infants born very preterm or of very low birth weight (VLBW) are prey to several adverse factors acting during the prenatal, perinatal, and neonatal periods, which may have a devastating effect on brain development. Indeed, among children born preterm or VLBW, brain damage is a significant problem, with parenchymal destruction, hypoxic–ischemic brain events and hemorrhages in the perinatal period strongly implicated in the development of cerebral palsy (CP) (Volpe, 1997). The advent of neuroimaging techniques has allowed researchers to examine brain abnormalities *in vivo*, rather than relying exclusively on the child's external symptomatology when diagnosing brain damage in newborn infants. Consequently, imaging procedures can be of great importance in guiding the clinical evaluation of children with CP (Hoon et al., 2003). Furthermore, neuroimaging techniques may play a vital role in identifying children who may benefit from neuroprotective interventions to prevent later motor impairment.

The accurate prediction of clinical outcome after neonatal brain damage has become increasingly important as the number of infants surviving such adversarial circumstances increases. Of interest is the accumulating literature on the motor deficits that frequently result from brain trauma. In a large prospective cohort study conducted by the Neonatal Brain Hemorrhage study group (Pinto-Martin et al., 1995), the investigators examined the relationship between abnormalities on neonatal US obtained at 4 and 24 hours and 7 days of age, and the subsequent development of CP at 2 years of age in low-birth-weight infants. Particularly noteworthy was the assessment of US-mediated risk factors for two levels of motor dysfunction, namely, disabling CP (DCP) and nondisabling CP (NDCP). Seven hundred and seventy-seven children were evaluated at follow-up, of which approximately 15% were classified as having CP. Of the children with CP, 8% had DCP, while 7% had NDCP. Although children with NDCP commonly exhibited neurological symptoms such as increased leg tone with an inability to dorsiflex at the ankle and/or difficulties with hip extension and adduction, these difficulties did not interfere with daily living. The authors suggested that this group of children could be best described as manifesting mild spastic diplegia. Children classified as having DCP also exhibited such neurological findings but in addition displayed significant impairment in their ambulatory abilities and markedly poorer motor performance on the Bayley Scales of Infant Development. Importantly, the investigators found that US revealed differences in the etiology of DCP and NDCP. Specifically, the most powerful risk factor for DCP was lesions of the white matter, as manifested by parenchymal echodensities/lucencies or ventricular enlargement. Matrix/intraventricular hemorrhage was also found to be a moderate risk factor for these children. In contrast, the only significant risk factor delineated on US for children with NDCP was parenchymal echodensities/lucencies or ventricular enlargement. Thus, these findings strongly suggest that US evidence of perinatal brain injury is a powerful predictor for the development of DCP, whereas NDCP appears to be less closely related to perinatal brain lesions.

Neuroimaging techniques such as CT and MRI have allowed investigators to examine in a more precise manner the relationship between brain abnormalities and developmental pathology. Studies have observed various structural and functional deviations in infants' brains and the consequent development of specific subtypes of CP among high-risk children (Aida et al., 1998; Hoon et al., 2003). Hoon and colleagues (2003) proposed that children with CP could be categorized into five distinct groups, spastic diplegia, spastic quadriplegia, spastic hemiplegia, extrapyramidal movement disorders (dystonia, athetosis, bradykinesia, chorea, and hemiballismus), and ataxia or hypotonia, each characterized by specific etiologies with characteristic findings on imaging.

Spastic diplegia is the most commonly described long-term motor sequelae of periventricular leukomalacia (PVL) (Aida et al., 1998), which is associated with prematurity (Volpe, 1995). PVL is characterized by multifocal zones of necrosis in the periventricular white matter that can be detected using both US and MRI and is associated with motor, cognitive and visual impairments in children with VLBW (Perlman, 1998; Stewart et al., 1999). In addition to necrosis and cysts, MRI may reveal abnormal intraventricular, germinal matrix, and parenchymal hemorrhages, ventricular dilatation, and diffuse and excessive signal intensity in the white matter (Maalouf et al., 1999). While US may show evidence of the aforementioned types of hemorrhages, an advantage of MRI is its ability to detect more subtle white matter deviations (Maalouf et al., 2001). Indeed, with preterm infants, parenchymal lesions that manifest as hemorrhage, leukomalacia, infarction, and a reduction in white matter on MRI at term have been reported to predict CP with a significantly higher sensitivity than US (100% vs. 67%, respectively). Recently, advanced quantitative volumetric three-dimensional MRI techniques have also revealed impaired cerebral cortical development in premature children with PVL, signified by a marked reduction in cerebral gray matter and a reduction in the volume of total brain myelinated white matter (Inder, Huppi, Warfield, et al., 1999).

An accumulating body of evidence suggests that some of the brain abnormalities characteristic of PVL that are detected during infancy may persist well into later childhood and adolescence. MRI correlates of PVL, specifically gliosis and ventricular dilatation, are common findings on cerebral MRI at 6 years of age in children with VLBW (Skranes, Nilsen, Smevik, Vik, & Brubakk, 1998). Follow-up MRI studies of adolescents 14 to 15 years of age who were born preterm have reported that these children continue to show excess ventricular dilatation, as well as thinning of the corpus callosum, intraparenchymal cysts, and white matter deficits (Stewart et al., 1999). In a more recent study by Nosarti and colleagues (2002), the MRI scans of adolescents 14–15 years of age, who were born prematurely, revealed a decrease in whole brain volume, gray matter volume, and bilateral hippocampal volumes at follow-up. An increase in the size of the lateral ventricles was also noted. Diffusion-weighted MRI has only begun to be applied to the detection of brain insult in the pediatric population. However, preliminary studies suggest that it shows great promise for the identification of the subtle white matter deviations characteristic of PVL in cases where neither CT nor conventional MRI detected any abnormality (Inder, Huppi, Zientara, et al., 1999). Given the strong relationship between many cases of PVL in the premature infant and the subsequent development of CP, in conjunction with the persistence of early brain injury, the early detection of white matter damage is vital in order to maximize healthy development of these infants, particularly their motor development.

A wide range of insults can be the basis for spastic quadriplegia, and MRI can be an important tool in establishing the etiology of this disorder. A history of prematurity, perinatal hypoxic–ischemic injury, infection, or nonaccidental trauma may provide the etiological basis for spastic quadriplegia; however, a range of unexpected causes may also be uncovered using MRI, such as congenital cytomegalovirus infection, agenesis of the corpus callosum, Dandy–Walker malformations, holoprosencephaly, and neuronal migration disorders (Hoon et al., 2003).

Children who present with hemiplegic CP represent a distinct group with characteristic neuroimaging findings. In the majority of these children the hemiplegia has a prenatal etiology; however, in a small number of children it is associated with neonatal cerebral infarction or childhood stroke (Hoon et al, 2003). Aida and colleagues (1998) found MRI indications of hemorrhagic venous infarction or grade IV hemorrhage in severe cases of subependymal hemorrhage (SEH) and extensive cerebral infarction, which resulted in the development of spastic hemiparesis in their sample of premature children. Children with evidence of end-stage PVL and periventricular parenchymal destruction associated with SEH or cerebral infarction displayed a combination of spastic diplegia and hemiparesis. Other neuroimaging studies of children with hemiplegia of a prenatal onset have observed brain malformations such as unilateral polymicrogyria (Pascual-Castroviejo, Pascual-Pascual, Viano, Martinez, & Palencia, 2001) and schizencephaly on MRI (Denis et al., 2000).

Extrapyramidal CP encompasses a variety of movement disorders that have abnormalities in the basal ganglia on MRI (Gururaj et al., 2002; Hoon et al., 1997; Johnston, Nishimura, Harum, Pekar, & Blue, 2001). There is, however, a subgroup of children who appear to have static extrapyramidal CP but in fact have underlying genetic–metabolic disorders (Hoon et al., 1997). Neuroimaging procedures have provided invaluable diagnostic clues in such cases and have assisted investigators in distinguishing the etiological substrate of the presenting symptoms. For example, one common cause of static extrapyramidal CP is hypoxic–ischemic encephalopathy at the end of a term gestation (Hoon et al., 1997). This type of CP displays a characteristic pattern of high-signal intensity in the putamen and thalamus on MRI (Hoon et al., 1997; Menkes & Curran, 1994), as well as atrophy in these two brain regions (Hoon et al., 1997). In contrast to children with this static form of extrapyramidal CP, children with genetic–metabolic diseases, such as mitochondrial and organic acid-related disorders, tend to manifest other signal abnormalities and atrophy in the globus pallidus, putamen, or caudate nucleus (Hoon et al., 1997).

Recent advances in neuroimaging have provided researchers and clinicians with *in vivo* information on brain structure and function, which has facilitated a better understanding of the underlying pathology of the motor disorders in children. Indeed, these imaging techniques have demonstrated a remarkable ability to determine etiological substrates of several pediatric movement disorders, especially CP.

NEUROIMAGING IN NEURODEVELOPMENTAL DISORDERS

Over the past 10 years, neuroimaging techniques have been increasingly used in the investigation of brain morphology and function among children presenting with complex neurodevelopmental disorders. No recent studies have specifically examined the brain structure and function of children with developmental coordination disorder (but see Bergstrom & Bille, 1978; Knuckley, Apsimin, & Gubbay, 1983). However, neuroimaging studies of children with developmental disorders such as autism, attention-deficit/hyperactivity disorder (ADHD), and reading disabilities (dyslexia), which are often accompanied by motor deficits, may provide some insight into the neural bases of developmental motor problems (also see Chapters 8, 15, and 19, this volume).

Autism

The core clinical features of childhood autism are significant impairments in social interaction, limited activities and interests, verbal and nonverbal communication deficits, and stereotypical behavior patterns (Rinehart, Bradshaw, Brereton, & Tonge, 2002). PET scans have found that children with autism display abnormal patterns of activation in the left temporal cortex (Boddaert, Belin, & Poline, 2001), an area heavily involved in language. In addition, cerebellar abnormalities have been consistently reported in this population (Carper & Courchesne, 2000; Pierce & Courchesne, 2001). Carper and Courchesne (2000) also reported that in at least some cases of autism, a correlation exists between the degree of frontal lobe abnormality and the degree of cerebellar abnormality, with excess neural tissue present in the frontal lobe and too little in the cerebellum. Although the cerebellum has long been known to be involved in motor coordination, recent research has also emphasized its involvement in cognitive, language, and sensory functioning (Eliez & Reiss, 2000). Interestingly, evidence from MRI studies has also revealed that reduced exploration and stereotyped behaviors, hallmark features of autism, may be inversely related to cerebellar size (Pierce & Courchesne, 2001). Thus, deviations in cerebellar development may have diverse and widespread effects on not only children's motor functioning but also their cognitive and behavioral functioning.

Many children with autism have also been found to display other motor symptoms (Green et al., 2002; Manjiviona & Prior, 1995) such as gait abnormalities and hypotonia (Vilensky, Damasio, & Maurer, 1981). Motor clumsiness has also been reported in these children (Bonnet & Gao, 1996; Gillberg & Kadesjo, 2003). Although no imaging studies have specifically investigated the brain mechanisms that may be responsible for these motor deficits, one recent study that used fMRI did report that individuals with autism exhibited less pronounced activation in the primary motor cortex and supplementary motor area during a simple finger-tapping test (Muller, Pierce, Ambrose, Allen, & Courchesne, 2001). Thus, evidence from neuroimaging research suggests that cerebellar abnormalities and abnormalities in the primary and supplementary motor areas may be associated with the impaired motor functioning noted in children with autism.

Attention-Deficit/Hyperactivity Disorder

ADHD is a heterogeneous disorder characterized by deficits in attention, impulse control, and motor regulation. Current neuroimaging studies of children with ADHD provide compelling evidence that abnormalities in the frontostriatal circuitry are implicated in the deficits associated with this syndrome. Studies using anatomical MRI have found the total brain volume of children with ADHD to be up to 5% smaller than that of normal children (Castellanos et al., 1996), and that a reduction in prefrontal volume, particularly in the right hemisphere, is evident in many of these children (Castellanos et al., 1996; Filipek et al., 1997). MR imaging also reveals reduced basal ganglia volume (Castellanos et al., 1996; Filipek et al., 1997). More recently, a study using fMRI found that children with ADHD (6–10 years of age) did not activate frontostriatal regions in the same manner as did their normally developing peers (Durston, 2003). In particular, during tasks that required cognitive control (i.e., the ability to suppress thoughts and actions), lower levels of activation were noted in the prefrontal cortex, the anterior cingulate gyrus, and basal ganglia regions of children with ADHD compared to normally developing children. Children with ADHD, however, were more likely to activate posterior regions of the parietal and occipital cortex. Rubia and colleagues (1999) also found that their sample of boys with ADHD, ranging in age from 12 to 18 years, displayed increased activation of posterior regions during a motor inhibition task. Thus, frontostriatal dysfunction may account for the deficits in executive functions in children with ADHD, including their difficulty in sustaining attention and their impaired ability to plan, organize, and sequence movements (Barkley, 1997). Less activation of the frontostriatal circuitry may also be implicated in their inability to inhibit certain behaviors (Durston, 2003). On tasks that require some degree of cognitive control, children with ADHD appear to rely on more diffuse brain areas, especially the posterior regions of the inferior parietal lobe and posterior cingulate, as well as the dorsolateral prefrontal regions (Durston, 2003).

Neuroimaging studies of ADHD have also focused on the basal ganglia, particularly the caudate nucleus, which is involved in attention, working memory, and executive function. The findings of these studies, however, have not been consistent. Some studies have reported reductions in left caudate volume (Filipek et al., 1997; Hynd et al., 1993; Semrud-Clikeman et al., 2000), whereas others have found reductions in right caudate volume (Castellanos et al., 1996, 2001). Smaller left globus pallidus and total globus pallidus volumes have also been observed in children with ADHD (Aylward et al., 1996).

In addition to deviations in frontostriatal circuitry, the size of the cerebellum has been found to be significantly smaller in children with ADHD, particularly the inferior posterior vermis (Mostofsky, Reiss, Lockhart, & Denckla, 1998). Mostofsky and colleagues (1998) suggested that this may contribute to the difficulties with timing that are often evident in children with ADHD. Comorbid motor impairments, which are commonly observed in children with ADHD (Gillberg & Kadesjo, 2003), may also be due to cerebellar dysfunction. It has also been suggested that the cerebellum may play an important role in modulating activity in the frontostriatal network (Giedd, Blumenthal, Molloy, & Castellanos, 2001). Cerebellar dysfunction, therefore, could influence the cognitive deficits and behavioral symptomatology associated with this disorder.

Learning Disabilities

The majority of the neuroimaging studies that have examined individuals with learning disabilities have focused on reading disability (dyslexia). These studies have attempted to identify the anatomic abnormalities that may underlie the language difficulties associated with this disorder. A variety of neuroimaging techniques have indicated that the planum temporale and angular gyrus are compromised in children with dyslexia (Semrud-Clikeman, 1997). SPECT studies have shown either an unusual or a reduced pattern of activation, predominantly in the left hemisphere, among children with dyslexia while performing reading tasks (Semrud-Clikeman, 1997). PET studies have observed increased regional cerebral blood flow in Broca's and Wernicke's area, but not in the insula, among individuals with dyslexia while performing rhyming tasks (Paulesu et al., 1996). These authors suggested that this finding could be indicative of a disconnection between anterior and posterior language areas, which are normally bridged by the insula.

In addition to their impairment in literacy-related skills, children and adults with dyslexia have also been found to exhibit deficits in balance, postural stability, coordination, muscle tone, and dexterity, which are largely thought to be due to cerebellar dysfunction (Fawcett & Nicolson, 1993, 1999; Fawcett, Nicolson, & Dean, 1996; Nicolson et al., 1999; Nicolson, Fawcett, & Dean, 1995). Recently, neuroimaging studies have attempted to directly examine the importance of the cerebellum in dyslexia; however, such studies have largely been confined to adults. For example, using PET, Nicolson and colleagues (1999) compared cerebellar activity in a group of young adult males (mean age 21 years), who were diagnosed with dyslexia before 10 years of age, and an age-matched control group. Compared with the control participants, individuals with dyslexia displayed significantly lower activation in the right cerebellar cortex when executing previously overlearned (i.e., automatic) motor sequence tasks and when learning a new sequence. Thus, the cerebellum may be implicated in the difficulties children with dyslexia have in automatizing skills in both literacy and nonliteracy (i.e., motor) domains (Nicolson & Fawcett, 1990).

NEUROIMAGING IN ADULT MOVEMENT DISORDERS

Changes in the basal ganglia in adult-onset movement disorders such as Parkinson's disease, Huntington's disease, and primary adult-onset dystonia, suggest that this brain structure plays a central role in their pathogenesis. A wide variety of neuroimaging methods have been used to examine the basal ganglia in these populations, including transcranial US, MRI, SPECT, and PET. In the following sections, we discuss the findings of these studies.

Parkinson's Disease

Parkinson's disease (PD) is a progressive neurodegenerative disorder that is characterized by rigidity, a shuffling walking style, and tremors of the hands, arms, and legs, which decrease when one is performing voluntary tasks (Cavanaugh & Blanchard-Fields, 2002). It has long been suggested from postmortem data and clinical evaluation that these symptoms are the result of a degeneration of dopaminergic neurons in the substantia nigra (SN). More recently, neuroimaging studies have allowed for *in vivo* examination of the SN and surrounding structures and have provided support for this hypothesis (Hutchinson & Raff, 2000; Seibyl et al., 1995).

Several imaging modalities have identified an important susceptibility marker for nigral injury (Becker, Seufert, Bogdahn, Reichmann, & Reiners, 1995; Hutchinson & Raff, 2000). In an initial study using transcranial US, 30 patients with PD and 30 healthy controls were compared. Becker and his colleagues (1995) reported that approximately 70% of the PD patients displayed a substantial increase in SN echogenicity. In contrast, this echo pattern was observed in only two of their control participants. Furthermore, the echogenicity characteristic of the PD patients corresponded to the severity of their motor deficits, with higher echogenicity associated with more severe motor impairment. Using MRI, Hutchinson and Ruff (2000) also reported marked degeneration of the SN in adults with PD, and that this deterioration preferentially occurred in a lateral-to-medial and in an anterior-to-posterior direction.

Several studies using SPECT and PET have reported a marked reduction in striatal uptake in individuals with PD compared to healthy controls, more so in the putamen than the caudate (Brucke et al., 1993; Innis et al., 1993). In addition, these studies have demonstrated that among PD patients, uptake appeared to be particularly lower in the putamen in comparison to that of the caudate. Moreover, the magnitude of striatal reduction was correlated with the severity of PD subject's motor symptoms, with a larger decrease associated with greater deficits in motor functioning.

Although the aforementioned studies have reported deviations in the SN in individuals with PD, other investigations have noted that many of these abnormalities are not unique to this population (Berg et al., 2002). Indeed, PET studies have shown that hyperechogenicity of the SN, characteristically seen in PD, can be seen in healthy young adults under 40 years of age, and that this may be associated with impairment of nigrostriatal pathways in some of these individuals (Berg et al., 2002). Therefore, hyperechogenicity in the SN has been proposed to be a potential susceptibility marker for nigral injury due to this striking similarly between symptomatic PD patients and a subgroup of healthy adults (Berg et al., 2002). Longitudinal follow-up studies, however, of healthy adults presenting with SN hyperechogenicity on imaging are clearly needed to determine whether these individuals do, in fact, manifest symptoms of the disease at a later time.

Huntington's Disease

Huntington's disease (HD) is a rare autosomal dominant disorder. Similar to PD, the course of HD is often progressive, with a gradual decrease in functional capabilities over time. HD generally manifests itself through choreiform movements (involuntary spasmodic jerking and twisting movements of the neck, trunk, and extremities), facial grimacing, and the inability to sustain a motor act such as sticking out one's tongue (Cavanaugh & Blanchard-Fields, 2002). Individuals with this disease eventually lose their ability to walk. They also exhibit a marked decline in cognitive functioning, coincident with emotional abnormalities such as mood swings and hallucinations (Cavanaugh & Blanchard-Fields, 2002).

The characteristic neuropathological features of HD are neostriatal atrophy and neuronal loss (Hedreen & Folstein, 1995). Neuroimaging studies have been used to quantify striatal atrophy, as well as decrements in striatal functioning, in HD patients. Indeed, compared to healthy controls, HD patients demonstrate increased echogenicity of the basal ganglia on transcranial US, especially in the caudate nucleus and substantia nigra (Postert et al., 1999). Transcranial US has also revealed ventricular enlargement in HD patients (Postert et al., 1999). Both SPECT and PET studies have shown decreased striatal blood flow and metabolism in HD (Harris et al., 1996; Kuwert et al., 1990). Moreover, a longitudinal study measuring changes in the basal ganglia on MRI in a sample of adult HD patients demonstrated a significant reduction in caudate, putamen, and total basal ganglia volume over time (Aylward et al., 1997). Adults with the genetic mutation for HD but showing no symptoms of the disease have also shown basal ganglia atrophy on MRI (Campodonico et al., 1998; Harris et al., 1999) and SPECT (Harris et al., 1999). In addition, reduced striatal volume is associated with several neurological abnormalities including greater motor impairment, slower mental processing speed, and poorer verbal learning (Campodonico et al., 1998).

MRI has also been used with adults with HD to document frontal lobe abnormalities (Aylward et al., 1998). Aylward and colleagues (1998) reported that moderately affected HD patients present with marked reduction in frontal lobe volume, particularly the volume of the white matter, whereas those only mildly symptomatic had frontal lobe volumes that were essentially identical to that of healthy control subjects. This difference between the groups remained even when both the mildly and moderately affected HD patients showed clear abnormalities in the basal ganglia. The reduction in frontal lobe volume was found to be related to measures of symptom severity and general cognitive functioning. However, this correlation did not remain significant when total brain atrophy was taken into consideration. Therefore, these findings suggest that the frontal lobe dysfunction may be implicated in the expression of symptoms characteristic of later stages of the disease, although this association may not be specific to the frontal lobes.

Primary Adult-Onset Dystonia

Dystonia is defined by involuntary muscular contractions that result in twitching movements and abnormal posturing (Ceballos-Baumann et al., 1995). Although the pathophysiology of dystonia remains unclear, recent PET studies have demonstrated abnormal activation of subcortical nuclei, the prefrontal cortex, and the supplementary motor areas, suggesting that dysfunction in the basal ganglia loop is implicated in the manifestation of dystonic movement disorders (Ceballos-Baumann et al., 1995). Basal ganglia abnormalities have also been detected using transcranial US (Naumann, Becker, Toyka, Supprian, & Reiners, 1996).

A coincident overactivity in prefrontal areas and underactivity in motor cortical areas has been reported in adults with idiopathic dystonia (Ceballos-Baumann et al., 1995). In a PET study involving six adults with idiopathic torsion dystonia (age range: 20–55 years) and six normal subjects (20–59 years of age), when performing a task that involved moving a joystick at paced intervals, those with dystonia showed significantly higher activity in the contralateral lateral premotor cortex, rostral supplementary motor area, and Brodmann area 8 (Ceballos-Baumann et al., 1995). The adults with dystonia also showed abnormally high activity in the anterior cingulate area, ipsilateral dorsolateral prefrontal cortex, and bilateral lentiform nucleus. Moreover, relative to controls, marked underactivity was observed in the caudal supplementary motor area, bilateral sensorimotor cortex, posterior cingulate, and mesial parietal cortex. The authors proposed that the overactivity associated with the striatum and frontal areas, and the underactivity of the aforementioned primary executive areas manifested by dystonic individuals during movement might account for the coexistence of involuntary posturing and bradykinesia in this disorder due to the intricate connections and feedback loops between these structures.

CONCLUSION

This chapter has provided an overview of the major imaging modalities. The advent of these techniques has resulted in invaluable insight into both normal and abnormal brain development. With these remarkable technological advancements, however, has come the increased recognition of the many unique challenges researchers and clinicians face when imaging children. Yet despite these challenges, neuroimaging techniques have allowed us to establish connections between etiological factors and disorders of early brain development.

More recently, researchers have used structural neuroimaging to explore the neurobiological substrates of neurodevelopmental disorders in children. The studies have suggested some common underpinnings in such complex disorders as autism, ADHD, and learning disabilities, and have revealed possible neuroanatomical bases for the relationship between these disorders and the motor deficits that are frequently associated with these disorders. Anatomical and functional imaging of adults presenting with cognitive and motor impairments have also improved our understanding of brain–behavior relationships. With the application of imaging techniques expanding at an unprecedented rate, great strides are certain to be made in our knowledge of the intricacies of the human brain. The ongoing development of advanced imaging techniques such as DWI and fMRI promises to further refine diagnostic and prognostic capabilities for affected children. The ability of imaging techniques to offer a more precise understanding of the etiological substrates implicated in childhood disorders could also be of great utility in the design of the more effective interventions for those at risk of maladaptive development.

ACKNOWLEDGMENTS

Grants from the Alberta Children's Hospital Foundation and the Canadian Institutes of Health Research supported the preparation of this chapter.

REFERENCES

Aida, N., Nishimura, G., Hachiya, Y., Matsui, K., Takeuchi, M., & Itani, Y. (1998). MR imaging of perinatal brain damage: Comparison of clinical outcome with initial and follow-up MR findings. *AJNR American Journal of Neuroradiology, 19,* 1909–1921.

Aylward, E. H., Anderson, N. B., Bylsma, F. W., Wagster, M. V., Barta, P. E., Sherr, M., et al. (1998). Frontal lobe volume in patients with Huntington's disease. *Neurology, 50,* 252–258.

Aylward, E. H., Li, Q., Stine, O. C., Ranen, N., Sherr, M., Barta, P. E., et al. (1997). Longitudinal change in basal ganglia volume in patients with Huntington's disease. *Neurology, 48,* 394–399.

Aylward, E. H., Reiss, A. L., Reader, M. J., Singer, H. S., Brown, J. E., & Denckla, M. B. (1996). Basal ganglia volumes in children with attention-deficit hyperactivity disorder. *Journal of Child Neurology, 11,* 112–115.

Barkley, R. A. (1997). Behavioral inhibition, sustained attention and executive functions: Constructing a unifying theory of ADHD. *Psychological Bulletin, 121,* 65–94.

Becker, G., Seufert, J., Bogdahn, U., Reichmann, H., & Reiners, K. (1995). Degeneration of substantia nigra in chronic Parkinson's disease visualized by transcranial color-coded real-time sonography. *Neurology, 45,* 182–184.

Berg, D., Roggendorf, W., Schroder, U., Klein, R., Tatschner, T., Benz, P., et al. (2002). Echogenicity of the substantia nigra: Association with increased iron content and marker for susceptibility to nigrostriatal injury. *Archives of Neurology, 59,* 999–1005.

Bergstrom, K., & Bille, B. (1978). Computed tomography of the brain in children with minimal brain damage: A preliminary study of 46 children. *Neuropadiaetrie, 9*, 378–384.

Boddaert, N., Belin, P., & Poline, J. B. (2001). Temporal lobe dysfunction in childhood autism: A PET auditory activation study. *Pediatric Radiology, 31*, S3.

Bonnet, K. A., & Gao, X. K. (1996). Asperger syndrome in neurologic perspective. *Journal of Child Neurology, 11*, 483–489.

Bookheimer, S. Y. (2000). Methodological issues in pediatric neuroimaging. *Mental Retardation and Developmental Disabilities, 6*, 161–165.

Boyer, R. S. (1994). Neuroimaging of premature infants. In A. J. Barkovich & T. P. Naidich (Eds.), *Neuroimaging clinics of North America: Pediatric neuroradiology* (Vol. 4, pp. 241–261). Philadelphia: Saunders.

Brucke, T., Kornhuber, J., Angelberger, P., Asenbaum, S., Frassine, H., & Podreka, I. (1993). SPECT imaging of dopamine and serotonin transporters with [^{123}I] beta-CIT. Binding kinetics in the human brain. *Journal of Neural Transmission. General Section, 94*, 137–146.

Campodonico, J. R., Aylward, E., Codori, A. M., Young, C., Krafft, L., Magdalinski, M., et al. (1998). When does Huntington's disease begin? *Journal of the International Neuropsychological Society, 4*, 467–473.

Carper, R. A., & Courchesne, E. (2000). Inverse correlation between frontal lobe and cerebellum sizes in children with autism. *Brain, 123*, 836–844.

Castellanos, F. X., Giedd, J. N., Berquin, P. C., Walter, J. M., Sharp, W., Tran, T., et al. (2001).Quantitative brain magnetic resonance imaging in girls with attention-deficit/hyperactivity disorder. *Archives of General Psychiatry, 58*, 289–295.

Castellanos, F. X., Giedd, J. N., Marsh, W. L., Hamburger, S. D., Vaituzis, A. C., Dickstein, D. P., et al. (1996). Quantitative brain magnetic resonance imaging in attention-deficit hyperactivity disorder. *Archives of General Psychiatry, 53*, 607–616.

Cavanaugh, J. C., & Blanchard-Fields, F. (2002). *Adult development and aging* (4th ed.). Belmont, CA: Thomson Learning.

Ceballos-Baumann, A. O., Passingham, R. E., Warner, T., Playford, E. D., Marsden, C. D., & Brooks, D. J. (1995). Overactive prefrontal and underactive motor cortical areas in idiopathic dystonia. *Annals of Neurology, 37*, 363–372.

Debillon, T., N'Guyen, S., Muet, A., Quere, M. P., Moussaly, F., & Roze, J. C. (2003). Limitations of ultrasonography for diagnosing white matter damage in preterm infants. *Archives of Disease in Childhood, Fetal and Neonatal Edition, 88*, F275–F279.

Denis, D., Chateil, J. F., Brun, M., Brissaud, O., Lacombe, D., Fontan, D., et al. (2000). Schizencephaly: Clinical and imaging features in 30 infantile cases. *Brain and Development, 22*, 475–483.

Durston, S. (2003). A review of the biological bases of ADHD: What have we learned from imaging studies? *Mental Retardation and Developmental Disabilities Research and Reviews, 9*, 184–195.

Eliez, S., & Reiss, A. L. (2000). MRI neuroimaging of childhood psychiatric disorders: A selective review. *Journal of Child Psychology and Psychiatry, 41*, 679–694.

Fawcett, A. J., & Nicolson, R. I. (1993). *Children with dyslexia show deficits on a range of primitive skills*. HIllsdale, NJ: Erlbaum.

Fawcett, A. J., & Nicolson, R. I. (1999). Performance of dyslexic children on cerebellar and cognitive tests. *Journal of Motor Behavior, 31*, 68–78.

Fawcett, A. J., Nicolson, R. I., & Dean, P. (1966). Impaired performance of children with dyslexia on a range of cerebellar tasks. *Annals of Dyslexia, 46*, 259–283.

Filipek, P. A., Semrud-Clikeman, M., Steingard, R. J., Renshaw, P. F., Kennedy, D. N., & Biederman, J. (1997). Volumetric MRI analysis comparing subjects having attention-deficit hyperactivity disorder with normal controls. *Neurology, 48*, 589–601.

Fox, P. T., & Raichle, M. E. (1986). Focal physiological uncoupling of cerebral blood flow and oxidative metabolism during somatosensory stimulation of human subjects. *Proceedings of the National Academy of Sciences USA, 83,* 1140–1144.

Frank, Y., & Pavlakis, S. G. (2001). Brain imaging in neurobehavioral disorders. *Pediatric Neurology, 25,* 278–287.

Giedd, J. N., Blumenthal, J., Molloy, E., & Castellanos, F. X. (2001). Brain imaging of attention deficit/hyperactivity disorder. *Annals of the New York Academy of Sciences, 931,* 33–49.

Gillberg, C., & Kadesjo, B. (2003). Why bother about clumsiness? The implications of having developmental coordination disorder (DCD). *Neural Plasticity, 10,* 59–68.

Green, D., Baird, G., Barnett, A. L., Henderson, L., Huber, J., & Henderson, S. E. (2002). The severity and nature of motor impairment in Asperger's syndrome: A comparison with specific developmental disorder of motor function. *Journal of Child Psychology and Psychiatry, 43,* 655–668.

Gururaj, A., Sztriha, L., Dawodu, A., Nath, K. R., Varady, E., Nork, M., et al. (2002). CT and MR patterns of hypoxic ischemic brain damage following perinatal asphyxia. *Journal of Tropical Pediatrics, 48,* 5–9.

Harris, G. J., Aylward, E. H., Peyser, C. E., Pearlson, G. D., Brandt, J., Roberts-Twillie, J. V., et al. (1996). Single photon emission computed tomographic blood flow and magnetic resonance volume imaging of basal ganglia in Huntington's disease. *Archives of Neurology, 53,* 316–324.

Harris, G. J., Codori, A. M., Lewis, R. F., Schmidt, E., Bedi, A., & Brandt, J. (1999). Reduced basal ganglia blood flow and volume in pre-symptomatic, gene-tested persons at-risk for Huntington's disease. *Brain, 122,* 1667–1678.

Hedreen, J. C., & Folstein, S. E. (1995). Early loss of neostriatal striosome neurons in Huntington's disease. *Journal of Neuropathology and Experimental Neurology, 54,* 105–120.

Hoon, A. H., Jr., Belsito, K. M., & Nagae-Poetscher, L. M. (2003). Neuroimaging in spasticity and movement disorders. *Journal of Child Neurology, 18*(Suppl. 1), S25–39.

Hoon, A. H., Jr., Reinhardt, E. M., Kelley, R. I., Breiter, S. N., Morton, D. H., Naidu, S. B., et al. (1997). Brain magnetic resonance imaging in suspected extrapyramidal cerebral palsy: Observations in distinguishing genetic-metabolic from acquired causes. *Journal of Pediatrics, 131,* 240–245.

Hutchinson, M., & Raff, U. (2000). Structural changes of the substantia nigra in Parkinson's disease as revealed by MR imaging. *AJNR American Journal of Neuroradiology, 21,* 697–701.

Hynd, G. W., Hern, K. L., Novey, E. S., Eliopulos, D., Marshall, R., Gonzalez, J. J., et al. (1993). Attention-deficit hyperactivity disorder and asymmetry of the caudate nucleus. *Journal of Child Neurology, 8,* 339–347.

Inder, T. E., Huppi, P. S., Warfield, S., Kikinis, R., Zientara, G. P., Barnes, P. D., et al. (1999). Periventricular white matter injury in the premature infant is followed by reduced cerebral cortical gray matter volume at term. *Annals of Neurology, 46,* 755–760.

Inder, T. E., Huppi, P. S., Zientara, G. P., Maier, S. E., Jolesz, F. A., di Salvo, D., et al. (1999). Early detection of periventricular leukomalacia by diffusion-weighted magnetic resonance imaging techniques. *Journal of Pediatrics, 134,* 631–634.

Innis, R. B., Seibyl, J. P., Scanley, B. E., Laruelle, M., Abi-Dargham, A., Wallace, E., et al. (1993). Single photon emission computed tomographic imaging demonstrates loss of striatal dopamine transporters in Parkinson disease. *Proceedings of the National Academy of Sciences USA, 90,* 11965–11969.

Johnston, M. V., Nishimura, A., Harum, K., Pekar, J., & Blue, M. E. (2001). Sculpting the developing brain. *Advances in Pediatrics, 48,* 1–38.

Just, M. A., Carpenter, P. A., Keller, T. A., Eddy, W. F. & Thulborn K. R. (1996). Brain activation modulated by sentence comprehension. *Science, 274,* 114–116.

Knuckley, N. W., Apsimin, T. T., & Gubbay, S. S. (1983). Computerized axial tomography in clumsy children with developmental apraxia and agnosia. *Brain and Development, 5,* 14–19.

Krasuski, J., Horwitz, B., & Rumsey, J. M. (1996). A survey of functional and anatomical neuroimaging techniques. In G. R. Lyon & J. M. Rumsey (Eds.), *Neuroimaging: A window to the neurological foundations of learning and behavior in children* (pp. 25–52). Baltimore: Brookes.

Kuwert, T., Lange, H. W., Langen, K. J., Herzog, H., Aulich, A., & Feinendegen, L. E. (1990). Cortical and subcortical glucose consumption measured by PET in patients with Huntington's disease. *Brain, 113,* 1405–1423.

Lammertsma, A. A. (2001). PET/SPECT: Functional imaging beyond flow. *Vision Research, 41,* 1277–1281.

Le Bihan, D. (1995). Molecular diffusion, tissue microdynamics and microstructure. *NMR in Biomedicine, 8,* 375–386.

Maalouf, E. F., Duggan, P. J., Counsell, S. J., Rutherford, M. A., Cowan, F., Azzopardi, D., et al. (2001). Comparison of findings on cranial ultrasound and magnetic resonance imaging in preterm infants. *Pediatrics, 107,* 719–727.

Maalouf, E. F., Duggan, P. J., Rutherford, M. A., Counsell, S. J., Fletcher, A. M., Battin, M., et al. (1999). Magnetic resonance imaging of the brain in a cohort of extremely preterm infants. *Journal of Pediatrics, 135,* 351–357.

Manjiviona, J., & Prior, M. (1995). Comparison of Asperger syndrome and high-functioning autistic children on a test of motor impairment. *Journal of Autism and Developmental Disorders, 25,* 23–39.

Menkes, J. H., & Curran, J. (1994). Clinical and MR correlates in children with extrapyramidal cerebral palsy. *AJNR American Journal of Neuroradiology, 15,* 451–457.

Ment, L. R., Bada, H. S., Barnes, P., Grant, P. E., Hirtz, D., Papile, L. A., et al. (2002). Practice parameter: Neuroimaging of the neonate: Report of the Quality Standards Subcommittee of the American Academy of Neurology and the Practice Committee of the Child Neurology Society. *Neurology, 58,* 1726–1738.

Mostofsky, S. H., Reiss, A. L., Lockhart, P., & Denckla, M. B. (1998). Evaluation of cerebellar size in attention-deficit hyperactivity disorder. *Journal of Child Neurology, 13,* 434–439.

Muller, R. A., Pierce, K., Ambrose, J. B., Allen, G., & Courchesne, E. (2001). Atypical patterns of cerebral motor activation in autism: A functional magnetic resonance study. *Biological Psychiatry, 49,* 665–676.

Naumann, M., Becker, G., Toyka, K. V., Supprian, T., & Reiners, K. (1996). Lenticular nucleus lesion in idiopathic dystonia detected by transcranial sonography. *Neurology, 47,* 1284–1290.

Nicolson, R. I., & Fawcett, A. J. (1990). Automaticity: A new framework for dyslexia research? *Cognition, 35,* 159–182.

Nicolson, R. I., Fawcett, A. J., Berry, E. L., Jenkins, I. H., Dean, P., & Brooks, D. J. (1999). Association of abnormal cerebellar activation with motor learning difficulties in dyslexic adults. *Lancet, 353,* 1662–1667.

Nicolson, R. I., Fawcett, A. J., & Dean, P. (1995). Time estimation deficits in developmental dyslexia: Evidence of cerebellar involvement. *Proceedings of the Royal Society of London, B (Biological Sciences), 259,* 43–47.

Nosarti, C., Al-Asady, M. H., Frangou, S., Stewart, A. L., Rifkin, L., & Murray, R. M. (2002). Adolescents who were born very preterm have decreased brain volumes. *Brain, 125,* 1616–1623.

Pascual-Castroviejo, I., Pascual-Pascual, S. I., Viano, J., Martinez, V., & Palencia, R. (2001). Unilateral polymicrogyria: A common cause of hemiplegia of prenatal origin. *Brain and Development, 23,* 216–222.

Paulesu, E., Frith, U., Snowling, M., Gallagher, A., Morton, J., Frackowiak, R. S., et al. (1996).

Is developmental dyslexia a disconnection syndrome? Evidence from PET scanning. *Brain, 119,* 143–157.

Perlman, J. M. (1998). White matter injury in the preterm infant: An important determination of abnormal neurodevelopmental outcome. *Early Human Development, 53,* 99–120.

Pierce, K., & Courchesne, E. (2001). Evidence for a cerebellar role in reduced exploration and stereotyped behavior in autism. *Biological Psychiatry, 49,* 655–664.

Pinto-Martin, J. A., Riolo, S., Cnaan, A., Holzman, C., Susser, M. W., & Paneth, N. (1995). Cranial ultrasound prediction of disabling and nondisabling cerebral palsy at age two in a low birth weight population. *Pediatrics, 95,* 249–254.

Postert, T., Lack, B., Kuhn, W., Jergas, M., Andrich, J., Braun, B., et al. (1999). Basal ganglia alterations and brain atrophy in Huntington's disease depicted by transcranial real time sonography. *Journal of Neurology, Neurosurgery, and Psychiatry, 67,* 457–462.

Raichle, M. E., Fiez, J. A., Videen, T. O., MacLeod, A. M., Pardo, J. V., Fox, P. T., et al. (1994). Practice-related changes in human brain functional anatomy during nonmotor learning. *Cerebral Cortex, 4,* 8–26.

Rinehart, N. J., Bradshaw, J. L., Brereton, A. V., & Tonge, B. J. (2002). A clinical and neurobehavioural review of high-functioning autism and Asperger's disorder. *Australian and New Zealand Journal of Psychiatry, 36,* 762–770.

Rubia, K., Overmeyer, S., Taylor, E., Brammer, M., Williams, S. C., Simmons, A., et al. (1999). Hypofrontality in attention deficit hyperactivity disorder during higher-order motor control: A study with functional MRI. *American Journal of Psychiatry, 156,* 891–896.

Seibyl, J. P., Marek, K. L., Quinlan, D., Sheff, K., Zoghbi, S., Zea-Ponce, Y., et al. (1995). Decreased single-photon emission computed tomographic [^{123}I]beta-CIT striatal uptake correlates with symptom severity in Parkinson's disease. *Annals of Neurology, 38,* 589–598.

Semrud-Clikeman, M. (1997). Evidence from imaging on the relationship between brain structure and developmental language disorders. *Seminars in Pediatric Neurology, 4,* 117–124.

Semrud-Clikeman M., Steingard, R.J., Filipek, P., Biederman, J., Bekken, K., & Renshaw, P.F., (2000). Using MRI to examine brain–behavior relationships in males with attention deficit disorder with hyperactivity. *Journal of the American Academy of Child and Adolescent Psychiatry, 39,* 477–84.

Skranes, J. S., Nilsen, G., Smevik, O., Vik, T., & Brubakk, A. M. (1998). Cerebral MRI of very low birth weight children at 6 years of age compared with the findings at 1 year. *Pediatric Radiology, 28,* 471–475.

Sowell, E., Thompson, R., Holmes, C. J., Jernigan, T. L., & Toga, A. W. (1999). In vivo evidence for post-adolescent brain maturation in frontal and striatal regions. *Nature Neuroscience, 2,* 859–861.

Stewart, A. L., Rifkin, L., Amess, P. N., Kirkbride, V., Townsend, J. P., Miller, D. H., et al. (1999). Brain structure and neurocognitive and behavioural function in adolescents who were born very preterm. *Lancet, 353,* 1653–1657.

Vilensky, J. A., Damasio, A. R., & Maurer, R. G. (1981). Gait disturbances in patients with autistic behavior: A preliminary study. *Archives of Neurology, 38,* 646–649.

Volpe, J. J. (1995). *Neurology of the newborn* (3rd ed.). Philadelphia: Saunders.

Volpe, J. J. (1997). Brain injury in the premature infant. Neuropathology, clinical aspects, pathogenesis, and prevention. *Clinics in Perinatology, 24,* 567–587.

CHAPTER 3

Approaches to Understanding the Neurobehavioral Mechanisms Associated with Motor Impairments in Children

ERIC A. ROY
SHAUNA BOTTOS
KELLY PRYDE
DEBORAH DEWEY

Several approaches to assessment have been developed for examining the motor impairments observed in neurodevelopmental disorders such as developmental coordination disorder (DCD). One approach involves the use of traditional neurological assessment measures. The general purpose of these measures is to provide information on the functional integrity of the central nervous system. These measures typically assume a sign or symptom-oriented approach to assessment. They examine "soft" signs, which have been defined as an abnormal motor or sensory performance in the absence of a localizable neurological disorder (Shafer, Shafer, O'Conner, & Stokman, 1983). A second assessment approach used to examine motor functioning in children involves the use of neuropsychological assessment batteries. A third approach we consider involves examining how movements are controlled. Here the space–time or kinematic features of movement are examined with a view to identifying deficits in movement control. Do children with DCD have difficulty in the on-line control of movement? Does this difficulty with on-line control vary with the type of feedback information (e.g., vision) or the complexity of the movement as reflected in measures such as the size of the target to which they are pointing.

In this chapter we explore each of these approaches. We begin with a description of the traditional neurological exams and the problems associated with their use in detecting and predicting motor impairment. This section is followed by a brief overview of the traditional neuropsychological batteries that have been used to assess children's motor status. In the third section, we review studies that have attempted to characterize the nature of motor control impairments in children with DCD. We end with some consideration of the relative merits of these approaches and of the need for assessments that integrate information provided by all three.

TRADITIONAL NEUROLOGICAL EXAMS

The topic of neurological subtle or "soft" signs and their clinical utility have been a subject of debate for several years. According to Deuel and Robinson (1987), these signs are commonly present in young children, and it is only when they persist into later years that their presence becomes *pathological*. The importance of a sign or symptom-oriented approach in both the clinical and research setting lies in its ability to aid in the diagnosis of a disorder and its ability to distinguish between normal and disordered groups of children. Although the results have been mixed, a number of studies have found that "soft" motor signs discriminate between typically developing children and children with cognitive disturbance or learning disabilities (Fellick, Thomson, Sills, & Hart, 2001; Huttenlocher, Levine, Huttenlocher, & Gates, 1990) and psychiatric disorders (Fellick et al., 2001). Fellick and colleagues (2001) found that the presence of soft signs had a sensitivity of 38% for detecting cognitive impairment, 42% for detecting problems in motor coordination, and 25% for detecting attention-deficit/hyperactivity disorder, in a sample of school-age children between the ages of 8 and 13 years. However, these authors also reported that assessment of subtle neurological signs was not sensitive or specific enough to detect children with impairment in other areas, such as visual–motor integration, suggesting that the utility in assessing these signs may be confined to a limited number of domains. In contrast, Nichols and Chen (1980) found that neurological soft signs did not discriminate between children with or without behavior or learning problems. Furthermore, it has been noted that soft neurological signs are often found among typically developing children (Marlow, Roberts, & Cooke, 1989) and, conversely, that their absence does not preclude learning problems or deviance in other areas of functioning (Huttenlocher et al., 1990).

Two of the most widely used measures of neurological functioning used with children are the Examination of the Child with Minor Neurological Dysfunction (Touwen, 1979) and the Physical and Neurological Examination for Soft Signs (PANESS) (Close, 1973) or the revised version entitled the Neurological Examination for Subtle Signs (NESS) (Denckla, 1985). The Examination of the Child with Minor Neurological Dysfunction was developed for children 3 to 12 years of age and contains 63 items divided into 10 categories: (1) sensorimotor apparatus, (2) posture, (3) balance of trunk, (4) coordination of extremities, (5) fine manipulative ability, (6) dyskinesia, (7) gross motor functions, (8) quality of motility, (9) associated movements, and (10) visual system (Touwen, 1979). The PANESS is a 43-item examination containing items that assess gross motor coordination, fine motor coordination, balance, persistence, optokinetic responses, cortical sensitivity, stereognosis, and graphesthesia.

Studies that have used these measures of neurological functioning to discriminate between normal developing children and children who are at risk for cognitive dysfunction, learning disabilities, or behavioral disorders have not reported consistent findings and have identified some methodological limitations. Marlow and colleagues (1989) using the Touwen neurological exam found that at 6 years of age subtle neurological signs were more common and more pronounced in the children with very low birth weight (VLBW) compared to children born at full term. In contrast, Huttenlocher and colleagues (1990) reported that many of the items of the Touwen neurological exam were less than satisfactory in differentiating between children at risk for learning disabilities and normal children. Specifically, Huttenlocher and colleagues noted that certain items, such as assessment for tremor and reflexes, were normal for most children, whereas other items, such as choreiform movements, evidenced poor interrater reliability. Research with the Touwen neurological exam has also found that some items are not appropriate for children of certain ages and that a ceiling effect was noted on certain items (i.e., alternating hand movements and tandem gait forward) at 5 years of age (Huttenlocher et al., 1990; Weisglas-Kuperus et al., 1994). Other criticisms of this neurological exam are that no normative data are available for either the total optimality scores or the category scores (Kakebeeke, Jongmans, Dubowitz, Schoemaker, & Henderson, 1993) and that the interrater reliability of this measure is highly variable even when the child's actual functioning has not changed (Kakebeekeet al., 1993).

Studies that have used the PANESS have also noted that it has some limitations. Werry and Aman (1976) examined whether the PANESS discriminated between groups of children with different disabilities. Their sample included children with hyperactivity and neurological impairment and typically developing children. They found that even though 75% of their sample was composed of children who might be expected to display signs of abnormality, only 12% of the signs occurred in as few as 50% of the children. They also noted that many of the neurological signs tested for were not present in any of the children. Furthermore, of seven items that were displayed in over 50% of the participants, five were present in more than 80%, suggesting that these items were unlikely to differentiate between groups. Camp, Bialer, Sverd, and Winsberg (1978) also found that the PANESS did not discriminate children with hyperactivity from typically developing children. They concluded that this measure lacked adequate clinical validity. A study conducted by Mikkelson, Brown, Minichiello, Millican, and Rappoport (1982) compared the PANESS scores of 30 boys with hyperactivity to those of 40 enuretic, 11 enuretic and encopretic, and 22 normal control children. Results revealed a strong negative correlation between age and PANESS scores with younger children obtaining higher scores. The authors also reported that the age-adjusted mean score of children with hyperactivity was significantly higher than that of the children in the enuretic and control groups. Further, of the two groups of children with enuretic problems, those who were also encopretic exhibited significantly more neurological soft signs than did those who were not. Mikkelson et al. concluded that the PANESS might be a valid measure of the level of *neurodevelopmental maturity* of children but it was not a useful diagnostic instrument. Indeed, this conclusion echoes that of other researchers who have stated that the presence of soft signs are indicative of delayed maturation rather than pathological functioning (Blondis, Snow, & Accardo, 1990).

The NESS is a revision of the PANESS (Denckla, 1985). Items that were difficult to administer or rarely scored were eliminated and new items were added. The normative data that are available for NESS are restricted to a few age groups and distinct motor tasks (Denckla, 1973, 1974). Examination of the reliability and stability of the various sensory and motor soft signs measured has produced mixed results. Vitiello, Ricciuti, Stoff, Behar, and Denckla (1989) estimated interobserver and test–retest reliability in 54 psychiatric patients and 25 normal children between the ages of 5 and 17 years. They reported acceptable interrater reliability for some of the tests, particularly those that were assessed on continuous scales, such as the time needed for 20 repetitive movements. In contrast, reliability was much lower for those signs that were categorically recorded and more dependent on subjective interpretation, including overflow movements and dysrhythmias. The stability of the soft signs, or test–retest reliability at 2 weeks was unsatisfactory for most of the categorically scored items (kappa and intraclass correlation coefficients < .50), including the presence of overflows, dysrhythmic movements, astereognosis, dysgraphesthesia, and inability to keep balance and hop on one foot. The poor stability of many of these signs over such a short period clearly brings into question their clinical significance.

In addition to the traditional measures of neurological assessment used with children, there are several measures of neurological functioning for preterm and term infants. These neonatal assessments are primarily used to predict neurological outcome at a later age, specifically cerebral palsy or other forms of motor impairment. Two main protocols exist for neonatal neurological evaluation, one devised by Dubowitz and Dubowitz (1981) for preterm and term infants and another by Prechtl (1977) for use with term infants. Abnormalities assessed using the Dubowitz evaluation include abnormal posture, generalized or segmental hypotonia or hypertonia, hypokinesis, abnormal head control, frequent tremors or startles, absent or abnormal responses or reflexes, hyporeactivity to stimulation, and irritability. Prechtl's examination classifies the infant's performance within the following categories: syndromes of abnormal posture, motility, motor system, symmetry, and reactivity.

Several studies have tried to correlate the presence of neurological abnormality in the newborn period with future motor outcome. Dubowitz and colleagues (1984) conducted a prospective study on the outcome at 1 year of 129 preterm infants. The infants underwent neurological assessment during the first week of life and again at 40 weeks postmenstrual age (PMA), and a comprehensive neurodevelopmental assessment was conducted at 1 year. The results of this study showed a good correlation between the neurological assessment at 40 weeks PMA and the outcome at 1 year of age. Ninety-one percent of the 69 infants considered neurologically normal at 40 weeks PMA were found to be neurologically normal at the 1-year follow-up. Of the 40 infants with an abnormal neurological examination at 40 weeks PMA, only 35% were considered normal at follow-up. Allen and Capute (1989) also reported a highly significant correlation between abnormal neonatal neurological assessment results in preterm infants and neuromotor outcome at 1–5 years of age. The neonatal assessment they used included items from both the Dubowitz assessment and the Prechtl examination but also contained neurological tests proposed by other investigators. Of the 125 preterm infants classified as normal in their sample, 81% had no motor abnormalities; 13% displayed minor neuromotor dysfunction characterized by lower extremity hypertonia and hyperreflexia, persistent toe walking, and/or hypotonia; and 6% developed cerebral palsy. In contrast, 38% of the infants classified as abnormal at initial assessment had cerebral palsy at follow-up, and 27% had minor neuromotor dysfunction. These two studies indicate that a relationship exists between preterm infants' performance on neonatal neurological examinations and future motor functioning, with those children showing abnormal results early having a greater likelihood of demonstrating motor dysfunction at a later age. However, one must be cautious when interpreting these findings as more than one-third of neonates in the Allen and Capute study whose neonatal neurodevelopmental assessment showed abnormal results had normal neuromotor outcomes. Further, a subgroup of infants who were classified as normal in the initial examination displayed adverse motor outcome at follow-up.

To address the poor sensitivity and specificity of these quantitative infant neurological assessments, new methods that emphasize qualitative assessment have been developed. Prechtl (1990) developed a method based on the qualitative observation of spontaneous motility of preterm and term infants. He described several types of spontaneous activity in the infant but found that the types of movements he termed *general movements* (GMs) were the most appropriate to observe when identifying abnormal behaviour. Normal GMs tend to be characterized by gross movements that involve the whole body and last from a few seconds to several minutes (Prechtl & Franzens, 2001). The GMs of abnormal infants lack complexity; they are slow and monotonous or brisk and chaotic, with dramatic reductions in subtle fluctuations of force, amplitude, and speed. Abnormal GMs may also appear rigid and lacking in normal smooth and fluent character. The quality of these GMs is assessed by viewing video recordings of the infant, with the analysis of the movements based on a global judgment of *normal* versus *abnormal* quality.

According to Prechtl and Franzens (2001) the observation of spontaneous movement of the neonate takes into account many of the inadequacies inherent in the quantitative approach to neurological assessment. Traditional quantitative measures have been faulted for their overemphasis on reflexes and stimulus–response relationships as signifying normality or pathology in the infant (Prechtl & Franzens, 2001). This reductionist approach fails to acknowledge the complexities of the infant nervous system. Observation of GMs, however, fully takes into account the intricacies of the young nervous system. Also, traditional neurological examinations are often unable to distinguish between brain-damaged and low-risk infants (Prechtl & Franzens, 2001). Indeed, the qualitative assessment of GMs in both preterm (Ferrari, Cioni, & Prechtl, 1990) and term infants (Prechtl, Ferrari, & Cioni, 1993) with brain damage has shown that it is not the incidence of GMs but the *quality* of their execution that is a good indicator of infant neurological status. Neurological examinations have also been relatively ineffective in detecting specific signs for the prediction of later cerebral palsy (Prechtl & Franzens, 2001). An extensive comparison between the results of traditional neurological examinations and the qualitative assessments of GMs in longitudinal studies on infants born preterm (Cioni, Ferrari, et al., 1997) and those born at term (Cioni, Prechtl, et al., 1997) revealed that GMs were better at predicting neurological outcome at 2 years of age, including cerebral palsy. The presence of consistent GM abnormalities was found to be a strong predictor of an unfavorable outcome (sensitivity 88.9%), whereas consistently normal or transiently abnormal GMs tended to predict normal development (specificity 95%). In contrast, the sensitivity of consistent neurological abnormalities was 72.5% and the specificity was 95%. Other investigators have found that two specific features of GMs, a persistent pattern of cramped-synchronized GMs and the absence of GMs of fidgety character, strongly predict cerebral palsy (Ferrari et al., 1990). In contrast, on neurological examinations no specific signs have been noted for the prediction of later cerebral palsy. Thus, qualitative assessment of GMs appears to be a more useful tool in predicting future neurological functioning in both preterm and term infants than are traditional infant neurological assessments.

Summary

The usefulness of traditional measures of neurological functioning in discriminating between normally developing children and children with or at risk for developmental disabilities remains controversial. The lack of normative data is a common criticism of these measures. Although some researchers endorse the reliability and validity of these measures in the assessment of children with, or at risk for, cognitive, learning, and behavioral difficulties, others argue that they fail to discriminate among such groups and their normally developing peers. Instead investigators have argued that the presence of soft signs should be viewed as evidence of delayed maturation as opposed to pathology. Comparison of the utility of the qualitative and quantitative methods for assessing the neurological status of preterm and term infants has also been a subject of debate in recent years. An accumulating body of research suggests that the qualitative assessment of general movements may be a more sensitive indicator of neurological dysfunction than the reflexes and responses that are typically assessed by traditional neonatal neurological examinations. Research has found that the qualitative approach to assessment exhibits a higher specific predictive value for later development of normalcy, minor neurological impairment, and cerebral palsy than traditional quantitative measures of neurological functioning. The traditional neurological examination of infants and children, however, remains an important component for the rapid diagnosis of a neurological disorder. It is also useful for monitoring the evolution of the disorder over time. Hence, both the traditional neurological examination and observation of the quality of GMs are important components of the assessment of motor functioning in infants and children.

NEUROPSYCHOLOGICAL ASSESSMENT

In addition to the traditional pediatric neurological assessment measures described previously, there exists a wide variety of neuropsychological assessment batteries that can be used to assess motor impairment in children. The typical neurological examination provides a broad overview of the child's neurological systems and essentially is more of a screening procedure, the results of which direct the nature and type of further investigations. Moreover, the pediatric neurological examination may provide only a hint that a neurological deficit may be present and, thus, other techniques are needed to determine the nature and degree of neurological impairment. Neuropsychological assessment provides insight into the functional integrity of basic cerebral processes, as well as a comprehensive evaluation of functions that are associated with or dependent on higher cerebral processes (Bigler, 1988). With children, the primary purpose of neuropsychological assessment is to document changes in behavior and development, which are the result of alterations in the functioning of the central nervous system (Hynd, Snow, & Becker, 1986). Therefore, although neurological and neuro-psychological examinations overlap to a certain extent, they are for the most part examining brain function at different levels. To date, the Halstead–Reitan Neuropsycho-logical Battery (HRNB) and the Luria–Nebraska Neuropsychological Battery (LNNB) have been the most widely used neuropsychological assessment approaches with children and are the primary focus of the discussion that follows.

There are two versions of the HRNB currently used with children. The first is the Halstead Neuropsychological Test Battery for Children, which is appropriate to use with children between the ages of 9 and 14 years, and the second is the Reitan–Indiana Neuropsychological Test Battery for Children, used with children 5–8 years of age. For the sake of simplicity, we refer to both of these versions as the HRNB. The HRNB is a comprehensive battery testing a range of abilities, with a small component devoted to the assessment of children's motor skills. There are three tests in this battery that are relevant to a discussion of motor functioning. They are the Finger-Tapping Test, the Trail Making Test, and the Grip Strength Test, all of which are used to assess subtle motor impairment (Spreen & Strauss, 1991). The Finger-Tapping Test is used to measure the motor speed of the index finger of both the preferred and nonpreferred hand (Spreen & Strauss, 1991). The Trail Making Test, also known as the Marching Test, assesses speed of visual search, attention, mental flexibility (Spreen & Strauss, 1991), and the coordinated function of the upper extremities (Reitan, 1971b). The Grip Strength Test, also known as the Hand Dynamometer Test, is used to assess the strength or intensity of the voluntary movements of each hand by having the child squeeze a hand dynamometer (Spreen & Strauss, 1991).

The HRNB has been most extensively used to discriminate between children with brain damage and normal children. Indeed, the validity of most of the tests incorporated within this battery has been established by comparing the performance of these two groups of children (Tramontana & Hooper, 1988). A series of investigations by Reitan (1971a, 1971b) suggest that the Finger-Tapping, Trail Making, and Grip Strength tests all reliably detect motor impairment in children with cerebral lesions between the ages of 5 and 8 and clearly distinguish them from normal children without evidence of cerebral injury. Although the results were somewhat variable for the individual tests, each of the measures of motor function classified 70–80% of the children into their appropriate groups (Reitan, 1971a). In a study of children between the ages of 9 and 14, Boll (1974) also found that these three tests detected motor impairment in children with brain damage.

Although not incorporated in the HRNB, the Purdue Pegboard Test is commonly used along with the Finger-Tapping and Grip Strength tests as part of the neuropsychological assessment of motor functioning. This test measures the finger and hand dexterity of the preferred and nonpreferred hands individually and then both hands together (Spreen & Strauss, 1991). It has typically been used in neuropsychological assessment to assist in localizing cerebral lesions and deficits (Spreen & Strauss, 1991); however, in recent years it has also been used to assess motor functioning in children at risk for developmental coordination disorder (Pitcher, Piek, & Hay, 2003).

A common practice in the neuropsychological assessment of children is the measurement of children's motor performance using both the preferred and nonpreferred hand in order to determine whether there is evidence of poor performance in one hand relative to the other. The debate surrounding the clinical significance, if any, of intermanual discrepancies on the Finger-Tapping, Grip Strength, and Purdue Pegboard tests has provided the impetus for much of the research in this area over the last two decades. What has become abundantly clear is that there is considerable variability in intermanual discrepancies in both individuals with brain damage, as well as normals (Bornstein, 1986). In general, children tend to display superior performance on these tasks with their preferred hand; however, it is not uncommon to find that the nonpreferred hand displays superior performance compared to the preferred hand (Bornstein, 1986). The test–retest reliability of the differences between hands has not been found to be highly reliable on the Finger-Tapping, Grip Strength, and Purdue Pegboard tests (Morrison, Gregory, & Paul, 1979; Reddon, Gill, Gauk, & Maerz, 1988). These inconsistencies make it difficult to accurately define a child's motor status, and they have diagnostic value only when differences are found on other tests. Indeed, it has been suggested that in order to gain a better understanding of any apparent motor dysfunction, it is necessary to assess the consistency of intermanual discrepancies across several motor tasks (Bornstein, 1986; Reddon et al., 1988). Because consistent intermanual discrepancies are rare in the normal population, motor impairment would be indicated in such circumstances.

The use of the HRNB to assess the motor functioning in children with minimal brain dysfunction (MBD) and learning disabilities (LD) has also received a great deal of attention in the research literature. Although a number of studies have reported that the HRNB distinguishes normal children from those with MBD and LD based on their motor performance (e.g., Rourke & Finlayson, 1978; Selz & Reitan, 1979), controversy surrounds how best to interpret the poorer performance of these two groups of children. It is not uncommon for children with MBD or LD to have attentional deficiencies (Hynd et al., 1986). Therefore, deficits among these children on measures of motor functioning may not reflect impaired neurological processes but, rather, impairment in the child's ability to sustain his or her attention over a lengthy period of time. Furthermore, many of the tests assessing motor function incorporated in the HRNB require the interplay of multiple abilities (Tramontana & Hooper, 1988), which require the child to draw on not only motor but also visual, tactile, and kinesthetic cues, making it difficult to determine the specific area in which the child is in fact deficient.

Similar to the HRNB, the Luria–Nebraska Neuropsychological Battery—Children's Revision (LNNB-CR) is designed to provide a comprehensive assessment of the neuropsychological functioning of children, and is used with children 8–12 years of age. The battery consists of 11 scales and has a total of 149 items. The scale assessing the children's motor skills predominantly measures motor speed, coordination, and ability to imitate motor movements. As is the case with the motor tests incorporated within the HRNB, the majority of studies using the LNNB-CR have focused on children with brain damage or learning disabilities (Hynd et al., 1986). Several studies that have used this battery to compare children with brain damage and normal children have noted significantly greater motor impairment in children in the former group (Gustavson et al., 1984). This test battery has also been reported to detect lower motor scores among learning disabled children relative to their nondisabled peers (Hynd et al., 1986).

Summary

Research with traditional neuropsychological assessment batteries suggests that the subset of tests used to assess motor functioning does detect motor impairment in some children. This research, however, has focused mainly on children with brain damage and/or learning disabilities. Research using these batteries and more recently developed neuropsychological assessment batteries such as the NEPSY (Korkman, Kirk, & Kemp; 1998) with other groups of children at risk for motor impairment is required. As is the case with the traditional neurological examinations, there are some methodological limitations with the motor tests included in the HRNB and LNNB-CR, such as questionable test–retest reliability and issues surrounding their validity. Further, the accumulating studies examining discrepancy scores between the preferred and nonpreferred hand suggest that it is imperative to examine the consistency of such discrepancies across a number of motor tasks before any conclusions are made about the child's motor status.

ANALYSES OF DEFICITS IN MOTOR CONTROL

This approach involves examining how children make reaching movements to objects/ targets in space (e.g., Pryde & Roy, 1999). In this work, which has focused on children with DCD, the temporal and spatial characteristics of their movements as described by movement kinematics are compared to those of children without DCD. Specifically, these studies have focused on reaction time (RT), movement time (MT), movement accuracy, and movement variability to examine how children with DCD plan, organize, and execute motor responses.

These studies of goal-directed arm movements have most often examined clumsy children's ability to use visual and kinesthetic feedback for movement control. Smyth (1991) examined the RT and MT of clumsy (school-screened) and control children for simple and complex pointing movements with vision either available or not. The simple pointing movements required a single vertical movement of 22 cm, while complex movements involved a sequence of three movements: a vertical movement of 22 cm, a horizontal movement of 25 cm to the right, and finally a horizontal movement of 50 cm to the left. Analyses revealed that the clumsy children exhibited significantly longer RTs overall, while the MT for the complex response only was found to be significantly longer for clumsy children. Interestingly, the removal of vision was found to increase MT by similar amounts for both groups indicating that clumsy and control children were equally able to use visual and kinesthetic feedback in controlling movement. Smyth concluded that clumsy children experience difficulty with the programming of longer, more complex movements resulting in a greater than normal dependence on feedback for movement control.

Rösblad and von Hofsten (1994) also examined the use of visual feedback in the control of goal-directed arm movements. In their study, children with and without DCD were required to pick up beads one at a time from a cup and place them into another cup. In one condition, vision of the targets (the cups) and the hand was prevented, while in the other this visual information was available. The results showed that children with DCD were consistently slower and much more variable than their peers. Similar to the findings of Smyth (1991), Rösblad and von Hofsten found that the withdrawal of visual information affected both groups of children in similar ways. In concert with Smyth (1991), they concluded that children with DCD have an impaired capacity to program their movements and, as a result, consistently move more slowly and variably due to their reliance on feedback control.

Interestingly, both of these studies concluded that the motor difficulties of clumsy children were due to an impaired capacity in movement programming arising from an increased reliance on feedback information. Both, however, failed to measure the end-point accuracy of the children's movements. It is possible that children with motor difficulties may have moved in the same time as their peers in the absence of vision, yet they may have been significantly less accurate. If children with DCD were less accurate in the absence of vision, this finding would suggest that they have difficulty controlling their movements based on kinesthetic feedback. A study conducted by van der Meulen, van der Gon, Gielen, Gooskens, and Willemse (1991) answered this shortcoming in that both end-point accuracy and movement kinematics were examined. Again, clumsy children (school-screened) and controls performed goal-directed arm movements with and without visual feedback. In this study, the group of clumsy children was selected based on ratings by school teachers and a test of motor impairment and were matched with a group of their peers on age and gender. Children were required to make horizontal aiming movements as quickly as possible to lighted targets positioned up to 24 cm away from the starting position. The authors found that the clumsy children differed from their peers in that they had longer overall MTs particularly in the presence of visual feedback and larger variability in the distance moved during the acceleration (preprogrammed) phase of the movement. They also found no significant differences between the groups for end-point accuracy regardless of visual feedback. On the basis of these results, van der Meulen and colleagues concluded that clumsiness is linked to an inaccuracy in the preprogrammed phase of the movement.

The findings of van der Meulen and colleagues (1991) are problematic in that the authors did not examine the number of corrective submovements in the deceleration phase of the movement. All the movements analyzed, then, consisted of one acceleration phase and one deceleration phase without prominent reaccelerations or redecelerations in the trajectory. This method of analysis is problematic because it precludes important information about the way in which children used sensory information to control their movements. This preclusion is especially troublesome in a study investigating the relationship between motor problems and sensory feedback as the use of feedback information is not examined. Studies of children and adults with various motor deficits have shown that the trajectories of visually guided aiming movements are often characterized by several acceleration and deceleration phases (Flowers, 1975, 1976; Forsstrom & von Hofsten, 1982; Schellekens, Scholten, & Kalverboer, 1983). These findings suggest that van der Meulen and colleagues did not examine an important aspect of the movement trajectory in clumsy children and renders the results of their study inconclusive.

The studies to this point have used largely discrete aiming movements. Geuze and Kalverboer (1988) used a continuous tapping task between two targets at a distance of 25 cm and examined the spatial and temporal parameters of performance in clumsy (school-screened) and control children. The results showed that both the preprogrammed phase and the feedback controlled correction phase contributed to the greater inaccuracy of clumsy children. The longer movement times and shorter, more variable acceleration phase indicate that clumsy children spend more time using feedback to correct the inaccuracy of the preprogrammed phase of their movements. Because visual feedback was not manipulated in this study, the origin of the programming problems of clumsy children (e.g., visual vs. nonvisual) could not be determined.

In a more recent study by Pryde and Roy (1999), two children with DCD-like characteristics (teacher-nominated) were examined on a manual aiming task and compared to a group of their same-age peers without motor difficulties. The aiming task was performed with and without visual feedback of the moving hand. The results revealed that the nature of the children's performance patterns were not only different from those of their peers but also from each other. Specifically, one child's movement problems did not dramatically affect his ability to produce aiming movements. The only difficulty was with respect to movement accuracy in the absence of vision, suggesting that his problems may lie at the perceptual stage of processing affecting his spatial localization abilities. In contrast, the findings for the other child indicated that his motor problems dramatically affected his ability to produce aiming movements. The nature of this child's difficulties suggested that his problems may lie more in the response programming and/or execution stages of processing affecting his ability to adjust the force parameters of movement. In concert with work on subtyping children with DCD based on their performance on a battery of tests, this study suggests that DCD may not result in a uniform change in movement control. Rather, DCD may involve somewhat heterogeneous subtypes of movement control problems.

Taken together these studies suggest that one mechanism underlying DCD is the impaired ability to accurately plan and organize a motor response, as revealed in studies showing longer total movement times and shorter inaccurate preprogrammed movements in children with motor difficulties characteristic of DCD (Geuze & Kalverboer, 1988; Rösblad & von Hofsten, 1994; Smyth, 1991; van der Meulen et al., 1991). Another mechanism proposed is a difficulty in using sensory feedback for motor control (Laslow, Bairstow, Bartip, & Rolfe, 1988; Missiuna, 1994; Rösblad & von Hofsten, 1994; Smyth & Glencross, 1988; Smyth & Mason, 1998). Although several researchers have concluded that the motor difficulties of children with DCD are due to an impaired capacity in motor programming, few detailed analyses have been conducted to specify the reasons. Furthermore, given the heterogeneity of DCD, few studies have performed within-group analyses to identify possible differences in individual patterns of performance.

In a recent study following on the work of Pryde and Roy (1999), Pryde (2000) investigated the movement planning and control strategies of children with DCD using detailed kinematic analyses in order to provide further insight into the mechanisms underlying these children's movement difficulties. A secondary aim of this study was to perform within-group analyses of performance within this population. In this study, the performance of 10, 7- to 9-year-old children identified as having the characteristics of DCD as defined by the fourth edition of *Diagnostic and Statistical Manual of Mental Disorders* (DSM-IV; American Psychiatric Association, 1994) was compared to that of 10 children without motor problems matched on gender and age. Participants performed a computer-based aiming movement that involved moving a cursor seen on the monitor from a start position located at the body midline to targets (1.25 cm or 2.25 cm in diameter) located at three distances (50 cm, 100 cm, and 150 cm) directly ahead of the start position. The participant moving a mouse on a graphics tablet with his or her unseen right hand affected cursor movement. Two vision conditions were included. In one, vision of the cursor was available throughout movement to the target. In the other vision of the cursor was not available during movement, but visual feedback as to the location of the cursor relative to the target was available once movement had stopped. Performance of the aiming movements was reflected in various kinematic measures of the movement trajectory to the target, as well as accuracy at peak velocity and at the end of the movement.

Looking first at the kinematic measures of performance, it is clear that the availability of visual feedback information is an important factor in defining how DCD affects movement control. Analyses of the overall time to execute each movement (MT) revealed that the children with DCD exhibited longer MTs only when vision was available. Further, the typical effect of target size on MT (movements to the smaller target took more time to complete) was seen for the control children regardless of the availability of vision. For the children with DCD this size effect was seen only when vision was available (see Table 3.1).

This interaction is important as it concurs with previous research (Rösblad & von Hofsten, 1994; Smyth, 1991; van der Meulen et al., 1991) revealing that the presence of visual feedback has a differential effect on the movement times of children with DCD. Specifically, relative to the controls, the DCD group demonstrated longer MTs overall and particularly with increases in movement complexity (smaller target or longer movement) only when vision was available.

Analyses of the kinematic components of MT reveal that the effects of the availability of vision in the children with DCD are seen primarily in the time spent in movement deceleration approaching the target. The children with DCD spent more time in deceleration but only when vision was available (see Table 3.1). Analyses of the number of corrective movements during this phase of the movement trajectory support this finding. The children with DCD exhibited a larger number of corrective movements, but again only when visual information relating to movement of the hand was available (see Table 3.1). These findings indicate that children with DCD do not benefit from visual feedback in the control of movement in the same way as their peers. They exhibit longer MTs, longer times in the feedback phase of the movement (i.e., time after peak velocity), and higher frequencies of corrective movements to control their hand toward the target.

TABLE 3.1. Performance of Groups on Aiming Task in Each Vision Condition

		Dependent measure		
Condition	Group	MT (msec)	TAPV (msec)	Number of subpeaks
Vision	DCD	1,275	900	2.6
	Control	525	500	1.9
No vision	DCD	1,250	625	2.2
	Control	1,150	633	1.8

Note. MT, movement time; TAPV, time after peak velocity.

Taken together these results reveal that the children with DCD generally program their movements in the same way as do their age-matched peers. Group differences appear primarily in the feedback-controlled phase of movement and are dependent on feedback availability, suggesting that the greater use of visual feedback in the DCD group is not related to a difficulty in movement programming but, rather, a difficulty in using or processing visual feedback information.

Analyses of these kinematic measures indicate that the differences between the children with DCD and their age-matched peers are seen primarily when visual information about hand movement is available. These findings would suggest that their relative performance did not differ when vision of the hand movement was unavailable. Analyses of movement accuracy, however, do reveal a difference. Movement accuracy for both the initial movement at peak velocity and at the end of the movement was lower for the children with DCD only when vision of the hand movement was not available.

These findings for accuracy are important in further understanding the impairments associated with DCD. The results for the time parameters, such as MT and time after peak velocity, suggest that there are no differences between the DCD and control groups in the no-visual-feedback condition. The findings for initial and final accuracy, however, indicate that this is not the case. In the absence of vision, children with DCD demonstrate significant difficulty generating spatially accurate movements. These findings then suggest that DCD may also involve a difficulty in integrating complex visual information about the target with proprioceptive feedback of the moving hand.

These findings concur with previous research in that the timing components of movements (e.g., MT) in children with DCD are differentially affected by the availability of visual feedback (e.g., Rösblad & von Hofsten, 1994; Smyth, 1991; van der Meulen et al., 1991). Moreover, we found that in the presence of visual feedback there were minimal differences between the DCD and control groups in the programming phases of movement (e.g., time to peak velocity) but significant differences in the feedback-controlled phases (e.g., time after peak velocity and number of subpeaks). These observations suggest that DCD likely involves a difficulty in processing sensory feedback rather than in motor programming. That DCD children's movements were significantly less accurate particularly for complex movements (smaller target size or larger movement amplitude) in the absence of visual feedback provides further support for this idea.

Analyses of the kinematic profiles provided further insight into the notion of a programming versus feedback deficit. Results revealed that the children used three different types of control for their manual aiming movements, a finding that is consistent with the findings of Pryde and Roy (1998, 1999) and Hay (1979, 1984). The three different kinematic profiles are described as follows:

1. "Step" movements involve several velocity peaks, accelerations, and decelerations and early braking activity without an initial ballistic movement (i.e., poorly programmed with a greater reliance on feedback). Young children with immature sensorimotor integration abilities typically exhibit these movements as adaptive strategies.
2. "Double peak" movements consist of gradual acceleration and deceleration phases and two velocity peaks with values within 5% of each other. These

movements appear to be a progression of immature step movements, yet they still lack the feedforward or programming capabilities associated with smooth single peak profiles (Pryde & Roy, 1998, 1999).

3. "Mature" movement patterns are characterized by a single velocity peak, an initial ballistic phase, and a smooth deceleration phase. These movements are typical of adult movement patterns.

Analyses (see Table 3.2) of the frequency of these profiles revealed that when visual feedback was available, DCD children exhibited significantly more double peak movements and significantly fewer mature movements than did the control children. When visual feedback was removed, children with DCD displayed significantly more step movements and significantly fewer mature profiles.

These findings indicate differences between the groups with respect to motor control strategies. Relative to the controls, children with DCD generally exhibited fewer mature and more immature movement profiles (e.g., step), indicating a difficulty in movement programming and an increased use of adaptive strategies to control their movements. Given these differences, it would seem important to investigate the relationship between the normal and abnormal movement profiles and the end-point accuracy of these movements. The question of interest here was whether the different control strategies led to differing degrees of accuracy in DCD and control children.

To examine the relationship between kinematic profiles and movement accuracy, individual movements were specified as accurate or inaccurate. Movements of the children with DCD were considered accurate if they were within 1.5 standard deviations of the mean of the age-matched peers in terms of end-point accuracy. Each movement then was categorized according to kinematic profile (i.e., mature or immature) and end-point accuracy (i.e., accurate or inaccurate) within each visual feedback condition, resulting in four kinematic/accuracy patterns: type I—mature, accurate; type II—mature, inaccurate; type III—immature, accurate; and type IV—immature, inaccurate.

Analyses of the frequency of each of these patterns (see Table 3.3) revealed that when visual feedback was available DCD children exhibited a higher frequency of Type III—immature, accurate movements. This finding is consistent with the findings for the comparison of the kinematic parameters, indicating that DCD children in this age range tend to have significant difficulty benefiting from visual feedback, spend more time in the feedback control phase, and make more corrections to control their movements.

TABLE 3.2. Percentage of Movement Patterns in Each Vision Condition

Condition	Group	Movement patterns		
		Mature	Two peaks	Step
Vision	DCD	80	10	10
	Control	98	1	1
No vision	DCD	70	11	19
	Control	81	10	9

TABLE 3.3. Percentage of Kinematic/Accuracy Patterns in Each Vision Condition

Condition	Group	Kinematic/accuracy pattern			
		Type I	Type II	Type III	Type IV
Vision	DCD	79	3	17	1
	Control	82	9	5	4
No vision	DCD	48	20	20	12
	Control	62	20	13	5

In the no-visual-feedback condition children with DCD exhibited significantly fewer type I patterns only, suggesting that there was no prevalence of any one kinematic/accuracy pattern beyond the type I pattern. DCD children exhibited a range of less efficient kinematic/accuracy patterns with considerable interindividual variability in the relative frequency of the more immature patterns (see Table 3.4 for the range of patterns).

These findings are consistent with previous research (Hay, 1979, 1984; Pryde & Roy, 1998, 1999) showing that children with DCD generally exhibited relatively fewer mature or "normal" movements and more immature or "abnormal" movements (e.g., step) relative to their peers. The higher frequency of irregular, multipeaked velocity profiles observed in children with DCD is consistent with the findings of the kinematic parameters, indicating that they experienced difficulty organizing and generating movements to contend with the demands of the manual aiming task.

The high frequency of abnormal, accurate movements for the children with DCD in the presence of visual feedback provides additional support for the notion that integration of visual information presents a processing challenge to children with DCD

TABLE 3.4. Percentage Distribution of Kinematic/Accuracy Patterns in the No-Vision Condition among the Children with DCD

Participant	Kinematic/accuracy pattern			
	Type I	Type II	Type III	Type IV
1	54	46	4	0
2	74	26	4	0
3	60	8	31	2
4	45	25	25	5
5	65	15	12	8
6	31	27	35	7
7	48	30	10	12
8	58	2	28	12
9	27	24	21	28
10	21	13	35	31

during movement execution. For these children to execute accurate movements, they rely more heavily on visual feedback for the on-line control of their hand toward the target. This increased dependence on feedback would lead to an increased prevalence of multipeaked, irregular movement profiles. Thus, it appears that visual feedback is somewhat of a "double-edged sword." Particularly when faced with complex target characteristics (i.e., targets that are small or far away) visual feedback presents a processing challenge for these children, yet visual feedback of their hand enables guidance to an accurate end point. When visual feedback was removed, the children with DCD demonstrated significantly fewer "perfect" movements—bell-shaped profiles with accurate end points—than exhibited by controls. This, too, is consistent with the results of the kinematic parameters analyses and further supports the idea that the removal of visual feedback poses a significant challenge to the programming and control of goal-directed movements in children with DCD. This challenge leads to a variety of poorly organized movement patterns.

What do these findings reveal about the deficit(s) underlying DCD? The comparisons between the DCD and control groups for the kinematic parameters and profiles in this study primarily lead to the kind of inconclusive results prevalent in the DCD literature. Children with DCD appear to have difficulty processing both visual and nonvisual feedback leading to longer MTs and/or decreased accuracy and a higher frequency of irregular velocity profiles. Considering models of sensorimotor functioning such as that proposed by Jeannerod (1988), several explanations of the findings could be postulated. One possibility is that the increased incidence of abnormal, multipeaked movements in the DCD group is the result of a generalized programming deficit (e.g., Geuze & Kalverboer, 1988; Rösblad & von Hofsten, 1994; Smyth, 1991; van der Meulen et al., 1991), causing children with this disorder to experience difficulty generating the normal, bell-shaped profiles predominantly exhibited by their peers. As a result, children with DCD spend more time using feedback to control their movements. However, the analyses of the kinematic parameters do not reveal significant differences between the DCD and control groups with respect to the TTPV—an indicator of the preprogrammed component of movement. Furthermore, some children with DCD executed movements with kinematic profiles comparable to those of controls. Given these latter findings, a generalized programming deficit in the DCD population seems unlikely.

Because children with DCD generally spend more time using feedback to control their movements, an alternative explanation could be that DCD is the result of a generalized deficit in feedback control, both visual and proprioceptive. This explanation would account for the longer MTs in the visual-feedback condition and the spatially inaccurate movements in the no-visual-feedback condition demonstrated by the DCD group. However, the higher frequency of abnormal, multipeaked movements and the variation in the kinematic/accuracy patterns in children with DCD relative to the controls indicates some signs of deficient programming and that some children are able to use feedback in ways comparable to their peers. Thus, these findings speak against the hypothesis of a generalized feedback deficit.

Interestingly, even a more detailed investigation of movement trajectories and movement accuracy (e.g., MT, velocity measures, accuracy, and kinematic profiles) in groups of children with and without DCD does not provide conclusive evidence explaining the deficient motor performance in DCD. It is only when analyses of movements in individual DCD children are examined that a more plausible explanation of the nature of the movement deficits in DCD is revealed. This alternative explanation stems from the assumption that DCD is a heterogeneous disorder and suggests that the disorder may be the result of a more global deficit in sensorimotor functioning characterized by variations in the expression of motor difficulties. This explanation suggests that the entire sensorimotor system may be implicated in DCD.

Support for such a generalized sensorimotor deficit comes from several findings in the data. First, children with DCD have often been found to perform significantly below average on standardized tasks requiring the integration of visual and proprioceptive information with motor functions. On the manual aiming task, this difficulty would have been exacerbated in the no-visual-feedback condition, which required children to integrate visual and proprioceptive information in a unique way (e.g., visual feedback of the target and proprioceptive feedback of the hand). Children with DCD reacted to this insecurity by using various adaptive strategies for movement execution. Some children primarily adopted a strategy of hesitant, on-line control leading to abnormal, multipeaked movements. For some, this strategy was successful and led to an accurate end point (e.g., type III—abnormal, accurate) while for other DCD children this strategy resulted in a significant spatial inaccuracy (e.g., type IV—abnormal, inaccurate). There was another subgroup of children with DCD who performed kinematically normal movements to inaccurate locations (e.g., type II—normal, inaccurate). Possibly these children are not aware of or underestimated their system's difficulty in integrating sensorimotor information for certain tasks. Finally, there was a subset of children with DCD who generated "perfect" movements with normal, bell-shaped profiles and a level of accuracy that was commensurate with their same-age peers (e.g., type I—normal, accurate). Their performance on the aiming task suggests that they adopted some effective strategies for coping with the deficiencies of their sensorimotor systems. Such a range of adaptive movement strategies due to central processing deficits has been previously described in the literature (Hermsdörfer et al., 1996).

Summary

In sum, the foregoing findings revealed that characterizing the effects of DCD on manual aiming involves a complex mix of kinematic and spatial accuracy data and depends on the demands of the aiming task (e.g., the availability of vision of the hand movement, target size, and movement amplitude). Our observations suggest that overall DCD does not affect the initial programming of movement but, rather, the processing of feedback information and the integration of feedback from vision and proprioception. However, large individual differences were apparent, suggesting that for some children the earlier programming stages were affected. In concert with much other work, then, DCD would appear to affect different processing stages in the unfolding manual aiming movement. As with our work on limb apraxia in stroke (e.g., Heath, Almeida, Roy, Black, & Westwood, 2003; Roy, 1996; Roy et al., 2000) that shows disruptions at different stages of gesture production depending on lesion location, so work on DCD may eventually reveal some such links between disruptions in processing stages in manual aiming and identifiable neurodevelopmental disorders.

GENERAL SUMMARY

In this chapter we have considered three approaches to examining the neurobehavioral mechanisms underlying neurodevelopmental disorders. The first involves assessing neurological functioning. The focus is on identifying neuromotor deficits linked to damage to brain regions arising from known neuropathological conditions. Finding such functional deficits in children with neurodevelopmental disorders such as DCD often leads to inferences that the disorder may be arising from damage to the brain areas known to subserve the affected functions. A similar assessment process is followed in the second approach, neuropsychological assessment. Similar inferences as to underlying neural correlates are also drawn using this approach. The primary difference between these approaches is the degree to which cognitive functioning can be evaluated in neuropsychological assessments. These two approaches to assessment, however, share the feature that they both involve relatively gross measures of performance such as overall time or accuracy. The third approach we have examined affords the opportunity to look at performance in more detail. This detail is seen through movement kinematics that reveal something about how the movement was controlled. Overall gross measures of performance similar to those used in the first two approaches, such as the time to complete a movement, can be partitioned into its temporal and spatial components. It is these components that provide insight into the processes involved in the control of movement. For example, in our work on DCD, analyses of these components revealed that feedback processing was one process affected in children with this disorder.

Another way of looking at these three approaches is to think about what neuropsychology has termed the *product* and the *process* dimensions of performance. The product dimension reflects the level of performance on a task such as accuracy or time with reference to some expected level of performance (e.g., norms). The process dimension refers to the means by which the performer achieves the product. The presence of certain types of error, the use of various types of strategy, or the analysis of the component processes underlying the product are often used as measures of the process dimension of performance. In a sense, the first two approaches focus largely on the product dimension, while the third is more focused on the process dimension. From this perspective one could envisage these approaches being on a continuum with the first two providing a broad-band analysis of the integrity of the neuromotor system and the third affording a more fine-grained analysis of what particular processes in the control of movement may be affected. This view would suggest the need for some integration of these approaches in order to clearly understand the nature of any neurodevelopmental disorder. In our work with adults with acquired brain disorders such as stroke, we have indicated the need to examine both of these dimensions of performance (Roy, 1990). As with these acquired neurological disorders so with neurodevelopmental disorders, the broad-band assessments serve as a means of diagnosing the presence of deficit (e.g., apraxia) or disorder (e.g., DCD) and the more fine-grained, process-oriented assessments afford insight into the potential neurobehavioral processes that are affected. A future goal for assessments of neurodevelopmental disorders may be to determine how best to integrate these approaches.

ACKNOWLEDGMENTS

Preparation of this chapter was partially funded through grants from the National Sciences and Engineering Research Council of Canada, the Ontario Mental Health Foundation, and the Heart and Stroke Foundation of Ontario to Eric A. Roy, and through grants from the Alberta Children's Hospital Foundation and the Canadian Institutes of Health Research to Deborah Dewey.

REFERENCES

Allen, M. C., & Capute, A. J. (1989). Neonatal neurodevelopmental examination as a predictor of neuromotor outcome in premature infants. *Pediatrics, 83,* 498–506.

American Psychiatric Association. (1994). *Diagnostic and statistical manual of mental disorders* (4th ed.). Washington, DC: Author.

Bigler, E. D. (1988). The role of neuropsychological assessment in relation to other types of assessment with children. In M. G. Tramontana & S. R. Hooper (Eds.), *Assessment issues in child neuropsychology* (pp. 67–91). New York: Plenum Press.

Blondis, T. A., Snow, J. H., & Accardo, P. J. (1990). Integration of soft signs in academically normal and academically at-risk children. *Pediatrics, 85,* 421–425.

Boll, T. J. (1974). Behavioral correlates of cerebral damage in children aged 9–14. In R. M. Reitan & L. A. Davison (Eds.), *Clinical neuropsychology: Current status and applications* (pp. 91–120). New York: Wiley.

Bornstein, R. A. (1986). Consistency of intermanual discrepancies in normal and unilateral brain lesion patients. *Journal of Consulting and Clinical Psychology, 54,* 719–723.

Camp, J. A., Bialer, I., Sverd, J., & Winsberg, B. (1978). Clinical usefulness of the NIMH physical and neurological examination for soft signs. *American Journal of Psychiatry, 135,* 362–364.

Cioni, G. C., Ferrari, F., Einspieler, C., Paolicelli, P. B., Barbani, T., & Prechtl, H. F. R. (1997). Comparison between observation of spontaneous movements and neurologic examination in preterm infants. *Journal of Pediatrics, 130,* 704–711.

Cioni, G., Prechtl, H. F. R., Ferrari, F., Paolicelli, P. B., Einspieler, C., & Roversi, M. F. (1997). Which better predicts later outcome in fullterm infants: Quality of general movements or neurological examination? *Early Human Development, 50,* 71–85.

Close, J. (1973). Scored neurological examination in pharmacotherapy of children. [Special issue—Pharmacotherapy of children]. *Psychopharmacology Bulletin, 9,* 142–148.

Denckla, M. B. (1973). Development of speed in repetitive and successive finger movements in normal children. *Developmental Medicine and Child Neurology, 15,* 635–645.

Denckla, M. B. (1974). Development of motor coordination in normal children. *Developmental Medicine and Child Neurology, 16,* 729–741.

Denckla, M. B. (1985). Revised neurological examination for subtle signs. *Psychopharmacology Bulletin, 21,* 773–800

Deuel, R. K., & Robinson, D. J. (1987). Developmental motor signs. In D. E. Tupper (Ed.), *Soft neurological signs* (pp. 95–129). Orlando, FL: Grune & Stratton.

Dubowitz, L. M. S., & Dubowitz, V. (1981). *The neurological assessment of the preterm and fullterm newborn infant.* London: Heinemann.

Dubowitz, L. M. S., Dubowitz, V., Palmer, P. G., Miller, G., Fawer, C. L., & Levene, M. I. (1984). Correlation of neurologic assessment in the preterm newborn infant with outcome at 1 year. *Journal of Pediatrics, 105,* 452–456.

Fellick, J. M., Thomson, A. P. J., Sills, J., & Hart, C. A. (2001). Neurological soft signs in mainstream pupils. *Archives of Disease in Childhood, 85,* 371–374.

Ferrari, F., Cioni, G., & Prechtl, H. F. R. (1990). Qualitative changes of general movements in preterm infants with brain lesions. *Early Human Development, 23,* 193–231.

Flowers, K. (1975). Ballistic and corrective movements on an aiming task: Intention and parkinsonian movement disorders compared. *Neurology, 25,* 413–421.

Flowers, K. (1976). Visual closed-loop and open-loop characteristics of voluntary movement in patients with parkinsonism and intention tremor. *Brain, 99,* 269–310.

Forsstrom, A., & von Hofsten, C. (1982). Visually directed reaching of children with motor impairments. *Developmental Medicine and Child Neurology, 24,* 653–661.

Geuze, R. H., & Kalverboer, A. F. (1988). Inconsistency and adaptation in timing of clumsy children. *Journal of Human Movement Studies, 13,* 421–432.

Gustavson, J. L., Golden, C. J., Wilkening, G. N., Hermann, B. P., Plaisted, J. R., MacInnes, W. D., et al. (1984). The Luria–Nebraska Neuropsychological Battery—Children's Revision: Validation with brain-damaged and normal children. *Journal of Psychoeducational Assessment, 2,* 199–208.

Hay, L. (1979). Spatial-temporal analysis of movements in children: Motor programs versus feedback in the development of reaching. *Journal of Motor Behavior, 11,* 189–200.

Hay, L. (1984) Discontinuity in the development of motor control. In W. Prinz & A. F. Sanders (Eds.), *Cognition and motor processes* (pp. 351–358). Berlin & Heidelberg: Springer-Verlag.

Heath, M., Almeida, Q. J., Roy, E. A., Black, S. E., & Westwood, D. (2003). Selective dysfunction of tool-use: A failure to integrate somatosensation and action. *Neurocase, 9,* 156–163.

Hermsdörfer, J., Mai, N., Spatt, J., Marquardt, C., Veltkamp, R., & Goldenberg, G. (1996). Kinematic analysis of movement imitation in apraxia. *Brain, 119,* 1575–1586.

Huttenlocher, P. R., Levine, S. C., Huttenlocher, J., & Gates, J. (1990). Discrimination of normal and at-risk preschool children on the basis of neurological tests. *Developmental Medicine and Child Neurology, 32,* 394–402.

Hynd, G. W., Snow, J., & Becker, M. G. (1986). Neuropsychological assessment in clinical child psychology. In B. B. Lahey & A. E. Kazdin (Eds.), *Advances in clinical child psychology* (Vol. 9, pp. 35–86). New York: Plenum Press.

Jeannerod, M. (1988). *The neural and behavioural organization of goal-directed movements.* Oxford, UK: Clarendon Press.

Kakebeeke, T. H., Jongmans, M. J., Dubowitz, L. M. S., Schoemaker, M. M., & Henderson, S. E. (1993). Some aspects of the reliability of Touwen's examination of the child with minor neurological dysfunction. *Developmental Medicine and Child Neurology, 35,* 1197–1205.

Korkman, M., Kirk, U, & Kemp, S. (1998). *NEPSY: A development neuropsychological assessment.* San Antonio, TX: Psychological Corp.

Laszlow, J. I., Bairstow, P. J., Bartrip, J., & Rolfe, V. T. (1988). Clumsiness or perceptuo-motor dysfunction? In A. M. Colley & J. R. Beech (Eds.), *Cognition and action in skilled motor behavior* (pp. 293–310). Amsterdam: North-Holland.

Marlow, N., Roberts, B. L., & Cooke, R. W. I. (1989). Motor skills in extremely low birth weight children at the age of 6 years. *Archives of Disease in Childhood, 64,* 839–847.

Mikkelsen, E. J., Brown, G. L., Minichiello, M. D., Millican, F. K., & Rappoport, J. L. (1982). Neurologic status in hyperactive, enuretic, encopretic, and normal boys. *Journal of the American Academy of Child Psychiatry, 21,* 75–81.

Missiuna, C. (1994). Motor skill acquisition in children with developmental coordination disorder. *Adapted Physical Activity Quarterly, 11,* 214–235.

Morrison, M. W., Gregory, R. J., & Paul, J. J. (1979). Reliability of the Finger Tapping Test and a note on sex differences. *Perceptual and Motor Skills, 48,* 139–142.

Nichols, P. L., & Chen, T. C. (1980). *Minimal brain dysfunction: A prospective study.* Hillsdale, NJ: Erlbaum.

Pitcher, T. M., Piek, J. P., & Hay, D. A. (2003). Fine and gross motor ability in males with ADHD. *Developmental Medicine and Child Neurology, 45,* 525–535.

Prechtl, H. F. R. (1977). *Neurological examination of the full-term newborn infant* (2nd ed.). London: Heinemann.

Prechtl, H. F. R. (1990). Qualitative changes of spontaneous movements in fetus and preterm infants are a marker of neurological dysfunction. *Early Human Development, 23,* 151–158.

Prechtl, H. F. R., Ferrari, F., & Cioni, G. (1993). Predictive value of general movements in asphyxiated fullterm infants. *Early Human Development, 35,* 91–120.

Prechtl, H. F. R., & Franzens, K. (2001). General movement assessment as a method of developmental neurology: New paradigms and their consequences. *Developmental Medicine and Child Neurology, 43,* 836–842.

Pryde, K. M. (2000). *Sensorimotor functioning in developmental coordination disorder: A kinematic and psychometric analysis.* Unpublished doctoral dissertation, University of Waterloo, Waterloo, Ontario, Canada.

Pryde, K. M., & Roy, E. A. (1998). Integrating vision and proprioception for manual aiming movements: A developmental study. *Journal of Sport and Exercise Psychology, 20,* s2.

Pryde, K. M., & Roy, E. A. (1999). Mechanism of developmental coordination disorder: Individual analyses and disparate findings. *Brain and Cognition, 40,* 230–234.

Reddon, J. R., Gill, D. M., Gauk, S. E., & Maerz, M. D. (1988). Purdue Pegboard: Test–retest estimates. *Perceptual and Motor Skills, 66,* 503–506.

Reitan, R. M. (1971a). Sensorimotor functions in brain-damaged and normal children of early school age. *Perceptual and Motor Skills, 33,* 655–664.

Reitan, R. M. (1971b). Trail making test results for normal and brain-damaged children. *Perceptual and Motor Skills, 33,* 575–581.

Rösblad, B., & von Hofsten, C. (1994). Repetitive goal-directed arm movements in children with developmental coordination disorders: Role of visual information. *Adapted Physical Activity Quarterly, 11,* 190–202.

Rourke, B. P., & Finlayson, M. A. J. (1978). Neuropsychological significance of variations in patterns of academic performance: Verbal and visual–spatial abilities. *Journal of Abnormal Child Psychology, 6,* 121–133.

Roy, E. A. (1990). The interface between normality and pathology in understanding movement control. In G. Reid (Ed.), *Advances in psychology: Vol. 47. Problems in movement control* (pp. 3–30). Amsterdam: North-Holland.

Roy, E. A. (1996). Hand preference, manual asymmetries and limb apraxia. In D. Elliott & E. A. Roy (Eds.), *Manual asymmetries in motor performance* (pp. 215–236) Boca Raton, FL: CRC Press.

Roy, E. A., Heath, M., Westwood, D., Schweizer, T. A., Dixon, M. J., Black, S. E., et al. (2000). Task demands in limb apraxia. *Brain and Cognition, 44,* 253–279.

Schellekens, J. M. H., Scholten, C. A., & Kalverboer, A. F. (1983). Visually guided hand movements in children with minor neurological dysfunction: Response time and movement organization. *Journal of Child Psychology and Psychiatry, 24,* 89–102.

Selz, M., & Reitan, R. M. (1979). Neuropsychological test performance of normal, learning disabled, and brain damaged older children. *Journal of Nervous and Mental Disease, 167,* 298–302.

Shafer, S. Q., Shafer, D., O'Conner, P. A., & Stokman, C. J. (1983). Hard thoughts on neurological "soft signs." In M. Rutter (Ed.), *Developmental neuropsychology* (pp. 133–143). New York: Guilford Press.

Smyth, M. M., & Mason, U. C. (1998). Use of proprioception in normal and clumsy children. *Developmental Medicine and Child Neurology, 40,* 672–681.

Smyth, T. R. (1991). Abnormal clumsiness in children: A defect of motor programming? *Child: Care, Health and Development, 17,* 283–294.

Smyth, T. R., & Glencross, D. J. (1988). Information processing deficits in clumsy children. *Australian Journal of Psychology, 38*, 13–22.

Spreen, O., & Strauss, E. (1991). *A compendium of neuropsychological tests: Administration, norms, and commentary*. New York: Oxford University Press.

Touwen, B. C. L. (1979). *Examination of the child with minor neurological dysfunction*. London: Spastics International Medical Publications.

Tramontana, M. G., & Hooper, S. R. (1988). Child neuropsychological assessment: Overview of current status. In M. G. Tramontana & S. R. Hooper (Eds.), *Assessment issues in child neuropsychology* (pp. 3–38). New York: Plenum Press.

van der Meulen, J. H. P., van der Gon, J. J. D., Gielen, C. C. A. M., Gooskens, R. H. J. M., & Willemse, J. (1991). Visuomotor performance of normal and clumsy children. I: Fast goal-directed arm-movements with and without visual feedback. *Developmental Medicine and Child Neurology, 33*, 40–54.

Vitiello, B., Ricciuti, A. J., Stoff, D. M., Behar, D., & Denckla, M. B. (1989). Reliability of subtle (soft) neurological signs in children. *Journal of the American Academy of Child and Adolescent Psychiatry, 28*, 749–753.

Weisglas-Kuperus, N., Baerts, W., Fetter, W. P. F., Hempel, M. S., Mulder, P. G. H., Touwen, B. C. L., et al. (1994). Minor neurological dysfunction and quality of movement in relation to neonatal cerebral damage and subsequent development. *Developmental Medicine and Child Neurology, 36*, 727–735.

Werry, J., & Aman, M. (1976). The reliability and diagnostic validity of the physical and neurological exam for soft signs (PANESS). *Journal of Autism and Childhood Schizophrenia, 6*, 253–262.

CHAPTER 4

Motor Proficiency Assessment Batteries

ANNA BARNETT
JUDITH PETERS

Assessment refers to the global process of synthesizing information about individuals in order to describe and better understand them. A variety of sources of information, both formal and informal, may be used to arrive at a description, including interviews, questionnaires, observation, or measurement. In this chapter, we focus primarily on formal measurement procedures using published assessment batteries.

A variety of motor disorders are examined throughout the chapters in this book. Some chapters discuss wide-ranging motor difficulties, whereas others focus on more specific problem areas, such as postural control or writing. There is also variation across and within the disorders described regarding severity of the condition, the nature of the difficulties experienced, and the impact it has on the child's day-to-day life. While there may be similar reasons for assessment, very different assessment tools are required to examine these disorders. What might be highly suitable for one condition will be totally inappropriate for another. For example, the assessment of a young child with cerebral palsy might involve traditional neurological measures of muscle tone and reflex activity together with an assessment of the child's ambulatory status and functional skills (see Roy, Bottos, Pryde, & Dewey, Chapter 3, this volume). However, there are many motor tasks that would be beyond the capability of a young child with severe cerebral palsy but would be appropriate to examine in children with conditions such as those described by Smith; Ahonen, Kooistra, Viholainen, & Cantell; and Wilson (in Chapters 7, 12, and 13, this volume, respectively). Children with developmental coordination disorder (DCD), for example achieve all the usual early motor milestones at some point in time but experience difficulty in learning more complex tasks such as skipping with a rope, catching a ball, or writing quickly and legibly. It is beyond the scope of this chapter to consider the full range of published instruments. Consequently, we have elected to concentrate on assessments designed for infants and those children who have developed basic movement skills (such as independent walking, reaching, and grasping) but who have difficulty learning more complex motor tasks. Before presenting reviews of some selected assessment tools, we first consider some general theoretical and practical issues concerning the assessment of motor proficiency. (For test reviews, see Appendices 4.1 to 4.13.)

THE PURPOSE OF ASSESSMENT

There are many reasons why an assessment of motor proficiency might be required. Although on occasion motor proficiency may be assessed by way of an isolated test at one point in time, it is usually more appropriate to consider assessment as an ongoing, cyclical process. Various stages within this process can be identified. For example, the starting point might be concern for a young child who is reluctant to join in physical play activities and appears socially isolated. In this case, an assessment of motor proficiency might be used to investigate whether or not motor difficulties play any role in the child's apparent problems and the extent and severity of any such problem. Sometimes pronounced difficulties can meet formal criteria, which may determine eligibility for extra support at school. Along with other relevant information, data from the motor assessment should lead to a specific plan of action for that child. Further assessment may be used to evaluate progress and achievement of goals and to plan further action. This example illustrates how the assessment of motor proficiency should be part of an ongoing process in the *identification, classification*, and *description* of motor difficulties, leading to the *planning and evaluation of intervention.*

THE PURPOSE OF A TEST

The reason for carrying out an assessment of motor proficiency needs to be carefully formulated. In making their choice of a suitable test, potential users need first to consider the purpose for which individual tests have been designed by consulting the formal statements of purpose made by test authors. We suggest that potential users familiarize themselves with five additional aspects of a test. These are (1) the professional background of the test author(s), (2) the terms used to describe the test and its components, (3) the range and nature of test items, (4) the way in which performance is measured, and (5) the extent to which nonmotor factors are considered in the assessment. Consideration of these five aspects will help the person carrying out the assessment establish the structure and purpose of a test and assist in determining if the test meets one's needs. Each of these aspects is discussed briefly here.

Professional Background

Professionals involved in developing tests of motor proficiency come from a variety of backgrounds, including occupational therapy, physiotherapy, special education, adapted physical activity, psychology, kinesiology, and medicine. Although personnel from these disciplines have an overlapping knowledge base and share many common interests, the training and focus of each is rather different. Potential test users need to be aware of the heterogeneous theoretical perspectives of these professional groups in order to understand the nature of the construct they set out to measure.

Terminology

Titles of assessment batteries reveal that a variety of terms are used to refer to the behavior that is being measured. Some tests use the term *movement* (e.g., the Movement Assessment Battery for Children [Movement ABC]; Henderson & Sugden, 1992), while others use the term *motor* (e.g., Bruininks–Oseretsky Test of Motor Proficiency [BOTMP], Bruininks, 1978; Test of Gross Motor Development—Second Edition [TGMD-2], Ulrich, 2000; Peabody Developmental Motor Scales—Second Edition [PDMS-2], Folio & Fewell, 2000). *Movement* refers to external, observable changes in body position, while the term *motor* usually refers to internal neuromuscular processes (Keogh & Sugden, 1985). The latter is sometimes preferred as we are concerned not only with the control of movement but also with the control of stabilization of the body, which is not always directly observable (Rosenbaum, 1991). In the assessment arena, however, the terms *motor* and *movement* often seem to be used interchangeably.

The interdependency of motor control and perceptual systems is widely acknowledged (Schmidt & Lee, 1999). However, it is clear that some of the tests make greater demands on the perceptual systems than others and this is directly reflected in their titles, for example, the Beery–Buktenica Developmental Test of Visual–Motor Integration Revised Fourth Edition (VMI-4; Beery, 1997) and the Sensory Integration and Praxis Tests (SIPT; Ayres, 1989). In the former, an attempt is made to assess perceptual and motor control skills separately; in the latter, the authors include overall planning and sequencing of actions. This higher-order skill is often referred to as praxis, although it is not uniformly defined in the literature.

Two other terms that have recently received much attention in the literature are *ability* and *skill*. An examination of recent textbooks indicates general agreement on the different constructs represented by these terms (Burton & Miller, 1998; Schmidt & Lee, 1999). Briefly, *ability* refers to the general capacity of an individual presumed to underlie performance on certain tasks, which is considered to remain relatively stable across an individual's lifetime. In contrast, *skill* refers to the capability to achieve a specific goal with maximum certainty, minimum energy, or minimum time, developed as a result of practice. Burton and Rodgerson (2001) report several inconsistencies in the way that these concepts have been applied in assessment tools.

Test manuals often use terms without accompanying definitions, making it difficult to appreciate the exact nature of the construct that tests are designed to measure and whether or not these are equivalent across different tools. If the terminology used does not clearly define the constructs, one needs to consider how they have been operationalized by consideration of tasks included in the test and how they are categorized.

Test Content

In our test reviews, the number of individual motor tasks on which a child's performance is measured varies enormously. Some tests allow for performance on each task to be considered separately. Most tests group tasks together into two or more subsections and consider the level of performance in each. The tasks included in a subsection are selected according to some criteria relating to categories of tasks. Inspection of the subsections included in our reviewed tests indicates variation in their number, the ways in which tasks have been categorized, and the labels assigned to these categories. This makes a comparison of tests very difficult and close scrutiny of the test manuals is required to appreciate fully the test content and nature of the items included.

Many of the tests reviewed here include tasks that involve balance and body transport in subsections labeled *gross motor* or *locomotor*. Most also include various tasks involving object manipulation in subsections receiving labels such as *fine motor, manual dexterity, upper limb speed and dexterity,* and *grasping*. Some tests have a separate subsection for tasks involving the reception and/or projection of a ball or other object, which may be referred to as ball skill or object control. Other subsections in tests include very specific categories of tasks, such as drawing, as well as broader categories concerned with the planning and organization elements of performance. In only one of the tests reviewed, the tasks are categorized according to the environmental context in which they are performed (Movement ABC Checklist; Henderson & Sugden, 1992).

The tasks selected for each subsection are judged by the test developers to represent distinct categories, a view that is sometimes supported by statistical methods such as factor analyses. In some tests, performance is also considered across all the tasks or subsections in terms of a single global measure or composite score. Burton and Rodgerson (2001) recommend that these global scores be considered to represent performance of the individual tasks tested rather than "performer attributes or abilities, which implicitly represent skills not even tested" (p. 357). In the same way that global IQ scores are debated, the meaning and use of composite scores is debated in the motor area.

Measurement Issues

Another aspect of a test that may illuminate the nature of the construct being measured relates to the way in which performance is assessed on individual tasks. Most of the tests we have reviewed use an *outcome* measure of speed or accuracy (e.g., time taken to complete a task, number of successful trials completed, or number of errors made). These provide an indication of how well a child completes a task, specified in terms of measures that are quantifiable and lend themselves to comparison with normative data. However, we have also included tests that focus on the nature or *quality* of performance (e.g., the Toddler and Infant Motor Evaluation [TIME], Miller & Roid, 1994; TGMD-2, Ulrich, 2000). Performance is assessed in relation to specified criteria, such as whether or not there is hip rotation and weight transference in ball throwing, rather than the distance thrown or whether a target is hit. Information on the nature of task performance and therefore a description of the difficulties that children encounter can be most valuable in planning instruction. Perhaps most useful is an approach that combines an analysis of the movement process with reference to outcome, or task achievement. Several tests attempt to combine these two types of information by encouraging the recording of descriptive data on task performance in a less formal way to complement strict measurements of performance outcome (Folio & Fewell, 2000; Henderson & Sugden, 1992; Miller, 1988).

Consideration of Nonmotor Factors

The now popular ecological perspective to the study of motor development stresses the relationship between the individual, the environment, and the task (Haywood & Getchell, 2001). One of the fundamental assumptions of dynamic systems theory is that individuals are composed of many complex, cooperative systems (Thelen & Spencer, 1998) that together are responsible for motor control. These include both motor and nonmotor factors, any one of which can facilitate or limit performance on a particular task. Burton and Miller (1998) refer to these as movement skill foundations and describe them as "all aspects of a person—physical, mental, and emotional" (p. 131). To interpret a child's performance on a motor test it is important to understand how their unique characteristics affect the child's behavior. It is well established that many children with motor disorders have concomitant perceptual, cognitive, social, emotional, behavioral, attentional, language, and other problems (Dewey, Crawford, Wilson, & Kaplan, Chapter 18, this volume; Frampton, Yude, & Goodman, 1998; Kaplan, Wilson, Dewey, & Crawford, 1998; Powell & Bishop, 1992), any one of which may influence performance on a motor task. Some tests allow the examiner flexibility to help a child display his or her optimal performance (e.g., by repeating instructions or describing a task in a different way rather than having to read instructions verbatim). Some tests also encourage the recording of nonmotor factors that are considered to influence performance (e.g., the Bayley Scales of Infant Development: Second Edition [BSID-II], Bayley, 1993; Miller Assessment for Preschoolers [MAP], Miller, 1988; Movement ABC Test and Checklist, Henderson & Sugden, 1992).

Tests designed to be used in infancy usually assess motor proficiency alongside other domains, such as cognitive, social, and language development (e.g., see our review of the Griffiths Mental Development Scales [GMDS; Griffiths & Huntley, 1996] and the BSID-II [Bayley, 1993]). This allows for the level of motor proficiency to be interpreted in a wider context and may have important implications for the understanding and management of the child's motor difficulties. Tests designed for older children, however, are usually concerned with a single domain of development and tend to be used by specialists in that field. Ideally, the results of a motor assessment should not be interpreted in isolation but in relation to a child's development in other domains. For the motor development specialist this can be achieved through collaboration with colleagues from different disciplines who are experienced in the assessment of development in other areas.

Environmental factors (both physical and sociocultural), as well as individual factors, may restrict or facilitate a child's performance. Most tests have standardized procedures for presenting the tasks and their manuals state the importance of testing in a quiet, distraction-free room that has adequate heating, lighting, ventilation, and so on. One of our reviewed tests invites users to record the testing conditions and the extent to which they are considered to interfere with the child's performance (the TGMD-2; Ulrich, 2000). In another it is suggested that performance on the same tasks might be systematically assessed in different contexts (Movement ABC Checklist; Henderson & Sugden, 1992). The effect of sociocultural factors on test performance is sometimes examined during the development phase of a test, with norms being compared from different sociocultural groups (e.g., see the TGMD-2; Ulrich, 2000). Another strategy used to investigate such factors is the careful comparison of performance on an established test of children from different socioeconomic or cultural groups (e.g., see developments of the Movement ABC Test; Henderson & Sugden, 1992).

PRACTICAL CONSIDERATIONS

In addition to considering the purpose for which individual tests have been designed, potential users must also consider several practical issues when choosing a test. Some of these are outlined next.

Experience Required

Carefully check in advance whether a test requires specialist qualifications or formal training or is restricted to certain professional groups (e.g., the SIPT; Ayres, 1989). Most tests specify that administrators should be familiar with the test procedures and materials and have experience of working with children with and without difficulties. To interpret the results of tests, sound knowledge and understanding of measurement concepts are essential and further qualification may be required.

Equipment

The test manual, record forms, and materials should be examined to ensure that they are suitable for one's needs, considering their format, length, content, and user-friendliness. Users should also carefully consider the range and type of materials needed to administer a test. The size and weight of the kit plus any extra materials required must be manageable if the test is to be carried regularly between sites. The space needed for testing should also be noted. Appropriately sized furniture should be provided for any items that involve tabletop activities. Items involving running, jumping, hopping, and so on demand considerable floor space, often with special floor markings or nonslip surfaces. Similarly, open space and/or a smooth wall may be needed for throwing and catching items. Standardized procedures may apply to the testing environment. Particularly when space is at a premium in the clinic or school setting, the test administrator will need to pay some attention to the selection of a suitable area that is free of furniture where he or she can work safely with the child. Many test manuals also specify the type of clothing, especially shoes, that the child should wear.

All the equipment needed for administration may or may not be included in the test kit. It is important that any items supplied or replaced by the test administrator comply with the specifications set out in the manual. The availability of replacement items when they become worn or broken should also be considered. Test users need to be confident that the test materials are appropriate for the children being tested, in relation to the child's age, cultural background, and so forth. A test must be appealing and motivating to a child and it must also meet local health and safety standards.

Administration Time

Some tests can be completed in a very short time (a few minutes) while others are lengthy (taking over 2 hours). The test administrator needs to select a test that will provide sufficient valid information for the purpose of the assessment within the time available. One needs to weigh the relevance of each part of the test for a particular child against how long he or she might take to complete it. A child with coordination or attention difficulties will take longer to complete tasks than a well-coordinated child and might need additional trials to pass items. On occasion administration of certain items will be inappropriate and therefore excluded (e.g., if a child has severe hemiplegia).

MEASUREMENT PRINCIPLES AND PSYCHOMETRIC PROPERTIES

For appropriate test selection, knowledge of basic measurement concepts is essential. Only then can one understand the principles behind construction and scoring, make responsible judgments about the usefulness of tests, and interpret results appropriately. Many texts provide detailed descriptions of the important measurement principles (for reviews, see Burton & Miller, 1998; Thomas & Nelson, 1996).

Norms

When using a norm-referenced test, the child's performance is compared to that of a "normative" (or "reference") group. When considering the use of this type of test, it is important to examine the appropriateness of the normative sample for the children being tested. Characteristics of the normative sample in terms of ethnicity, cultural background, socioeconomic status, and geographical location should be noted, as should the age of the children, the number of boys and girls, and the date of data collection. Many test developers use national census data to select and carefully match the normative sample to a given population. However, if there is any doubt about the suitability of the published test norms, users should seriously consider collecting their own normative data. In our reviews, we outline the composition of the normative sample for the various tests and also note who examined the children in the collection of normative data.

Raw scores of children in the normative sample are collected to establish the usual pattern and range of performance in a defined population. These data are then used as a standard against which the performance of other children is measured. To compare a child's performance to that of the normative group, performance scores are usually converted into relative scores, such as standardized scores or percentiles. This may be at the level of individual items of the test and/or composite scores. Tests that encompass the entire range of performance have sometimes been treated as equivalent to a standard intelligence test and the composite score as the motor equivalent of an IQ (intelligence quotient). Other tests do not span the entire range of performance and focus on the identification only of those children experiencing difficulties (e.g., the MAP; Miller, 1988).

An alternative to norm-referencing is to use criterion-referenced tests. In this case the child's performance is compared to some predetermined criterion, indicating what the child can and cannot do (e.g., Clinical Observation of Motor and Postural Skills [COMPS]; Wilson, Pollock, Kaplan, & Law, 1994).

Scoring

The test administrator needs to be clear about the type of scores yielded, whether and how they are converted, and how they may be interpreted. Some tests involve very simple procedures, such as the summing of raw scores and comparison to a single cut off point (e.g., Developmental Coordination Disorder Questionnaire [DCDQ], Wilson, Kaplan, Crawford, Campbell, & Dewey, 2000; Movement ABC Checklist, Henderson & Sugden, 1992). In other tests the procedure is much more complex, involving the weighting of items and use of tables to convert scores several times (e.g., BOTMP, Bruininks, 1978; COMPS, Wilson et al., 1994).

To make performance data meaningful, raw scores are usually converted into numbers that provide comparison to the normative sample. Commonly, raw scores are expressed in terms of the number of standard deviation units (Z-scores) that lie above or below the mean. In most tests these are transformed to "standard" scores, with arbitrary numbers chosen as the mean and standard deviation. For composite scores, a mean of 100 and a standard deviation of 15 are usually chosen (e.g., BSID-II, Bayley, 1993; BOTMP, Bruininks, 1978; TGMD-2, Ulrich, 2000; VMI-4, Beery, 1997). Subtest scores may have a mean of 15 and a standard deviation of 5 (e.g., the BOTMP, Bruininks, 1978) or a mean of 10 and a standard deviation of 3 (e.g., TIME, Miller & Roid, 1994; TGMD-2, Ulrich, 2000). In some tests, scores are converted to percentiles. These represent the percentage of scores that fall below or are equal to a particular score and are often used to specify cutoff points, or scores that are considered to designate the point of motor impairment (e.g., the 5th, 10th, or 15th percentile point). Some tests, including the TIME (Miller & Roid, 1994) and VMI-4 (Beery, 1997), express data as stanines (short for "standard nine"). Here raw scores are first converted to percentiles, then according to the corresponding Z-score range, assigned a value from 1 to 9 (with a mean of 5 and a standard deviation of 1.96).

Reliability

Reliability refers to the consistency or repeatability of a measure. A reliable test will yield more or less the same scores across time and across different examiners. Test users need to know how much variability can be expected from a test and should decide whether that amount of variability is acceptable for their purpose. In addition to noting overall reliability statistics reported, one should also determine the population on which these aspects of the test were examined and the methods used. In our review of the tests we note whether three aspects of reliability have been reported in the test manuals. First, we report on the *internal consistency* of scores within a test, showing the extent to which the items reflect one basic dimension. Second, we consider the *stability* of the test between different performances separated in time (measured by the test–retest method). Third, we consider the *objectivity* of tests by reporting the extent to which different testers obtain the same score on the same children (referred to as intertester or interrater reliability). Given the reliability coefficients of a test (which may be obtained in various ways), users need to evaluate the extent to which they allow them to use a test with confidence. One helpful concept, which is noted in our reviews, is the standard error of measurement (SEM). This expresses variation in terms of a standard deviation and estimates the range of scores within which an obtained score might actually fall when using a test with a certain reliability coefficient value. Further information is described in detail in books devoted to research methods and statistics (e.g., Howell, 1992).

Validity

Validity of measurement indicates the degree to which a test does what it is supposed to do. This is difficult to demonstrate, as it is a relative rather than an absolute concept. A test's validity will vary according to the purpose for which the results are being used and the types of individuals tested. It is widely agreed that test developers should provide evidence of different types of validity including *content relevance, criterion related*, and *construct identification*. Different terms are sometimes employed to refer to these concepts, and they can be examined in a variety of ways.

The content relevance of a test concerns whether the measure obviously reflects the meaningful elements of the construct being measured. Although it is not possible to supply statistical evidence for this, it can be judged by consulting relevant literature and experts in the field. Criterion-related validity concerns the degree to which scores on a test are related to some recognized standard or criterion. Most commonly this involves a test being correlated with some criterion that is administered at about the same time (i.e., concurrently) and is thus referred to as concurrent validity. Popular criterion measures include tests that have already been widely used (such as the BOTMP, Bruininks, 1978), but judge's ratings may also serve as criterion measures. When the criterion measure is some later behavior that is predicted by performance on the test, it is referred to as predictive validity.

The third type of validity commonly reported relates to construct identification, or the degree to which the test measures the hypothetical construct of concern. In our reviews we note whether any of the following three methods have been reported in the test manuals: (1) factor-*analytic* methods to determine how many factors (or dimensions) are included within a construct, and which tasks best represent those factors; (2) a known *group-difference* method, in which the test scores of groups that should differ on the behaviour being measured are compared; and (3) *age-difference* methods, which demonstrate the relationship of age to performance on the test.

The accumulation of evidence for a test's reliability and validity is an ongoing process. Users need to examine the contents of a test manual in the first instance but should also consult other published material describing ways in which clinicians and researchers have gained extra information about the test. In addition, when working over time with a particular test, users can accumulate their own body of data.

TEST REVIEWS

Our reviews (Appendices 4.1–4.13 [pages 84–109]) consider a selection of assessment instruments that can loosely be described as tests of motor proficiency. We have included instruments that represent a range of perspectives, designed for different purposes and for children of different ages. Broadly speaking, the instruments fall into four groups. Those included in the first group are designed for infants and young children. They assess motor proficiency alongside other developmental domains, such as cognition or language and social skills. Our reviews focus primarily on those parts of the tests that assess motor skill, although it is not recommended to use these in isolation. In this section we include the GMDS (Griffiths & Huntley, 1996), the BSID-II (Bayley, 1993), and the MAP (Miller, 1988). The GMDS can be used from birth, the BSID-II from 1 month and the MAP from 2 years (see Appendices 4.1, 4.2, and 4.3).

Tests included in our second group focus on the motor domain, and include instruments designed for infants and older children (up to the age of 14 years). Here we have reviewed the PDMS-2 (Folio & Fewell, 2000), the TIME (Miller & Roid, 1994), the TGMD-2 (Ulrich, 2000), the Movement ABC Test (Henderson & Sugden, 1992), and the BOTMP (Bruininks, 1978) (see Appendices 4.4, 4.5, 4.6, 4.7, and 4.8). The third group contains two observational checklists to be completed by teachers and/or caregivers: the Movement ABC checklist (Henderson & Sugden, 1992) and the DCDQ (Wilson, Kaplan, Crawford, Campbell, & Dewey, 2000) (see Appendices 4.9 and 4.10). The fourth group contains tests that focus on specific areas of motor proficiency. Here we have included the VMI-4 (Beery, 1997), the SIPT (Ayres, 1989), and the COMPS (Wilson et al., 1994) (see Appendices 4.11, 4.12, and 4.13).

The format of each review is identical. Each provides information on the purpose of the test (as stated in the manual), the professional background of the test author(s), and a note on the development of the test, indicating previous editions where applicable. The level of experience and the time required to administer the test are then provided, as well as comments on the test equipment. This is followed by an outline of the test structure, content and administration, and scoring procedures. The composition of the normative sample is noted. We also indicate whether certain aspects of reliability and validity are reported in the test manual. An indication of the countries in which the tests are most used is given if available and any translations of the manuals into languages other than English are recorded. Current developments of the test are also noted. Each review ends with our general comments on the limitations and strengths of the test.

FUTURE ISSUES

We now consider some issues that might influence future test use and development.

Increasing Demands for Formal Assessment

Increasing demands are being placed on those working in health and education sectors by government legislation, professional codes of practice, and insurance companies to account for their service delivery (NHS Centre, 1999; Sackett, Straus, Richardson, Rosenberg, & Haynes, 2000). There is increasing demand for standardized, norm-referenced assessment procedures and increasing responsibility of test users to produce information that is reliable and meaningful. It is important to recognize that staff members will need considerable training and support to enable them to select appropriate assessment tools, administer and score items, interpret results, and communicate these results effectively to all stakeholders.

Increasing Recognition of the Importance of Motor Development

The topic of motor development has extended beyond the medical domain and now receives much broader attention. There is increasing recognition in psychology and education of the importance of the development of motor skill. Alongside interest in the typical and atypical development of motor skills, there is growing focus on the relationship with development in cognitive, social, emotional, and other domains. This increased awareness, together with recognition that developmental disorders of movement, reading, attention, and so forth, commonly co-occur, means that more and more, motor proficiency batteries are becoming part of general neuropsychological and developmental assessments. Instruments such as those reviewed in this chapter are increasingly administered alongside tests of cognitive function in order to obtain a comprehensive picture of a child's development. The inclusion of a reliable and valid assessment of motor proficiency provides a more holistic understanding of the child's profile of performance and may assist in planning intervention programs.

The Application of New Approaches

In this chapter, we have made reference to the ecological perspective on the development of motor proficiency and, more specifically, to the increasingly popular dynamic systems approach. This reference stresses the dynamic interrelationship between factors concerned with the individual, the environment, and the task (Kamm, Thelen, & Jensen, 1990). No motor proficiency assessment batteries have yet been developed entirely around dynamic systems principles, although some do contain elements of this approach.

Frequently the tasks or movement patterns performed by the child at assessment are rigidly specified. However, some tests also include suggestions for clinical exploration with less formal procedures. These range from the innovative notion of using parents as partners during test administration (Miller & Roid, 1994) to encouragement of the test administrator to use "expert scaffolding" to develop and adapt the test tasks (Henderson & Sugden, 1992, p. 118). This general approach is formalized and referred to by others as Ecological Task Analysis (Burton & Davis, 1996; Davis & Burton, 1991). This first involves the identification of the movement skill and skill patterns for a particular functional task (e.g., walking along a line). Then the effect of systematic changes to task, performer, and environment variables (e.g., widening the line, holding the child's hand, and giving praise for effort) are examined. The changes being made and their effect on performance are formally recorded to reveal the precise set of conditions under which the individual can complete a task (for an example, see Burton & Miller, 1998, p. 313).

This approach to assessment can incorporate the measurement of performance in relation to normative data but also has the advantage of going beyond this to explore broader aspects of the child's skills and the contextual factors that influence performance. Extended exploration of this type begins the process of instruction and can yield rich information for future planning.

A Focus on Function

Many now recognize the importance of assessing everyday life motor skills that allow a child to function at home, at school, and at play. Standardized measures of motor proficiency have been criticized for poor ecological validity. Assessment of performance areas that do not reflect daily play activity may force clinicians to seek their own supplementary checklists of activities of daily living (ADL). We have reviewed two formal observation checklists in which parents and/or teachers assess motor skills within the context of the home and school environment. Watkinson and colleagues (2001) employed another technique and examined the use of a self-report measure to determine the frequency with which children in a specific context normally engage in various everyday playground activities. Limited space here has prevented inclusion of several tests that focus specifically on functional aspects of performance (e.g., the Pediatric Evaluation of Disability Inventory, Haley, Coster, Ludlow, Haltiwanger, & Andrellos, 1992; the Gross Motor Function Measure, Russell, Rosenbaum, Avery, & Lane, 2002; the Gross Motor Performance Measure, Boyce et al., 1995; the Assessment of Motor and Process Skills, Fisher, 2003; and broader Quality of Life Measures, Eiser & Morse, 2001). Such tests, however, may be a useful adjunct to standardized measures of motor proficiency.

The Influence of Technological Advances

Recent advances in technology have produced new methods for quantifying and describing quality of movement that are now regularly applied in both research and clinical settings. The increased use of digital video recording allows for performance to be viewed repeatedly and at various speeds, enabling detailed and accurate observations to be noted and analyzed. Sophisticated movement analysis systems are available that can digitize the position of joints, limbs, and other body parts in two or three dimensions (see Roy et al., Chapter 3, this volume, for a more detailed discussion). Calculations of distance, time, velocity, and acceleration are automatically computed, allowing for a very detailed analysis and description of movement. This technology has been used extensively in the analysis of gait patterns (Gage & Koop, 1995) and reaching and grasping (Rösblad & von Hofsten, 1994; Sugden & Utley, 1995). Drawing and writing have also been analyzed by digitizing the position of the pen using a graphics tablet (e.g., Smits-Engelsman, Niemeijer, & van Galen, 2001; Tucha & Lange, 2001). Force transducers are sometimes used alongside motion analysis techniques to measure changes in the amount of force exerted by particular body parts. They can be placed under the feet in the study of balance and gait (Browne & O'Hare, 2000) and between the thumb and fingers to examine grip (Hill & Wing, 1998). These sophisticated technologies quantify movement patterns and evaluate progress but may provide little information about functional performance.

Other emerging technologies, such as virtual reality systems, can simulate three-dimensional environments. These have been used in the laboratory to explore the use of visual information in the control of movement (Wann, Mon-Williams, McIntosh, Smyth, & Milner, 2001) and although regularly used for skill training in certain careers (e.g., pilots and drivers), their value in the therapeutic environment is only just emerging. Currently, costs prohibit more general use; however, in the future this technology may offer affordable applications to assessment.

Advances in technology have led to innovative approaches to assessment at a distance (Elford et al., 2000) and new ways of managing data. Computer software is used in the scoring, analysis, and reporting for some tests (e.g., the SIPT; Ayres, 1989). Although scoring time and errors may be reduced, computer programs cannot replace some aspects of assessment. Expert knowledge will always be required for the valid interpretation of results.

The Impact of Ethical and Legal Reviews

New human rights laws have an impact on the assessment process and test users will need to carefully consider issues concerning informed consent (from the caregiver and the child) when administering a test. In the context of current child abuse issues, sensitivity is needed to ensure that caregivers and children are aware of the degree of undressing and handling that may be involved for test administration. The tester must take care to avoid any situation that might be open to criticism. New data protection laws including patient data and accessibility of patient records need to be considered. Changes in health and safety legislation must also be taken into account when using tests of motor proficiency. These affect a range of issues, including the type of materials and manipulables that are used, how they are cleaned, and the lifting and handling of heavy assessment kits (Mandelstam, 2001).

The Assessment of Different Populations

The use of tests of motor proficiency with populations of children that differ in some way from those on which a test was standardized and normed is a further important issue. Most assessment batteries of motor proficiency have been developed in North America, Australasia, or Europe, yet there is growing demand for their use worldwide. Recent studies suggest that although some test items are appropriate for children from different cultures, others are culture-dependent, with very different norms (Chow, Barnett, & Henderson, 2001; Miyahara et al., 1998). If tests are to be used outside the culture in which they were developed, the appropriateness of test items and norms must be examined prior to their use in clinical settings.

Even within the same cultural setting, there may be populations that are not represented in the original normative data of a test. Normative samples often include only a very small number or totally exclude children with obvious sensory or physical impairments. However, there may well be a particular need to assess the motor proficiency of children from these populations. Test items may be appropriate if modifications are made to the way in which instructions and demonstrations are provided (e.g., adaptation for sign language and simplifying directions) and while some tests allow for such flexibility, others have strict rules for administration. Some test items will obviously be inappropriate for such populations and will need to be either modified or excluded all together. Any deviations from the normal test procedure and scoring must be recorded and the results interpreted with caution. The formal adaptation of existing test items and the collection of normative data for children with specific impairments are only just beginning to be considered.

CONCLUDING REMARKS

The proliferation of motor assessment batteries may lead one to question why there cannot be one agreed measure of motor proficiency. However, when we consider the vast range of motor skills, the number of different disciplines concerned with motor development, and their diverse reasons for undertaking assessment in this area, it soon becomes obvious why this could never be the case. The large number of published tests may make choice bewildering but also provide opportunity to closely match an instrument to one's needs. There are many reports describing the value of using two or more instruments in a stepwise procedure—for example, to identify children with motor difficulties (Wright & Sugden, 1996). The relationship between different assessment batteries also continues to help inform test users about the extent to which different tests appear to measure the same or different skills (e.g., Crawford, Wilson, & Dewey, 2001). Often a combination of different test batteries is found to yield the most useful information about a range of skills that make up a child's motor proficiency (e.g., Jongmans, Mercuri, Dubowitz, & Henderson, 1998).

At the beginning of this chapter, we outlined some of the different purposes of assessment. The purpose of any assessment that is undertaken needs to be clearly formulated in order that an appropriate instrument is selected, as the selection of the instrument drives the whole assessment process.

REFERENCES

American Psychiatric Association. (1994). *Diagnostic and statistical manual of mental disorders* (4th ed.). Washington, DC: Author.

Ayres, A. J. (1962). *The Ayres Space Test.* Los Angeles: Western Psychological Services.

Ayres, A. J. (1964). *Southern California Motor Accuracy Test.* Los Angeles: Western Psychological Services.

Ayres, A. J. (1968). *Southern California Perceptual–Motor Tests.* Los Angeles: Western Psychological Services.

Ayres, A. J. (1972). *Southern California Sensory Integration Tests.* Los Angeles: Western Psychological Services.

Ayres, A. J. (1989). *Sensory Integration and Praxis Tests.* Los Angeles: Western Psychological Services.

Bayley, N. (1936). *California Infant Scale of Mental Development.* Berkeley: University of California Press.

Bayley, N. (1969). *Bayley Scales of Infant Development.* New York: Psychological Corp.

Bayley, N. (1993). *Bayley Scales of Infant Development* (2nd ed.). San Antonio, TX: Therapy Skill Builders.

Bayley, N. (2001). *Bayley Scale of Infant Development. Second Edition. Motor Scale Kit.* New York: Psychological Corp.

Beery, K. E. (1967). *The Developmental Test of Visual–Motor Integration.* Cleveland, OH: Modern Curriculum Press.

Beery, K. E. (1997). *The Beery–Buktenica Test of Visual–Motor Integration with supplemental Developmental Tests of Visual Perception and Motor Coordination.* Parippany, NJ: Modern Curriculum Press.

Boyce, W., Gowland, C., Rosenbaum, P., Lane, M., Plews, N., Goldsmith, C., et al. (1995). The

Gross Motor Performance Measure: Validity and responsiveness of a measure of quality of movement. *Physical Therapy, 75,* 603–613.

Browne, J., & O'Hare, N. (2000). A quality control procedure for force platforms. *Physiological Measurement, 21,* 515–524.

Bruininks, R. H. (1978). *Bruininks–Oseretsky Test of Motor Proficiency examiner's manual.* Circle Pines, MN: American Guidance Service.

Burton, A. W., & Davis, W. E. (1996). Ecological task analysis: Theoretical and empirical foundations. *Human Movement Science, 15,* 285–314.

Burton, A. W., & Miller, D. E. (1998). *Movement skill assessment.* Champaign, IL: Human Kinetics.

Burton, A. W., & Rodgerson, R. W. (2001). New perspectives on the assessment of movement skills and motor abilities. *Adapted Physical Activity Quarterly, 18,* 347–365.

Chow, S., Barnett, A. L., & Henderson, S. E. (2001). The Movement Assessment Battery for Children: A comparison of 4-year-old to 6-year-old children from Hong Kong and the United States. *American Journal of Occupational Therapy, 55,* 55–61.

Crawford, S. G., Wilson, B. N., & Dewey, D. (2001). Identifying developmental coordination disorder: Consistency between tests. *Physical and Occupational Therapy in Pediatrics, 20,* 29–50.

Croce, R. V., Horvat, M., & McCarthy, E. (2001). Reliability and concurrent validity of the Movement Assessment Battery for Children. *Perceptual and Motor Skills, 93,* 275–280.

Crowe, T. K. (1989). Pediatric assessments: A survey of their use by occupational therapists in northwestern school systems. *Occupational Therapy Journal of Research, 9,* 273–286.

Davis, W. E., & Burton, A. (1991). Ecological task analysis: Translating movement behavior theory into practice. *Adapted Physical Activity Quarterly, 8,* 154–177.

Doll, E. A. (Ed.). (1946). *The Oseretsky Tests of Motor Proficiency: A translation from the Portuguese translation.* Circle Pines, MN: American Guidance Service.

Eiser, C., & Morse, R. (2001). A review of measures of quality of life for children with chronic illness. *Archives of Disease in Childhood, 84,* 205–211.

Elford, R., White, H., Bowering, R., Ghandi, A., Maddiggan, B., St. John, K., et al. (2000). A randomized, controlled trial of child psychiatric assessments conducted using videoconferencing. *Journal of Telemedicine and Telecare, 6,* 73–82.

Fisher, A. G. (2003). *Assessment of motor and process skills* (5th ed.). Fort Collins, CO: Three Star Press.

Folio, M., & Fewell, R. (1983). *Peabody Developmental Motor Scales. Second edition.* Austin, TX: Pro-Ed.

Folio, M. R., & Fewell, R. R. (2000). *Peabody Developmental Motor Scales. Second edition.* Austin, TX: Pro-Ed.

Frampton, I., Yude, C., & Goodman, R. (1998). The prevalence and correlates of specific learning difficulties in a representative sample of children with hemiplegia. *British Journal of Educational Psychology, 68,* 39–51.

Gage, J. R., & Koop, S. E. (1995). Clinical gait analysis: Application to management of cerebral palsy. In P. Allard, I. A. F. Stokes, & J. P. Blanchi (Eds.), *Three dimensional analysis of human movement* (pp. 349–362). Champaign, IL: Human Kinetics.

Geuze, R. H., Jongmans, M. J., Schomaker, M. M., & Smits-Engelsman, B. C. M. (2001). Clinical and research diagnostic criteria for developmental coordination disorder: A review and discussion. *Human Movement Science, 20,* 7–47.

Griffiths, R. (1984). *The abilities of young children.* High Wycombe, UK: ARICD.

Griffiths, R. (1986). *The abilities of babies.* New York: McGraw-Hill.

Griffiths, R., & Huntley, M. (1996). *The Griffiths Mental Development Scales from birth to 2 years. The 1996 Revision.* High Wycombe, UK: ARICD.

Haley, S. M., Coster, W. J., Ludlow, L. H., Haltiwanger, J., & Andrellos, P. J. (1992). *Pediatric Evaluation of Disability Inventory*. Boston: New England Medical Center Hospitals.

Hattie, J., & Edwards, H. (1987). A review of the Bruininks–Oseretsky Test of Motor Proficiency. *British Journal of Educational Psychology, 57*, 104–113.

Haywood, K., & Getchell, N. (2001). *Life span motor development*. Champaign, IL: Human Kinetics.

Henderson, S. E., & Barnett, A. L. (2001) *Assessment of motor competence in the teenage years: Revision of age band 4 of the Movement ABC*. Paper presented at the conference proceedings of the 13th International Symposium for Adapted Physical Activity, Vienna, Austria.

Henderson, S. E., & Sugden, D. A. (1992). *Movement Assessment Battery for Children*. New York: Psychological Corp.

Hickey, A., Froude, E. H., Williams, A., Hart, T., & Summers, J. (2001). Performance of Australian children on the Miller Assessment for Preschoolers compared to USA norms. *Australian Journal of Occupational Therapy, 47*, 86–94.

Hill, E., & Wing, A. (1998). Developmental disorders and the use of grip force to compensate for inertial forces during voluntary movement. In K. J. Connolly (Ed.), *The psychobiology of the hand* (pp. 199–212). London: MacKeith Press.

Howell, D. C. (1992). *Statistical methods for psychology* (3rd ed.). Belmont, CA: Duxbury Press.

Jongmans, M. J. (1993). *Perceptuo-motor competence in prematurely born children at school age: Neurological and psychological aspects*. Unpublished doctoral thesis, Institute of Education, University of London.

Jongmans, M., Mercuri, E., Dubowitz, L., & Henderson, S. (1998). Perceptual–motor difficulties and their concomitants in six-year-old children born prematurely. *Human Movement Science, 17*, 629–653.

Kamm, K., Thelen, E., & Jensen, J. L. (1990). A dynamical systems approach to motor development. *Physical Therapy, 70*, 763–75.

Kaplan, B., Wilson, B., Dewey, D., & Crawford, S. (1998). DCD may not be a discrete disorder. *Human Movement Science, 17*, 471–490.

Keogh, J., & Sugden, D. (1985). *Movement skill development*. New York: Macmillan.

Lawlor, M. C., & Henderson, A. (1989). A descriptive study of the clinical practice patterns of occupational therapists working with infants and young children. *American Journal of Occupational Therapy, 43*, 755–764.

Mandelstam, M. (2001). Safe use of disability equipment and manual handling: Legal aspects—Part 2, manual handling. *British Journal of Occupational Therapy, 64*, 73–80.

Miller, L. (1988). *Miller Assessment for Preschoolers*. San Antonio, TX: Therapy Skill Builders.

Miller, L. J. (1993). *FirstSTEP: Screening test for evaluating preschoolers*. San Antonio, TX: Therapy Skill Builders.

Miller, L. J., & Roid, G. H. (1994). *The T.I.M.E. Toddler and Infant Motor Evaluation: A standardized assessment*. Tucson, AZ: Therapy Skill Builders.

Miyahara, M., Tsujii, M., Hanai, T., Jongmans, M., Barnett, A., Henderson, S. E., et al. (1998). The Movement Assessment Battery for Children: A preliminary investigation of its usefulness in Japan. *Human Movement Science, 17*, 679–697.

NHS Centre of Reviews and Dissemination. (1999). Getting evidence into practice. *Effective Health Care, 5*, 1–16.

Powell, R., & Bishop, D. (1992). Clumsiness and perceptual problems in children with specific language impairment. *Developmental Medicine and Child Neurology, 34*, 755–765.

Reynard, C. L. (1975). *The nature of motor expectancies and difficulties in kindergarten children*. Unpublished master's thesis, University of California at Los Angeles.

Rodger, S. (1994). A survey of assessments used by paediatric occupational therapists. *Australian Occupational Therapy Journal, 41*, 137–142.

Rösblad, B., & Gard, L. (1998). The assessment of children with developmental coordination disorders in Sweden: A preliminary investigation of the suitability of the Movement ABC. *Human Movement Science, 17*, 711–719.

Rösblad, B., & von Hofsten, C. (1994). Repetitive goal-directed arm movements in children with developmental coordination disorder: Role of visual information. *Adapted Physical Activity Quarterly, 11*, 190–202.

Rosenbaum, D. (1991). *Human motor control.* San Diego, CA: Academic Press.

Russell, D., Rosenbaum, P., Avery, L., & Lane, M. (2002). The Gross Motor Function Measure (GMFM-66 and GMFM-88) user's manual. *Clinics in Developmental Medicine No. 159.* Cambridge, UK: McKeith Press.

Sackett, D., Straus, S., Richardson, W., Rosenberg, W., & Haynes, R. (2000). *Evidence-based medicine: How to practice and teach evidence based medicine.* London: Churchill Livingstone.

Schmidt, R., & Lee, T. (1999). *Motor control and learning. A behavioral analysis* (3rd ed.). Champaign, IL: Human Kinetics.

Schneider, E., Parush, S., Katz, N., & Miller, L. J. (1995). Performance of Israeli versus US preschool children on the Miller Assessment for Preschoolers. *American Journal of Occupational Therapy, 49*, 19–23.

Schouten, P. W., & Kirkpatrick, L. A. (1993). Questions and concerns about the Miller Assessment for Preschoolers. *Occupational Therapy Journal of Research, 13*, 7–28.

Sherill, C. (1998). *Adapted physical activity, recreation and sport: Cross disciplinary and life-span* (5th ed.). Boston: McGraw-Hill.

Smits-Engelsman, B., Niemeijer, A., & van Galen, G. (2001). Fine motor deficiency in children diagnosed as DCD based on poor grapho-motor ability. *Human Movement Science, 20*, 161–182.

Stott, D., Moyes, F., & Henderson, S. E. (1972). *Test of Motor Impairment.* San Antonio, TX: Psychological Corp.

Stott, D. H., Moyes, F. A., & Henderson, S. E. (1984). *The Test of Motor Impairment—Henderson revision.* San Antonio, TX: Psychological Corp.

Sugden, D. A. (1972). *Incidence and nature of motor problems in kindergarten school children.* Unpublished master's thesis, University of California at Los Angeles.

Sugden, D. A., & Chambers, M. E. (2003). Intervention in children with developmental coordination disorder: the role of parents and teachers. *British Journal of Educational Psychology, 73*, 545–561.

Sugden, D., & Sugden, L. (1991). The assessment of movement skill problems in 7- and 9-year old children. *British Journal of Educational Psychology, 61*, 329–345.

Sugden, D., & Utley, A. (1995). Interlimb coupling in children with hemiplegic cerebral palsy. *Developmental Medicine and Child Neurology, 37*, 293–309.

Thelen, E., & Spencer, J. P. (1998). Postural control during reaching in young infants: A dynamic systems approach. *Neuroscience Behavioral Review, 22*, 507–14.

Thomas, J., & Nelson, J. (1996). *Research methods in physical activity.* Champaign, IL: Human Kinetics.

Tucha, O., & Lange, K. (2001). Effects of methylphenidate on kinematic aspects of handwriting in hyperactive boys. *Journal of Abnormal Child Psychology, 29*, 351–356.

Tyler, B., & Miller, K. (1986). The use of tests by psychologists: Report on a survey of BPS members. *Bulletin of the British Psychological Society, 39*, 405–410.

Ulrich, D. A. (1981). The standardization of a criterion-referenced test in fundamental motor and physical fitness skills. *Dissertation Abstracts International, 43*, 146A–147A.

Ulrich, D. A. (1982). *The Objectives-Based Motor Skill Assessment Instrument.* Unpublished manuscript, Southern Illinois University, Carbondale.

Ulrich, D. A. (1985). *Test of gross motor development*. Austin, TX: Pro-Ed.

Ulrich, D. A. (2000). *Test of gross motor development* (2nd ed.). Austin, TX: Pro-Ed.

Wallen, M., & Walker, R. (1995). Occupational therapy practice with children with perceptual motor dysfunction: Findings of a literature review and survey. *Australian Occupational Therapy Journal, 42,* 15–25.

Wann, J., Mon-Williams, M., McIntosh, R., Smyth, M., & Milner, A. (2001). The role of size and binocular information in guiding reaching: Insights from virtual reality and visual form agnosia III (of III). *Experimental Brain Research, 139,* 143–150.

Watkinson, E. J., Causgrove Dunn, J., Cavaliere, N., Calzonetti, K., Wilhelm, L., & Dywer, S. (2001). Engagement in playground activities as a criterion for diagnosing developmental coordination disorder. *Adapted Physical Activity Quarterly, 18*(1), 18–34.

Wilson, B. N., Kaplan, B. J., Crawford, S. G., Campbell, A., & Dewey, D. (2000). Reliability and validity of a parent questionnaire on childhood motor skills. *American Journal of Occupational Therapy, 54,* 484–493.

Wilson, B. N., Kaplan, B. J., Crawford, S. G., & Dewey, D. (2000). Interrater reliability of the Bruininks–Oseretsky Test of Motor Proficiency—Long Form. *Adapted Physical Activity Quarterly, 17,* 95–110.

Wilson, B., Pollock, N., Kaplan, B.J., & Law, M. (1994). *Clinical Observation of Motor and Postural Skills.* San Antonio, TX: Psychological Corp.

Wilson, B., Pollock, N., Kaplan, B. J., Law, M., & Faris, P. (1992). Reliability and construct validity of the Clinical Observations of Motor and Postural Skills. *American Journal of Occupational Therapy, 46,* 775–783.

Wright, H., & Sugden, D. (1996). A two-step procedure for the identification of children with developmental co-ordination disorder in Singapore. *Developmental Medicine and Child Neurology, 38,* 1099–1105.

Wright, H. C., & Sugden, D. A. (1998). A school based intervention programme for children with developmental coordination disorder. *European Journal of Physical Education, 3,* 35–50.

Wright, H. C., Sugden, D. A., Ng, R., & Tan, R. (1994). Identification of children with movement problems in Singapore: Usefulness of the Movement ABC checklist. *Adapted Physical Activity Quarterly, 11,* 150–157.

Age: 0–2 yr. *Purpose:* To establish the level at which a child is performing across different developmental domains.

Background and development: Devised by Ruth Griffiths, a psychologist. First published as "The Abilities of Babies" (Griffiths, 1954, revised 1986). Current version revised and published by Association for Research in Infant and Child Development (ARICD). An extension of the scales, for ages 2–8 yr, was published as The Abilities of Children (Griffiths, 1970, revised 1984). The 2- to 8-yr scale is undergoing revision in the U.K.

Experience required: Restricted to use by pediatricians and psychologists with accredited training.

Manual: Contains description of items, psychometric information and norm tables. The Huntley (1996) edition concerns revision only. Original must be consulted for background information.

Record forms: Single form for any age. Test items clearly listed for each scale alongside age in months.

Materials: Most items in case or additional bag. Stairs and space to kick a ball also needed.

Administration time (min): 30–45

Domains: (A) locomotor; (B) personal/social; (C) hearing and language; (D) eye and hand coordination; (E) performance. There are 54–58 items in each scale (35 in 1st year, 19–23 in 2nd year).

*Examples of **motor content:*** (A) roll, sit, stand, walk, run; (B) hold spoon, drink from cup, take off shoes and socks; (C) making sounds; (D) reach, grasp, throw, scribble, build with bricks; (E) manipulate cube, complete form boards.

Administration. Items evaluated by observing child perform set tasks under standard conditions, performing freely with the test materials, or from information supplied by parent/caregiver. Scoring usually begins on items 2 mo below child's chronological age and continues up and down scale until child has 6 successive passes and 6 successive failures.

Scoring: Items are listed against age in months at which they were passed by 50% of normative sample. Items scored as pass (1) or fail (0) and summed for each domain. Raw scores converted to age equivalents and sub- and general quotients (mean 100, *SD* 15). Subquotients can also be converted into percentile equivalents.

Norms: 665; U.K. Selected according to age, gender and geographical region. Sample composition is also described in terms of residence (urban/rural), social class, and ethnic grouping.

Exclusions: Known severe disability, severe adverse social conditions, or mother did not use English.

Examiners: Doctors and psychologists experienced in using previous edition of test.

*Psychometric information **printed in manual** (users should also consult subsequent publications):*

Reliability	**Validity** (Griffiths, 1986, only)	
Internal consistency: Yes	*Content:* No	*Construct:*
Stability: Yes	*Criterion-related:*	Factor analysis: No
Objectivity: No	Concurrent: No	Group differentiation: No
SEM: Yes	Predictive: No	Age differentiation: No

(continued)

Current use and development: Previous edition used extensively by doctors and psychologists in U.K. (Tyler & Miller, 1986). Griffiths and Huntley (1996) report it is used in much of the English-speaking world and on the continent of Europe. They also note it is available in Italian, Swedish, Spanish, and German.

Limitations: No evidence of test validity reported in manual and as there is overlap in content between the scales, they cannot be considered as independent. All scales include some items that involve motor control and coordination and there is also overlap in the type of items included within the three scales specifically concerned with motor skill (locomotor, eye/hand, and performance).

Strengths: Although now considered rather old-fashioned, the original manuals provide a wealth of information on the testing of babies and young children. Training ensures high standards of administration. The test as a whole provides a useful assessment of performance on a wide range of motor items.

APPENDIX 4.2. Bayley Scales of Infant Development (Bayley, 1993)

Age: 1 mo–3 yr, 6 mo: *Purpose:* To identify infants with developmental delays and to be used as a basis for planning intervention and evaluating outcome.

Background and development: The author has a background in psychology. This battery, with a pedigree stemming from tests developed by Bayley in the 1930s (e.g., California Infant Scale of Motor Development, 1936), is the updated edition of the BSID (Bayley, 1969).

Experience required: Formal graduate or professional training in individual assessment required.

Manual: Clear and comprehensive with good illustrations, photographs and instructions for test administration. Also includes psychometric information, norms and case studies.

Record forms: One for each scale. Cues for start position, materials needed, start and finish items, and drawing items are clearly printed on the forms.

Materials: Most items contained in large case. Stairs also needed.

Administration time (min): Under 15 mo: 25–35; over 15 mo: 60

Domains (no. items): Mental (178); motor (111); behavior rating (30). Items from Mental and Motor scales divided into four domains: cognitive, language, motor, social/personal

*Examples of **motor content:*** Body control, coordination of large muscles, fine manipulation, dynamic movement, postural imitation, stereognosis. Includes rolling, crawling and creeping, sitting, standing, walking, running, and jumping. Fine motor manipulations involved in prehension, adaptive use of writing implements and imitation of hand movements are included.

Administration: Cue sheets indicate relevant items according to age. Explicit instructions must be followed for positioning the child and tester, presenting the stimulus, and timing and scoring the response. Basal rules apply when credits achieved on four items and ceiling after two or more items failed.

Scoring: Each item credited if criteria are achieved. Credits summed, including those below basal. Raw scores converted to standard scores (Mental Development Index [MDI] or Psychomotor Development Index [PDI], with mean 100, $SD = 15$), percentiles, stanines, and age equivalents. Developmental age can also be determined for four domains: cognitive, language, motor and personal/social.

Norms: 1,700; U.S. in 1991–1992. Stratified according to gender, race/ethnicity, geographic region and parent education to represent U.S. population of infants ages 1–42 mo, based on 1988 U.S. Census.

Exclusions: Significant medical complications, mental, physical, or behavioral problems.

Examiners: 340 with extensive testing experience, trained in BSID-II administration.

*Psychometric information **printed in manual** (users should also consult subsequent publications):*

Reliability	*Validity*	
Internal consistency: Yes	*Content:* Yes	*Construct:*
Stability: Yes	*Criterion-related:*	Factor analysis: Yes
Objectivity: Yes	Concurrent: Yes	Group differentiation: Yes
SEM: Yes	Predictive: No (reported in BSID only)	Age differentiation: No

(continued)

Current use and development: Widely used in U.K. and U.S. by pediatricians and therapists. Motor Section has been repackaged as BSID-II Motor Scale Kit (Bayley, 2001), for therapists who require a motor assessment only. The kit includes the Bayley Manual and pack of record forms (identical to full kit), a manual of Motor Scale Administration Directions and all necessary Motor Scale manipulables. It covers age range 1–42 mo and norms are from the Psychomotor Index of the BSID-II. Administration time is 10 min for the youngest babies to 20 min at > 9 months.

Limitations: Considerable skill required in administration and the full test is lengthy. The many materials included result in a large and heavy kit bag.

Strengths: Can be used in a flexible manner to explore child's strengths and weaknesses and the Behavior Rating Scale is particularly useful. Guidance is included in the manual for testing children with physical or perceptual problems. A comprehensive test that gives in depth information on motor skills.

Age: 2 yr, 9 mo–5 yr, 8 mo. *Purpose:* To evaluate a broad range of skills and detect strengths and weaknesses. Provides a structured clinical framework to identify mild, moderate, and severe developmental delay and offers pointers for further evaluation.

Background and development: The author has a background in occupational therapy and early childhood special education. This is one of a series of test batteries developed over the past 20 yr. A shorter screening test, FirstSTEP (Miller, 1993) is available, taking 15 min to administer (plus time to score the Social–Emotional, Adaptive Behavior, and optional Parent/ Teacher Scales). The Toddler and Infant Motor Evaluation (Miller & Roid, 1994), reviewed in this chapter, completes this trio of tests devised by Miller, all of which reflect the construct of sensory integration contributing to movement proficiency.

Experience required: No specialist training required, except for supplemental observation sheet.
Manual: Comprehensive with clear instructions for administration and scoring, guidance for qualitative observations and detailed psychometric information.
Record forms: Single form with cue sheets filed alongside clear item score sheets for each age band.
Materials: All items contained in a case, including mat, walking line, and small stimulus items. Space also needed for walking item.

Administration time (min): 25–35

Domains (no. items): Foundations (10), coordination (7), verbal (4), nonverbal (5), complex tasks (4) Seven 6-monthly age bands with age-appropriate items. *Additional features:* Behavior checklist, guidelines for qualitative observation.

*Examples of **motor content**:* Fine manipulation, block construction, drawing, stereognosis, articulation, static balance, walking, postural imitation and control, sequencing.

Administration: All children perform the same number of items, presented as a series of "games." Cue sheets indicate items according to age with explicit instructions read or demonstrated. Test can be adapted to yield information for planning intervention.

Scoring: Raw scores for individual items entered onto score sheet into series of colored boxes: red (potential problem, bottom 5th percentile); yellow (possible problem, 6th to 25th percentile); green (above 25th percentile). Total number of red and yellow scores used to provide an overall total score and performance index scores, expressed in percentiles.

Norms: 1,204; U.S. in 1980. Stratified according to age, gender, community size, and socioeconomic factors.

Exclusions: Physical, mental or emotional impairment, not fluent in English/living at home with a parent.

Examiners: Under supervision of a registered occupational therapist.

*Psychometric information **printed in manual** (users should also consult subsequent publications):*

Reliability	Validity	
Internal consistency: Yes	*Content:* Yes	*Construct:*
Stability: Yes	*Criterion-related:*	Factor analysis: Yes
Objectivity: Yes	Concurrent: Yes	Group differentiation: Yes
SEM: Yes	Predictive: Yes	Age differentiation: Yes

(continued)

Current use and development: Has been widely used in U.S. and U.K. by therapists and pediatricians (Lawlor & Henderson, 1989). Has also been used with Israeli and Australian populations (Hickey, Froud, Williams, Hart, & Summers, 2001; Schneider, Parush, Katz, & Miller, 1995), with some differences to U.S. norms noted. A Japanese and Chinese version is also available. FirstSTEP has extensive reliability and validity data and includes novel simple motor items that tap both execution and planning of movement (e.g., games using string, sequenced jumping patterns, and graded balance items).

Limitations: Concerns about the predictive validity of the test have been expressed (Schouten & Kirkpatrick, 1993). Some language reflects the U.S. origin (e.g., cookie, mom, and inclusion of cents), which compromises its use worldwide.

Strengths: Covers comprehensive range of skills considered to underlie motor performance, including tasks tapping tactile and proprioceptive skill, alongside tasks that combine muscle power and planning, such as kneel stand and supine flexion. A wide range of objective and subjective observation is undertaken in tasks requiring oral motor function, upper limb gesture, manual dexterity, and graphomotor skill.

Age: Birth–6 yr. *Purpose:* To estimate a child's motor competence relative to his or her peers. Qualitative and quantitative aspects of individual skills are assessed which is valuable for educational and therapy intervention planning. Designed to be used to evaluate a child's progress and also as a research tool.

Background and development: Both authors have a background in physical education and special education. This test is a modification of the original PDMS (Folio & Fewell, 1983).

Experience required: No formal training specified.

Manual: "Examiners' Manual" provides instructions for administration, scoring and interpretation of results. Also includes psychometric information, including norm tables. "Guide to Item Administration" gives detailed instructions on procedure. "Motor Activities Program Manual" introduces activities to facilitate development. A Motor Development Chart gives a quick reference to normative skills.

Record forms: Single form lists all test items with abbreviated administration instructions. Each form may be used to test a child on four occasions.

Materials: Some items supplied in case, including form board, pegboard, button strip, and laces. Examiner must supply 20 common objects, including ball, cup, scissors, and also stairs, rope, and sturdy object (e.g., stool). Large space needed for running and jumping. Examiner must prepare some taped lines or targets.

Administration time (min): Either gross or fine motor section: 20–30; Whole test: 45–60.

Domains (no. items): Gross motor section: Reflexes (8 items for birth–11 mo), stationary (30) measures equilibrium and balance, locomotion (89) includes crawling, walking, running, hopping, and jumping, Object manipulation (24 items for children over 11 mo) includes catching, throwing, and kicking. Fine motor section: Grasping (26) comprises one hand grasp and progresses to bilateral manipulation; Visual–motor integration (72) includes reaching and grasping, building with blocks, and copying designs.

Administration: Instructions, either read out or demonstrated, are repeated up to three times for each item. Entry points, based on age are clearly indicated, as are basals and ceiling levels. Information is included on adapting instructions for children with hearing or other specific difficulty related to understanding, although this affects the interpretation of test results.

Scoring: Each item has specific criteria scored on a point system: 2 = performance meets criteria, 1 = does not fully meet criteria, and 0 = attempt does not show skill is emerging. Any item omitted or not attempted is scored zero. Raw scores summed to give subtest scores and converted to standard scores (mean 10, *SD* 3). Scores from gross and fine motor subtests summed to give gross motor quotient (GMQ) and fine motor quotient (FMQ), respectively. GMQ and FMQ form the total motor quotient (all with mean 100, *SD* 15). Percentiles are also provided for subtests and quotients as well as age equivalents. *T*-scores, *s*-scores, or stanines may also be obtained. (PDMS-2 Software Scoring and Report System are available.)

Norms: 2003, from U.S. and Canada in 1997–1998. Stratified according to age, gender, geographic region, community, race, ethnicity, and social economic status based on data from the 1997 U.S. Census.

Exclusions: None reported.

Examiners: Purchasers of PDMS and occupational/physiotherapists.

(continued)

*Psychometric information **printed in manual** (users should also consult subsequent publications):*

Reliability	Validity	
Internal consistency: Yes	*Content:* Yes	*Construct:*
Stability: Yes	*Criterion-related:*	Factor analysis: Yes
Objectivity: Yes	Concurrent: Yes	Group differentiation: Yes
SEM: Yes	Predictive: No	Age differentiation: Yes

Current use and development: A recent update of the PDMS, which was widely used in the U.S.

Limitations: Some weaknesses of the PDMS still hold for this version (e.g., poor specification of equipment, organization of items, and scoring procedures) (see Burton & Miller, 1998). There are also problems with the intervention section. It is difficult to provide precise, structured activity programs without running into problems of misinterpretation by inexperienced users.

Strengths: This user-friendly test has detailed instructions and good reliability. It includes a good range of fine and gross motor items and covers a wide age range.

Age: 4 mo–3 yr, 6 mo. *Purpose:* To provide a comprehensive evaluation of motor proficiencies and difficulties, identify motor delay/deviation, develop remediation programs, and evaluate efficacy of treatment.

Background and development: One of a trio of tests by Lucy Miller, who has a background in occupational therapy and early childhood special education. Gale Roid has a background in psychology.

Experience required: May be administered at two competency levels: Primary subtests require moderate training and clinical expertise (although Functional Performance subtest requires specialized interview technique). The three clinical subtests require advanced training with in-depth knowledge of typical and atypical movement. Neurodevelopmental therapy (Bobath) and/or SI certification is likely to help understanding of the Motor Organization subtest.

Manual: Comprehensive administration directions with clear pictures. Contains details of development, psychometrics and norms.

Record forms: Single form, clearly set out with illustrations.

Materials: Most items in small bag, including toy car, balls, shoelaces, rattle, squeaky toy, small cubes etc. Examiner must prepare markings and supply a blanket and small cereal pieces.

Administration time (min): Youngest: 10–20, older: 20–40 (additional 15 for Functional Performance subtest).

Domains: Primary subtests (5): Mobility (moving in/out of postures, e.g., supine, sit, and stand), stability (positional stability of postures), motor organization (movements to interact with toys, e.g., reach and grasp), social–emotional (level of attention, activity, etc.), and functional performance (self-care, feeding, dressing, etc.). Additional clinical subtests (3): atypical positions, quality rating, and component analysis.

Administration: Parent/caregiver is involved as partner in assessment process. Variety of procedures used including prompting parent to position or interact with child, observing child in free play, and interviewing parent. Administered with flexibility to account for different styles of parent–child interaction. Experienced testers can record and rate movement patterns against pictures or verbal description of atypical positions.

Scoring: Raw scores from primary subtests converted to standard scores (mean 10, *SD* 3). An appendix gives *z* scores, percentiles, and stanines. Component analysis and Quality Rating subtests at present provide raw scores only but may be used to demonstrate change in performance over time. The Atypical Positions subtest norms are based only on children with motor delays or deviations and it is therefore interpreted differently from a traditional scaled score. Scoring options also provided for out-of-age norms and atypical motor patterns.

Norms: 731; U.S. in 1992–1993. Stratified according to age, gender, ethnicity, and socioeconomic status, based on data from the 1990 U.S. Census.

Exclusions: For standardized scores, children with motor delays or deviations who were biologically or environmentally at risk.

Examiners: 75 examiners experienced in motor assessment of young children and most were neurodevelopmental (Bobath) and/or sensory integration (SIPT) trained/certified.

(continued)

*Psychometric information **printed in manual** (users should also consult subsequent publications):*

Reliability	*Validity*	
Internal consistency: Yes	*Content:* Yes	*Construct:*
Stability: Yes	*Criterion-related:*	Factor analysis: Yes
Objectivity: Yes	Concurrent: No	Group differentiation: Yes
SEM: Yes	Predictive: No	Age differentiation: Yes

Current use and development: This test is gaining popularity. A glossary is provided in which very specific terminology used in the descriptions is defined. The authors identify this as an area for further development and request feedback in an effort to gain greater clarity in this notoriously difficult domain.

Limitations: Considerable expertise is required to use all aspects of the test. It may be hard for some professionals to allow parents freedom to initiate assessment handling.

Strengths: Provides a comprehensive assessment of motor skill for infants and young children. Parental involvement in the assessment is innovative and appealing. The manual has an excellent section on parents as partners in test administration.

Age: 3 –10 yr. *Purpose:* To identify children who are significantly behind their peers in gross motor development, plan an instructional program in gross motor development, to assess individual progress and evaluate intervention programs.

Background and development: The author has a background in adapted physical education and works in special education. This was originally developed as a criterion-referenced test in fundamental motor and physical fitness skills (Ulrich, 1981). The fundamental motor skills part became the Objective-Based Motor Skill Assessment Instrument (Ulrich, 1982). This was modified and published as the TGMD (Ulrich, 1985) and is now in its second edition.

Experience required: No specific qualifications stipulated.

Manual: Extremely clear and comprehensive, including psychometric information and norm tables. Appendices provide an illustrated guide for administration and scoring.

Record forms: Single form on which materials required, directions for administration and performance criteria are listed for each item. There are also sections in which to record the profile of standard scores and notes on the testing conditions.

Materials: There is no test kit. Examiner must supply the materials depicted in a figure (six types of ball, a beanbag, tape, traffic cones, a bat, and a batting tee). A clear space (maximum of 60 feet) is needed as well as a wall against which a ball can be kicked. Examiner must prepare floor markings.

Administration: Verbal description and accurate demonstration given for each task, followed by a practice trial and additional demonstration if needed. Two trials are performed.

Domains (no. items): Locomotor (6): run, gallop, hop, leap, horizontal jump and slide. Object control (6): striking a stationary ball, stationary dribble, catch, kick, overhand throw, underhand roll.

Administration time (min): 15–20

Scoring: 3–5 performance criteria, which represent a mature pattern of the skill, are listed for each item. Criteria are scored 1 if met and 0 if not. Raw scores are summed over two trials for each task. These are summed to give raw scores for locomotor and object control subtests, with a maximum value of 48. Subtest raw scores can be converted to standard scores with a (mean 10, *SD* 3) and to percentiles. Separate norms for girls and boys are provided for object control but are combined for locomotor subtest. Subtest standard scores can be combined and converted to percentiles and a composite standard score (mean 100, SD 15). Raw scores from the two subtests can also be converted to age equivalents.

Norms: 1,208, U.S. in 1997–1998. Stratified according to geographic region, gender, race, rural or urban residence, parent education, and disability to represent U.S. population based on 1997 U.S. Census. Children with learning disabilities and other handicaps were included in the sample.

Exclusions: None reported.

Examiners: Physical educators and individuals who had purchased the first edition of the test.

(continued)

*Psychometric information **printed in manual** (users should also consult subsequent publications):*

Reliability	*Validity*	
Internal consistency: Yes	*Content:* Yes	*Construct:*
Stability: Yes	*Criterion-related:*	Factor analysis: Yes
Objectivity: Yes	Concurrent: No	Group differentiation: Yes
SEM: Yes	Predictive: Yes	Age differentiation: Yes

Current use and development: The first edition of this test has been widely used in the U.S. The test is gaining popularity in Europe.

Limitations: Specific focus on gross motor skill may be too narrow for needs of some clinicians. Skill is required to consider performance criteria while observing the child. May be best suited to children over 5 yr as it focuses on mature performance and does not allow for assessment of change below this level. Does not allow for the notion that a task may be achieved in many different ways.

Strengths: Relatively inexpensive and quick to administer. Has good reliability and validity that has been demonstrated for different subgroups as well as the entire normative sample. Samples a good range of functional gross motor tasks. Focus on movement patterns aids in understanding of poor performance.

Age: 4–12 yr. *Purpose:* To identify children with motor difficulties, to help describe these, to plan appropriate intervention and to document change when evaluating intervention.

Background and development: The authors have a background in physical education and psychology. The complete Movement ABC package has three components: this standardized test, a teacher checklist (reviewed separately), and guidelines for intervention. The test has its origins in Denis Stott's modifications of the Oseretsky tests. It was first published as the Test of Motor Impairment (Stott, Moyes, & Henderson, 1972) and revised by Henderson (TOMI-R; Stott, Moyes, & Henderson, 1984).

Experience required: No specific qualifications stipulated.

Manual: Single manual covers all components of Movement ABC package. Photographs and clear instructions are provided for administration. Psychometric information is provided together with percentile norms for total scores and the 5th and 15th percentile points for total and subscores.

Record forms: Separate forms for each of four age bands (4–6 yr, 7–8 yr, 9–10 yr, 11–12 yr). Scaled scores for single age years are set out clearly for each item, with observation checklists printed alongside.

Materials: All items supplied in case. Examiner must prepare wall and floor markings.

Administration time (min): 20–40

Domains (no. items): Manual dexterity (3), ball skill (2), balance (3). Each age band contains age-appropriate items. *Additional feature:* rating of behaviors that might influence a child's performance.

Administration: A demonstration and practice phase is given, with extra trials allowed on some tasks. Test can be used formally to yield scores to determine child's status in relation to norms or used for clinical exploration to yield information for planning intervention. In the latter case adaptations to test administration and qualitative observations of performance are recommended.

Scoring: Raw scores are converted to scaled scores, which can be summed to give three subscores (for manual dexterity, ball skill, and balance) and a total score. 5th and 15th percentile points are provided for the subscores and total score. Total scores < 5th percentile are considered as indicative of a definite motor problem, scores between 5th–15th percentile suggest a degree of difficulty that is borderline.

Norms: 1,234, U.S. in 1990. Selected to be representative in terms of gender, geographical region and ethnic origin, according to 1983 U.S. Census.

Exclusions: Children with obvious physical handicaps.

Examiners: Had a special interest in either adapted physical activity or motor development.

Psychometric information **printed in manual** *(users should also consult subsequent publications):*

Reliability	Validity	
Internal consistency: No	*Content:* Yes	Construct:
Stability: Yes	*Criterion-related:*	Factor analysis: No
Objectivity: No (TOMI-R	Concurrent: Yes	Group differentiation: Yes
only)	Predictive: No	Age differentiation: No
SEM: No		

(continued)

Current use and development: Used mainly in the U.K. and other parts of Europe (with publications in six languages). One of the most commonly used tests in research on DCD (Crawford et al., 2001; Geuze, Jongmans, Shoemaker, & Smits-Engelsman, 2001). A revision of age band 4 and extension of norms for children over 12 yr is underway at the time of writing (Henderson & Barnett, 2001). Data collected in Europe closely resembles the U.S. standardization sample (Jongmans, 1993; Rösblad & Gard, 1998), while differences have been found with data from Asia (Chow et al., 2001; Miyahara et al., 1998).

Limitations: Information in the manual on the reliability and validity of the current version are limited and methods for obtaining this data have been criticized (Burton & Miller, 1998). Recent work, however, reports favorably on the psychometric properties of the test (Croce, Horvat, & McCarthy, 2001).

Strengths: The test covers a broad range of skills. Scoring procedures allow for the identification of small changes in performance for children with movement difficulties. Positive reports on the cognitive-motor approach to intervention are emerging (Sugden & Chambers, 2003; Wright & Sugden, 1998).

Age: 4–14 yr. *Purpose:* For screening, placement, planning of instruction/intervention, evaluation of progress/training, and diagnosis of developmental problems.

Background and development: At the time of publication the author was a professor of psychoeducational studies. The test was based partly on the U.S. adaptation of the Oseretsky Tests of Motor Proficiency (Doll, 1946), published in Russian in 1923 and later translated into Portuguese and then English. No revisions have taken place since its publication in 1978.

Experience required: No specific training or qualifications stipulated

Manual: Directions are clearly set out with diagrams to help the administration and scoring of some items Psychometric information and norm tables are also provided.

Record forms: Single form for long or short form of the test, for a child of any age. It is clearly set out although rather long.

Materials: Most items supplied in very large case. Examiner must supply two chairs, a table, gym mat, or carpeted surface and large space for running.

Administration time (min): 45–60 (long form), 15–20 (short form).

Domains (no. items): Gross motor (20), fine motor (17), upper-limb coordination (9). Gross motor has four sections: running speed and agility (1), balance (8), bilateral coordination (8), strength (3). Fine motor has three sections: response speed (1), visual–motor control (8), upper-limb speed and dexterity (8). Upper-limb coordination has one section (9). A short form is also available with 14 items, including at least one from each of the eight subtests.

Administration: A wide range of items is administered to children of all ages. Specific instructions for each task are given; some are also demonstrated or have a practice trial.

Scoring: The scoring is complicated, involving nine separate steps and the weighting and rescaling of scores three times. Raw scores for each item are converted to point scores to appropriately weight the difficulty of each item. Point scores are summed for each of the eight subtests and converted to subtest standard scores (which can be converted to age equivalents). Subtest standard scores are converted to gross motor and fine motor composite standard scores (mean 50, SD 10). Summing the gross motor composite, fine motor composite, and upper-limb coordination standard score gives the battery composite (mean 100, SD 15). The composite standard scores may be converted to percentiles, stanines and age equivalents.

Norms: 676 and 89, U.S. and Canada, respectively. Stratified according to age, gender, race, community size, and geographic region to represent U.S. population based on 1970 U.S. Census.

Exclusions: Children with severe physical impairments.

Examiners: Trained and supervised.

*Psychometric information **printed in manual** (users should also consult subsequent publications):*

Reliability	Validity	Construct:
Internal consistency: Yes	*Content:* Yes	Factor analysis: Yes
Stability: Yes	*Criterion-related:*	Group differentiation: Yes
Objectivity: Yes	Concurrent: *No*	Age differentiation: Yes
SEM: Yes	Predictive: *No*	

(continued)

Current use and development: Has had sustained popularity throughout Canada and U.S. with therapists and other professionals (Burton & Miller, 1998; Crowe, 1989; Rodger, 1994; Sherrill, 1998). To our knowledge, there are no plans to revise the test or gather new normative data.

Limitations: Lengthy to administer. Validity and reliability have been questioned (Burton & Miller, 1998; Hattie & Edwards, 1987; Wilson, Kaplan, Crawford, Campbell, & Dewey, 2000). The lack of recent normative data is a major cause for concern.

Strengths: The broad range of items included and their progression within subtests (particularly in the balance section) provide the clinician with a comprehensive assessment tool. Allows for measurement across the entire range of performance and benefits from having a single set of items for all ages.

Age: 5–11 yr. *Purpose:* Screening or identifying children for special services, clinical exploration, intervention planning, and program evaluation.

Background and development: Both authors have a background in physical education and psychology. The complete Movement ABC package has three components: this checklist, a standardized test (reviewed separately), and guidelines for intervention. The original version of the checklist evolved from the work of Jack Keogh and his students as the University of California checklist (Reynard, 1975; Sugden, 1972). It was later rewritten and used as the Motor Competence Checklist (Sugden & Sugden, 1991) before being published as part of the Movement ABC.

Experience required: Primarily intended for teachers but may be used by other professionals and parents.

Manual: Single manual covers all components of Movement ABC package. Includes details on administration, psychometric properties and 5th/15th percentile points for total "motor" scores of checklist.

Record forms: Single form. Items listed with space alongside for recording rating.

Materials: No materials provided. Children are observed using equipment usually available in school.

Administration time: Completed over 1–2-week period of observation.

Domains (no. items): Four sections: (1) child stationary/environment stable (12), (2) child moving/environment stable (12), (3) child stationary/environment changing (12), (4) child moving/environment changing (12). *Additional feature:* Section 5 to rate behaviors that might interfere with movement performance.

Administration: Child observed in natural contexts. Each item rated on 4-point scale (0–3), showing how child deals with the task (very well–not close).

Scoring: Ratings for each task summed for each section. Section scores summed to give total "motor" score. 5th and 15th percentile points for total scores are provided in manual for ages 6, 7, 8 and 9+ yr. Scores below 5th percentile are considered to reflect movement problems that require special consideration and a full assessment with the Movement ABC test is recommended. Children with scores < 15th percentile considered "at risk" for movement problems. Items in section 5 scored on 3-point scale, indicating frequency with which child displays the described behavior. The authors recommend that interpretation of the scores in this section should be qualitative rather than quantitative.

Norms: 298; U.K. Randomly chosen from classes in rural and urban schools selected from a defined geographical area.

Exclusions: None reported.

Examiners: Classroom teachers are shown how to use the checklist.

*Psychometric information **printed in manual** (users should also consult subsequent publications):*

Reliability	**Validity**	
Internal consistency: No	*Content:* Yes	*Construct: Yes*
Stability: Yes	*Criterion-related:*	Factor analysis: No
Objectivity: No	Concurrent: Yes	Group differentiation: Yes
SEM: No	Predictive: No	Age differentiation: Yes

(continued)

Current use and development: Mainly used in U.K. and some other European countries. Has also been employed in series of studies in Singapore and reported to be suitable for use there (Wright & Sugden, 1996; Wright, Sugden, Ng, & Tang, 1994). As part of the Movement ABC package it has been translated into several languages other than English (see review of Movement ABC Test).

Limitations: Psychometric information in the manual is limited, but as the test is used more, further information may be published. In our experience, some teachers find the checklist rather long and difficult to complete in full.

Strengths: Provides a way of quantifying performance in natural settings. The categorization of tasks is unlike that in other tests and provides useful information on the pattern of performance. When used in combination with the Movement ABC Test, this is reported to be a useful tool for the identification of children with movement difficulties. The checklist and test combined provide useful information for planning intervention, evaluations of which are beginning to emerge (Sugden & Chambers, 2003).

APPENDIX 4.10. Developmental Coordination Disorder Questionnaire (Wilson, Kaplan, Crawford, Campbell, & Dewey, 2000)

Age: 8–14 yr. *Purpose:* To identify children with motor problems, with a specific focus on developmental coordination disorder (DCD).

Background and development: The authors have backgrounds in occupational therapy and psychology. This is the first version of the questionnaire to be produced.

Experience required: No specific qualifications or experience stipulated.

Manual: There is no manual but development of the questionnaire and its psychometric properties are detailed in Wilson, Kaplan, Crawford, Campbell, and Dewey (2000).

Record forms: A single form lists items with the rating scale alongside. A separate sheet is provided, onto which item scores are transferred and summed for each of four subsections.

Materials. No materials needed.

Administration time: Takes a few minutes to complete by someone who knows the child well.

Domains (no. items): Control during movement (6), fine motor/handwriting (4), gross motor/planning (4), general coordination (3)

Administration: May be completed by the parent/caregiver or presented as an interview. The items refer to general impressions of how a task is performed (e.g., item one: "Throws a ball in a controlled and accurate fashion, compared to other children the same age as your child") rather than performance on specific tasks. For each item, parents are asked to compare the degree of coordination of their child with other children of the same age and to rate this on a 5-point scale ranging from "Not at all like your child" (1) to "Extremely like your child" (5). The questionnaire contains a mixture of positively and negatively worded items.

Scoring: Individual scores for each item are transferred to a scoring sheet, reversing scores for negatively worded items. Scores from each of the four sections are summed and a total score computed. The maximum total score is 85. Scores from 0–48 fall in the 0–10th percentile and indicate DCD. Scores of 49–57 fall in the 11–24th percentile and indicate suspect DCD and scores of 58–85 fall in the 25–100th percentile and indicate that there is probably no DCD.

Norms: 306, Canada (two-thirds with learning/attention problems). One-third matched for age but did not have such problems. The sample was divided into three groups based on the children's performance on the BOTMP and the Movement ABC Test: a DCD group (38), suspect DCD (45), and non-DCD group (223).

Exclusions: Children over age 14 yr, 6 mo. No other exclusions reported.

Examiners: Not applicable. Questionnaires either completed at home and returned by mail or completed through telephone interview.

Psychometric information printed in manual (users should also consult subsequent publications):

Reliability	*Validity*	
Internal consistency: Yes	*Content:* Yes	*Construct:*
Stability: No	*Criterion-related:*	Factor analysis: Yes
Objectivity: No	Concurrent: Yes	Group differentiation: Yes
SEM: No	Predictive: No	Age differentiation: No

(continued)

Current use and developments: A newly developed instrument currently used in Canada, the Netherlands, and U.K. At the time of writing the authors are investigating the use of an amended version for children ages 5–7 yr.

Limitations: In our view, use of the term *DCD* in the title and as assigned to those scoring below the 25th percentile is inappropriate, as movement difficulties identified may not meet the strict criteria for a diagnosis of DCD (American Psychiatric Association, 1994). One item contains a Canadian term (*birdie*) that may not be appropriate to use in other countries

Strengths: This recently developed questionnaire is quick and easy to use and score and it covers a range of motor skills.

APPENDIX 4.11. Beery–Buktenica Developmental Test of Visual–Motor Integration—Revised Fourth Edition (Beery, 1997).

Age: 3–18 yr. *Purpose:* To identify, through early screening, children who may need special assistance. To test the effectiveness of intervention and to advance research.

Background and development: The author has a background in child development and clinical psychology. The test was first published as the VMI in 1967 (Beery, 1967) and revised in 1982 and 1989. The 1997 publication includes two supplementary tests.

Experience required: No specific requirements are stipulated.

Manual: Contains details of administration and scoring, and psychometric information with norm tables.

Record forms: Full and short format test booklets contain 27 and 18 items, respectively. A recording and scoring sheet are provided on the inside cover. The geometric forms are presented at the top of horizontally oriented pages. There are blank squares beneath, in which the child makes his/her attempt. There are separate forms for the supplementary tests. *Materials:* None provided. The examiner must supply a soft pencil or ballpoint pen. A ruler and protractor may be needed when first scoring the test.

Administration time (min): 10–15, an additional 3 for visual perception test and 5 for motor coordination test.

Domains (no. items): Visual–motor integration (18 or 27, depending on age). Supplemental tests: Visual Perception (27), Motor Coordination (27).

Administration. May be administered to an individual or group. Directions are read from the manual. A sequence of 27 geometric forms is copied with paper and pencil (18-item version is available for children ages 3–7 yr). The supplemental tests use the same stimulus forms and should be used with those who have scored below the average range on the VMI. In the visual perception test the child chooses one geometric form that is exactly the same as each stimulus from among others that are not the same. As many of the 27 stimuli as possible are to be identified in 3 min. In the motor coordination test the stimulus forms are traced with a pencil without going outside the double-lined paths.

Scoring: In the VMI one point is awarded for each correct item up to three consecutive incorrect items. In the visual perception and motor coordination subtests all forms attempted within a specified period are scored. The maximum score is 27. Criteria are provided for each form, together with scoring examples. Raw scores can be converted to standard scores (mean 100, *SD* 15) or to age equivalents. Standard scores can be further converted to scaled scores with (mean 10, *SD* 3). Other scores including *T*-scores (mean 50, *SD* 10) and percentiles are provided.

Norms: 2,614; U.S. in 1995–1996. Stratified according to age, gender, ethnicity, socioeconomic status, residence (urban, suburban, rural) and geographic location to represent data from the 1990 U.S. Census. Included those with "disabling conditions." *Exclusions:* None reported.

Examiners: School psychologists and learning disability specialists. Scored by author and research assistants.

(continued)

*Psychometric information **printed in manual** (users should also consult subsequent publications):*

Reliability	*Validity*	
Internal consistency: Yes	*Content:* Yes	*Construct:*
Stability: Yes	*Criterion-related:*	Factor analysis: Yes
Objectivity: Yes	Concurrent: Yes	Group differentiation: Yes
SEM: Yes	Predictive: Yes	Age differentiation: Yes

Current use and development: A popular tool worldwide. Surveys have found previous versions of the test to be frequently used (e.g., Rodger, 1994; Wallen & Walker, 1995).

Limitations: Test administrators need practice to score the test items reliably. The test is limited to an examination of only one area of motor skill, requiring the control of a pencil. The supplementary motor coordination test would benefit from further development.

Strengths: Quick and easy to administer, providing a more detailed measure of graphic skill than other tests. The addition of the supplementary visual and motor tests provides a useful extension of the test, allowing for a more detailed examination of a child's visual–perceptual and perceptual–motor skills.

Age: 4 yr–8 yr, 11 mo. *Purpose:* A diagnostic and descriptive tool to assess several different practic abilities, aspects of sensory processing of vestibular, proprioceptive, kinesthetic, tactile and visual systems, and behavioral manifestations purported to be connected with sensory integrative dysfunction. Designed for use in both clinical and research settings. The test is not suitable for children with a severe neuromotor problem (such as spasticity or athetosis).

Background and development: The author has a background in occupational therapy. The test was developed from a group of perceptual–motor tests published in 1960s (e.g., Ayres, 1962, 1964, 1968). The SIPT is a revision of the Southern California Sensory Integration Tests (Ayres, 1972).

Experience required: Formal training is recommended in SI theory, SIPT test administration, and interpretation. Interpretation should be by individuals with sound theoretical knowledge and understanding of sensory integration (SI) and praxis (e.g., therapists, mainly occupational and physiotherapists).

Manual: Comprehensive, containing information on psychometrics and instructions for administration and scoring.

Record forms: Computer-scannable record sheets reiterate concise details from the manual, of the administration protocol for each item.

Materials: All items are provided in a very large case on wheels, including a postrotary nystagmus board, and wooden constructional praxis form. A large floor space is required for some items.

Administration time (min): 120 (over two sessions)

Domains (no. items): Form and Space Perception (4), Somatic and Vestibular Sensory Processing Tests (6), Praxis Tests (6), Bilateral Integration and Sequencing Tests (1 subtest plus 4 included from other domains). Items include manual dexterity, balance, a comprehensive set of praxis subtests and items tapping sensory processing.

Administration: Each task is taught following a standardized verbal and demonstration protocol. Practice items are included.

Scoring: Raw or scaled scores are recorded onto record form (or computer disc) and sent to Western Psychological Services (WPS) in U.S. with a fee for scanning and marking. WPS returns an extensive test report for professionals and description of the SIPT for parents. The report includes Z score (SD), SEM, percentile score for each item and a breakdown of subscores such as right and left hand function. A visual and written profile compares the child's result with six SI diagnostic prototypes.

Norms: 1997, U.S. in 1984–1995. Representative in terms of gender, community (rural/urban), school type, geographic region and ethnic origin according to the 1980 U.S. Census. Included children receiving special services such as remedial reading or speech therapy.

Exclusions: Children with identified motor or sensory impairment.

Examiners: 100 trained examiners who met defined accuracy criteria.

(continued)

*Psychometric information **printed in manual** (users should also consult subsequent publications):*

Reliability	*Validity*	
Internal consistency: No	*Content:* Yes	*Construct:*
Stability: Yes	*Criterion-related:*	Factor analysis: Yes
Objectivity: Yes	Concurrent: Yes	Group differentiation: Yes
SEM: No	Predictive: No	Age differentiation: Yes

Current use and development: Used extensively in U.S. Trained SIPT testers are practicing internationally, including in Europe, South Africa, Australia, and Japan. There has been increased training and use of the test in the U.K. with the collection of U.K. norms starting at the time of writing.

Limitations: Training and practice are essential for it to be valid. Lengthy and complex to administer and score, relying heavily on expertise of the examiner. Interpretation of reports requires careful translation from SI jargon to be understood transprofessionally. Equipment is very heavy and there is emphasis on the upper limb. There is no throwing, aiming, or explosive lower-limb action, such as jumping.

Strengths: The range of sensory/perceptual and movement items provide interest and variety for the child. This is one of the few standardized objective measures of aspects of praxis. Several of its unique subtests have good reliability and the test has value as a specialized research tool.

APPENDIX 4.13. Clinical Observation of Motor and Postural Skills (Wilson, Pollock, Kaplan, & Law, 1994)

Age: 5–9 yr. *Purpose:* To identify motor problems associated with underlying postural control and stability components of movement. Also to help determine the type of intervention approach that is indicated for a specific child. The authors emphasize that it should be interpreted in combination with a functional performance measure. The test is aimed at the student with suspected motor problems (e.g., DCD) but without neuromotor problems (e.g., cerebral palsy, epilepsy, or with general intellectual delay).

Background and development: The authors have a background in occupational therapy and psychology. COMPS was developed from clinical observation protocols based on the work of Jean Ayres, author of the SIPT (Ayres, 1989). There was concern that many occupational and physical therapists use these clinical observations informally in a non-standardized manner and their clinical practice may consequently be guided by invalid interpretation. An important stated objective in developing the test included standardization of administration procedures and the development of objective criteria for scoring purposes.

Experience required: Designed for use by pediatric occupational and physiotherapists. Others with less specific experience should check scoring against a more experienced tester. Its similarity to clinical observation used in the SI model makes it especially useful for anyone who has training in SI methods.

Manual: Contains illustrations and instructions for administration of each item, scoring and limited psychometric detail.

Record forms: A single form for all ages. Point scores are provided on the form but the manual must be consulted for additional weighting of some scores.

Materials: A pair of asymmetric tonic neck reflex (ATNR) measurement tools contained in a small folder. The tester must provide a floor mat and two chairs. An area of 2½ × 3 meters is required.

Administration time (min): 15–20

Domains: Six clinical observations: slow movements of the arms, rapid forearm rotation (diadokokinesis), finger–nose touching, prone extension posture, ATNR, supine flexion.

Administration: The child carries out each item following demonstration, verbal instruction, and/or physical prompt by the examiner but no practice is allowed.

Scoring: Quantitative and/or qualitative measures are scored and summed for each item. Some scores have to be transformed from a 0–12-point raw score to a 0–3-point scale. Item scores are then weighted and summed. The total is then adjusted for age. A final weighted total score < 0 indicates problems in motor and postural skills and a score of > 0 is indicative of normal function in this area.

Norms: None available, this is a criterion-referenced test.

Psychometric information **printed in manual** *(users should also consult subsequent publications):*

Reliability	*Validity*	
Internal consistency: Yes	*Content:* Yes	*Construct:*
Stability: Yes	*Criterion-related:*	Factor analysis: Yes
Objectivity: Yes	Concurrent: Yes	Group differentiation: Yes
SEM: No	Predictive: No	Age differentiation: No

(continued)

108

Current use and development: Used in the U.S. and Canada and recently it is becoming more familiar in the U.K. mainly to SI trained occupational and physiotherapists. It is used both for assessment in clinical practice and as a research tool. There are plans to extend the test for older children.

Limitations: The joint measure tools are awkward to use and may compromise the result in a ticklish (tactile defensive) child. Combining the six scores to give a total may not give a valid reflection of the clinical picture.

Strengths: A quick, straightforward screening test, which includes physical activities that are fun for the child and is readily usable in the clinic setting. A very useful attempt to make clinical observation more objective and this test has potential for further development.

PART II
CLINICAL DISORDERS

CHAPTER 5

Neurodevelopmental Motor Disorders

CEREBRAL PALSY AND NEUROMUSCULAR DISEASES

THOMAS A. BLONDIS

All aspects of the spectrum of developmental disabilities present the handicapped individual with major challenges throughout life. Milder disabilities and sometimes seemingly subclinical disabilities are chronic lifelong conditions. Chronic conditions that affect the motor functioning of a child have an effect not only on the individual but also on every person who is within his or her family. Subclinical forms such as mild cerebral palsy, coordination disorders, and Asperger syndrome are often ignored because they do not require orthopedic or physical medicine specialists. Other chapters in this book focus on these conditions. This chapter focuses on more severe forms of neurodevelopmental disability, such as cerebral palsy, muscular dystrophy, and ataxia.

CEREBRAL PALSY

Cerebral palsy (CP) represents the prototypical disability because of the wide continuum of comorbidity associated with this condition. Orthopedic, neuromuscular limitations, visual deficits, seizures, cognitive deficiencies, and psychiatric conditions are among the areas that interfere with accessibility for persons with CP (Blondis, 1996; Capute & Accardo, 1996). Other major disabilities that have an underlying neuromuscular, metabolic, or degenerative etiology can mimic CP. Therefore, it is important that CP be differentiated from these other disorders.

CP is a disorder of movement and posture secondary to a static encephalopathy. CP is a broad-spectrum term that defines a number of nonprogressive syndromes or motor disorders. It occurs in about 1 in 500 liveborn children (Hagberg, Hagberg, Olow, & van Wendt, 1996; Tomlin, 1995). It is not a disease and does not imply a specific cause (Capute & Accardo, 1996); the impairments are secondary to lesions or malformations usually of the pyramidal or extrapyramidal tracks. The insult to the brain occurs during the early stages of development and may occur during the prenatal period, labor, and birth or the early postnatal period.

Clinical manifestations of CP include persisting primitive reflexes, abnormalities in tone, inability to move against gravity, and poor variability of movement. CP is a nonprogressive neurological disorder, although inadequate intervention can result in a progressive musculoskeletal disability. Detection of CP at an early age may avoid complications such as weakness, skeletal deformity, and medical interventions. It also may lead to the recognition of hereditary metabolic or neurodegenerative diseases that mimic CP (Pellegrino, 2002; Taft, Matthews, & Molnar, 1983).

Classification

CP can be classified in three ways: (1) clinically, (2) pathophysiologically, and (3) topographically. The following sections present these three different approaches to classifying CP.

Clinically

CP is typically classified according to the clinical presentation (i.e., spasticity, tone, and ataxia) of the primary motor deficits. The most commonly used classifications are spastic CP (which includes spastic diplegia, spastic quadriplegia, and spastic hemiplegia), extrapyramidal CP, hypotonic CP, and ataxic CP. Spastic CP is associated with dysfunction in the corticospinal tracts that results in increased muscle tone, increased or hyperreflexia and the persistence of primitive reflexes (Tomlin, 1995). It has been reported to account for between 66 and 82% of CP cases (Menkes & Sarnat, 2000). Extrapyramidal CP (i.e., dyskinetic CP), which accounts for between 5 and 22% of cases, results from dysfunction in the basal ganglia and extrapyramidal pathways. It is characterized by a variety of abnormal motor patterns and postures such as involuntary athetoid movements of the limbs or dystonic posturing of the trunk and limbs (Menkes & Sarnat, 2000; Prechtl & Stemmer, 1962; Tomlin, 1995). Hypotonic CP is characterized by a generalized decrease in muscle tone that persists from infancy to beyond 3 years of age. Many children with this type of CP develop cerebellar symptoms, including incoordination, gait disturbances, and impairments in rapid coordination of successive movements (Menkes & Sarnat, 2000). Although the etiology of this form of CP is not clear, there is some suggestion that it might be due to delayed development of the cerebellum or in maturation of type 1 and type 2 muscle fibers (Menkes & Sarnat, 2000).

When *ataxia* is of the congenital and nonprogressive type, it is termed *ataxic CP*. Typical signs of ataxia arising from cerebellar dysfunction include wide-based gait, limb dysmetria, tremor, dysarthria, and nystagmus. As ataxic CP is uncommon, possible metabolic disease, an acute infectious process, or an associated mental retardation syndrome should be considered as possible differential diagnoses.

Pathophysiological

Involvement of the pyramidal tracts causes spastic forms of cerebral palsy, whereas involvement of the basal ganglia causes involuntary movement disorders (e.g., choreoathetosis and dystonia). It is possible to have both the pyramidal tract and extrapyramidal tract involved in mixed CP, and in this case, one clinical scenario usually predominates over the other.

The most common form of CP in Europe, the United States, and Canada is spastic diplegia due to periventricular leukomalacia occurring in preterm infants born prior to 32 weeks of gestation (Hagberg, Hagberg, Beckung, & Uvebrant, 2001). Periventricular leukomalacia is thought to be caused by an ischemic insult to the periventricular white matter (Volpe, 1989).

CP can also be the result of perinatal ischemic injury in the term infant, which is usually the result of hypoxic–ischemic injury most likely mediated by glutamate toxicity. These hypoxic–ischemic injuries can result in (1) border zone infarctions, which are limited to border zone regions between arterial distributions; (2) global necrosis, which may cause microcephaly and cystic necrosis of the brain; and (3) involvement of the basal ganglia and the thalamus. If children suffer intrapartum infarction they may develop choreoathetosis CP due to damage to the basal ganglia (Menkes & Curran, 1994). Kernicterus, which is due to excessive bilirubin, destroys the basal ganglia and can also result in choreoathetoid CP. In Western countries, however, this form of CP has been drastically reduced with the use of double-exchange transfusion to decrease bilirubin levels when they approach dangerous levels. Infarction of the middle cerebral artery distribution late in the third trimester often results in congenital hemiplegia, with right hemiplegia occurring twice as often as left hemiplegia.

Ataxic CP in the most pure sense of the term is caused by a hypocerebellum or may be the result of brain damage following a traumatic brain injury. A form of CP resembling ataxic CP can be caused by metabolic abnormalities, and there are some syndromes associated with mental retardation that have motor involvement resembling ataxia. CP can also be due to congenital malformations such as neuronal migration anomalies (schizencephaly, lissencephaly, polymicrogyria, hydranencephaly, hypocerebellum, Dandy–Walker malformation). Congenital infections during the first trimester can also cause severe to profound forms of CP—that is, cytomegalovirus (periventricular calcifications), toxoplasmosis (calcifications in the periventricular area, basal ganglia, and cortex), and herpes simplex types 1 and 2 (predominantly type 2).

Topographical

Topographical classification of CP relates to those body structures in which posture and/or movement are compromised. Following are the topographical forms of CP (Capute & Accardo, 1996; Crothers & Paine, 1988; Prechtl & Stemmer, 1962; Scherzer & Tchamuter, 1990).

- *Spastic diplegia.* Lower extremities are the most dysfunctional extremities. Upper extremities may appear completely normal, but they may be somewhat compromised.
- *Asymmetric spastic diplegia.* Lower extremity is more involved on one side than the other. It is possible that the side less affected appears totally normal.
- *Spastic hemiplegia.* One side of the pyramidal tract of the brain is affected causing the opposite side of the body to be impaired. The upper extremity is more involved than the lower extremity.
- *Double spastic hemiplegia.* This term applies to a person in whom both upper extremities are more involved than the lower extremities. This is rare, and the term used is confusing because hemiplegia means one side of the brain/body.

- *Spastic quadriplegia (triplegia)*. All four extremities are involved. Usually, each of the extremities is equally involved, but in some instance one extremity may be less involved. Oral–motor structures are usually involved, and this is termed *pseudobulbar palsy* (indicating that much of the impairment is due to neurological overflow due to the brain injury).
- *Dyskinetic cerebral palsy*. All four extremities and the oral pharyngeal musculature are involved. The oral–motor involvement is termed bulbar palsy.
- *Ataxic cerebral palsy*. All four extremities are involved and the oral musculature is also involved.

Early Clues to Cerebral Palsy

Clinical research suggests that the early neurological signs associated with CP may not be sensitive enough by themselves to apply the diagnosis of CP (Nelson & Ellenberg, 1982). A "focal" neurological finding, however, increases the clinician's suspicion regarding the diagnosis. During the first year, findings such as "sustained clonus" or extensor plantar reflexes can be markers of concern, but they do not confirm a diagnosis.

The classic study and resulting paper "Children who 'Outgrew' Cerebral Palsy" (Nelson & Ellenberg, 1982) demonstrated that early motor signs of CP at 1 year of age can resolve. In this study, a neurological examination was performed by neurologists from 12 cooperating teaching hospitals on 37,000 children who were enrolled in the National Collaborative Perinatal Project (NCPP) of the National Institute of Neurological and Communicative Disorders and Stroke. At the age of 1 year, 229 children were diagnosed with "definite" CP. Two hundred twenty-three of 229 were reexamined at 7 years and also received vision, hearing, speech, and psychological evaluations. Some 51.1% of those diagnosed with CP at 1 year of age lost the diagnosis at 7 years of age. The majority of children who lost this diagnosis were diagnosed with other neurological problems at 7 years of age. Notable diagnoses applied to the children who lost the diagnosis of CP were mental retardation (22.3%), speech motor abnormalities (12.8%), reduced visual acuity (50%), abnormal extraocular movements (22.3%), and hyperactivity (19.1%).

Examination and Diagnosis of Cerebral Palsy

Elsbeth Kong (1991) proposed that "tables of reflexes" and "motor milestones" should be used as guidelines to determine if there is a problem, but observation of movements in various positions are essential for a valid diagnosis of CP. The components of proposed observation include variability of movement, the use of accessory muscles, movement against gravity, and changes in tone according to position. Although much information can be gained from such lengthy clinical observations, they do not ensure a diagnosis of CP.

The traditional neurological exam can also be useful with modifications in making a valid diagnosis of CP. However, because of the evolving nature of CP and particularly in the case of spastic diplegia, different neurological signs need to be examined as the infant develops and matures. In early exams, infants with spastic diplegias display hypotonia especially in the axis of the body. This results in the inability to maintain head or body in the midline position and inability to right the head and neck. In prone, these infants are unable to lift their head off the surface of a table or crib during the first half of the first year. Infants with CP continue into the second half of the first year to have "head lag" when pulled to a sitting position. Postural, equilibrium, and righting responses are delayed and are in competition with whole-body brain stem reflexes (primitive reflexes). The infants are unable to develop a downward parachute by 4 months and fail to develop a positive support. They "sit in air" if an attempt is made to get them to bear weight on extended lower extremities during the first 6 months of age. It is common to see sustained clonus (six or more beats of clonus) when elicited; spontaneous clonus of the lower extremities is a common sign of pathology. During the transition phase at about 6 months chronological age or for the premature infant 6 months adjusted age, infants with CP display less hypotonia and some subtle signs of hypertonia appear. The hypertonic phase usually begins at 9 months to 1 year of age.

Neuropsychological Functioning

With the improved survival in preterm infants, the interest in tracking the cognitive and neuropsychological outcome of CP and especially spastic diplegia has increased. The incidence of major disabilities (moderate/severe mental retardation, seizures) associated with CP has remained constant, but an increasing number of children with CP display learning disabilities, attention-deficit/hyperactivity disorder, and borderline intelligence (Aylward, 2002).

The literature on the cognitive and neuropsychological functioning of children with CP is sparse and often does not differentiate between types of CP (Fennell & Dikel, 2001). The few studies that have investigated children with different types of CP have found that individuals with spastic quadriplegia are in most cases severely intellectually impaired, whereas half of the children with spastic hemiplegia obtain IQ scores in the average range (Nelson & Ellenberg, 1982). Research on children with spastic diplegia has shown that performance IQs are significantly lower than verbal IQs, which are in the average range (Fedrizza et al., 1993, 1996; Goto, Ota, Iai, Sugita, & Tanabe, 1994). A recent study that investigated the mental processing of children with spastic diplegia found that (1) sequential processing scores were superior to simultaneous processing scores on the Kaufman Assessment Battery for Children; (2) half of the children with spastic diplegia received high scores in sequential processing; and (3) the areas of inferior processing were visuomotor coordination and spatial arrangement (Shimizu, 1999). Similar findings have been reported by other investigators (Olsen, Vainionpaa, Paakko, Pyhtinen, & Jarvelin, 1998). Thus, this form of CP appears to be characterized by specific impairments in visual–perceptual–motor functions (Fedrizza et al., 1996; Goto et al., 1994; Koeda & Takeshita, 1992).

A study that investigated neuropsychological functioning in children with hemiplegic CP found that right-hemiplegic children (left lateralized brain lesion) displayed deficits on measures of syntactic awareness and sentence repetition, and higher-order language functions; however, receptive vocabulary was intact. Left-hand function was correlated with math achievement scores, which supports the idea that mathematical ability requires good visual–spatial skills (Kiessling, Denckla, & Carlton, 1983).

Children with extrapyramidal CP have been found to display a wide range of intellectual abilities, with many of these individuals scoring in the normal range (Lou, 1998). Because of severe dysarthria of the muscles involved in speech, some of these children may have delays or deficits in language skills (Fennell & Dikel, 2001).

In children with hypotonic CP, intellectual functioning is rarely impaired. However, this type of CP is associated with learning disabilities (Tomlin, 1995). The specific subtypes of learning disabilities have not been described in detail; however, Fennell and Dikel (2001) stated that these children displayed deficits in motor programming for handwriting, attentional dysfunction, and motor output.

Studies have also examined the relationship between handedness and cognitive functioning in children with CP. It has been suggested that early left-hemisphere lesions are associated with pathological left-handedness and a shift of language to the right hemisphere (Rasmussen & Milner, 1977). Carlson and colleagues (1994) compared 18 children with right- and 13 children with left-sided congenital hemiplegia to normal age-matched controls on measures of verbal and nonverbal function. CT scans were performed on 27/31 hemiplegic children. All children with left-sided hemiplegia (right-hemispheric-index group) were right-handed. In the children with right-sided hemiplegia (left-hemispheric-index group), 16/18 were left-handed, and all 18 children preferred the left foot. In the normal control group, 16 children preferred the right hand and 3 children displayed a left-hand preference. The two hemiplegic groups were impaired on nonverbal functions compared with controls. The right-hemiplegic group was more impaired on verbal functions than the left-hemiplegic group and the controls; however, these impairments were restricted to girls.

In summary, there remains a significant lack of precise information on the cognitive and neuropsychological functioning of children with different types of CP. The limited research that has been done suggests that children with different types of CP display different patterns of deficits in neuropsychological functioning and that preterm children with spastic diplegia are at particular risk for visual perceptual deficits.

In terms of psychosocial outcome, children with CP and average intelligence have been found to have poor self-esteem, poor self-concept, and delayed social adjustment in a longitudinal study that followed the children from adolescence into adulthood (Magill-Evans & Restall, 1991) (see Miyahara & Cratty, Chapter 19, this volume, for a more detailed discussion of the psychosocial adjustment of children with disabilities). Limited research however, has directly investigated the psychosocial outcomes of children with CP. Further, with the studies that have been conducted, there are questions regarding the methodologies used. Thus, there is a need for more and better investigations of the factors affecting psychosocial adjustment in children with CP.

Management

Significant progress has been made in the treatment of CP. New technology such as gait analyses can be helpful in making decisions with regard to intervention. In addition, a number of medications can be used to treat individuals with CP. The use of Botox (botulinum toxin) has been found to be safer than motor point blocks (Bhakta, Cozens, Alastair, Chamberlain, & Banford, 2000; Ubhi, Bhakta, Ives, Allgar, & Rousounis, 2000). Small amounts have been found to reduce spasticity for 3 to 6 months. Baclofen pumps are an advance over oral antispasticity medication because they maintain an effect over longer periods of time; however, unpleasant side effects are problematic.

It is very important that children with CP receive adequate nutrition; that orthotics, prosthetics, and antispasticity medication are suppressing contractures; that equipment such as wheelchairs are appropriate for their size; and that adequate equipment is provided as this will prevent bone and muscle wasting (i.e., for the non-ambulatory child with CP). The demands of the child on the caregiver(s) must also be taken into account and caregivers should be provided with assistance in dealing with the stresses associated with caring for the child.

Because of the high incidence of visual disturbances, children with CP need an initial eye exam and follow-up if called for. Also, investigations for seizure disorders may be needed. Multidisciplinary intervention is important and both occupational and physical therapy are essential to improving motor function, delaying the development of musculoskeletal contractures, and furthering adaptive skills and hand use. Neuro-development therapy (NDT), however, has never been shown to be useful. In a ran-domized, masked, controlled study of infants and toddlers with CP, those assigned to infant stimulation made significantly better progress on both the Bayley Mental and Motor scales than did the group receiving NDT (Palmer et al., 1989) (see Polatajko, Rodger, Dhillon, & Hirji, Chapter 21, this volume, for a more detailed discussion of treatment interventions).

NEUROMUSCULAR DISEASES

Neuromuscular diseases are usually progressive disorders, but sometimes they are acute disorders that can be corrected. There are countless muscular disorders and rare subtypes of the same disorders. This chapter discusses the more common forms that can present during childhood (Gupta & Appleton, 2001). Table 5.1 outlines the neuromuscular disorders that are discussed and describes the muscle groups involved and the genetic markers. Some neuromuscular diseases are not progressive. In the case of progressive neuromuscular diseases, however, the course may quickly lead to death or may be slowly progressive and not lead to death. The time of onset and the developmental evolution of these diseases are of primary importance to both the clinician and the family. Many of these diseases have defined genetic etiologies, and if this is the case, the parent(s) need to receive genetic counseling. Onset of these diseases is variable, some occurring in childhood and some in adulthood. This chapter focuses only on the neuromuscular diseases that have an onset during early childhood, middle childhood, and adolescence.

Duchenne Muscular Dystrophy

Duchenne muscular dystrophy (DMD) is an X-linked recessive genetic disease and is the most common hereditary neuromuscular disease. It is characterized by progressive weakness and degeneration of skeletal muscles, which is associated with pathological changes in the muscles, due to deficiency of the protein dystrophin (Dubowitz, 1995). Children with this condition lose previously acquired gross and fine motor skills such as the ability to walk and write. Normally, the X-linked recessive type of inheritance confines the disorder to males, but carrier women may show a variety of minor muscle abnormalities and are occasionally symptomatic. The disease is not limited to a spe-

TABLE 5.1. The Muscular Dystrophies and Peripheral Neuropathies

Disease	Onset	Muscle groups affected	Inheritance	Gene/ protein
Duchenne	2–4 years	Proximal	X-linked recessive	Xp21/ dystrophin
Becker	11 years (mean)	Mainly limb girdle and proximal	X-linked recessive	Xp21/ dystrophin
Limb-girdle group	Child to adolescent	Mainly limb girdle and proximal	Autosomal recessive	13q12, 17q12– q21,15q, 2p, 5q/ various proteins
Congenital muscular dystrophy	Infancy	All	Autosomal recessive	
Merosin deficient				6q
Merosin normal				?
Plus central nervous system abnormality				
Fukuyama				9q31-33/ fukutin
Walker–Warberg				?
Muscle–eye–brain				POMGnT1?
Facioscapulohumeral	Adolescent and adult	Initially proximal and later distal	Autosomal dominant	4q35
Myotonic dystrophy (Steinert)	Wide variance	Distal	Autosomal dominant 19q13 expands	
Spinal muscular atrophy	Childhood	Proximal	Autosomal recessive	5q12.2– 13.3

cific race. The most comprehensive monograph on this disorder to date is that of Emery (1998).

DMD has a lifetime incidence of approximately 1:3,500 in male infants (Roland, 2000). Early development is normal, although the average age of walking is delayed (20 months). The onset of the disease occurs between 2 and 4 years of age. Clinical onset is marked by weakness and wasting of proximal muscles. Pseudohypertrophy of the calf muscles is a characteristic finding. Proximal muscle wasting occurs in the upper and lower extremities, shoulders, and pelvic girdles. There is no involvement of facial muscles. These children develop musculoskeletal contractures (e.g., equinovarus). Most children are wheelchair bound by age 12, and subsequently develop progressive scoliosis and respiratory problems. Cardiac involvement is common, and the EKG (electrocardiogram) is almost always abnormal by late childhood. Death usually occurs by the early 20s and is often the result of a respiratory infection (Dubowitz, 1995).

The most comprehensive text with regard to the molecular genetics of this disorder was published in 1998 by Emery. In individuals with DMD, serum creatine phosphokinase (CPK) activity is very high, particularly in the early stages of the disease before clinical signs are evident. The X-linked recessive gene for this disorder is located at the middle of the short arm of the X chromosome (Xp21), and it is one of the largest base pairs in length containing around 60 coding regions. A deletion in the dystrophin gene is identified in 60% of the cases. Dystrophin is a cytoskeletal protein, which is largely specific to skeletal, cardiac, and smooth muscle. Assessment of dystrophin in a muscle biopsy is an essential part of the examination for DMD, as absence of dystrophin confirms the diagnosis (Dubowitz, 1995; Mendel et al., 2001). If the dystrophin protein is present in reduced amount and size, a milder form of Xp21 dystrophy (i.e., Becker type) is suggested (Dubowitz, 1995).

Neuropsychological Functioning

The prevalence of mental retardation in individuals with DMD has been reported to range from 20 to 50% (Benson & Hunter, 1987; Rapaport et al., 1992). A recent meta analysis of intellectual functioning in 1,146 individuals with DMD reported that 34.8% of the children had a Full Scale intelligence quotient (FIQ) of less than 70 (Cotton, Voudouris, & Greenwood, 2001). After reviewing the literature on intellectual functioning in children with DMD, Dubowitz (1995) concluded that the mean IQ of children with DMD in most of the studies was in the region of 85 and that the range of IQ seemed to follow a normal distribution with some skewing to the left. Studies have shown that in DMD, the cognitive impairment is not progressive and is not correlated with the duration or severity of the muscle disease or the age of the child (Prosser, Murphy, & Thompson, 1969; Worden & Vignas, 1962; Zellweger & Hanson, 1968). Recent molecular and neuropsychological analyses have suggested that deletions and duplications located in the distal part of the dystrophin gene appear to be associated with cognitive impairment (Moizard et al., 1998).

Studies that have examined the neuropsychological functioning of children with DMD have focused on the verbal deficits displayed by these children; few have examined the exact nature of the nonverbal (i.e., visual–perceptual and visual–motor) deficits. Studies that have investigated Verbal IQ (VIQ)–Performance IQ (PIQ) discrepancies have reported that VIQ tends to be lower (Appleton, Bushby, Gardner-Medwin, Welch, & Kelly, 1991; Dorman, Hurley, & D'Avogon, 1988; Karagan, Richman, & Sorensen, 1980). Investigations of verbal functioning in individuals with DMD have reported impairments in verbal fluency (Billard, Gillet, Barthez, Hommet, & Bertrand, 1998; Dorman et al., 1988), reading (Billard et al., 1992, 1998), phonological production (Billard et al., 1998; Dorman et al., 1988), receptive language (Smith, Sibert, & Harper, 1990), expressive language (Karagan et al., 1980), verbal learning and attention (Billard et al., 1998; Hinton, De Vivo, Nereo, Goldstein, & Stern, 2000; Savage & Adams, 1979), and working memory (Hinton et al., 2000).

A number of early studies of children with DMD reported that verbal abilities were more adversely affected than nonverbal abilities (Karagan & Zellweger, 1978; Leibowitz & Dubowitz, 1981). The recent meta analysis by Cotton and colleagues (2001) examined this and found that that the mean VIQ for their sample ($N = 881$) was 80.4 and the mean PIQ ($N = 878$) was 85.4. They asserted that a 5-point VIQ–PIQ discrepancy was not clinically significant. They also reported that not all the children who participated in their study displayed deficits in VIQ and that some of the children had PIQs that were significantly less than their VIQs.

It has been argued that in children with DMD, PIQ declines with age and the pro-gression of the disease (Black, 1973). As these nonverbal tasks require speed, as well as accuracy, it is not surprising that individuals with DMD would evidence a decline in PIQ as the disease becomes more severe and the motor skills decline. More research that investigates the exact nature of nonverbal (i.e., visual–perceptual and visual–motor) deficits in children with DMD is needed. Further, the influence of factors such as age and severity of the disease on the expression of these nonverbal impairments is essential.

Management

Care for children with DMD should be provided by a multidisciplinary team consist-ing of a pediatrician, physiatrist, pediatric neurologist, genetic counselor, physical therapist, occupational therapist, orthopedic surgeon, respiratory therapist, and social worker. Various interventions can be used in the habilitation of children with this pro-gressive disease such as physical and occupational therapy. Medications such as pred-nisone have been found to prolong walking ability in children with DMD; however, significant side effects, including excessive weight gain, have been noted (Dubowitz, 1995). Transplantation of myoblasts (muscle stem cells) from a healthy donor has also been used as a treatment but with limited success. In most cases, immunological rejec-tion of the tissue and limited ability of the transplanted cells to migrate into other mus-cle tissues have resulted in the failure of this treatment. Current research is focusing on muscle transplantation and gene therapy.

Becker Muscular Dystrophy

Becker muscular dystrophy (BMD) is like DMD but milder with a later onset and pro-gression of the disease (Dubowitz, 1995). The incidence of BMD is around 1 in 30,000 to 40,000 male births (Garner-Medwin, 1980). The mean age of clinical onset of BMD is 11 years of age with the lower limbs being affected first. Following the initial presen-tation, the limb girdle and proximal limb muscles become clinically affected. Like DMD, pseudohypertrophy of the calves develops. Facial muscles are not affected. Se-rum CPK is usually elevated. The mean age for needing a wheelchair is 27 years, and the mean age of death is 42 years (range is 23–63 years) (Emery & Skinner, 1976).

BMD is also an X-linked recessive disease and recent studies with recombinant DNA techniques have shown that it has the same location as the Duchenne gene. The relationship between DMD and BMD has been demonstrated through molecular ge-netic studies (Dubowitz, 1995). In BMD, however, the deletion of the gene is small in comparison to the DMD gene (Dubowitz, 1995; Norman, Thomas, Coakley, & Harper, 1980). The protein dystrophin is absent in DMD, but normal or reduced amounts of an altered protein are seen in BMD (Dubowitz, 1995; Hoffman et al., 1988). The habilitation approach for BMD is similar to that for DMD.

Neuropsychological Functioning

Few studies have investigated the neurocognitive functioning of individuals with BMD; yet there are some suggestions in the early literature that BMD may be associated with mental retardation (Emery & Skinner, 1976; Zellweger & Hanson, 1967). However, a more recent study by Karagan and Sorensen (1981) reported that their subjects with BMD had a mean Verbal IQ of 89.94 and a mean Performance IQ of 94.19, and that there was a significant discrepancy between VIQ and PIQ with patients with BMD obtaining significantly lower VIQ scores. Melo et al. (1995) in their study of 22 patients with BMD did not find a significant discrepancy between VIQ and PIQ (VIQ = 87.6; PIQ = 85.4). Furthermore, only one of their patients evidenced mild mental retardation. Thus, the limited evidence to date suggests that BMD may be associated with lowered cognitive functioning relative to the normal population; however, whether individuals with BMD evidence lower VIQ relative to PIQ is open to question.

Autosomal Limb-Girdle Dystrophies

This disorder, like BMD and DMD, is a limb-girdle muscular dystrophy (LGMD); however, it is an autosomal recessive disease and so both sexes are affected equally. In most families, weakness usually develops in late childhood, but it can develop earlier. Some affected patients do not present until early adult life. Weakness can begin either in the shoulder or in the pelvic girdle. As the disease progresses, proximal limb weakness progresses. Distal strength is spared. Facial weakness can occur, but it does not cause the significant weakness seen in facioscapulohumeral dystrophy. Progression in patients that present in childhood may be quick or it may be slow and progressive. Cardiac involvement is not a usual feature of LGMD, but abnormal EKG patterns are found in some cases. Defects in a range of muscle specific proteins (e.g., adhalin, sarcoglycans, and calpain) have been noted in individuals who suffer from this disorder (Dubowitz, 1995; Emery, 1998).

To make this diagnosis, the late-onset Kugelberg–Welander form of spinal muscular atrophy must be ruled out, as well as specific congenital myopathies and metabolic myopathies. An electromyographic (EMG) is useful to rule out spinal muscular atrophy. However, to rule out other possible diseases (glycogenosis and chronic polymyositis), muscle biopsy is recommended.

Neuropsychological Functioning

In terms of neurocognitive outcomes, few studies were found in the literature. Melo and colleagues (1995) examined intellectual functioning in 22 individuals with LGMD using the Wechsler Adult Intelligence Scale. Mean FIQ was found to be 87.8; no significant discrepancy was noted between VIQ and PIQ. The distribution of IQ scores was quite wide and ranged from 59 to 113. In contrast to the findings of Melo and colleagues, Miladi, Bourguignon, and Hentati (1999) reported that the mean nonverbal IQ (as measured by The Test of Nonverbal Intelligence, 2nd Edition) of a Tunisian population suffering from LGMD was 102. Their results also indicated that this population did not display a deficit in basic perceptual skills. The large differences between these two studies in reported mean IQ could be due to a number of factors, including (1) differences in the measures used to assess intelligence, (2) differences in the socioeconomic and education profiles of the samples, and (3) differences in the type(s) of LGMD found in these two populations, one from Brazil and the other from Tunisia.

Thus, at this point it would be premature to draw any conclusions regarding the neurocognitive functioning of individuals with LGMD.

Congenital Muscular Dystrophy

Congenital muscular dystrophy (CMD) refers to a group of disorders in which infants present with muscle weakness at birth or within the first few months of life; hypertonia is often associated with this condition. These disorders are associated with a dystrophic pattern on muscle biopsy. The condition tends to remain relatively static; however, some children may show slow progression, whereas others may have actual functional improvement and achieve the ability to walk. There may be respiratory and swallowing problems at the time of presentation and the diaphragmatic involvement may lead to respiratory failure in later childhood and adolescence (Dubowitz, 1995).

In 1993, an International Consortium on CMD separated a pure form of CMD, without structural brain changes, from three other forms of CMD (Fukuyama, Walker–Warburg, and muscle–eye–brain disease), which were associated with structural brain changes (Dubowitz, 1993–1994). The pure form of CMD has also been separated into two forms: merosin-positive and merosin-negative. Imaging studies have found that children with pure CMD show some changes of signal on magnetic resonance imaging (MRI) and that these changes are localized in the white matter, affect both hemispheres, spare the corpus callosum and the brain stem, and are related to merosin deficiency (Dubowitz, & Fardeau, 1993–1994; Philpot, Sewry, Pennock, & Dubowitz, 1995; Vainzof et al., 1995; Van der Knaap, & Valk, 1995). Recent studies have also found cortical dysplasia on brain MRI in infants with merosin deficiency, suggesting that in some cases neuronal migration disorder could be a feature of merosin-deficient CMD (Brett et al., 1998; Sunada, Edgar, Lotz, Rust, & Campbell, 1995; Trevisan et al., 1996). Mild to moderate cerebellar hypoplasia has also been reported in a significant proportion of children with merosin-deficient CMD (Philpot et al., 1999; Trevisan et al., 1996; Voit, 1997–1998) but also in children with merosin-positive CMD (Echenne, Rivier, Jellali, et al., 1997; Echenne, Rivier, Tardieu, Brive, & Mornet, 1997).

Neuropsychological Functioning

In terms of neurocognitive functioning, severe mental retardation is a consistent feature of the forms of CMD associated with structural brain changes (i.e., Fukuyama, Walker–Warburg, and muscle–eye–brain disease) but has not been associated with merosin-positive and merosin-deficient CMD (Dubowitz, 1993–1994; Dubowitz & Fardeau, 1993–1994; Philpot et al., 1995). A number of case reports have found some degree of cognitive impairment in children with CMD (Echenne, Rivier, Jellali, et al., 1997; Trevisan et al., 1996) and a recent review reported that 20% of patients with CMD showed cognitive impairment and/or epilepsy (Voit, 1997–1998). In a recent study by Mercuri and colleagues (1999), the relationship between cognitive impairment and merosin status in 22 children with pure CMD was investigated. The results indicated that the spectrum of cognitive abilities of children with pure CMD was very wide with FIQ ranging from 51 to 134. No consistent association was found between cognitive abilities and merosin status. When the merosin-positive and merosin-negative groups were subdivided according to MRI findings, it was noted that diffuse white matter changes localized to the periventricular regions did not seem to increase the risk of cognitive difficulties compared to children with CMD who had normal MRIs. The presence of cerebellar hypoplasia ($N = 4$) in addition to these white matter changes was associated with lower PIQ. Furthermore, the one child with cortical dysplasia had severe mental retardation. On the basis of these results, Mercuri and colleagues (1999) concluded that although severe cognitive impairment was relatively rare in children with pure CMD, the spectrum of cognitive abilities was quite wide and that there was no association between cognitive abilities and merosin status.

Facioscapulohumeral Dystrophy

Facioscapulohumeral dystrophy (FSHD) is extremely variable in its presentation. Mild cases are often undetected. Onset usually occurs in late childhood and adolescence. The neck muscles and shoulder girdle are the muscle groups that present the earliest. Winging of the scapula is often also seen in asymptomatic and mild cases. Facial muscles are significantly affected, and the patient is often unable to smile. The patient has weak eye closure. Loss of distal power in the upper extremities occurs late in the course of the disease. The pectoralis major muscle may be absent. Problems with upper extremity functions can be significant. Serum creatinine phosphokinase is usually not elevated. Early signs of this disease can be confirmed by an EMG. The disease progresses very slowly, and severe disability does not occur before middle age. The lifespan of adults with FSHD is usually normal. There is no associated cardiac or intellectual involvement (Dubowitz, 1995).

Myotonic Dystrophy

Myotonic dystrophy (DM) is a progressive multisystem disease with a population incidence of 1:8000 (Wieringa, 1994). Its prominent feature is myotonia, a form of dystonia involving increased muscular contractility. It is perhaps the most variable of all muscular disorders. Even though myotonia is considered a prominent feature, only 36% of patients present with myotonia. Muscle weakness is a presenting symptom in 60% of patients suffering with DM. Somnolence is present in the majority of symptomatic carriers. Initial behavioral signs may be a lack of alertness and activity intermittently throughout the day. It affects multiple organ systems including the following: smooth muscle (frequent problems with constipation), cardiac muscle (cardiac arrhythmias), skeletal muscle (weakness of distal muscles), peripheral nerve, endocrine (associated with diabetes, hypothyroidism), eye (usually cataracts), lungs, skin, hair (frontal baldness), and brain (learning disabilities have been demonstrated, as well as psychiatric problems in later life). Earlier onset is associated with more system involvement. The disorder is usually looked on as a disease of adult life and the classical form has its onset in adolescence or adulthood; however, it may present at birth or during childhood and adolescence (Dubowitz, 1995; Emery, 1998; Harper, 2001a, 2001b, 2001c).

Family studies done in the 1940s (Thomasen, 1948; Thomsen, 1876) clearly showed an autosomal dominant pattern. Recognition that the mutational defect in DM was an unstable trinucleotide repeat expansion on chromosome 19 came in 1992.

This became clear when unusual DNA fragments, variable within a family, were detected in patients affected with DM on chromosome 19 (Buxton et al., 1992; Harley et al., 1992). Six key papers were published that confirmed that the instability was due to a specific trinucleotide (CTG) repeat (Alamadis et al., 1992; Brook et al., 1992; Buxton et al., 1992; Fu et al., 1992; Harley et al., 1992; Mahadevan et al., 1992). In addition, these papers provided sequence data on the gene involved. The study of the gene showed that it had predicted properties of a serine-threonine protein kinase (Harper, 2001a).

In patients with DM, serum CPK is usually elevated. The dystrophic changes are indicators of muscle damage and are seen in other muscular dystrophies. The EMG shows two abnormalities; myotonia potentials show little or no decline in amplitude, and they have a long duration (Dubowitz, 1995; Harper, 2001c).

Harley and colleagues (1993) proposed a classification of four different categories of DM in relation to age of onset and clinical symptoms: (1) the congenital form with clinical symptoms present from birth on (i.e., hypotonic cerebral palsy, and respiratory and/or feeding problems), and mild to moderate developmental delay; (2) the juvenile or childhood form with symptoms present in childhood before the age of 10 years; learning disabilities are often prominent, while neuromuscular symptoms are mild or sometimes even absent; (3) the classical or adult form with typical neuromuscular symptoms in adolescence or early adult life; and (4) the mild form with minimal or no neuromuscular symptoms in middle or older age.

Studies have shown that the congenital form requires approximately 1,000 CTG repeats. In the congenital form, the neonate is extremely hypotonic at birth and numerous systematic involvements can be expected. The childhood form usually requires approximately 200–800 CTG repeats. With this number of repeats, the symptoms can occur anywhere from several months of age up to adolescence. A patient with 100–200 CTG repeats usually presents in early adulthood. The initial carrier in most cases has approximately 50 repeats and may or may not develop symptoms until later in life (Dubowitz, 1995; Emery, 1998; Harper, 2001a, 2001b, 2001c).

Neuropsychological Functioning

Congenital DM is usually associated with in cognitive impairment (Dubowitz, 1995; Harper, 2001c; Martinello, Piazza, Pastorello, Angelini, & Trevisan, 1999; Roig, Balliu, Navarro, Brugera, & Losada, 1994; Steyaert et al., 1997). Martinello and colleagues (1999) reported that in their study, the IQs of children with congenital DM ranged from 52 to 79 and Roig and colleagues (1994) reported that all of their patients had IQs under 65. MRI studies of children with congenital DM have shown ventricular dilation, hypoplasia of the corpus callosum, and mild abnormalities of the supratentorial white matter (Martinello et al., 1999).

As noted previously, children with the juvenile form of DM do not display any significant neurological or motor symptoms before adulthood; learning disabilities are the most prominent feature of this type of DM (Steyaert, de Die Smulders, Fryns, Goosens, & Willekens, 2000). Two studies by Steyaert and colleagues (1997, 2000) found that the FIQ of children with childhood DM were below 100 ranging from 50 to 97. Lower IQ was correlated with longer expansion in the DM gene. Furthermore, the expansion lengths correlated with the transmitting parent's sex with inheritance from the mother associated with longer expansion length than from the father.

Steyaert and colleagues (2000) also reported that DM was frequently associated with a psychiatric diagnosis. Fifteen of the 24 children (63%) obtained a diagnosis on a structured psychiatric interview. The most frequent diagnoses were attention-deficit/hyperactivity disorder (ADHD) (33%) and anxiety disorder (25%). The finding that the most frequent psychiatric diagnosis was ADHD is consistent with the findings by van Spaendonck, Ter Bruggen, Weyn-Banningh, and Maassen (1995) that in adult-onset DM, executive functions can be impaired. This suggests that the frontal areas of the brain may be involved in the pathophysiology of DM (Steyaert et al., 2000).

Adult-onset DM appears to be associated with normal intelligence (Rubinsztein, Rubinsztein, McKenna, Goodburn, & Holland, 1997; Turnpenny, Clark, & Kelly, 1994). However, studies that have investigated specific neuropsychological functions have reported that individuals with adult-onset DM show difficulties with memory (Rubensztein et al., 1997), executive functions (van Spaendonck et al., 1995), attention and concentration (Woodward, Heaton, Simon, & Ringel, 1982), abstraction and new concept formation (Bird, Follett, & Griep, 1983; Woodward et al., 1982), and visual–spatial tasks (Bird et al., 1983; Censori, Danni, Del Pesce, & Provinciali, 1990).

Spinal Muscular Atrophy

Spinal muscular atrophy (SMA) is a genetically heterogeneous group of disorders characterized by loss of motor function, muscular atrophy, and degeneration of the anterior horn cells in the spinal cord and brain stem. SMA has an incidence exceeding 1:10,000 and is one of the most common autosomal recessive diseases in childhood and adolescence. Patients with SMA present with muscle weakness affecting the proximal limb muscles more than distal muscles and the lower limb muscle more than upper limb muscles, hypotonia, and hyporeflexia or no deep tendon reflexes. They develop fasciculations that are usually noted in the tongue. The inheritance of most forms of SMA is autosomal recessive. In most patients a deletion in chromosome 5q has been detected. There are three possible genes that have been described that exist in this region of chromosome 5: the survival motor neuron gene, the neuronal apoptosis inhibitory protein gene, and the p44 gene. Commercial gene testing is available, but the complex genetic organization of this region has made molecular analysis very difficult (Dubowitz, 1995; Emery, 1998; Wirth, 2000).

Three subtypes of SMA can be differentiated according to the age of onset, severity of symptoms, and motor milestones. SMA type 1 patients have the onset of symptoms during the first 6 months of life and typically have a lifespan of less than 2 years of age. SMA type 2 has its onset during the first 18 months. These patients may sit unassisted but do not develop walking and typically survive into adulthood. With individuals with type 2 SMA, the single most important factor determining prognosis is respiratory function. Those cases with more in intercostal involvement have a poorer outlook. SMA type III has its onset after 18 months of age. These patients develop walking and have a nearly normal life expectancy (International SMA Consortium, 1999).

Neuropsychological Functioning

Studies that have investigated the neurocognitive functioning of children with SMA have reported that these children display normal intelligence (e.g., Billard et al., 1992; von Gontard et al., 2002; Whelan, 1987). In fact, von Gontard and colleagues (2002) in the largest study of children with SMA types 1–III ($N = 96$) to date reported no significant differences in IQ, as assessed by the Raven Colored and Standard Progressive Matrices, between the children with SMA (mean IQ = 109.6) and healthy controls (mean IQ = 104.1). Furthermore, they found no significant differences in IQ among the different types of SMA. Thus, it can be concluded that the IQs of children with SMA fall in the normal range.

METABOLIC DISEASES

It is important to briefly mention metabolic diseases that can be confused with CP or with muscular diseases. Table 5.2 contains a list of some metabolic disorders and the movement problems with which they can present. They can be divided into various categories: leukodystrophies, gray matter diseases, amino acid disorders, organic acid disorders, lysosomal enzyme deficiencies, genetic syndromes, and mitochondrial diseases. This information is included to give the reader an idea of the multitude of diseases one must consider when evaluating a child who presents with motor deficits.

NEURODEVELOPMENTAL ASSESSMENT

Children who present with motor problems typically undergo a neurodevelopmental assessment. The following sections discuss the essential components of such an assessment.

Medical History

The medical history is a very important component of the neurodevelopmental assessment. It should include information on antecedents and family genetics as these may

TABLE 5.2. Metabolic Diseases Associated with Movement Disorders

Disease	Age of onset	Abnormal movement
Metachromatic leukodystrophy	2–3 years	Loss of gait
Adrenoleukodystrophy	8–9 years	Spasticity
Neuropathy–ataxia–retinitis pigmentosa	Variable	Ataxia
Kearne–Sayre syndrome	Variable	Ophthalmoplegia
Type I glutaric aciduria	Variable	Choreoathetosis
Propionic acadimia	Variable	Choreoathetosis
Lesch–Nyhan disease	First year	Dystonia or chorea
Batten's disease	Second year	Spasticity
Wilson's disease	Childhood	Dystonia
Friedreich's ataxia	Before puberty	Gait and limb ataxia
Spinocerebellar ataxia 1–14	Various	Various
Machado–Joseph disease	Depends on penetrance	Ataxia

TABLE 5.3. Frequent Causes of Neuromotor Disabilities

- Fetal teratogens
  - Cytomegalovirus
  - Toxoplasmosis
- Fetal passage through the birth canal
  - Herpes simplex virus
  - Group B streptococcal meningitis
- Germinal matrix events in premature infants
  - Periventriucular leukomalacia (PVL) due to poor autonomic regulation of blood pressure in premature neonates of ±30 weeks' gestation or less
  - Intraventricular hemorrhage associated with PVL
- Perinatal strokes
  - Associated with meconium aspiration
  - Associated with persistent fetal circulation or chronic hypoxemia
- Very hyperbilirubinemia (kernicterus)
  - Early discharge of full-term infants without follow-up by parent
  - Very quick rise in Hyperbilirubin in a neonate with very low birth weight

provide clues to the cause of the disability. Information on motor and developmental milestones may also be useful in developing some hypotheses regarding the child's difficulties. It is also important to establish whether or not the child has evidenced a loss of motor and/or developmental abilities. A complete pregnancy and birth history, which includes information on problems that occurred during the pregnancy, prescription and nonprescription medications (anticonvulsants, antidepressants, antipsychotic, lithium, etc.) taken, other drugs and substances consumed that are potentially teratogenic (cigarettes, alcohol, cocaine, heroin, marijuana, hallucinogens, etc.), and the time during the pregnancy and the frequency with which they were taken should be obtained. Birth weight in comparison to gestational age should be considered. The clinician should also inquire about factors that could have affected the child's development (e.g., early childhood head injury). The medical history should also include information on medical diseases and conditions that the child has experienced, previous hospitalizations, and medications. A genetic family tree of both the father and mother's relatives should also be obtained. This knowledge base can assist in linking antecedents to potential causes of developmental disabilities. Table 5.3 lists some frequent causes of static encephalopathy from the perinatal period that are associated with impaired motor development.

Physical Examination

The physical exam includes a general exam of all systems. It may elucidate both the cause of neuromotor delay and possible associated conditions (e.g., cardiac conditions). The examination should test for joint limitation and contractures, note muscular hypertrophy, hemihypertropy, pseudohypertrophy, muscular wasting, and differences in the length of either upper or lower extremities. Anthropometric measurements should also be taken. In addition, dysmorphologies should be noted and laboratory investigations that could elucidate the basis for the motor deficits should be ordered.

Neurodevelopmental Examination

Delayed motor milestones throughout the first year of life are a marker for neuro-motor or muscular deficits (see Table 5.4 for a list of motor milestones and the average age of attainment). The neurodevelopmental exam, which includes both a neurological exam and an assessment of neurocognitive functioning, is an essential component in the identifying motor deficit, elucidating the basis for these motor problems and determining the functional level of the child. The neurological exam requires an assessment of cranial nerve function, tone, reflexes, involuntary movements (i.e., dystonia, choreiform movements, athetoid movements, tremors, and nystagmus), strength, and gait. During the first 3 years, neurological development undergoes rapid development and changes; therefore, the tasks used to assess neurological functioning change as the child matures and develops. For example, the tasks used to assess cranial nerve function in the infant change significantly over the first year of life. Beginning at 1 month of age the normal infant can follow an object horizontally. At 2 months of age, the infant can follow an object vertically, and at 3 months of age the infant can follow an object moving in a circular fashion. By 4 months of age, the infant will blink if an ob-

TABLE 5.4. Average Ages of Motor Milestones

Gross motor milestones	Fine motor milestones	Mean age of attainment
Rolls over prone to supine	Hands open; hands to midline; reach	4 months
Rolls over supine to prone; sits (supported)	Obtains object	5 months
Sits (alone)	Transfers object; unilateral reach; radial rake	6 months
Creeps (prone locomotion)		7 months
Comes to sit; crawls; stands		8 months
Immature cruise	Scissors grasp (three-finger grasp)	9 months
Mature cruise	Immature (inferior) pincer grasp	10 months
Walks few steps or one hand held	Mature (overhand) pincer grasp	11 months
Walks (independently)	Voluntary release (opens pincer)	12 months
Runs	Scribbles spontaneously; uses spoon without spilling	18 months
Walks up and down stairs one step at a time	Imitates stroke with a pencil; hand preference	24 months
Alternates feet going up stairs; pedals tricycle	Copies a circle	3 years
Alternates feet going down stairs	Copies a square; buttons	4 years
Stand on one foot 15 seconds; hops 15 times	Draws a triangle; static tripod pencil grasp	5 years
Rhythmic skipping	Catches a ball on a bounce; ties shoes	5½ years
Pedals bicycle	Spreads with a knife; catches ball on fly	6 years

ject moves close toward the infant's eye. The infant first "orients" or turns his or her head toward a voice at 4 months of age. At 5 months of age, the infant turns his or her head toward sound. By 7 months of age, if a bell is rung to one side and above eye level, the infant will first turn to the side of the sound and then up to find the bell. At 9 months, the infant will look directly at the bell that is located to one side and above eye level.

In children who are 4 years of age and older, in addition to the an assessment of cranial nerve function, tone, reflexes, involuntary movement, strength, and gait, the neurological exam should also include observations of the behavior of the child, such as his or her responses to interactions, level of activity, temperament, and undressing and dressing. Hand preference or the lack of preference should be noted and vision and hearing should be screened. The child's standing posture should also be observed. Having the child come to stand from a prone position on the floor could also shed insight into his or her strength and posture.

The neurocognitive assessment involves an assessment of cognitive, developmental, and adaptive functioning. Measures appropriate for the child's age and level of motor impairment need to be used in order to obtain an accurate picture of the child's level of functioning. Some of the standardized tests that can be used to assess cognitive functioning in children with motor difficulties include the Bayley Scales of Infant Development—II, the Wechsler Preschool and Primary Scales of Intelligence—3rd Edition (WPPSI-III), The Wechsler Intelligence Scale for Children—4th Edition (WISC-IV), The Vineland Adaptive Behavior Scales, The Fagan Test, the Ravens Colored/Progressive Matrices, and the Test of Nonverbal Intelligence, Second Edition. In addition to standardized assessment cognitive function, the neurocognitive assessment could also include other measures of neuropsychological function and a standardized assessment of motor function (see Barnett & Peters, Chapter 4, this volume, for a detailed discussion of standardized motor assessment measures). These measures may provide additional information concerning specific areas of neurocognitive impairment, which may be useful in habilitation.

ACKNOWLEDGMENTS

I wish to thank the late Arnold J. Capute, MD, for his very helpful suggestions in the preparation of this chapter. Dr. Capute, who passed away on November 30, 2003, held an endowed chair at Johns Hopkins School of Medicine and was a Professor of Pediatrics at the Kennedy Krieger Institute. Dr. Capute was the person responsible for making neurodevelopmental disabilities a new subspecialty in pediatrics. He will be greatly missed by all of us who work in the field of developmental disabilities.

REFERENCES

Alamdadis, C., Jansen, C., Amemiya, C., Shutler, G., Tsilfidis, C., Mahadevan, M., et al. (1992). Cloning of the essential myotonic dystrophy region: Mapping of the putative defect. *Nature, 355,* 548–551.

Appleton, R. E., Bushby, K., Gardner-Medwin, D., Welch, J., & Kelly, P. J. (1991). Head circumference and intellectual performance of patients with Duchenne muscular dystrophy. *Developmental Medicine and Children Neurology, 33,* 884–890.

Aylward, G. P. (2002). Cognitive and neuropsychological outcomes: More than IQ scores. *Mental Retardation and Developmental Disabilities Research Reviews, 8*, 234–240.

Benson, B. A., & Hunter, B. (1987). Physical handicaps. In C. L. Frame & J. L. Matson (Eds.), *Handbook of assessment of childhood psychopathology* (pp. 121–134). New York: Plenum Press.

Bhakta, B. B., Cozens, J. A., Alastair, J., Chamberlain, M. A., & Bamford, J. M. (2000). Impact of botulinum toxin type A on disability and carer burden due to arm spasticity after a stroke: A randomised double blind placebo controlled trial. *Journal of Neurology, Neurosurgery and Psychiatry, 69*(2), 217–221.

Billard, C., Gillet, P., Barthez, M., Hommet, C., & Bertrand, P. (1998). Reading ability and processing in Duchenne muscular dystrophy and spinal muscular atrophy. *Developmental Medicine and Child Neurology, 40*, 12–20.

Billard, C., Gillet, P., Signoret, J. L., Uicaut, E., Bertrand, P., Fardeau, M., et al. (1992). Cognitive functions in Duchenne muscular dystrophy: A reappraisal and comparison with spinal muscular atrophy. *Neuromuscular Disorders, 2*, 371–378.

Bird, T. D., Follett, C., & Griep, E. (1983). Cognitive and personality function in myotonic muscular dystrophy. *Journal of Neurology, Neurosurgery and Psychiatry, 46*, 971–980.

Black, F. W. (1973). Intellectual ability as related to age and stage of disease in muscular dystrophy: A brief note. *Journal of Psychology, 84*, 333–334.

Blondis, T. A. (1996). The spectrum of mild neuromotor disabilities. In A. J. Capute & P. J. Accardo (Eds.), *Developmental disabilities in infancy and childhood* (Vol. II, 2nd ed., pp. 199–208). Baltimore: Brookes.

Brett F. M., Costigan, D., Farrell, M. A., Heaphy, P., Thornton, J., & King, M. D. (1998). Merosin-deficient congenital muscular dystrophy and cortical dysplasia. *European Journal of Paediatric Neurology, 2*, 77–82.

Brook, J. D., McCurrach, M. E., Harley, H. G., Buckler, A. J., Church, D., Aburatani, H., et al. (1992). Molecular basis of myotonic dystrophy: Expansion of a trinucleotide (CTG) repeat at the 3'end of a transcript encoding a protein kinase family member. *Cell, 68*, 799–808.

Buxton, J., Shelbourne, P., Davies, J., Jones, C., Van Tongeren, T., Aslandis, C., et al. (1992). Deletion of an unstable fragment of DNA specific to individuals with myotonic dystrophy, *Nature, 355*, 547–548.

Capute, A. J., & Accardo, P. J. (1996). Cerebral palsy: The spectrum of motor dysfunction. In A. J. Capute & P. J. Accardo (Eds.), *Developmental disabilities in infancy and childhood* (Vol. II, 2nd ed., pp. 81–94). Baltimore: Brookes.

Carlson, G., Uvebrant, P., Hugdahl, K., Arvidsson, J., Wiklund, L. M., & von Wendt, L. (1994). Verbal and non-verbal function of children with right versus left-hemiplegic cerebral palsy of pre- and perinatal origin. *Developmental Medicine and Child Neurology, 36*, 503–512.

Censori, B., Danni, M., Del Pesce, M., & Provinciali, L. (1990). Neuropsychological profile in myotonic dystrophy. *Journal of Neurology, 237*, 251–256.

Cotton, S., Voudouris, N. J., & Greenwood, K. M. (2001). Intelligence and Duchenne muscular dystrophy: Full-Scale, Verbal, and Performance intelligence quotients. *Developmental Medicine and Child Neurology, 43*, 497–501.

Crothers, B., & Paine, R. S. (1988). *The natural history of cerebral palsy.* Cambridge, UK: Cambridge University Press.

Dorman, C., Hurley, A. D., & D'Avogon, J. (1988). Language and learning disorders of older boys with Duchenne Muscular Dystrophy. *Developmental Medicine and Child Neurology, 30*, 315–327.

Dubowitz, V. (1993–1994). Workshop report on 22nd ENMC-sponsored meeting on congenital muscular dystrophy held in Baarn, The Netherlands, May 14–16. *Neuromuscular Disorders, 4*, 75–81.

Dubowitz, V. (1995). *Muscle disorders in childhood.* London: Saunders.

Dubowitz, V., & Fardeau, M. (1993–1994). Workshop report on 27nd ENMC-sponsored meeting on congenital muscular dystrophy held in Baarn, The Netherlands, April 22–24. *Neuromuscular Disorders, 4*, 253–258.

Echenne, B., Rivier, F., Jellali, A. J., Azais, M., Mornet, D., Pons, F., et al. (1997). Merosin positive congenital muscular dystrophy with mental deficiency, epilepsy, and MRI changes in the cerebral white matter. *Neuromuscular Disorders, 7*, 187–190.

Echenne, B., Rivier, F., Tardieu, M., Brive, M., & Mornet, D. (1997). Merosin positive congenital muscular dystrophy and cerebellar hypoplasia: An original ceregro-muscular syndrome. *Neuromuscular Disorders, 7*, 432.

Emery, A. E. H. (Ed.). (1998). *Neuromuscular disorders: Clinical and molecular genetics*. New York: Wiley.

Emery, A. E. H., & Skinner, R. (1976). Conical studies in benign (Becker type) X-linked muscular dystrophy. *Clinical Genetics, 10*, 189–201.

Fedrizza, E., Iverno, M., Botteon, G., Anderloni, A., Filippine, G., & Farinotti, M. (1993). The cognitive development of children born preterm and affected by spastic diplegia. *Brain Development, 15*, 428–432.

Fedrizza, E., Iverno, M., Bruzzone, M. G., Botteon, G., Salette, V., & Farinotti, M. (1996). MRI features of cerebral lesions and cognitive functions in preterm spastic diplegia children. *Pediatric Neurology, 15*, 207–212.

Fennell, E. B., & Dikel, T. N. (2001). Cognitive and neuropsychological functioning in children with cerebral palsy. *Journal of Child Neurology, 16*, 58–63.

Fu, Y.-H., Pizziti, A., Fenwick, R. G. Jr., King, J., Rajnarayan, S., Dunne, P. W., et al. (1992). An unstable triplet repeat in a gene related to myotonic muscular dystrophy. *Science, 255*, 1256–1258.

Gardner-Medwin, D. (1980). Clinical features and classification of muscular dystrophies. *British Medical Bulletin, 36*, 109–115.

Goto, M., Ota, R., Iai, M., Sugita, K., & Tanabe, Y. (1994). MRI changes and deficits of higher brain functions in preterm diplegia. *Acta Paediatrica, 83*, 506–511.

Gupta, R., & Appleton, R. E. (2001). Cerebral palsy: Not always what it seems. *Archives of Diseases in Childhood, 85*, 356–360.

Hagberg, B., Hagberg, G., Beckung, E., & Uvebrant, P. (2001). Changing panorama of cerebral palsy in Sweden. VIII. Prevalence and origin in the the birth year period 1991–94. *Acta Paediatrica, 90*, 271–277.

Hagberg, B., Hagberg, G., Olow, I., & van Wendt, L. (2001). The changing panorama of cerebral palsy in Sweden. VII. Prevalence and origin in the in the birth year period 1987–90. *Acta Paediatrica, 85*, 954–960.

Harley, H. G., Brook, J. D., Rundle, S. A., Crow, S., Reardon, W., Buckler, A. J., et al. (1992). Expansion of an unstable DNA region and phenotypic variation in myotonic dystrophy. *Nature, 355*, 545–546.

Harley, H. G., Rundle, S. A., McMillan, J. C., Myring, J., Brook, J. D., Crow, S., et al. (1993). Size of the unstable CTG repeat sequence in relation to phenotype and parental transmission of myotonic dystrophy. *American Journal of Human Genetics, 52*, 1164–1174.

Harper, P. S. (2001a). The genetic basis of myotonic dystrophy. In P. S. Harper (Ed.), *Myotonic dystrophy* (3rd ed., pp. 307–363). New York: Saunders.

Harper, P. S. (2001b). Myotonic dystrophy. *Major Problems in Neurology, 37*, 139–167.

Harper, P. S. (2001c). Myotonic dystrophy in infancy and childhood. In P. S. Harper (Ed.), *Myotonic dystrophy* (3rd ed., pp. 223–263). New York: Saunders.

Hinton, V. J., De Vivo, D. C., Nereo, N. E., Goldstein, E., & Stern, Y. (2000). Poor verbal working memory across intellectual level in boys with Duchenne muscular dystrophy. *Neurology, 54*, 2127–2132.

Hoffman, E. P., Fischbeck, K. H., Brown, R. H., Johnson, M., Medori, R., Loike, J. D., et al. (1988). Characterization of dystrophin in muscle-biopsy specimens from patients with Duchenne's or Becker's muscular dystrophy. *New England Journal of Medicine, 318,* 1363–1368.

International SMA Consortium. (1999). 1998 Meeting Report. *Neuromuscular Disorders, 9,* 272–278.

Karagan, N. J., Richman, L. C., & Sorensen, J. P. (1980). Analysis of verbal disability in Duchenne muscular dystrophy. *Journal of Nervous and Mental Disease, 168,* 419–423.

Karagen, N. J., & Sorensen, J. P. (1981). Intellectual functioning in non-Duchenne muscular dystrophy. *Neurology, 31,* 448–452.

Karagen, N. J., & Zellweger, H. U. (1978). Early verbal disability in children with Duchenne muscular dystrophy. *Developmental Medicine and Child Neurology, 20,* 435–441.

Kiessling, L. S., Denckla, M. B., & Carlton, M. (1983). Evidence for differential hemispheric function in children with hemiplegic cerebral palsy. *Developmental Medicine and Child Neurology, 25,* 727–734.

Koeda, T., & Takeshita, K. (1992). Visuo-perceptual impairment and cerebral lesions in spastic diplegia with preterm birth. *Brain Development, 14,* 239–244.

Kong, E. (1991). Fruherfassung von Zerebralparesen [Early diagnosis of cerebral paresis]. *Kinderkrankenschwester, 10,* 395–397.

Leibowitz, D., & Dubowitz, V. (1981). Intellect and behaviour in Duchenne muscular dystrophy. *Developmental Medicine and Child Neurology, 23,* 577–590.

Lou, H. C. (1998). Cerebral palsy and hypoxic-hemodynamic brain lesions in the newborn. In C. E. Coffey & R. A. Brumback (Eds.), *Textbook of pediatric neuropsychiatry* (pp. 1073–1092). Washington, DC: American Psychiatric Association.

Magill-Evans, J. E., & Restall, G. (1991). Self-esteem of person with Cerebral Palsy: From adolescence to adulthood. *American Journal of Occupational Therapy, 45,* 819–825.

Mahadevan, M., Tsilfidis, C. Sabourin, L., Shutler, G., Amemiya, C., Jansen, G., et al. (1992). Myotonic dystrophy mutation: An unstable CTG repeat in the 3' untranslated region of the gene. *Science, 255,* 1253–1255.

Martinello, F., Piazza, A., Pastorello, E., Angelini, C., & Trevisan, C. P. (1999). Clinical and neuroimaging study of central nervous system in congenital myotonic dystrophy. *Journal of Neurology, 246,* 186–192.

Mele, M., Laurianno, V., Gentil, V., Eggers, S., Del Bianco, S. S., Gemenez, P. R., et al. (1995). Becker and limb–girdle muscular dystrophies: A psychiatric and intellectual level comparative study. *American Journal of Medical Genetics, 60,* 33–38.

Mendell, J. R., Buzin, C. H., Feng, J., Yan, J., Serrano, C., Sangani, D. S., et al. (2001). Diagnosis of Duchenne dystrophy by enhanced detection of small mutation. *Neurology, 57,* 645–650.

Menkes, J. H., & Curran, J. (1994). Clinical and MR correlates in children with extrapyramidal cerebral palsy. *AJNR American Journal of Neuroradiology, 15,* 451–477.

Menkes, J. H., & Sarnat, H. B. (2000). Perinatal asphyxia and trauma. In J. H. Menkes & H. B. Sarnat (Eds.), *Child neurology* (pp. 401–466). Philadelphia: Lippincott, Williams & Wilkins.

Mercuri, E., Gruter-Andrew, J., Philpot, J., Sewry, C., Counsell, S., Henderson, S., et al. (1999). Cognitive abilities in children with congenital muscular dystrophy: Correlation with brain MRI and merosin status. *Neuromuscular Disorders, 9,* 383–387.

Miladi, N., Bourguigon, J-P., & Hentati, F. (1999). Cognitive and psychological profile of a Tunisian population of limb girdle muscular dystrophy. *Neuromuscular Disorders, 9,* 352–354.

Moizard, M-P., Billard, C., Toutain, A., Berret, F., Nadine, M., & Morain, C. (1998). Are Dp71 and Dp140 brain dystrophin isoforms related to cognitive impairment in Duchenne muscular dystrophy? *American Journal of Medical Genetics, 80,* 32–41.

Nelson, K. B., & Ellenberg, J. H. (1982). Children who "outgrew" cerebral palsy. *Pediatrics,* *69,* 529–53.

Norman, A., Thomas, N., Coakley, J., & Harper, P. (1980). Distinction of Becker from limb–girdle muscular dystrophy by means of dystrophin cDNA probes, *Lancet,* *41,* 466–468.

Olsen, P., Vaintonapaa, L., Paakko, E., Pyhtinen, J., & Jarvelin, M. R. (1998). Psychological findings in preterm children related to neurologic status and magnetic resonance imaging. *Pediatrics,* *102,* 329–336.

Palmer, F. B., Shapiro, B. K., Wachtel, R. C., Allen, M. C., Hiller, J. E., Harryman, S. E., et al. (1989). The effects of physical therapy on cerebral palsy: A controlled trial in infants with spastic diplegia. *New England Journal of Medicine,* *318,* 803–808.

Pellegrino, L. (2002). Cerebral palsy. In M. L. Batshaw (Ed.), *Children with disabilities* (5th ed., pp. 443–466). Baltimore: Brookes.

Philpot, J., Cowan, F., Pennock, J., Sewry, C., Dubowitz, V., Bydder, G., et al. (1999). Merosin deficient congenital muscular dystrophy: The spectrum of brain lesions on magnetic resonance imaging. *Neuromuscular Disorders,* *9,* 81–85.

Philpot, J., Sewry, C., Pennock, J., & Dubowitz, V. (1995). Clinical phenotype in congenital muscular dystrophy: Correlations with expression of merosin in skeletal muscle. *Neuromuscular Disorders,* *5,* 301–305.

Prechtl, H. F. R., & Stemmer, C. J. (1962). The choreiform syndrome in children. *Developmental Medicine and Child Neurology,* *4,* 119–127.

Prosser, E. J., Murphy, E. G., & Thompson, M. W. (1969). Intelligence and the gene for Duchenne muscular dystrophy. *Archives of Disease in Childhood,* *44,* 221–230.

Rapaport, D., Passos-Bueno, M. R., Takata, R. I., Campiotto, S., Eggers, S., Vainzof, M., et al. (1992). A deletion including the brain promoter of the Duchenne muscular dystrophy gene is not associated with mental retardation. *Neuromuscular Disorders,* *2,* 117–120.

Rasmussen, T., & Milner, B. (1977). The role of early left-brain injury in determining lateralization of cerebral speech function. In S. J. Dimond & D. Blizzard (Eds.), *Evolution and lateralization of the brain* (pp. 355–369). New York: Annals of the New York Academy of Sciences.

Roig, N., Balliu, P. R., Navarro, C., Brugera, R., & Losada, M. (1994). Presentation, clinical course, and outcome of the congenital form of myotonic dystrophy. *Journal of Pediatric Neurology,* *11,* 208–213.

Roland, E. H. (2000). Muscular dystrophy. *Pediatrics in Review,* *27,* 1–7.

Rubinsztein, J. S., Rubinsztein, D. C., McKenna, P. J., Goodburn, S., & Holland, A. J. (1997). Mild myotonic dystrophy is associated with memory impairment in the context of normal general intelligence. *Journal of Medical Genetics,* *34,* 229–233.

Savage, R. D., & Adams, M. (1979). Cognitive functioning and neurological deficit: Duchenne muscular dystrophy and cerebral palsy. *Australian Psychologist,* *14,* 59–75.

Scherzer, A. L., & Tschamuter, I. (1990). *Early diagnosis and therapy in cerebral palsy: A primer on infant developmental problems.* New York: Marcel Dekker.

Shimizu, M. (1999). Features of mental processing spastic diplegia. *Japanese Journal of Special Education,* *37,* 61–67.

Steyaert, J., de Die-Smulders, D., Fryns, J. P., Goossens, E., & Willekens, D. (2002). Letter to the editor: Behavioral phenotype in childhood type of dystrophia myotonica. *American Journal of Medical Genetics,* *96,* 888–889.

Steyaert, J., Umans, S., Willekens, D., Legius, E., Pijkels, E., de Die-Smulders, C., et al. (1997). A study of the cognitive and psychological profile in 16 children with congenital or juvenile myotonic dystrophy. *Clinical Genetics,* *52,* 135–141.

Sunada, Y. Edgar, T. S., Lotz, B. P., Rust, R. S., & Campbell, K. P. (1995). Merosin-negative congenital muscular dystrophy associated with extensive brain abnormalities. *Neurology,* *45,* 2084–2089.

Taft, L. T., Matthews, W. S., & Molnar, G. E. (1983). Pediatric management of the physically handicapped child. *Advances in Pediatrics, 30,* 13–60.

Thomasen, E. (1948). *Myotonia: Thomsen's disease (myotonia congenita), paramyotonia and dystrophia myotonica.* Copenhagen: Universitetsforlaget I Aahus.

Thomsen, J. (1876). Tonische krampfe in Wilkrulich beweg lichen muskeln infolge von erebter psychischer disposition (ataxia muscularis). *Archiv fur Psychiatrie und Nervenkrankheiten, 6,* 702–718.

Tomlin, P. I. (1995). The static encephalopathies. In R. W. Newton (Ed.), *Color atlas of pediatric psychiatry* (pp. 203–216). London: Times-Wolfe International.

Trevisan, C. P., Martinello, F., Feruzza, E., Fanin, M., Chevallay, M., & Tome, F.M. (1996). Brain alterations in the classical form of congenital muscular dystrophy. Clinical and neuroimaging follow-up of 12 cases and correlation with the expression of merosin in muscle. *Childs Nervous System, 12,* 604–610.

Turnpenny, P., Clark, C., & Kelly, K. (1994). Intelligence quotient profile in myotonic dystrophy, intergenerational deficit, and correlation with CTG amplification. *Journal of Medical Genetics, 31,* 300–305.

Ubhi, T., Bhakta, B. B., Ives, H. L., Allgar, V., & Rousounis, S. H. (2000). Randomized double blind placebo controlled trial on the effect of botulinum toxin on walking in cerebral palsy. *Archives of Diseases in Children, 83*(6), 481–487.

Van der Knaap, M. S., & Valk, J. (1995). *Magnetic resonance of myelin, myelination and myelin disorders* (2nd ed.). New York: Springer.

van Spaendonck, K. P. M., Ter-Bruggen, J. P., Weyn-Banningh, E. W. A., & Maassen, B. M. (1995). Cognitive function in early adult and adult onset myotonic dystrophy. *Acta Neurologica Scandinavica, 6,* 456–461.

Vainzof, M., Marie, S. K. N., Reed, U. C., Schwartzman, J. S., Pavanello, R.C., Passos-Bueno, M.R., et al. (1995). Deficiency of merosin (laminin M or 2) in congenital muscular dystrophy associated with cerebral white matter alterations. *Neuropediatrics, 26,* 293–297.

Volpe (2001). Neurobiology of periventricular leukomalaicia in the premature infant. *Pediatric Research, 50*(5), 553–562.

Voit, T. (1997–1998). Congenital muscular dystrophies: Update. *Brain and Development, 20,* 65–74.

von Gontard, A., Zerres, K., Backes, M., Laufersweiler-Plass, C., Wendland, C., Melchers, et al. (2002). Intelligence and cognitive function in children and adolescents with spinal muscular atrophy, *Neuromuscular Disorders, 12,* 130–136.

Whelan, T. B. (1987). Neuropsychological performance of children with Duchenne muscular dystrophy and spinal muscle atrophy. *Developmental Medicine and Child Neurology, 29,* 212–220.

Wieringa, B. (1994). Commentary. Myotonic dystrophy is reviewed: Back to the future? *Human Molecular Genetics, 3,* 1–7.

Wirth, B. (2000). An update of the mutation spectrum of the survival motor neuron gene (SMN1) in autosomal recessive spinal muscular atrophy (SMA). *Human Mutation, 15,* 229–237.

Woodward, J. B., Heaton, R. K., Simon, D. B., & Ringel, S. A. (1982). Neuropsychological findings in myotonic dystrophy. *Journal of Clinical Neuropsychology, 4,* 335–342.

Worden, D. K., & Vignos, P. J. Jr. (1962). Intellectual function in childhood progressive muscular dystrophy. *Pediatrics, 29,* 968–977.

Zellweger, H., & Hanson, J. W. (1967). Slowly progressive X-linked recessive muscular dystrophy (type IIIb). *Archives of Internal Medicine, 120,* 525–536.

Zellweger, H., & Hanson, J. W. (1968). Psychometric studies in muscular dystrophy type IIIa (Duchenne). *Developmental Medicine and Child Neurology, 9,* 576–581.

CHAPTER 6

Motor Disorders in Children with Intellectual Disabilities

DIGBY ELLIOTT

LINDSAY BUNN

In this chapter, we deal with the perceptual–motor problems and rehabilitation issues associated with intellectual impairment. One of the difficulties inherent in our task is the diverse set of circumstances that can lead to an intellectual impairment. From a functional point of view, mental retardation is defined on the basis of three criteria (American Association on Mental Retardation, 1997). An individual must exhibit significant subaverage intellectual functioning as well as limitations in adaptive life skill. These first two shortcomings must be manifested before the individual reaches 18 years of age.

If one assumes that intelligence is normally distributed and subaverage intelligence predisposes an individual to limitations in adaptive behavior, then our group of interest should include between 2 and 2.5% of the population. Interestingly, there appears to be a larger proportion of the population, approximately 3%, with intelligence quotients of 70 and below than predicted by the normal distribution (Dingman & Tarjan, 1960).

Several decades ago, Zigler (1967) suggested that this overrepresentation at the low end of the distribution exists because there are two fundamental groups of people with intellectual impairment. As with any distribution of human characteristics, there are people who, by definition, must fall at the low end (i.e., 2.28 %). For these individuals, there is no specific known cause. Both heredity and environment have been hypothesized to affect their placement on the intelligence distribution. These individuals are often described as having a cultural–familial or sociocultural intellectual impairment. The remainder of the population, with intelligence quotients of 70 and below, in theory, has a known cause for their intellectual handicap. This group is not a single group at all but is made up of people with metabolic, chromosomal, and other acquired disorders (anoxia, closed-head injury, exposure to environmental toxins, etc.; see Grossman, 1977, for medical classification system).

Many of the studies designed to examine perceptual–motor behavior in children with intellectual impairment have involved participants with diverse etiologies. In spite of this problem, there appear to be some characteristics of motor control and learning that generalize to this large heterogeneous group. In this chapter, we first discuss the perceptual–motor and learning problems encountered by children with intellectual impairment of a variety of etiologies before focusing our attention on children with specific syndromes. Partly because of our own research history, we pay special attention to research involving children with Down syndrome. We then turn our attention to some recent research involving children with Williams syndrome.

GENERAL PERCEPTUAL–MOTOR PROBLEMS ASSOCIATED WITH INTELLECTUAL IMPAIRMENT

One of the most established findings in the motor control literature is that children with intellectual impairments are slower at both initiating and executing goal-directed movements than other persons of a similar chronological age (Hoover & Wade, 1985). As well as exhibiting longer mean reaction times and movement times, individual reaction time distributions are characterized by greater variability and a marked positive skew (Baumeister & Kellas, 1968). This disadvantage in speeded movement initiation becomes even more pronounced with an increase in the number of stimulus–response alternatives (Vernon, 1986). Children and adults who are intellectually impaired also exhibit greater movement time disadvantages as the accuracy demands of the movement goal are increased (Wade, Newell, & Wallace, 1978). Thus, they have particular difficulty when making large amplitude movements to small objects/targets (see Hodges, Cunningham, Lyons, Kerr, & Elliott, 1995).

In an attempt to understand the relation between reaction time and mental age (Eysenck, 1967), research in the 1960s and 1970s was concerned with isolating particular sensory, decision-making, and response events that might explain perceptual–motor slowness in children and adults with intellectual impairment (Hoover & Wade, 1985). Interestingly, perceptual, decision-making and motor processes have all been implicated in the slowness associated with intellectual impairment (Nettlebeck & Brewer, 1981). Probably the most powerful account of psychomotor slowness and intellectual impairment was originally developed to explain increased reaction time associated with aging. The basic idea is that mean slowness, as well as reaction time variability and skewness, can be explained by the way a person with intellectual impairment approaches the overall reaction time task (Brewer & Smith, 1982, 1984).

In a typical two-choice reaction time situation a participant is told to respond "as quickly as possible" to the appropriate stimulus, but to "avoid making mistakes." In this situation, participants must discover how fast they are able to respond without making a mistake. For the average participant, this discovery process takes only 20 or 30 trials (see Welsh & Elliott, 2000). The first reaction time is relatively long, and then over several trials the reaction times become shorter until an error is made. The trial following an error is usually longer, but the participant quickly works his or her way toward establishing a reaction time bandwidth for responding that optimizes speed and accuracy. Long reaction times following an error contribute to the slight positive skew evident in most reaction time distributions.

Brewer and Smith (1982) hypothesized that children and adults with intellectual impairments may have difficulty finding and tracking this bandwidth. In a series of experiments, involving trial-to-trial analyses of serial, two-choice reaction times, Brewer and Smith (1984) found that participants with undifferentiated intellectual impairments were able to recognize decision-making errors, as evidenced by longer reaction times following an error. However, they were less able to use error and performance feedback over a series of trials to quickly zero in on the safe–fast performance zone. For example, while fast reaction times for the intellectually impaired participants were just as fast as reaction times for control participants, reaction times remained elevated for more trials after an error, thus not only contributing to long mean reaction times but also creating more variability and positive skewness. This pattern of results suggests that perceptual–motor slowness in this group may be more a function of strategic difficulties than a weak link in the information-processing chain of events.

Like the reaction time research, studies designed to examine the execution of simple goal-directed movements have focused on identifying the specific processes that contribute to the slowness of these movements. For example, by manipulating the accuracy requirements associated with simple aiming movements, researchers have attempted to determine whether movement execution problems can be attributed to difficulty with advance planning or the on-line processing of response-produced feedback during the actual execution of a movement (e.g., Wade et al., 1978). The assumption has usually been that smaller targets and movements over greater amplitudes require more feedback-based control.

Although young adults with intellectual impairment have been shown to take more time to complete even simple movements than do other persons of a similar chronological age, their disadvantage increases with the accuracy demands of the task. While it is tempting to suggest that this difficulty reflects problems using response-produced feedback, it could also be that less effective advance planning contributes to a greater need for feedback-based control. When visual feedback is withdrawn during a movement, the performance of intellectually challenged people is no more disrupted than the performance of their chronological and mental age-matched peers (Hodges et al., 1995). Overall, however, the typical movement trajectory of a person with an intellectual impairment is associated with far more discontinuities in acceleration than that of his or her peers. These discontinuities are usually taken to reflect feedback-based modification to the movement. Although these "corrections" certainly contribute to a longer movement time, the aiming movements of people with intellectual impairments are also characterized by lower peak velocities and accelerations. Peak velocity and peak acceleration are usually associated with the movement planning processes that occur prior to movement initiation. Perhaps children and adults with intellectual impairments have difficulty in selecting the appropriate muscular forces for optimizing speed and accuracy in goal-directed aiming. It may also be the case that, like reaction time, some of the movement execution differences between people with and without an intellectual impairment reflect the absence of an effective strategy for making rapid error-free movements. We know, for example, that when visual feedback about rapid limb movements is available, children and adults without intellectual impairment gradually learn to produce high velocities early in the movement so that they have more real time to use visual feedback late in the movement (see Elliott,

Helsen, & Chua, 2001, for a review). It still remains to be determined whether or not persons with intellectual impairment adopt this strategy.

The type of strategic problem that affects the organization, and possibly the execution, of rapid limb movements also has an impact on other types of perceptual–motor behaviors (Hoover & Wade, 1985). For example, in a study that involved remembering simple linear upper-limb movements, Reid (1980b) demonstrated that adolescents who are intellectually challenged failed to adopt a rehearsal strategy to prevent the deterioration of movement related information over a retention interval. This failure to spontaneously use a strategy for remembering is characteristic of chronologically younger children (Brown, 1974). Interestingly however, when Reid (1980a) taught participants with an intellectual impairment a simple visualization strategy, recall of the movement improved substantially. Although this provides some optimism for the development of instructional protocols that involve both basic skill instruction and the development of metacognitive strategies for practicing and performing a skill, research on metacognition with intellectually impaired children and adults indicates that strategies do not generalize well between learning situations (Brown & Campione, 1986).

Bouffard (1990) has suggested that while teaching an effective strategy is important, instructional protocols should also incorporate the development of a skill-specific knowledge base, metacognitive knowledge, executive procedures for problem solving, and adequate motivation and practice. Although intriguing, his approach to teaching intellectually impaired children needs to be put to the empirical test.

MOTOR LEARNING IN INDIVIDUALS WITH INTELLECTUAL IMPAIRMENT

Because children with intellectual impairment fail to spontaneously adopt cognitive strategies designed to facilitate skill acquisition, it is all the more important to structure skill acquisition sessions to optimize the processing of task-relevant information. Perhaps one of the most entrenched myths about people with and without intellectual impairments is that repetition facilitates motor learning. This view is in sharp contrast to a rich motor learning literature indicating that both within- and between-task variability contribute to the long-term retention and generalizability of skill (see Schmidt & Lee, 1999).

For example, if one is teaching a child to add, it is ineffective to ask the same question two times in a row (e.g., "What is 31 plus 4?") because when the question is asked the second time, the child does not need to solve the problem—he or she simply repeats the answer (e.g., "35"). Learning to solve the problem, not just remembering the answer, contributes to skill retention and transfer. When learning to throw a ball, it is better to practice a variety of distances and throwing speeds in a mixed-up order than to practice one speed or distance at a time (Schmidt, 1975). Variability in the learning situation requires the performer to solve a different movement problem on each attempt. This type of learning generalizes to new and unique throwing situations.

Porretta (1982) examined variability of practice in the acquisition of a ball-kicking skill in a group of intellectually handicapped 10-year-old boys, as well as boys of a similar chronological and mental age. All the children benefited more from an instructional protocol that involved kicking the ball in four different incline conditions than practicing in a single situation when they were required to perform a novel kicking task. Presumably the more variable practice experience facilitated the development of movement schema appropriate for a diverse class of kicking behaviors.

Although practicing different variations of a task appears to be more effective than constant practice for both children with and without intellectual impairment, studies involving variability in the order of task instruction have produced mixed results. For example, in a study involving intellectually challenged adolescents, Edwards, Elliott, and Lee (1986) found that randomizing task order (e.g., A, C, B, C, A . . .) produced better transfer to a novel variation of the task than blocked practice (e.g., A, A, A, B, B, B, C . . .). Heitman and Gilley (1989) found no reliable difference between the two types of practice schedule. Given that children with intellectual handicaps often fail to adopt appropriate problem-solving strategies, perhaps the benefits of a more variable practice experience will be realized best when the interval between trials is used to direct the performers attention to task specific information processing. This instructional approach also allows persons with intellectual handicaps to reap the skill acquisition benefits typically associated with distributed, as opposed to massed practice (Lee & Genovese, 1988).

Consistent with the notion that persons with intellectual handicaps benefit from instructional approaches that combine physical practice with cognitive training, Surburg, Porretta, and Sutlive (1995) found that mental imagery was an effective tool in teaching a throwing task to a group of adolescents with mild intellectual impairment. Specifically, participants who were taught to imagine throwing a ball to a target between actual throwing trials exhibited superior throwing accuracy to people receiving only physical practice. Although this study did not include a control group of individuals without intellectual impairment, instructional protocols involving mental practice may provide greater benefits to intellectually challenged children than to others. This is because the protocol introduces a strategy that may not be adopted spontaneously (Brown, 1974).

In summary, many of the motor control and learning problems exhibited by persons with intellectual impairments stem from the absence of strategic behavior in skill acquisition and performance rather than motor deficits per se. Although some researchers have associated these sorts of information-processing problems with frontal lobe dysfunction (e.g., Luria, 1973), a developmental model probably provides the best framework for describing the motor behavior of most children with undifferentiated intellectual impairments. That is, both the cognitive and motor performance of these children reflects their mental, as opposed to chronological, age. For cases in which an intellectual impairment is associated with a particular chromosomal, metabolic, or acquired etiology, more specific patterns of perceptual–motor function/dysfunction may be expected. In what follows, we discuss two particular etiologies that have been of interest to researchers in our lab.

DOWN SYNDROME

Down syndrome (DS) is a chromosomal anomaly that leaves the individual affected with an extra 21st chromosome. The syndrome is associated with approximately 1 in every 800 live births and is one of the leading causes of intellectual impairment. Although children with DS exhibit many of the same intellectual and perceptual–motor problems described in the previous section, they also display a number of information-processing strengths and weaknesses unique to the syndrome.

Infants with DS are usually born with hypotonia. This is a condition associated with reduced levels of electrical activity or "tone" in the skeletal muscles. Whether or not there is a causal relation between hypotonia and perceptual–motor slowness in children with DS is controversial (see Anwar & Hermelin, 1979). Studies on joint stiffness and stretch reflex activity in children and young adults with DS argue against the notion that individuals with DS are disadvantaged by poor muscle tone (Davis & Kelso, 1982; Davis & Sinning, 1987; Shumway-Cook & Woollacott, 1985). Moreover, long reaction times in persons with DS are associated more with central processing time than with the mechanical properties of the muscle (Davis, Sparrow, & Ward, 1991). Although poor muscle tone does not seem to explain limb control problems in children with DS (see Latash, 1992), there is evidence to indicate that children and adults with DS display a different pattern of muscle activation in the initiation of rapid limb movements (Anson & Mawston, 2000). Specifically, while most people exhibit a proximal-to-distal pattern of muscle activation when initiating rapid upper-limb movements, persons with DS exhibit electrical activity in their distal muscles before the proximal muscles become active (Anson & Davis, 1988). These findings and other work on the time course and amplitude of agonist and antagonist activity (see Anson & Mawston, 2000, for a review) indicate that children, adolescents, and young adults with DS may achieve the same movement goal as other intellectually challenged persons in an entirely different way.

Some of the most detailed work on the control of limb movements in children with DS has been conducted by using optoelectric technology to examine limb trajectories under different sensory and task conditions. For example, Charlton, Ihsen, and Oxley (1996, 1998) had 8- to 10-year-old children with DS and children without DS of a similar mental and chronological age reach and grasp objects that were either placed in another position or thrown into a container. Their goal was to determine whether the children were able to develop a movement strategy specific to the task requirements. The children with DS completed their movements to the objects more slowly than did children of the same chronological age. Despite the fact that their mean performance was similar to that of the chronologically younger participants, children with DS exhibited greater trial-to-trial variability. Although the movement trajectories of all the children were affected by the characteristics of the object and the task requirements, the children with DS and their developmentally younger counterparts spent more time decelerating the movement as they approached the object than did the chronologically older children. There were also more discontinuities in the movement trajectories of the children with DS (see also Kulatunga-Moruzi & Elliott, 1999). This was particularly true when the task required precision (Charlton, Ihsen, & Lavelle, 2000). As mentioned earlier, movement trajectories with these characteristics are often associated with the use of visual and kinesthetic feedback to correct error inherent in the initial movement impulse. This dependence on feedback could reflect either a difficulty in planning and programming a movement prior to movement initiation (Frith & Frith, 1974) or inefficient on-line control. Interestingly, in aiming experiments with adult participants, persons with DS are no more disrupted than other participants by the removal of response-produced visual feedback at movement initiation (Hodges et al., 1995). In fact, participants with DS were more accurate in their target aiming under no-vision conditions than were other intellectually challenged persons of a similar mental age. Perhaps as Henderson, Morris, and Frith (1981) have suggested, persons with DS have relatively intact spatial abilities but have trouble timing the onset and offset of muscular force. This idea is consistent with research involving ball catching which indicates that children with DS position their hands appropriately but are slow in timing the ball-grasping movements (Savelsbergh, van der Kamp, Ledebt, & Planinsek, 2000).

Although there is some indication that children and adults with DS have difficultly with the preparation and timing of upper-limb movements, they generally perform as well as other intellectually challenged individuals when they are able to regulate their movements on the basis of kinesthetic and/or visual information. However, persons with DS exhibit very specific movement problems when they are required to organize a sequence of movements on the basis of verbal information (see Heath, Elliott, Weeks, & Chua, 2000, for a review). Work from our lab indicates that these specific movement problems may be related to an atypical pattern of brain organization unique to persons with DS.

A number of studies using dichotic listening procedures have demonstrated that both children and young adults with DS exhibit a reversed ear advantage for the perception of speech sounds (see Elliott, Weeks, & Chua, 1994, for a review and meta-analysis). This ear advantage, as well as several neuroimaging studies (see Weeks, Chua, Weinberg, Elliott, & Cheyne, 2002), indicate that most people with DS are right-hemisphere specialized for the perception of speech. Persons with DS, however, do not exhibit reversed cerebral specialization for all language function. We have demonstrated, using several different paradigms, that young adults with DS are left-hemisphere specialized for speech production (Elliott, Edwards, Weeks, Lindley, & Carnahan, 1987; Heath & Elliott, 1999) and the control of other oral and manual movements (e.g., Elliott & Weeks, 1990). We have proposed that this biological dissociation between the functional systems responsible for speech perception and the systems important for the organization and control of movement (including speech movements) leads to problems with verbal–motor integration. Specifically, people with DS will have problems with tasks that require the organization and control of limb and oral movements on the basis of verbal direction.

Consistent with our model of brain organization, we have shown that young adults with DS make more errors performing sequences of simple gestures on the basis of verbal direction than do other people of a similar mental age (Elliott, Weeks, & Gray, 1990). This problem becomes more pronounced as the number of gestures in the sequence increases. When the sequence of gestures is demonstrated instead of verbally cued, however, persons with DS perform as well as, or better than, their mental age counterparts. We have also shown that adolescents and young adults with DS make more speech production errors than do control participants when they are required to repeat, as opposed to read, a list of one-syllable words (Bunn, Simon, Welsh, Watson, & Elliott, 2002). Once again, we attribute these specific problems to the need for interhemispheric integration when an individual with DS must structure a movement sequence on the basis of verbal information. The degradation of information during interhemispheric transfer may be more pronounced than for other individuals because of commissural anomalies associated with DS (Raz, Torres, & Briggs, 1995).

The specific verbal–motor difficulties experienced by persons with DS have implications for motor skill instruction. For example, Elliott, Gray and Weeks (1991) demonstrated that young adults with DS had more difficulty learning to perform a simple sequence of movements than did other individuals of a similar mental age when the instructions were given verbally. More recently, Maraj, Li, Hillman, Johnson, and Ringenbach (2003) found that a visual instructional protocol was more effective than a verbal protocol for teaching children and young adults with DS a novel computer task. Chronometric work, in which advance information about an upcoming movement is provided either visually or verbally, indicates that the verbal–motor difficulties experienced by persons with DS are related to the movement planning process (LeClair & Elliott, 1995).

Although we have just scratched the surface of the literature on perceptual–motor behavior in children with DS (for a more extensive review, see Weeks, Chua, & Elliott, 2000), it should be clear that, in some movement contexts, persons with DS can be expected to behave like other persons with intellectual impairment, while in other situations they will exhibit a unique pattern of function/dysfunction. Work in our laboratory has been motivated not only by an interest in DS but also because DS provides a model for examining the interaction between complex perceptual–motor systems. This second motivation is now providing a basis for the development of a research program involving children with Williams syndrome.

WILLIAMS SYNDROME

Williams syndrome (WS) is a rare, neurodevelopmental disorder with an incidence of 1 in 25,000–50,000 live births. Genetic in origin, this syndrome is caused by the submicroscopic deletion of a region on the long arm of chromosome 7, which contains both the LIM kinase 1 gene (LIMK1) and the gene that codes for elastin (Bellugi, Lichtenberger, Mills, Galaburda, & Korenberg, 1999; Ewart et al., 1993). The deletion of genes in this region is thought to be responsible for many of the characteristics associated with WS.

The first gene identified to be associated with WS is the gene that codes for elastin. Elastin is usually found in the connective tissue of many important parts of the body including the skin, ligaments, organs, and artery walls. Most important to researchers and clinicians interested in the control of movement, individuals with WS also often experience joint hypermobility during childhood because elastin is not present in their connective tissue. To combat joint instability, children with WS often develop atypical postures. These adaptive strategies often lead to contractures in adulthood (Morris & Mervis, 1999). Individuals with WS can also experience abnormal curvatures of the spine, such as kyphosis and lordosis, which again may be related to their elastin deficiency (Morris & Mervis, 1999). Abnormal curvatures of the spine, joint hypermobility and the eventual tightening of tissues surrounding the joint often seen in individuals with WS can lead to abnormal gait patterns and postures that may affect participation in various types of physical activity.

Although a deficiency in elastin explains some of the physical features and medical problems associated with WS, it does not account for the neurocognitive profile associated with this syndrome (Mervis, Morris, Bertrand, & Robinson, 1999). In 1996, Frangiskakis and colleagues linked the deletion of one copy of LIMK1 with a very specific aspect of the WS phenotype—a weakness in visuospatial cognition. This observed weakness in visuospatial cognition for individuals with WS has implications for a multitude of tasks requiring gross or fine motor control.

Although most individuals with WS have a mild to moderate intellectual impairment, tests of overall cognitive function do not tell the full story (Bellugi, Lichtenberger, Jones, Lai, & St. George, 2000). A closer look at tasks that target language, face recognition and visuospatial processing give us a more accurate picture of the strengths and weaknesses associated with WS. For example, tasks requiring expressive language, grammar, and the use of affective devices in storytelling are performed with little difficulty by older children and adults with WS (Bellugi et al., 2000). On the other hand tasks that require visuospatial processing are problematic for children with WS. One exception to this general rule is in the recognition and identification of faces. Children and adults with WS perform significantly better than IQ-matched participants with DS on tests targeting face processing. Many perform at levels similar to chronological age–matched participants without intellectual impairment (Bellugi et al., 2000).

Our initial interest in WS was motivated by their neurocognitve profile which shows a pattern of strengths and weaknesses often described by researchers as opposite that of individuals with DS. For example, when Bellugi and colleagues (Bellugi, Wang, & Jernigan, 1994; Wang, Doherty, Rourke, & Bellugi, 1995) tested children and adults with WS and DS using the Block Design subtest of the Wechsler Intelligence Scale for Children—Revised (WISC-R), results indicated that although both groups scored very similarly, the pattern of their responses were quite different. Participants with WS tended to have difficulty producing the overall arrangement of the blocks, a square, whereas participants with DS had difficulty reproducing the internal pattern of the block arrangement.

In addition to performance on a block task, Bellugi and colleagues compared drawing in children and adults with WS and DS. After examining the drawings by both groups, researchers concluded that while individuals with DS produced cohesive, yet simple, drawings that lacked detail, participants with WS produced comprehensive but disorganized illustrations (Bellugi et al., 2000). Bellugi and colleagues concluded that individuals with WS might have a local processing bias, whereas participants with DS tend to organize perceptual information globally.

The drawing and block design studies were not developed to specifically examine local–global processing and thus the "global–local" conclusions drawn from these between-task comparisons were post hoc. Bihrle, Bellugi, Delis, and Marks (1989) developed a hierarchical processing task with a standard scoring system to further study visuospatial processing in WS and DS. In this experiment, adolescents with WS and DS were asked to copy a large global figure made of smaller local forms (e.g., a "D" made out of "Ys"). Although both groups had difficulty, participants with WS tended to haphazardly produce the local forms all around the page, while age- and IQ-matched participants with DS omitted the local detail but replicated the global forms. The same pattern of results emerged whether participants were asked to copy the figure from memory or a card that lay in front of them. Birhle and colleagues likened the local processing bias observed in the participants with WS to that seen in individuals with right-hemisphere damage and the global processing bias observed in the participants with DS to that often seen in individuals with left-hemisphere brain damage.

Pani, Mervis, and Robinson (1999) suggested that the primary problem with visuospatial construction in individuals with WS was not a local organizational bias. Rather, they have difficulty changing from a global to local processing perspective. In a study by Pani and colleagues, participants with WS completed a visual search task, susceptible to global spatial processing, in which they were required to locate a "T" or an "F" in five visual displays of similar figures. Both the control group and the group with WS had shorter response times for Display 2 than for Display 1. This indicates that they were spontaneously organizing the figures globally rather than locally. Participants with WS had more difficulty, when compared to a control group, responding to visual search Display 1. This display required a switch in processing level, as evidenced by a substantially longer mean response time, relative to the overall distribution of times for each group. Therefore, it may be that people with WS are able to globally process the figures. However, they have difficulty switching from one level of processing to another.

Wang and colleagues (1995) administered the Visual–Motor Integration Test (Beery, 1982), which requires participants to copy 24 drawings of increasing complexity, to a group of adolescents with WS and a group with DS to verify earlier findings of difficulties in visuospatial awareness. They found that whereas participants with both WS and DS scored equally poorly on the test, the qualitative differences reported were similar to that found by Bellugi and colleagues. Wang and colleagues also administered a group of tests that were sensitive to right-hemispheric damage (RHD) in order to investigate the suitability of the RHD model of cognitive function in WS. The performance of the participants with WS on the Benton Faces (Benton, Hamsher, Varney, & Spreen, 1983) and Noncanonical Views (Carey & Diamond, 1990), along with the absence of evidence for any type of neglect, indicated that contrary to the comparison drawn by Birhle and colleagues (1989), a RHD model is not an appropriate description of cognitive function in WS. Wang and colleagues suggested that the neurocognitive strengths and weaknesses of children and adults with WS may be best understood by considering the dissociation between the ventral and dorsal streams of the visual system (Milner & Goodale, 1995).

Projections that make up the ventral stream traverse from the primary visual cortex to the inferotemporal cortex. The dorsal stream, however, receives projections from not only the primary visual cortex but also other visual systems, such as the superior colliculus. It terminates in the posterior parietal cortex. The ventral and dorsal streams appear to be functionally distinct. The ventral stream is specialized for pattern recognition, whereas the dorsal stream is largely responsible for the control of goal-directed movement (Milner & Goodale, 1995). Wang and colleagues (1995) suggested that the visuospatial problems associated with WS were more associated with dorsal stream function.

Atkinson and colleagues (1997) examined the ventrodorsal hypothesis using two visuospatial tasks that have been employed to dissociate the two systems in persons with brain injury (Milner & Goodale, 1995). The first task involved posting a card into a mail slot. The slot could be positioned in a number of orientations. Posting the card into the mail slot required on-line, visual–manual control to bring the card to the proper position. The second task required participants to simply match the orientation of a card in a mannequin's hand to the orientation of the mail slot. This pattern recognition task has been shown to be sensitive to ventral stream function. Approximately half the children with WS performed the matching task within the same range of the children without WS. The rest of the children with WS performed the task with errors greater than did the control group. Children with WS had more difficulty than children without WS on the posting task. Atkinson and colleagues (1997) concluded that a deficit in dorsal stream function might help explain difficulties in visuospatial awareness in children with WS. Although the authors believe that a dorsal stream deficit exists and may help to explain the on-line visual control problems associated with drawing, block construction tasks, and even walking over uneven ground, they acknowledge that not all aspects of visuospatial impairment may be associated with this neural pathway.

Although children with WS do exhibit marked visuospatial and visual–motor problems compared to other children of the same chronological age, it is encouraging to note that these difficulties appear to diminish with age and/or experience. For example, Mervis and colleagues (1999) reported a strong positive correlation between chronological age and performance on the Pattern Construction subtest of the Differential Ability Scales (Elliott, 1990) in a group of children, adolescents, and adults with WS. Thus, at least some of the difficulties experienced by children with WS may be related to a slower pattern of visual–motor development than a permanent neurological difference. Although this notion is also consistent with the work of Bertrand, Mervis, and Eisenberg (1997) on the copying of complex figures, more detailed developmental work needs to be done in which the relative contributions of age and experience can be explored.

A better understanding of the visual–motor problems associated with WS will help improve the quality of life of individuals with WS and their families. For example, research into how visual–motor problems affect physical activity, activities of daily living, and play will help physical educators, physiotherapists, occupational therapists, and parents provide individuals with WS the tools to better navigate their environments. Preliminary research in perceptual–motor control will set the stage for research designed to facilitate participation in physical activity programs and sports and the development of instructional protocols to improve daily living and self-help skills. By optimizing motor skill acquisition, children with WS will achieve a greater sense of independence, self-efficacy and self-esteem.

SUMMARY AND CONCLUSIONS

In this chapter, we have attempted to provide a basic framework for understanding the perceptual–motor problems associated with intellectual impairment. Although it is clear that a developmental model explains some of the metacognitive and strategic problems associated with deficits in perceptual–motor speed and skill acquisition, it is also the case that different subgroups of children with intellectual impairment can be expected to show unique patterns of function/dysfunction. As an example, we have detailed some of the specific perceptual–motor strengths and weakness associated with DS and WS. What we have failed to emphasize is that even within a distinct group of children with intellectual impairment, one should always expect at least as much interindividual variability as in the general population. This, of course, highlights the importance of individual assessment as well as educational and rehabilitation planning.

REFERENCES

American Association on Mental Retardation. (1997). *Mental retardation: Definition, classification, and systems of support* (9th ed.). Washington, DC: Author.

Anson, J. G., & Davis, S. A. (1988). Neuromotor programming and Down syndrome. *International Journal of Neuroscience, 40*, 82.

Anson, J. G., & Mawston, G. A. (2000). Patterns of muscle activation in simple reaction time tasks. In D. J. Weeks, R. Chua, & D. Elliott (Eds.), *Perceptual motor behavior in Down syndrome* (pp. 3–24). Champaign, IL: Human Kinetics.

Anwar, F., & Hermelin, B. (1979). Kinesthetic movement after-effects in children with Down's syndrome. *Journal of Mental Deficiency Research, 23*, 287–297.

Atkinson, J., King, J., Braddick, O., Nokes, L., Anker, S., & Braddick, F. (1997). A specific deficit of dorsal stream function in Williams' syndrome. *Neuroreport, 8*, 1919–1922.

Baumeister, A. A., & Kellas, G. (1968). Distribution of reaction times of retardates and normals. *American Journal of Mental Deficiency, 72*, 715–718.

Bellugi, U., Lichtenberger, L., Jones, W., Lai, Z., & St. George, M. (2000). The neurocognitive profile of WS: A complex pattern of strengths and weaknesses. *Journal of Cognitive Neuroscience, 12*, 7–29.

Bellugi, U., Lichtenberger, L., Mills, D., Galaburda, A., & Korenberg, J. (1999). Bridging cognition, the brain and molecular genetics: Evidence from WS. *Trends in Neurosciences, 22*, 197–207.

Bellugi, U., Wang, P. P., & Jernigan, T. L. (1994). Williams syndrome: An unusual neuropsychological profile. In S. H. Bromand & Grafman, J. (Eds.), *Atypical cognitive deficits in developmental disorders: Implications for brain function* (pp. 23–56). Hillsdale, NJ: Erlbaum.

Benton, A. L., Hamsher, K. de S., Varney, N. R., & Spreen, O. (1983). *Contributions to neuropsychological assessment*. New York: Oxford University Press.

Bertrand, J., Mervis, C. B., & Eisenberg, J. D. (1997). Drawing by children with WS: A developmental perspective. *Developmental Neuropsychology, 13*, 41–67.

Bihrle, A. M., Bellugi, U., Delis, D., & Marks, S. (1989). Seeing either the forest or the trees: Dissociation in visuospatial processing. *Brain and Cognition, 11*, 37–49.

Bouffard, M. (1990). Movement problem solutions by educable mentally handicapped individuals. *Adapted Physical Activity Quarterly, 7*, 183–197.

Brewer, N., & Smith, G. A. (1982). Cognitive processes for monitoring and regulating speed and accuracy of responding in mental retardation: A methodology. *American Journal of Mental Deficiency, 87*, 211–222.

Brewer, N., & Smith, G. A. (1984). How normal and retarded individuals monitor and regulate speed and accuracy of responding in serial choice tasks. *Journal of Experimental Psychology: General, 113*, 71–93.

Brown, A. L. (1974). The role of strategic behavior in retardate memory. In N.R. Ellis (Ed.), *International review of research in mental retardation* (Vol. 7, pp. 55–111). New York: Academic Press.

Brown, A. L., & Campione, J.C. (1986). Training for transfer: Guidelines for promoting flexible use of trained skills. In M. G. Wade (Ed.), *Motor skill acquisition of the mentally handicapped* (pp. 257–271). Amsterdam: North-Holland.

Bunn, L., Simon, D. A., Welsh, T. N., Watson, C., & Elliott, D. (2002). Speech production errors in adults with and without Down syndrome following verbal, written and pictorial cues. *Developmental Neuropsychology, 21*, 157–172.

Carey, S., & Diamond, R. (1990). *Canonical–noncanonical views test*. Unpublished manuscript, Harvard University.

Charlton, J. L., Ihsen, E., & Lavelle, B. M. (2000). Control of manual skills in children with

Down syndrome. In D. J. Weeks, R. Chua, & D. Elliott (Eds.), *Perceptual–motor behavior in Down syndrome* (pp. 25–48). Champaign, IL: Human Kinetics.

Charlton, J. L., Ihsen, E., & Oxley, J. (1996). Kinematic characteristics of reaching and grasping in children with Down syndrome. *Human Movement Science, 15*, 727–743.

Charlton, J. L., Ihsen, E., & Oxley, J. (1998). The influence of context in the development of reaching and grasping: Implications for assessment of disability. In J. P. Piek (Ed.), *Motor behavior and human skill. A multidisciplinary approach* (pp. 283–302). Champaign, IL: Human Kinetics.

Davis, W. E., & Kelso, J. A. S. (1982). Analysis of "invariant characteristics" in the motor control of Down's syndrome and normal subjects. *Journal of Motor Behavior, 14*, 194–212.

Davis, W. E., & Sinning, W. E. (1987). Muscle stiffness in Down syndrome and other mentally handicapped subjects: A research note. *Journal of Motor Behavior, 19*, 130–144.

Davis, W. E., Sparrow, W. A., & Ward, T. (1991). Fractionated reaction times and movement times of Down syndrome and other adults with mental retardation. *Adapted Physical Activity Quarterly, 8*, 221–233.

Dingman, H. F., & Tarjan, G. (1960). Mental retardation and the normal distribution curve. *American Journal of Mental Deficiency, 64*, 991–994.

Edwards, J. M., Elliott, D., & Lee, T. D. (1986). Contextual interference effects during skill acquisition and transfer in Down's syndrome adolescents. *Adapted Physical Activity Quarterly, 3*, 250–258.

Elliott, C. D. (1990). *Differential ability scales.* San Antonio, TX: Harcourt Brace.

Elliott, D., Edwards, J. M., Weeks, D. J., Lindley, S., & Carnahan, H. (1987). Cerebral specialization in young adults with Down syndrome. *American Journal of Mental Deficiency, 91*, 480–485.

Elliott, D., Gray, S., & Weeks, D. J. (1991). Verbal cuing and motor skill acquisition for adults with Down syndrome. *Adapted Physical Activity Quarterly, 8*, 210–220.

Elliott, D., Helsen, W. F., & Chua, R. (2001). A century later: Woodworth's (1899) two-component model of goal-directed aiming. *Psychological Bulletin, 127*, 342–357.

Elliott, D., & Weeks, D. J. (1990). Cerebral specialization and the control of oral and limb movements for individuals with Down's syndrome. *Journal of Motor Behavior, 22*, 6–18.

Elliott, D., Weeks, D. J., & Chua, R. (1994). Anomalous cerebral lateralization and Down syndrome. *Brain and Cognition, 26*, 191–195.

Elliott, D., Weeks, D. J., & Gray, S. (1990). Manual and oral praxis in adults with Down's syndrome. *Neuropsychologia, 28*, 1307–1315.

Ewart, A. K., Morris, C. A., Atkinson, D., Jin, W., Sternes, K., Spallone, P., et al. (1993). Hemizygosity at the elastin locus in a developmental disorder, WS. *Nature Genetics, 5*, 11–16.

Eysenck, H. J. (1967). Intelligence assessment: A theoretical and experimental approach. *British Journal of Educational Psychology, 37*, 81–98.

Frangiskakis, J. M., Ewart, A. K., Morris, C. A., Mervis, C. B., Bertrand, J., Robinson, B. F., et al. (1996). LIM-kinase 1 hemizygosity implicated in impaired visuospatial constructive cognition. *Cell, 86*, 59–69.

Frith, U., & Frith, C. D. (1974). Specific motor disabilities in Down's syndrome. *Journal of Child Psychology and Psychiatry, 15*, 293–301.

Grossman, H. (1977). *Manual on terminology and classification in mental retardation.* Washington, DC: American Association on Mental Deficiency.

Heath, M., & Elliott, D. (1999). Cerebral specialization for speech production in persons with Down syndrome. *Brain and Language, 69*, 193–211.

Heath, M., Elliott, D., Weeks, D. J., & Chua, R. (2000). A functional systems approach to movement pathology in persons with Down syndrome. In D. J. Weeks, R. Chua, & D.

Elliott (Eds.), *Perceptual–motor behavior in Down syndrome* (pp. 305–320). Champaign, IL: Human Kinetics.

Heitman, R. J., & Gilley, W. F. (1989). Effects of blocked versus random practice by mentally retarded subjects on the learning of a novel skill. *Perceptual and Motor Skills, 69,* 443–447.

Henderson, S. E., Morris, J., & Frith, U. (1981). The motor deficit in Down's syndrome children: A problem of timing? *Journal of Child Psychology and Psychiatry, 22,* 223–245.

Hodges, N. J., Cunningham, S. J., Lyons, J., Kerr, T. L., & Elliott, D. (1995). Visual feedback processing and goal-directed movement in adults with Down syndrome. *Adapted Physical Activity Quarterly, 12,* 176–186.

Hoover, J. H., & Wade, M. G. (1985). Motor learning theory and mentally retarded individuals: A historical review. *Adapted Physical Activity Quarterly, 2,* 228–252.

Kulatunga-Moruzi, C., & Elliott, D. (1999). Manual and attentional asymmetries in goal-directed movements in adults with Down syndrome. *Adapted Physical Activity Quarterly, 16,* 138–154.

Latash, M. L. (1992). Motor control in Down syndrome: The role of adaptation and practice. *Journal of Developmental and Physical Disabilities, 4,* 227–261.

LeClair, D. A., & Elliott, D. (1995). Movement preparation and the costs and benefits associated with advance information for adults with Down syndrome. *Adapted Physical Activity Quarterly, 12,* 238–249.

Lee, T. D., & Genovese, E. D. (1988). Distribution of practice in motor skill acquisition: Learning and performance effects are considered. *Research Quarterly for Exercise and Sport, 59,* 277–287.

Luria, A. R. (1973). *The working brain.* New York: Penguin.

Maraj, B. K. V., Li, L., Hillman, R., Johnson, J., & Ringenbach, S. D. (2003). Verbal and visual instruction in motor skill acquisition for persons with and without Down syndrome. *Adapted Physical Activity Quarterly, 20,* 57–69.

Mervis, C. B., Morris, C. A., Bertrand, J., & Robinson, B. F. (1999). WS: Findings from an integrated program of research. In H. Tagar-Flusberg (Ed.), *Neurodevelopmental disorders: Contributions to a new framework from the cognitive neurosciences* (pp. 65–110). Cambridge, MA: MIT press.

Milner, A. D., & Goodale, M. A. (1995). *The visual brain in action.* New York: Oxford University Press.

Morris, C. A., & Mervis, C. B. (1999). Williams syndrome. In S. Goldstein & C. R. Reynolds (Eds.), *Handbook of neurodevelopmental and genetic disorders in children* (pp. 555–590). New York: Guilford Press.

Nettlebeck, T., & Brewer, N. (1981). Studies of mild mental retardation and timed performance. In N. R. Ellis (Eds.), *International review of research in mental retardation* (Vol. 10, pp. 62–106). New York: Academic Press.

Pani, J. R., Mervis, C. B., & Robinson, B. F. (1999). Global spatial organization by individuals with WS. *Psychological Science, 10,* 453–458.

Porretta, D. L. (1982). Motor schema formation by EMR boys. *American Journal of Mental Deficiency, 87,* 164–172.

Raz, N., Torres, I. J., & Briggs, S. D. (1995). Selective neuroanatomical abnormalities in Down's syndrome and their cognitive correlates: Evidence from MRI morphometry. *Neurology, 45,* 356–366.

Reid, G. (1980a). The effects of memory strategy instruction in the short-term motor memory of the mentally retarded. *Journal of Motor Behavior, 12,* 221–227.

Reid, G. (1980b). Overt and covert rehearsal in short term motor memory of mentally retarded and nonretarded persons. *American Journal of Mental Deficiency, 85,* 69–77.

Savelsbergh, G., van der Kamp, J., Ledebt, A., & Planinsek, T. (2000). Information coupling in children with Down syndrome. In D. J. Weeks, R. Chua, & D. Elliott (Eds.), *Perceptual–motor behavior in Down syndrome* (pp. 251–275). Champaign, IL: Human Kinetics.

Schmidt, R. A. (1975). A schema theory of discrete motor learning. *Psychological Review, 82,* 225–260.

Schmidt, R. A., & Lee, T. D. (1999). *Motor control and learning: A behavioral emphasis* (3rd ed.). Champaign, IL: Human Kinetics.

Shumway-Cook, A., & Woollacott, M. H. (1985). Dynamics of postural control in the child with Down syndrome. *Physical Therapy, 65,* 1315–1322.

Surburg, P. R., Porretta, D. L., & Sutlive, V. (1995). Use of imagery practice for improving a motor skill. *Adapted Physical Activity Quarterly, 12,* 217–227.

Vernon, P. A. (1986). Speed of information-processing, intelligence, and mental retardation. In M. G. Wade (Ed.), *Motor skill acquisition of the mentally handicapped* (pp. 113–129). Amsterdam: North-Holland.

Wade, M. G., Newell, K., & Wallace, S. A. (1978). Decision time and movement time as a function of response complexity in retarded persons. *American Journal of Mental Deficiency, 83,* 135–144.

Wang, P. P., Doherty, S., Rourke, S. B., & Bellugi, U. (1995). Unique profile of visuoperceptual skills in a genetic syndrome. *Brain and Cognition, 29,* 54–65.

Weeks, D. J., Chua, R., & Elliott, D. (Eds.). (2000). *Perceptual–motor behavior in Down syndrome.* Champaign, IL: Human Kinetics.

Weeks, D. J., Chua, R., Weinberg, H., Elliott, D., & Cheyne, D. (2002). A preliminary study using magnetoencephalography to examine brain function in Down's syndrome. *Journal of Human Movement Studies, 42,* 1–18.

Welsh, T. N., & Elliott, D. (2000). The preparation and control of goal-directed limb movements in persons with Down syndrome. In D. J. Weeks, R. Chua, & D. Elliott (Eds.), *Perceptual–motor behavior in Down syndrome* (pp. 49–70). Champaign, IL: Human Kinetics.

Zigler, E. (1967). Familial mental retardation: A continuing dilemma. *Science, 155,* 292–298.

CHAPTER 7

Motor Problems in Children with Autistic Spectrum Disorders

ISABEL M. SMITH

The goal of this chapter is to introduce autistic spectrum disorders (ASD) and some of the key issues related to motor and perceptual–motor functions in these conditions. Autism has been the focus of increasing attention from researchers in diverse areas of the cognitive and neurological sciences. Individuals with autism display marked patterns of affected and spared abilities, the study of which has not only advanced our knowledge of autism but also made significant contributions to the understanding of normal development. The history of research on the development of social understanding (Baron-Cohen, Tager-Flusberg, & Cohen, 1999) is a good example of the reciprocal benefits for understanding autism and normal cognitive development. A recent surge in motor and perceptual–motor skill research has similar potential to inform our understanding of autism and other disorders of development, as well as of normal functioning. It also highlights the importance of investigating the role of lower-level processes, including motor skills, in the development of higher-order functions such as communication and social interaction.

Following a short introduction to the autistic spectrum, I address the first of my two main objectives, which is to provide a current perspective on the issue of whether motor problems characterize a particular subtype of ASD, as is often asserted. This discussion updates that of Smith (2000). The second aim is to highlight some evidence of basic differences in the interaction of attentional, perceptual, and motor systems in autism that have implications for the performance of motor tasks and for understanding some fundamental psychological aspects of this complex and challenging disorder. Again, my focus is on selected recent work rather than an exhaustive review of motor phenomena. For detailed discussion of stereotyped motor behavior in autistic spectrum disorders, consult Lewis and Bodfish (1998), as well as Turner's (1999) fine treatment of the range of repetitive behavior in autism.

AUTISTIC SPECTRUM DISORDERS: DEFINITION AND DESCRIPTION

I will use the term *ASD* in preference to the DSM-IV (American Psychiatric Association, 1994) categorical label of "pervasive developmental disorder" (or PDD; see also ICD-10 [World Health Organization, 1992]) to subsume prototypical autism (DSM-IV, autistic disorder), and the range of conditions with similar phenotypes (DSM-IV, Asperger disorder and pervasive developmental disorder—not otherwise specified [PDD-NOS][1]), except when giving details of specific study criteria or when otherwise required for clarity. Although there are several reasons for preferring ASD to PDD terminology, the most important for the present purpose is that it remains controversial whether the DSM-IV subgroupings within the PDD category reflect clinically or theoretically meaningful distinctions (Fein et al., 1999). As elaborated later, the issue of differential motor skill patterns illustrates the complexity of this broader debate. Readers who wish a more comprehensive treatment of the characteristics of autism are referred to Wing (1997). Here I only briefly highlight the developmental pattern that characterizes ASD, which entails abnormalities in three major defining domains: social development, communication, and cognitive and behavioral style.

First, social development is atypical in ASD. Early in life, this is most commonly manifested as a lack of interest in people, and a failure to show the well-integrated use of eye gaze, facial expressions, and "body language" by which even very young babies engage, or are engaged by, other people (Mundy, Sigman, & Kasari, 1994). These basic skills may never develop in the more impaired individuals with autism, whose social interactions remain very limited. More able people with ASD continue to experience difficulty with the complex and subtle rules of verbal and nonverbal behavior that govern social behavior and may appear disinterested, conspicuously naïve, or extremely awkward in their social relationships.

Communication is the second domain affected by ASD. Both verbal and nonverbal routes of communication, at whatever levels achieved, are impaired. A substantial minority of people with ASD do not develop spoken language (Bryson & Smith, 1998); significantly, some of these individuals also have difficulty acquiring gestural communication systems (Seal & Bonvillian, 1997). Most people with ASD have substantially delayed and disordered language, evident in both their receptive and expressive abilities. The language of even the most verbally capable individuals with ASD tends to be literal, pedantic, and repetitive, although vocabulary and syntax may be entirely intact. Pragmatic skills are universally affected, with limited reciprocity in the exchange of ideas and limited appreciation of other people's points of view.

Finally, ASD is also characterized by a rigid cognitive and behavioral style. Delays in the development of play skills are among the first signs of difficulty in this domain. Stereotyped handling or arranging of objects, such as flipping of string or lining up of toys, tends to predominate over imaginative play. Preoccupations with particular objects or topics may develop, as may repetitive motor mannerisms or adherence to rigid

---

[1]The DSM-IV categories of Rett's disorder and childhood disintegrative disorder are much rarer (and less well studied) than the other PDDs. Both are distinguished by a deteriorating developmental course. For Rett's disorder, there is also a specific pattern of motor loss and an identified genetic substrate (Mount, Hastings, Reilly, Cass, & Charman, 2003). These disorders are outside the scope of this chapter and are not discussed further.

behavioral routines. Often, a person with ASD becomes distressed by changes in physical surroundings or departures from a familiar schedule of events.

Even this brief rendering of some of the key features of ASD invites speculation about the role of motor functions in many of the described phenomena. This is perhaps most evident in the domain of repetitive and inflexible behavior. However, the lack of appropriate modulation and integration of nonverbal behaviors such as gaze and gesture that characterizes the impaired socialization and communication skills in autism also deserves emphasis. Only relatively recently have various researchers begun to integrate these disparate phenomena into a more cohesive picture (e.g., Rogers & Bennetto, 2000; Russell, 1998; Smith & Bryson, 1994). A concomitant research trend, to which I return, is renewed interest in the effects of ASD on more basic information-processing mechanisms such as perception of visual motion (Spencer et al., 2000) or face recognition (Joseph & Tanaka, 2003), as contrasted with an emphasis on higher-level social–cognitive functions. Both of these trends have contributed to increased emphasis on motor and perceptual–motor phenomena in the autism literature.

SUBTYPES WITHIN THE AUTISM SPECTRUM

As previously stated, the subtypes within the autistic spectrum that are of interest for this chapter are autism in its prototypical form (DSM-IV, autistic disorder; ICD 10, childhood autism), subthreshold or atypical autism (DSM-IV, PDD-NOS; ICD 10, atypical autism), and Asperger syndrome (DSM-IV, Asperger's disorder; ICD-10, Asperger's syndrome). Other than the number and severity of core autistic symptoms, the major differentiating features among these subtypes are the presence or absence of concomitant mental retardation and of significant language impairment. Mental retardation is present in approximately 75% of people with prototypical autism and in a smaller proportion of those with subthreshold/atypical presentations (Bryson & Smith, 1998). In clinical practice, a diagnosis of Asperger syndrome is usually given only for persons whose intellectual abilities are at least in the borderline range (but see Gillberg, 1998). Asperger syndrome (AS) is also defined by a lack of significant delay in early language development.

Differentiation between AS and the minority of cases of prototypical autism who present without mental retardation ("high-functioning" autism, hereafter HFA) has been controversial (Schopler, 1998; Szatmari, 1998; Volkmar & Klin, 2000). Although AS was incorporated into DSM with the fourth edition (American Psychiatric Association, 1994), and clinical use of the diagnosis has increased dramatically since, opinion remains divided as to whether this is a distinct syndrome with respect to etiology, natural history, or response to treatment. It is particularly interesting that in the early accounts of autism, motor skills were frequently described not only as unimpaired but as strengths (e.g., Kanner, 1943/1973). In contrast, motor clumsiness was described in several of Asperger's (1944/1991) original cases and proposed as a feature of AS by Wing (1981) when she brought the syndrome to the English scientific literature. These clinical impressions might be attributable to the fact that so many developmental domains are impaired in the classic presentation of autism that relative strengths in motor skills were highly salient. This uneven profile sets these children apart from many others with developmental disabilities. Conversely, among those individuals with the Asperger presentation (i.e., without early language delay or mental retardation), relative sparing of verbal and intellectual abilities may make poor motor skills more evident. It may be relevant to consider that the peer group of a child with AS is more likely to consist of typical children, whereas children with autism may be compared more often with those with developmental disabilities. Thus, for children at either end of the autistic spectrum, motor skills may stand in contrast to those of their peers but in different directions. It is worth bearing this point in mind as the evidence for differential motor involvement in AS and HFA is reviewed in the next section.

MOTOR IMPAIRMENT IN ASPERGER SYNDROME VERSUS HIGH-FUNCTIONING AUTISM

Studies have indicated that the reliability of the differential diagnosis of AS and HFA is not strong, especially relative to the excellent reliability associated with distinguishing ASD from non-ASD diagnoses (Volkmar & Klin, 2000; but see Mahoney et al.,1998). Furthermore, much of the research that compares these putative subgroups has been criticized on the basis that diagnostic criteria are inconsistent across studies. Methodological weaknesses have been a particular problem in studies of motor and perceptual–motor skills in AS and HFA (Ghaziuddin, Tsai, & Ghaziuddin, 1992; Smith, 2000). Various refinements of Asperger's (1944/1991) and Wing's (1981) diagnostic criteria have either retained clumsiness (or poor motor skills) as a defining feature of AS (e.g., Gillberg, 1989; Klin, Volkmar, Sparrow, Cicchetti, & Rourke, 1995) or as an associated feature (e.g., DSM-IV [American Psychiatric Association, 1994]; ICD-10 [World Health Organization, 1992]; Szatmari, Bartolucci, & Bremner, 1989; Szatmari, Tuff, Finlayson, & Bartolucci, 1990). Earlier work on this issue has been reviewed in detail by Ghaziuddin et al. (1992) and Smith (2000), both concluding that comparative studies of motor skills in AS and HFA were unlikely to be productive until the same diagnostic criteria were used across studies and "clumsiness" was operationally defined. Smith (2000) argued further that a different, analytic approach would be required to understand motor and perceptual–motor skills and their associations with other features across the autistic spectrum. For example, the use of better-controlled experimental tasks that isolate components of movement preparation and execution might differentiate individuals within the spectrum and provide an empirical basis for subgroups such as Asperger syndrome.

Data continue to accumulate that are relevant to this debate regarding motor skills in AS versus HFA. Ghaziuddin and Butler (1998) compared performance on the Bruininks–Oseretsky test of motor functions in three groups of 12 participants with (1) autism, (2) AS, or (3) another ASD (i.e., PDD-NOS). Participants were recruited from a clinical series; no matching for IQ was attempted. All those with AS had Full Scale IQs above 70, and none of the participants met criteria for autistic disorder. Results showed that all groups were impaired relative to norms on the standardized motor battery, with the poorest performance noted in the group with autistic disorder. There were no differences between the other two groups. When IQ was covaried, no group differences remained, suggesting that motor impairments in ASD may be associated with intellectual level rather than subtype differences.

The same point was made more definitively by Miller and Ozonoff (2000). In a study designed to clarify the neuropsychological distinctions between AS and HFA, they tested 40 children with ASD, ages 6–13 years. Their careful group assignment procedure is noteworthy. Information from research "gold standard" measures, the Autism Diagnostic Interview—Revised (ADI-R; Lord, Rutter, & LeCouteur, 1994) and the Autism Diagnostic Observation Schedule (ADOS; Lord, Rutter, & DiLavore, 1998) were used to determine whether participants met DSM-IV criteria. All participants had Full Scale IQs above 70. Those with AS ($N = 14$) had intact early language and never met criteria for autism. The remaining 26 participants met criteria for autism (HFA). The children's motor abilities were assessed using the Movement Assessment Battery for Children (M-ABC; Henderson & Sugden, 1992), a standardized assessment that yields Manual Dexterity, Ball Skills, and Balance subscores, as well as a Total Impairment score. Results indicated that only the Manual Dexterity score differentiated the AS and HFA groups, with AS children showing more impairment; this result was obtained only when IQ scores were covaried in the analysis. Test performance was supplemented by parental reports of the children's developmental histories from the ADI-R. While 66% of parents reported that their AS children were clumsy, so did 85% of parents of children with HFA. The authors repeated all of their analyses with IQ-matched subgroups of their sample (13 children with HFA and 14 with AS), and the pattern of results was unchanged. In addition, motor skills did not contribute significantly to a discriminant function analysis, intelligence measures being the most discriminating contributors to group assignment. Based on their comprehensive analyses, Miller and Ozonoff concluded that there is little evidence that AS is neuropsychologically distinct from HFA. Instead, they argued that AS represents the most intellectually able end of the autistic spectrum. With specific reference to motor skills, they noted that their results indicate some tendency to weaker performance specific to the fine motor domain for children with AS, when IQ differences between AS and HFA are controlled. However, they note further that no particular motor difficulties are universal or specific in AS and therefore are not diagnostic.

One study that focused on younger children reached a similar conclusion. Iwanaga, Kawasaki, and Tsuchida (2000) compared the profiles of 10 preschoolers with AS and 15 with HFA, selected from a clinical series. Diagnosis followed DSM-IV criteria; the authors state that no child with AS had delayed language at age 3. Measures of motor function were from a Japanese adaptation of the Miller Assessment for Preschoolers (JMAP). The JMAP yields a 10-item "Foundation Index," based on "sense of position and movement, sense of touch, and development of the basic components of movement" (Iwanaga et al., 2000). The "Coordination Index" consists of seven items (three of which overlap with Foundation items) assessing gross, fine, and oral motor skills. There are three additional JMAP indices: Verbal, Nonverbal, and Complex Tasks. With respect to the motor measures, these authors reported that the AS group differed significantly from the HFA group on the Foundation Index, with all AS individuals falling at or below the fifth percentile; 67% of HFA scores were in this range, with an additional 20% in the 6–25th percentiles. Despite the overlap with the Foundation Index, scores on the Coordination Index did not distinguish the groups, with 50 and 53% of the AS and HFA groups, respectively, placing at or below the fifth percentile, and 70 (AS) and 80% (HFA) between the 6th and 25th percentiles. No specific items differentiated the groups. Iwanaga and colleagues concluded that clumsiness cannot serve as a diagnostic feature to distinguish AS from autism, given the high prevalence of motor problems in both the AS and HFA groups.

The preceding discussion makes it clear that any simple characterization of AS as involving reduced motor skills relative to HFA is not supported by the evidence. Instead, results of these recent investigations reinforce the points previously made by Ghaziuddin and Butler (1998) and Smith (2000). While the AS–HFA distinction does not hold up in the motor domain, this is not to say that *patterns* of motor performance, including developmental variations in motor abilities and associations with other characteristics, may not vary across the spectrum of autism. More studies are appearing that test specific hypotheses about motor and perceptual–motor impairments in ASD.

MOTOR IMPAIRMENTS IN AUTISTIC SPECTRUM DISORDERS

Aside from the questions of whether AS and HFA are distinguishable, and whether motor skills contribute to such a distinction, various aspects of motor functioning in individuals with disorders on the autistic spectrum have been the focus of recent work. These studies have used standardized and/or experimental motor and perceptual–motor tasks. In addition, recent research that has employed functional neuroimaging to examine the neural substrate of motor skills in autism is beginning to bear fruit.

As indicated in the foregoing section on ASD subtypes, earlier claims that even high-functioning ASD is associated with poor performance on standardized motor skill assessments have generally been confirmed, and increased interest in these findings is apparent in the number of recent studies. In spite of the lack of diagnostic specificity of motor problems for AS, a focus on AS continues to be apparent in the literature. Gunter, Ghaziuddin, and Ellis (2002) tested a group of eight individuals with AS (mostly adolescents; seven males), compared with verbal IQ-matched typically developing controls (sex of controls not given). Unlike most studies, Gunter and colleagues did not observe deficits on simple motor tasks. AS participants threaded beads as rapidly as normal controls on a nonstandardized task. A novel line-tracing task using an "Etch-a-Sketch" toy was used to assess bimanual coordination and visual–motor control, again with no differences obtained between the AS and normal control groups. Finally, Luria's reciprocal coordination task (bimanual alternation of making and releasing a fist) was administered, with six of eight AS participants and all eight controls obtaining "passing" scores. In their discussion, Gunter and colleagues described these results as suggesting that "motor problems are a characteristic, but not an essential, feature of AS." This study is limited by a small sample, nonstandard tasks, minimal information about the scoring of performance, and a relatively uninformative (normal) control group.

Weimar, Schatz, Lincoln, Ballantyne, and Trauner (2001) also pursued the issue of motor impairment in AS. Their AS group of 10 male children and adolescents was matched on a case-control basis to a typically developing group on verbal IQ, as well as age, sex, and socioeconomic status. Diagnoses of AS were based on DSM-IV criteria; therefore, participants were not selected on the basis of motor skills. Full-Scale IQs appear to be in the normal range, and no children with evidence of language delay were included. Measures included finger tapping, Grooved Pegboard, Trail Making, finger–thumb apposition, the Developmental Test of Visual–Motor Integration, a 26-item apraxia assessment, and tests of ataxia (balance and gait while walking a line heel-to-toe, static balance). No impairments were found (for AS or controls) on simple

manual motor tasks such as finger tapping or pegboards. However, Weimar and colleagues obtained significant differences on their apraxia measures, especially an increase in posture errors (i.e., inaccurate hand configurations during testing of manual
gesture imitation). This result is consistent with previous findings in non-Asperger
ASD (e.g., Rogers, Bennetto, McEvoy, & Pennington, 1996; Smith & Bryson, 1998).
Problems with balance during the eyes-closed condition were also observed, again
confirming previous work with participants with non-Asperger ASD (Kohen-Raz,
Volkmar, & Cohen, 1992). Finally, the authors reported poor finger–thumb apposition performance, which they attributed to the failure by AS individuals to watch their
hands during the task. Weimar et al. summarized these observations by noting the role
of proprioception (perceptual awareness of body position) in each of the tasks in
which deficits were found. They concluded that impaired proprioceptive rather than
motor abilities appeared characteristic of AS.

Weimar and colleagues' (2001) failure to find motor problems in children with AS
is somewhat surprising, as most previous studies have found deficits on comparable
tasks in individuals with ASD, including AS (Smith, 2000, and above). On the other
hand, Weimar and colleagues' speculations regarding the use of visual and proprioceptive information by individuals with ASD are interesting and are elaborated on
later. The inconsistencies in the findings of these studies underscore yet again the difficulties in the literature on motor problems in AS versus HFA, both with sample selection and the conceptualization of clumsiness or motor problems. Investigators' choices
of control groups are also clearly critical. Both Gunter and colleagues (2002) and
Weimar and colleagues compared the motor skills of children with AS to those of typically developing children. The more important question, given what we understand of
the heterogeneity of motor skills within the autistic spectrum, is whether the profile of
skills differs from that seen in children with other developmental disorders. The issue
of individual differences also bears attention in the context of this heterogeneity.

Green and colleagues (2002) have made a more substantial contribution to the issue of syndrome specificity of motor problems in ASD. Green and colleagues set out to
determine whether motor impairment was present in a carefully diagnosed group of
children with AS, and whether the nature or extent of motor problems differentiated
these children from a matched group with a specific developmental disorder of motor
function (SDD-MF). This ICD-10 diagnosis is similar to DSM-IV's developmental coordination disorder and is used to categorize children who present with marked specific motor problems in the absence of mental retardation, language problems, or
other neurodevelopmental disorder. The ADI-R was used to probe for autistic symptoms in the AS group, and to rule out ASD in the SDD-MF sample. The M-ABC and a
test of praxis (specifically, imitation of meaningless movements, and object use pantomime) were used to measure motor functions in the two groups (11 boys with AS, 9
boys with SDD-MF, all with verbal IQs of at least 80). The results indicated that the
AS group obtained a mean M-ABC score somewhat higher than the SDD-MF mean
(indicative of greater impairment). Furthermore, all AS participants met the cutoff for
motor impairment used to select the SDD-MF group. These findings confirm that
clumsiness is indeed characteristic of children with AS, leaving the question of whether
the pattern of impairment differed from that in SDD-MF. Only the Ball Skills subtest
appeared to distinguish the groups, with AS boys showing poorer scores. Deficiencies
in such skills may be exacerbated for individuals with AS in part because their social

deficits limit their experiences with ball games (Tantum, 1991). Performance on the Manual Dexterity and Balance subtests was equally impaired for the two groups. On the test of praxis, the AS group performed more poorly than did controls, with no significant effect of gesture type (meaningless vs. symbolic) or any significant interaction. However, there were no differences in the error patterns observed for the two groups on these manual gesture tasks. The authors therefore concluded that clumsy motor performance was characteristic of children with AS. More important, they demonstrated that the clumsiness of these children was not qualitatively distinct from that seen in children with specific motor problems unaccompanied by either autistic symptoms or language problems.

Green and colleagues' (2002) study is a significant contribution to our understanding of motor phenomena in ASD. Surprisingly, the broader literature on developmental motor problems has seldom been referred to in the debate regarding motor skills in autism, and as indicated previously, clinical controls have not always been employed. The demonstration that children selected on the basis of their motor difficulties alone show a comparable pattern of impairment to those with AS provides a cautionary tale regarding the necessity of careful control group choices. Those involved in research on ASD must remain cautious about inferring autism-specific dysfunction. This has been an issue especially in studies comparing the performance of individuals with AS and HFA to that of typically developing IQ-matched controls.

Motor skills in children with ASD who are not "high functioning" have received little recent attention. An exception is the study by Hauck and Dewey (2001), which examined the relationship between ambiguous hand preference and motor skills in children with autism. Specifically, the investigators sought evidence to evaluate three theories that have been proposed to account for the increased prevalence of ambiguous/inconsistent-handedness reported in autism. Participants were 20 children, ages 2½ to 7 years, who met criteria for autistic disorder. Two control groups were matched on mental age to the children with autism. The first control group consisted of children with nonspecific developmental delays; they were also matched on chronological age to the group with ASD. The typically developing children in the second mental-age-matched group were, on average, 8 months younger than the children with autism. The Motor Domain of the Battelle Development Inventory (Newborg, Stock, Wnek, Guibaldi, & Svinicki, 1984) was administered, yielding age-equivalent scores for Fine Motor and Gross Motor skills. The results confirmed that ambiguous-handedness is observed more frequently in children with autism than in matched developmentally delayed controls. The fine and gross motor skills of the developmentally delayed group were significantly higher than those of the typical controls (who were younger, and whose scores were at expected levels for their age). Neither the fine nor gross motor scores of the children with autism differed significantly from either control group. Analysis of trends suggested that for the children with autism only, those who had not developed a hand preference showed relatively poor fine motor skills. Thus, there appears to be a complex relationship between the development of hand preference and motor skill in autism that is unlike that observed in other children with developmental delays. The implications of these findings remain to be explored. In particular, these findings raise questions about the developmental course of motor skill acquisition that may be important as we advance our understanding of possible subtypes.

The previous studies have used global measures of performance on complex tasks such as those in clinical test batteries to examine the motor and perceptual–motor skills of children with ASD. We now turn our discussion to studies that have examined component processes of motor and perceptual–motor tasks.

SPECIFIC MOTOR FUNCTIONS IN AUTISTIC SPECTRUM DISORDERS

Rinehart, Bradshaw, Brereton, and Tonge (2001) articulated the need to determine whether motor dysfunction in autism was primarily attributable to deficits in motor execution or to motor planning. They hypothesized a deficit in movement preparation, based on Hughes's (1996) work that demonstrated problems with movement planning. Rinehart and colleagues contrasted the performance of 5- to 19-year-olds with AS ($N = 12$) or HFA ($N = 11$). Diagnoses were made according to DSM-IV criteria, using procedures that included the ADI-R. Each group was matched to a typically developing control group for age, sex, and Full Scale IQ. Rinehart and colleagues employed a motor reprogramming task to examine separately the preparation and execution of movements. The task required participants to alternate repeatedly between left and right button presses, in response to a light cue at the base of each button. On "oddball" trials, the participant was cued to move in an unexpected direction to another adjacent button (a movement of equal distance). The results indicated that speed of motor execution in this movement reprogramming task resembled that of controls for both HFA and AS groups. However, both clinical groups differed from their controls on the movement preparation parameters, but in different ways. Children with HFA showed fast movement preparation across trials and were unaffected by the oddball trial. Controls were slower to prepare "pre-oddball" movements but responded faster on the trials immediately following the oddball. On the other hand, participants with AS were slower than their controls to prepare the first movement following oddball trials, thus demonstrating a response time cost where controls showed a benefit. The authors concluded that high-functioning persons with ASD show deficits in movement preparation rather than execution. The differences between AS and HFA in the pattern of impaired movement preparation were interpreted as evidence of differential neuropsychological mechanisms operating in the two forms of ASD, specifically the extent of frontostriatal involvement (postulated to be more extensive in AS than HFA).

While movement preparation abnormalities are consistent with some findings of motor planning deficits in autism (e.g., Hughes, 1996), these findings require additional study, particularly in light of such factors as the attentional demands of Rinehart et al.'s paradigm. As the authors acknowledge, abnormalities in the modulation of spatial attention have been demonstrated in ASD (Bryson, Landry, & Wainwright, 1997; Burack, Enns, Stauder, Mottron, & Randolph, 1997). However, again, comparisons to the performance of typically developing controls are not sufficient, given the evidence that motor difficulties are widespread among children with a variety of developmental disorders (Wilson & MacKenzie, 1998). Much remains to be learned about the interaction of attentional, sensory–perceptual, and motor systems in autism and related conditions.

NEURAL CORRELATES OF MOTOR FUNCTIONING
IN AUTISTIC SPECTRUM DISORDERS

Another rapidly expanding area of research is examining the neural substrates of motor and other functions in individuals with autism using neuroimaging techniques such as those discussed in detail by Dewey and Bottos (Chapter 2, this volume). Müller, Pierce, Ambrose, Allen, and Courchesne (2001) have conducted functional magnetic resonance imaging (fMRI) studies exploring such issues as whether people with autism show different patterns of localized neural activation during motor tasks. Their findings include evidence of atypical cortical activation during the performance of simple visually paced finger movements by eight adolescents and adults with autism, compared with normal controls. In addition, individuals with autism showed more variability in their motor responses. Müller and colleagues interpret these results as being consistent with their previous findings of abnormalities in both the anatomy and function of the cerebellum and related structures in individuals with autism (Courchesne, 1997). These findings, obtained with a small sample, bear replication as well as fuller exploration of their significance.

Mostofsky and colleagues (2002) have also reported fMRI findings that indicate abnormalities in the neural underpinnings of motor control. In their experiment, 13 children with HFA (ages 8–13 years) showed reduced patterns of activation in posterior cortex while performing serial finger-tapping movements. Controls were 20 typically developing children. Mostofsky and colleagues also suggested that abnormalities in parietal–cerebellar circuitry that subserve motor learning are responsible for the deficits in rotary pursuit learning in children with ASD noted in a preliminary report by his group (Mostofsky, Goldberg, & Denckla, 2001).

These lines of inquiry show promise in establishing underlying neurological abnormalities that may give rise to atypical motor performance in autism. It will be necessary to heed the lessons of clinical studies and to compare the performance of research participants with autism with that of other clinical groups, rather than only typically developing controls, in order to establish whether these motor abnormalities are autism-specific. These early findings also need to be merged with continued careful analytic studies that document the nature of abnormalities in motor performance in autism, their interactions with sensory–perceptual and/or attentional differences and their implications for real-world phenomena, such as praxic impairments (i.e., disorders of learned movements). A great deal of excitement has been generated recently by the identification of a candidate neural substrate for the ability to imitate movements. The discovery of a cell population that responds to both the performance of actions and the sight of cospecifics performing those actions in monkeys (Gallese, Fadiga, Fogassi, & Rizzolatti, 1996) and in humans (Iacoboni et al., 1999) has been considered particularly important for its potential for explaining the specifically impaired development of imitation abilities in autism (e.g., Williams, Whiten, Suddendorf, & Perrett, 2001). Several research groups are pursuing work relating neural imaging of the relevant areas to various aspects of behavior (e.g., Rizzolatti, Fadiga, Fogassi, & Gallese, 2002), including imitation in autism. Preliminary results (e.g., Williams, Whiten, Perrett, Murray, & Gilchrist, 2003) suggest different patterns of activation during simple motor tasks in response to visual cues in individuals with autism. These findings need to be extended and integrated with the results of other neuroimaging work, such as that cited previously that implicates cerebellar abnormalities (Müller et al., 2001). Given the level of interest these studies have generated, rapid advances can be anticipated.

PRAXIS AND PERCEPTUAL–MOTOR DYSFUNCTION IN AUTISTIC SPECTRUM DISORDERS

There is a consensus that imitation of body movements is specifically impaired in ASD, based on comprehensive reviews by Rogers (1999; Rogers & Bennetto, 2000) and Smith (2000; Smith & Bryson, 1994). Compared with both typical and clinical controls, individuals with autism tend to imitate less, to produce poorer approximations of manual and body postures, and to commit specific types of errors more frequently (although see Green et al., 2002, discussed previously). For example, when imitating a gesture in which the palm of the hand "faces" the viewer, the person with ASD may reverse the palm. While not unique to ASD, this error has now been observed significantly more often in ASD than controls in several studies (Ohta, 1987; Smith & Bryson, 1998; Whiten & Brown, 1999). This finding has been interpreted as an indication that, even on the level of action (vs. thought), people with autism have difficulty integrating information specifying first- and third-person perspectives (Barresi & Moore, 1996). In my lab, we have also observed that when children with ASD have learned an arm movement sequence, a similarly telling error occurs after the model is shown unexpectedly from a novel perspective. Our preliminary data suggest that the children have difficulty recognizing that the familiar movements are unchanged when presented from a different view (Smith, 2002). These data are consistent with the view that imitation may be a challenge in part because the information specifying "other" is not readily available for translation into movement of the self. It remains to be determined whether there is a general problem with perceptual–motor interactions or the construction of amodal representations in autism. An alternative possibility is a specific abnormality in the construction of the body schema, which may in turn be related to deficient functioning of a mirror neuron system.

Additional evidence is needed regarding whether integration of information across perceptual modalities is atypical in ASD, a possibility that has been suggested by both anecdotal and experimental evidence (O'Neill & Jones, 1997; Smith, 2000). Specifically, the interaction of visual and proprioceptive/kinesthetic input in the control of actions in autism deserves close attention. In many circumstances the behavior of people with ASD tends to be "visually driven," that is, dictated by the immediacy of visual stimuli (e.g., Fox & Tallis, 1994). Perhaps this is most apparent in situations in which visual and proprioceptive sources of information are in conflict (Hermelin & O'Connor, 1970; Masterton & Beiderman, 1983). This phenomenon may help to account for the extent to which behavior is context-bound in autism. That is, concrete visual similarities, rather than amodal or conceptual relationships, may determine the individual's responses.

Perceptual–motor difficulties in autism have also long been recognized in the occupational therapy literature, well-reviewed by Anzalone and Williamson (2000). These descriptive studies contribute observations that beg exploration, for example, the tendency of people with autism to engage in stereotypical "self-stimulatory" motor behaviors or to manipulate objects to afford close visual scrutiny. Empirical tests of the perceptual–motor mechanisms underlying these phenomena are challenges for future research. The possible roles of abnormalities in the modulation of spatial attention (Bryson et al., 1997) and inhibition (Brian, Tipper, Weaver, & Bryson, 2002) need to be considered in an adequate account of intermodal processing and perceptual–motor functioning in autism. Should distinctive patterns of abnormal information processing and motor performance be found to characterize older individuals with ASD, identification of these patterns may also lead to new hypotheses about the origins and natural history of the disorder. Increasingly there is evidence that very early in life, differences in motor and sensory behaviors may indicate risk for autism.

EARLY SIGNS OF AUTISM: ATYPICAL MOTOR AND PERCEPTUAL–MOTOR DEVELOPMENT?

There are two sources of evidence that children with ASD show motor and sensory differences as infants, well prior to diagnosis of the disorder. First are retrospective analyses of videotapes recorded during the infancies of children later diagnosed with ASD. Teitelbaum, Teitelbaum, Nye, Fryman, and Maurer (1998), using a detailed movement coding system, reported a variety of motor disturbances for 17 children who later received ASD diagnoses. These infants' symptoms included unusual oral–motor movements and atypical acquisition of motor milestones. Unfortunately, no control data were presented, which raises the now familiar question of whether a comparable group of children with other developmental disabilities would show similar atypical behaviors.

In the context of the critical need for earlier diagnosis of ASD, and retrospective reports of the early development of children later diagnosed with autism (Adrien et al.,1992; Baranek, 1999; Dawson, Osterling, Meltzoff, & Kuhl, 2000; Osterling, Dawson, & Munson, 2002), Bryson and her collaborators (2001) have developed the Autism Observation Scale for Infants (AOSI). The AOSI includes items intended to elicit motor and sensory behaviors that have been observed in infants later diagnosed with autism, as well as items sensitive to differences in early social and communicative behaviors that are associated with autism. Bryson and colleagues (Zwaigenbaum et al., 2002) are administering the AOSI prospectively to a large group of high-risk infants (those who have an older sibling with ASD). Preliminary data suggest that sensory and motor phenomena may be important predictors of an autism diagnosis (Zwaigenbaum et al., 2002). As with other findings discussed in this chapter, discriminant validation with groups of children with other developmental disabilities will be essential, and these studies are in progress.

SUMMARY

Motor problems are common in individuals with ASD, but all available evidence confirms that they do not differentiate reliably among ASD subtypes, as currently defined. From a practical standpoint, this means that clumsiness should not be considered as a criterion for AS. The possibility remains, however, that specific patterns of motor or perceptual–motor differences may be associated with particular constellations of ASD symptoms, and that these relationships may be uncovered with additional research.

Studies using neuroimaging techniques promise to enrich our understanding of the roots of these differences, particularly in light of indications that abnormal functioning of the "mirror neuron" system may provide a neural substrate for the well-established imitation deficits in ASD. However, a focus on the nature and quality of motor performance, in addition to the neurological localization of deficits, remains important. How, as well as whether, a child performs a task is important, as our knowledge of individual differences and of patterns of association among motor and other symptoms is still limited. The most critical variables continue to be a careful description of the participant characteristics, a hypothesis-driven and componential approach to the choice of tasks and use of appropriate controls.

I have emphasized that basic processes contribute to the development of higher functions. A corollary is that a cascade of developmental consequences may follow from an initial disruption of one or more fundamental processes (cf. Dawson & Lewy, 1989a, 1989b). In this vein, the possible role of perceptual–motor differences in the genesis of autism is another area of inquiry that has the potential to assist in the pressing clinical need for earlier identification. Major tasks ahead include the documentation of the growth of motor and perceptual–motor skills in autism, from prospective studies of both at-risk and early-identified children, compared with controls with other forms of developmental disorder, as well as typically developing children. Much work is needed for us to better understand how well-integrated perceptual–motor functioning enables early social–cognitive development. Models are needed that account for normal acquisition of these skills, and for the specific patterns of motor skill differences that can be observed in disorders of development that are also empirically dissociable in other respects. This volume stands to advance this cause and, ultimately, to benefit the clinical agenda.

REFERENCES

Adrien, J. L., Perrot, A., Sauvage, D., Leddet, I., Larmande, C., Hameury, L., et al. (1992). Early symptoms in autism from family home movies: Evaluation and comparison between 1st and 2nd year of life using IBSE scale. *Acta Paedopsychiatrica, 55*, 71–75.

American Psychiatric Association. (1994). *Diagnostic and statistical manual of mental disorders* (4th ed.). Washington, DC: Author.

Anzalone, M. E., & Williamson, G. G. (2000). Sensory processing and motor performance in autism spectrum disorders. In A. M.Wetherby & B. M. Prizant (Eds.), *Autism spectrum disorders: A transactional developmental perspective* (pp.143–166). Baltimore: Brookes.

Asperger, H. (1991). "Autistic psychopathy" in childhood. In U. Frith (Ed. & Trans.), *Autism and Asperger syndrome* (pp. 37–92). Cambridge UK: Cambridge University Press. (Original work published 1944)

Baranek, G. (1999). Autism during infancy: A retrospective video analysis of sensory-motor and social behaviors at 9–12 months of age. *Journal of Autism and Developmental Disorders, 29*, 213–224.

Baron-Cohen, S., Tager-Flusberg, H., & Cohen, D. J. (Eds.). (1999). *Understanding other minds: Perspectives from developmental cognitive neuroscience* (2nd ed.). Oxford, UK: Oxford University Press.

Barresi, J., & Moore, C. (1996). Intentional relations and social understanding. *Brain and Behavioral Sciences, 19,* 107–122.

Brian, J. A., Tipper, S. P., Weaver, B., & Bryson, S. E. (2002, November). *Inhibitory control in autism spectrum disorders: Hyper-processing of color versus normal inhibition of location.* Poster presented to the International Meeting for Autism Research, Orlando, FL.

Bryson, S. E., Landry, R., & Wainwright, J. A. (1997). A componential view of executive dysfunction in autism: Review of recent evidence. In J. A. Burack & J. T. Enns (Eds.), *Attention, development, and psychopathology* (pp. 232–262). New York: Guilford Press.

Bryson, S. E., Rombough, V., McDermott, Wainwright, A., Szatmari, L., & Zwaigenbaum, L. (2001, November). *Autism Observation Scale for Infants: Scale development and preliminary reliability data.* Paper presented to the International Meeting for Autism Research, San Diego, CA.

Bryson, S. E., & Smith, I. M. (1998). Epidemiology of autism: Prevalence, associated characteristics, and implications for research and service delivery. *Mental Retardation and Developmental Disabilities Research Reviews, 4,* 97–103.

Burack, J. A., Enns, J. T., Stauder, J. E. A., Mottron, L., & Randolph, B. (1997). Attention and autism: Behavioral and electrophysiological evidence. In D. J. Cohen & F. R. Volkmar (Eds.), *Handbook of autism and pervasive developmental disorders* (2nd ed., pp. 226–247). New York: Wiley.

Courchesne, E. (1997). Brainstem, cerebellar, and limbic neuroanatomical abnormalities in autism. *Current Opinion in Neurobiology, 7,* 269–278.

Dawson, G., & Lewy, A. (1989a). Arousal, attention, and the socioemotional impairments of individuals with autism. In G. Dawson (Ed.), *Autism: Nature, diagnosis, and treatment* (pp. 49–74). New York: Guilford Press.

Dawson, G., & Lewy, A. (1989b). Reciprocal subcortical–cortical influences in autism: The role of attentional mechanisms. In G. Dawson (Ed.), *Autism: Nature, diagnosis, and treatment* (pp. 144–173). New York: Guilford Press.

Dawson, G., Osterling, J., Meltzoff, A. N., & Kuhl, P. (2000). Case study of the development of an infant with autism from birth to two years of age. *Journal of Applied Developmental Psychology, 21,* 299–313.

Fein, D., Stevens, M., Dunn, M., Waterhouse, L., Allen, D., Rapin, I., et al. (1999). Subtypes of pervasive developmental disorder: Clinical characteristics. *Child Neurology, 5,* 1–23.

Fox, N. S., & Tallis, F. (1994). Utilization behaviour in adults with autism: A preliminary investigation. *Clinical Psychology and Psychotherapy, 1,* 210–218.

Gallese, V., Fadiga, L., Fogassi, L., & Rizzolatti, G. (1996). Action recognition in the premotor cortex. *Brain, 119,* 593–609.

Ghaziuddin, M., & Butler, E. (1998). Clumsiness in autism and Asperger syndrome: A further report. *Journal of Intellectual Disability Research, 42,* 43–48.

Ghaziuddin, M., Tsai, L. Y., & Ghaziuddin, N. (1992). A reappraisal of clumsiness as a diagnostic feature of Asperger syndrome. *Journal of Autism and Developmental Disorders, 22,* 651–656.

Gillberg, C. (1989). Asperger syndrome in 23 Swedish children: A clinical study. *Developmental Medicine and Child Neurology, 31,* 520–531.

Gillberg, C. (1998). Asperger syndrome and high-functioning autism. *British Journal of Psychiatry, 172,* 200–209.

Green, D., Baird, G., Barnett, A. L., Henderson, L., Huber, J., & Henderson, S. E. (2002). The severity and nature of motor impairment in Asperger's syndrome: A comparison with specific developmental disorder of motor function. *Journal of Child Psychology, 43,* 655–668.

Gunter, H. L., Ghaziuddin, M., & Ellis, H. D. (2002). Asperger syndrome: Tests of right hemisphere functioning and interhemispheric communication. *Journal of Autism and Developmental Disorders, 32,* 263–282.

Hauck, J. A., & Dewey, D. (2001). Hand preference and motor functioning in children with autism. *Journal of Autism and Developmental Disorders, 31,* 265–278.

Henderson, S. E., & Sugden, D. A. (1992). *Movement Assessment Battery for Children.* San Antonio, TX: Psychological Corporation.

Hermelin, B., & O'Connor, N. (1970). *Psychological experiments with autistic children.* Oxford, UK: Pergamon Press.

Hughes, C. (1996). Planning problems in autism at the level of motor control. *Journal of Autism and Developmental Disorders, 26,* 90–107.

Iacoboni, M., Woods, R. P., Brass, M., Bekkering, H., Mazziotta, J. C., & Rizzolatti, G. (1999). Cortical mechanisms of human imitation. *Science, 286,* 2526–2528.

Iwanaga, R., Kawasaki, C., & Tsuchida, R. (2000). Brief report: Comparison of sensory–motor and cognitive function between autism and Asperger syndrome in preschool children. *Journal of Autism and Developmental Disorders, 30,* 169–174.

Joseph, R. M., & Tanaka, J. (2003). Holistic and part-based face recognition in children with autism. *Journal of Child Psychology and Psychiatry, 44,* 529–542.

Kanner, L. (1973). Autistic disturbances of affective contact. In *Childhood psychosis: Initial studies and new insights.* Washington, DC: V.H. Winston. (Original work published 1943)

Klin A., Volkmar, F. R., Sparrow, S. S., Cicchetti, D. V., & Rourke, B. P. (1995). Validity and neuropsychological characterization of Asperger syndrome: Convergence with nonverbal learning disabilities syndrome. *Journal of Child Psychology and Psychiatry, 36,* 1127–1140.

Kohen-Raz, R., Volkmar, F. R., & Cohen, D. J. (1992). Postural control in children with autism. *Journal of Autism and Developmental Disorders, 22,* 419–432.

Lewis, M. H., & Bodfish, J. W. (1998). Repetitive behavior disorders in autism. *Mental Retardation and Developmental Disabilities, 4,* 80–89.

Lord, C., Rutter, M., & DiLavore, P. (1998). *The Autism Diagnostic Observation Schedule—Generic.* Chicago: Department of Psychiatry, University of Chicago.

Lord, C., Rutter, M., & LeCouteur, A. (1994). Autism Diagnostic Interview—Revised: A revised version of a diagnostic interview for caregivers of individuals with possible pervasive developmental disorders. *Journal of Autism and Developmental Disorders, 24,* 659–685.

Mahoney, W. J., Szatmari, P., MacLean, J. E., Bryson, S. E., Bartolucci, G., Walter, S. D., et al. (1998). Reliability and accuracy of differentiating pervasive developmental disorder subtypes. *Journal of the American Academy of Child and Adolescent Psychiatry, 37,* 278–285.

Masterton, B. A., & Biederman, G. B. (1983). Proprioceptive versus visual control in autistic children. *Journal of Autism and Developmental Disorders, 13,* 141–152.

Miller, J. N., & Ozonoff, S. (2000). The external validity of Asperger disorder: Lack of evidence from the domain of neuropsychology. *Journal of Abnormal Psychology, 109,* 227–238.

Mostofsky, S., Goldberg, M., & Denckla, M. (2001, November). *Impaired learning of rotary pursuit in children with autism.* Paper presented to the International Meeting for Autism Research, San Diego.

Mostofsky, S., Goldberg, M., Schafer, J. G., Boyce, A., Flower, A., Denckla, M., et al. (2002, November). *Differences in posterior cortical fMRI activation during finger sequencing in children with autism.* Paper presented to the International Meeting for Autism Research, Orlando, FL.

Mount, R. H., Hastings, R .P., Reilly S., Cass, H., & Charman, T. (2003). Towards a behavioural phenotype for Rett syndrome. *American Journal of Mental Retardation, 108,* 1–12.

Müller, R. A., Pierce, K., Ambrose, J. B., Allen, G., & Courchesne, E. (2001). Atypical patterns of cerebral motor activation in autism: A functional magnetic resonance study. *Biological Psychiatry, 49,* 665–676.

Mundy, P., Sigman, M., & Kasari, C. (1994). Joint attention, developmental level, and symptom presentation in autism. *Development and Psychology, 6,* 389–401.

Newborg, J., Stock, J. R., Wnek, L., Guidubaldi, J., & Svicki, J. (1984). *The Battelle Development Inventory.* Chicago: Riverside.

Ohta, M. (1987). Cognitive disorders of infantile autism: A study employing the WISC, spatial relationship conceptualization and gesture imitations. *Journal of Autism and Developmental Disorders, 17,* 45–62.

O'Neill, M., & Jones, R. S. P. (1997). Sensory-perceptual abnormalities in autism: A case for more research? *Journal of Autism and Developmental Disorders, 27,* 283–294.

Osterling, J. A., Dawson, G., & Munson, J. A. (2002). Early recognition of 1–year-old infants with autism spectrum disorder versus mental retardation. *Development and Psychopathology, 14,* 239–251.

Rinehart, N. J., Bradshaw, J. L., Brereton, A. V., & Tonge, B. J. (2001). Movement preparation in high-functioning autism and Asperger Disorder: A serial choice reaction time task involving motor reprogramming. *Journal of Autism and Developmental Disorders, 31,* 79–88.

Rizzolatti, G., Fadiga, L., Fogassi, L., & Gallese, V. (2002). From mirror neurons to imitation: Facts and speculation. In A. N. Meltzoff & W. Prinz (Eds.), *The imitative mind: Development, evolution, and brain bases* (pp. 247–266). Cambridge, UK: Cambridge University Press.

Rogers, S. (1999). An examination of the imitation deficit in autism. In J. Nadel & G. Butterworth (Eds.), *Imitation in infancy.* Cambridge, UK: Cambridge University Press.

Rogers, S. J., & Bennetto, L. (2000). Intersubjectivity in autism. In A. M. Wetherby & B. M. Prizant (Eds.), *Autism spectrum disorders: A transactional developmental perspective* (pp. 79–107). Baltimore: Brookes.

Rogers, S. J., Bennetto, L., McEvoy, R. E., & Pennington, B. F. (1996). Imitation and pantomime in high-functioning adolescents with autism spectrum disorders. *Child Development, 67,* 2060–2073.

Russell, J. (Ed.). (1998). *Autism as an executive disorder.* Oxford, UK: Oxford University Press.

Schopler, E. (1998). Premature popularization of Asperger syndrome. In E. Schopler, G. Mesibov, & L. J. Kunce (Eds.), *Asperger syndrome or high-functioning autism?* (pp. 385–399). New York: Plenum Press.

Seal, B. C., & Bonvillian, J. D. (1997). Sign language and motor functioning in students with autistic disorder. *Journal of Autism and Developmental Disorders, 27,* 437–466.

Smith, I. M. (2000). Motor functioning in Asperger syndrome. In A. Klin, F. R. Volkmar, & S. S. Sparrow (Eds.), *Asperger syndrome* (pp. 97–124). New York: Guilford Press.

Smith, I. M. (2002, November). *Observational learning of motor sequences in autism.* Poster presented at the International Meeting for Autism Research, Orlando, FL.

Smith, I. M., & Bryson, S. E. (1994). Imitation and action in autism: A critical review. *Psychological Bulletin, 116,* 259–273.

Smith, I. M., & Bryson, S. E. (1998). Gesture imitation in autism I: Nonsymbolic postures and sequences. *Cognitive Neuropsychology, 15,* 747–770.

Spencer, J., O'Brien, J., Riggs, K., Braddick, O., Atkinson, J., & Wattam-Bell, J. (2000). Motion processing in autism: Evidence for a dorsal stream deficiency. *NeuroReport, 11,* 2765–2767.

Szatmari, P. (1998). Differential diagnosis of Asperger disorder. In E. Schopler, G. Mesibov, & L. J. Kunce (Eds.), *Asperger syndrome or high-functioning autism?* (pp. 61–76). New York: Plenum Press.

Szatmari, P., Bartolucci, G., & Bremner, R. (1989). Asperger's syndrome: Comparison of early history and outcome. *Developmental Medicine and Child Neurology, 31,* 709–720

Szatmari, P., Tuff, L., Finlayson, A. J., & Bartolucci, G. (1990). Asperger's syndrome and autism: Neurocognitive aspects. *Journal of the American Academy of Child and Adolescent Psychiatry, 29,* 130–136.

Tantam, D. (1991). Asperger syndrome in adulthood. In U. Frith (Ed.), *Autism and Asperger syndrome* (pp. 147–183). Cambridge, UK: Cambridge University Press.

Teitelbaum, P., Teitelbaum, O., Nye, J., Fryman, J., & Maurer, R. G. (1998). Movement analysis in infancy may be useful for early diagnosis of autism. *Proceedings of the National Academy of Science USA, 95,* 13982–13987.

Turner, M. (1999). Annotation: Repetitive behaviour in autism: A review of psychological research. *Journal of Child Psychology and Psychiatry, 40,* 839–849.

Volkmar, F. R., & Klin, A. (2000). Diagnostic issues in Asperger syndrome. In A. Klin, F. R. Volkmar, & S. S. Sparrow (Eds.), *Asperger syndrome* (pp. 25–71). New York: Guilford Press.

Weimer, A. K., Schatz, A. M., Lincoln, A., Ballantyne, A. O., & Trauner, D. A. (2001). "Motor" impairment in Asperger syndrome: Evidence for a deficit in proprioception. *Developmental and Behavioral Pediatrics, 22,* 92–101.

Whiten, A., & Brown J. D. (1999). Imitation and the reading of other minds: Perspectives from the study of autism, normal children and non-human primates. In S. Bråten (Ed.), *Intersubjective communication and emotion in ontogeny: A sourcebook* (pp. 260–280). Cambridge, UK: Cambridge University Press.

Williams, J. H., Whiten, A., Perrett, D. I., Murray, A., & Gilchrist, A. (2003, April). *Imitation in autism: A systematic review and a neuro-imaging study.* Paper presented at the annual meeting of the Society for Research in Child Development, Tampa, FL.

Williams, J. H., Whiten, A., Suddendorf, T., & Perrett, D. I. (2001). Imitation, mirror neurons and autism. *Neuroscience Behavioural Review, 25,* 287–95.

Wilson, P. H., & McKenzie, B. E. (1998). Information processing deficits associated with developmental coordination disorder: A meta-analysis of research findings. *Journal of Child Psychiatry, 39,* 829–840.

Wing, L. (1981). Asperger's syndrome: A clinical account. *Psychological Medicine, 11,* 115–129.

Wing, L. (1997). Syndromes of autism and atypical development. In D. J. Cohen & F. R. Volkmar (Eds.), *Handbook of autism and pervasive developmental disorders* (2nd ed., pp. 148–172). New York: Wiley.

World Health Organization. (1992). *International classification of mental and behavioural disorders* (10th ed.). *Clinical descriptions and diagnostic guidelines.* Geneva: Author.

Zwaigenbaum, L., Bryson, S. E., Brian, J., McDermott, C., Rombough, V., Roberts, W., & Szatmari, P. (2002, November). *Predicting social–communication impairments in young siblings of children with autism.* Poster presented at the International Meeting for Autism Research, Orlando, FL.

CHAPTER 8

Acquired Childhood Conditions
with Associated Motor Impairments

DEBORAH DEWEY
SHAUNA BOTTOS
DAVID E. TUPPER

Acquired cerebral disorders in children have been associated with intellectual impairment and developmental disability. However, children with many acquired conditions also display varied problems in the motor domain. In this chapter, we discuss the motor and perceptual–motor problems associated with a number of acquired childhood conditions. Specifically, we examine the motor and perceptual–motor difficulties encountered by children who have experienced pediatric head injury, childhood stroke, acute lymphoblastic leukemia, pediatric HIV, meningitis, hydrocephalus, exposure to toxins, and malnutrition. These are by no means the only acquired conditions that result in perceptual–motor impairments in children. The discussion, however, highlights the fact that a number of acquired childhood conditions result in motor impairments.

TRAUMATIC BRAIN INJURY

Traumatic brain injury (TBI) is a major cause of disability in children. The incidence of head trauma has been estimated to be 200 per 100,000 children per year (Kraus, 1995). Head trauma during childhood is most frequently a result of falls, motor vehicle accidents, sports-related injuries, or child abuse (Spreen, Risser, & Edgell, 1995). Boys are more commonly injured than girls, a gender discrepancy that emerges in infancy and becomes even more pronounced during the school-age years (Kraus, 1995).

The movement disorders associated with TBI are frequently the result of damage to the basal ganglia or nigrostriatal pathways (Guthrie, Mast, Richards, McQuaid, & Pavlakis, 1999). Research has shown that there is a strong dose–response relationship between the severity of the brain trauma and the degree of impairment, with posttraumatic movement disorders more commonly seen among children with severe brain trauma (Jaffe et al., 1992; Krauss, Trankle, & Koop, 1996). In fact, motor impairment is often a predictor or correlate of longer-term outcome from pediatric TBI (Klonoff, Clark, & Klonoff, 1993; Papero, Snyder, Gotschall, Johnson, & Eichelberger, 1997).

Lesions of the nervous system sustained during acquired craniocerebral trauma include diffuse axonal injury, multifocal contusional or vascular pathology, and possible hypoxia or secondary cellular dysfunction. Resulting movement disorders may include restricted or excessive limb motion, balance disturbances, or impairments in the timing and control of actions.

Acquired Neurological Motor Symptoms

Children with TBI display numerous neurologically mediated motor symptoms that may interfere with day-to-day functioning. Spasticity, a condition characterized by increased tone associated with hyperreflexia, is often the result of lesions at the cortical level or in its projections to the corticospinal tracts. It is frequently observed in children with TBI, particularly those with severe brain trauma (Costeff, Groswasser, & Goldstein, 1990; Wallen, Mackay, Duff, McCartney, & O'Flaherty, 2001) and accounts for many of the impairments in gross and fine motor coordination and dexterity evident among children with brain injury (Guthrie et al., 1999).

Another commonly encountered motor disability among children with TBI is ataxia (Brink, Imbus, & Woo-Sam, 1980; Costeff et al., 1990). Ataxia results in an inability in the effective control of the speed, range, force, and direction of movement and consequently difficulties with balance and the performance of precise movements are often evident (Spreen et al., 1995). A recent prospective study of children ranging in age up to 14 years in Australia provides compelling evidence that ataxia is far more characteristic of children suffering severe TBI than of children who sustain mild brain injury (Wallen et al., 2001). Results indicated that only children with severe TBI displayed ataxia (20% of the left upper limb and 6% of the right upper limb) on a baseline screening assessment. Although some of the children with mild TBI did manifest signs of ataxia at a 6-month follow-up, children with severe TBI were still significantly more likely to display this condition. Moreover, at a 2-year follow-up, 7% of the children who sustained severe TBI continued to display ataxia of the upper limbs, whereas no children who suffered mild TBI showed any lasting signs of ataxia.

Dysarthria is a motor speech disorder that can be the result of developmental or acquired conditions. Alajouanine and Lhermitte (1965) and Guttmann (1942) reported that dysarthria occurs frequently following the initial period of mutism in children with acquired brain lesions. Dysarthria may be due to central or peripheral nervous system damage and may affect phonation, respiration, articulation, feeding, swallowing, and intelligibility of speech. The incidence of dysarthria in TBI is unclear, although it is fairly common, and it would appear that the recovery from dysarthria is greater in children than in adults. Preliminary evidence also suggests that the severity of dysarthria may not be as great in children as in adults with similar lesions (Levin & Chapman, 1998; Murdoch, Ozanne, & Cross, 1990).

Following basal ganglia injury, choreoathetosis has been observed in many children with TBI (Guthrie et al., 1999). Chorea is manifest as involuntary, irregular, jerky and brisk movements, while athetosis involves slow, writhing movements (Spreen et al., 1995). Basal ganglia injury may also result in dystonia, a condition characterized by abnormal posturing and movement due to the simultaneous contraction of agonist and antagonist muscles (Spreen et al., 1995). Athetosis, ataxia, and dystonia often coexist with spasticity, a combination that greatly decreases graded muscle control (Guthrie et al., 1999).

Posttraumatic tremor has also been recognized as a complication of head injury in children (Obeso & Narbona, 1983), and appears to be associated with midbrain trauma (Johnson & Hall, 1992). In a survey of 289 children with severe TBI, the prevalence of significant tremor was reported to be at least 45% (Johnson & Hall, 1992). For the majority of the children, the onset of the tremor was within 2 months of the accident (49%), 40% showed onset between 2 and 12 months, and 2–3% in the second year following injury. In most children, the tremor occurred when a static posture was maintained and was exacerbated by activity. Although in the majority of cases, tremor subsided over time (54%), for many children it remained unchanged (31%), and for some children, it progressively worsened for a period of up to 3 years after the injury (5%).

Neuropsychological Motor Characteristics

One of the most commonly observed motor skill impairments evident among children with TBI, especially those with severe TBI, is a slowed response on a variety of timed motor tasks (Ewing-Cobbs, Fletcher, & Levin, 1995). Indeed, children with severe brain trauma have been found to exhibit significantly poorer performance on speeded motor response tasks such as coding, name writing, and finger tapping compared to children with mild or moderate TBI (Bawden, Knights, & Winogron, 1985; Jaffe et al., 1992). Consistent with these findings, Knights and colleagues (1991) found that there was a significant difference on timed tests of visual–motor speed and coordination between children with severe TBI and children with mild and moderate TBI; the latter two groups showing little difference in their performance and few deficits on motor tasks.

In a study conducted by Chaplin, Deitz, and Jaffe (1993), children with TBI were compared with normal controls on both gross and fine motor tasks. The authors found that children with TBI scored significantly lower than did their counterparts without TBI on the gross motor composite of the Bruininks–Oseretsky Test of Motor Proficiency (BOTMP). On all the specific gross motor subtests (i.e., running speed and agility, balance, bilateral coordination, and strength), children with TBI performed significantly worse than did those in the control group. In contrast, there was no difference between children with TBI and control children on the fine motor composite of the BOTMP; however, children with TBI did score significantly lower on the fine motor subtest measuring upper-limb speed and dexterity. One commonality of all of the aforementioned subtests is that they were timed. This suggests that poorer performance on motor tests for individuals with TBI is highly related to the speed of the motor response required. This is consistent with previous research that suggests that the speed of visual–motor responses is especially affected by TBI (Knights et al., 1991).

Although a number of studies have examined the impact of TBI on mobility and general motor skill functioning, few have focused specifically on the posttraumatic sequelae of TBI on upper-limb function. The one study that examined upper-limb performance found that in contrast to children with mild TBI, the most severely injured children had abnormal tone (dystonia) and motor control (Wallen et al., 2001). In particular, upper-limb dysfunction in the severe TBI group was marked by spasticity, hypotonia, and ataxia. Similarly, while no mild TBI subjects had difficulty with arm or hand control, most of the participants with severe TBI had some abnormalities in these areas as a consequence of their brain injuries. Importantly, the upper-limb function difficulties were still present at 2-year follow-up in children with severe TBI; 25–50% of these children had abnormal muscle tone, impaired arm and hand control, difficulty with tasks that required bilateral activity, and an abnormal or delayed handwriting grasp or poor handwriting, which in some cases required them to use a keyboard. In contrast, children in the mild TBI and the non-TBI control groups, displayed no persisting impairments.

With regard to more complex perceptual–motor skills, Yeates, Patterson, Waber, and Bernstein (2003) examined the constructional skills of children with closed head injury (CHI) using the Rey–Osterrieth Complex Figure (ROCF). Participants were 37 children, 6–14 years of age, with a history of CHI and 430 normative controls. Results indicated that the CHI group performed more poorly than did the comparison group on all measures. Performance was inversely related to severity of injury, and it varied qualitatively as a function of age at injury. Relative to the normative controls, children with CHI included fewer parts of the stimulus, made more errors, and organized their drawings less well. The authors concluded that CHI during childhood and adolescence is associated with subsequent deficits in constructional skills, over and above any declines in cognitive or motor speed.

Frontal lobe lesions are common in TBI and both higher cognitive and motoric sequelae are often related to anterior cerebral lesion localizations. It is therefore likely that children with TBI-related motor dysfunction also commonly show associated impairment in these higher cognitive or executive functions (Ewing-Cobbs et al., 1995; Ewing-Cobbs, Levin, & Fletcher, 1998). To date, the relationship between motor performance deficits and measures of executive functioning has not been studied extensively. It has been proposed, however, that measures of executive motor functioning, particularly assessment of motor sequencing, motor fluency, and overflow and inhibitory motor control, should routinely be included in evaluations of children with TBI (Denckla, 1994).

Although children with mild TBI have been described as showing few lasting motor performance deficits, recent evidence suggests that these children may display subtle changes in balance, response speed, and running speed (Gagnon, Forget, Sullivan, & Friedman, 1998). Gagnon and colleagues (1998) examined 28 children ages 5–15 years who had sustained a mild TBI (Glasgow Coma Scale score 13–15) with the BOTMP after they had been discharged from the hospital. Although all the children demonstrated normal functioning on a standard neurological examination, when compared to published norms on the BOTMP, the children's motor performance was significantly lower in the domains of balance, response speed, and running speed and agility.

The foregoing findings support the growing body of evidence that suggests that as the severity of head injury increases, more pronounced motor and perceptual–motor deficits are evident, and that these deficits tend to persist in many children with severe brain injury. Children with mild and moderate TBI, however, show no or few lasting motor performance deficits (O'Flaherty et al., 2000). As a result, the outcome of TBI can range from complete recovery of normal motor functioning to persistent impairment on many tasks, especially those requiring speeded responses, coordination, and gross and fine motor skills. Because of these persisting motor deficiencies in pediatric TBI, a school-based physical and motor treatment program is often necessary following outpatient rehabilitative treatment (Russell, Krouse, Lane, Leger, & Robson, 1998), and utilization of a kinesiology-based perspective may be particularly beneficial in working with such children (DePaepe & Lange, 1994).

CHILDHOOD STROKE

Cerebrovascular accidents (CVA, "strokes") are rare in children. They occur when the blood supply to a part of the brain is suddenly interrupted (ischemic), or when a blood vessel in the brain bursts, leaking blood into the spaces surrounding the brain cells (hemorrhagic). The reported incidence of stroke in children (birth to 14 years) is 2.5 to 2.7 cases per 100,000 children (Schoenberg, Mellinger, & Schoenberg, 1978). The causes of pediatric stroke are diverse (see Trauner, 1998); however, children with cardiovascular disease and sickle cell disease appear to be particularly vulnerable (Carlin & Chanmugam, 2002).

Evidence from studies focusing on motor functioning after childhood stroke suggest a wide spectrum of motor impairments, with the most common being hemiparesis (paralysis on one side of the body), often resulting from infarction in the territory of the middle cerebral artery (Giroud et al., 1997). The outcome of such damage has been found to be variable, ranging from normal functioning to severe impairment. An examination of the severity of hemiparesis in 42 children who experienced an early unilateral stroke sustained *in utero* or perinatally revealed that motor impairment was present in 33 children; nine children showed no motor deficits (Lanska, Lanska, Horwitz, & Aram, 1991). Among those children with motor dysfunction, two showed subclinical levels of functioning manifest as abnormal reflexes or tone asymmetry, yet displayed normal coordination and strength; one patient had an action tremor without hemiparesis; seven children had mild hemiparesis, which was characterized by mild weakness or incoordination with close to normal functional use of the involved extremities; 12 patients had moderate hemiparesis presenting as significant functional loss, such as pathological early hand preference or delayed gross motor skill acquisition, but retained assistive hand use; and 11 children had severe hemiparesis in which a severe gait disorder or a nonfunctional hand was evident.

In contrast to strokes that occur during the prenatal and neonatal periods, the clinical presentation of stroke later in childhood appears to be marked by significantly more overt signs of motor dysfunction immediately following the CVA. For instance, older infants and toddlers with stroke commonly present with abrupt onset of a hemiparesis, with or without seizures (Lanska et al., 1991), difficulty using one hand, or dragging of one leg (deVeber, 2002). In these children, the motor deficit is noted to be the most pronounced at the onset and tends to improve with time. Moreover, Lanska and colleagues (1991) reported that among the sample of older children in their study (median age 42 months), those children who improved the most tended to do so relatively quickly following their stroke, usually within 2 weeks. In comparison, children who continued to exhibit a major functional disability at discharge from the hospital, usually a nonfunctional upper limb, did not recover significant functional use in the long term. Thus, although the majority of children were found to regain some strength and ambulated independently, many of the children continued to have severe functional disability.

Consistent with the findings by Lanska and colleagues (1991), other investigators have reported hemiparesis as a common outcome following stroke in children beyond the neonatal period. Keidan, Shahar, Barzilay, Passwell, and Brand (1994) found that 40% of the infants and children in their study (mean age 6 years) exhibited acute hemiplegia or monoplegia. More recently, Mancini and colleagues (1997) observed hemiparesis in 45% of a sample of children who suffered a stroke between 2 months and 17 years of age. These findings demonstrate the consistency in outcome following CVA among children and adolescents (deVeber, 2002).

Although the prognosis for full functional recovery of the side(s) of the body affected by paralysis may appear poor for many children following a CVA, this is not always the case. Wulfeck, Trauner, and Tallal (1991) found that despite the presence of hemiparesis in infants who suffered early localized, unilateral cerebral infarction within the first 2 months of life, functional motor development was not significantly delayed. Furthermore, in many of the children, the hemiparesis resolved or was markedly diminished by 2 years of age, with all the children being capable of independent ambulation. Studies of children who experienced stroke pre- or perinatally have also reported that some of these children acquired motor milestones at nearly expected times, even in the presence of hemiparesis (Trauner, Chase, Walker, & Wulfeck, 1993). The majority, however, still continued to exhibit at least mild residual motor impairment (Trauner et al., 1993).

In addition to hemiparesis, child survivors of stroke may experience many other motor deficits that may be a significant source of disability. Neurological examinations often reveal that the infant or child has persistent difficulty with tasks involving fine and gross motor skills, in addition to impaired motor tone, strength, reflexes, and involuntary movements (deVeber, MacGregor, Curtis, & Mayank, 2000). Indeed, deVeber and colleagues (2000) reported that more than 70% of the children with stroke had such residual motor deficits. In a more recent study, Gordon, Ganesan, Towell, and Kirkham (2002) also observed activity limitation due to impairment in both gross and fine motor functioning in children following stroke.

Disturbances in voluntary movements have also been reported in children with pediatric stroke. Dusser, Goutieres, and Aicardi (1986) found that of 22 cases of idiopathic strokes, permanent motor handicap persisted in 18 children. After an average follow-up duration of 48 months, disturbances of voluntary movement were evident and were thought to be due to the frequent occurrence of basal ganglia infarctions in this sample. In addition, residual dystonia or dyskinesia, often a result of striato-capsular infarcts, was observed in 14 children. Dystonia has also been reported to appear several months or years after the actual stroke (Demierre & Rondot, 1983; Mancini et al., 1997).

As noted previously, children with sickle cell disease may be at particular risk for stroke. Sickle cell anemia is an inherited hemoglobulinopathy that is characterized by an abnormally high amount of hemoglobin S (rather than the normal hemoglobin A) in the blood, resulting in the more viscous, sickled red blood cells that aggregate and slow blood flow. Thus, individuals with sickle cell disease are predisposed to blockage of vessels and possible infarction (Trauner, 1998). It is estimated that stroke may occur in 7–24% of children younger than 15 years of age with sickle cell disease. Most of the strokes occur via large-vessel occlusion, and distal branches of the internal carotid system are particularly common sites. Some children with sickle cell disease may have recurrent strokes in different cerebral blood vessels. Intracranial hemorrhages are far less common but have been described (Van Hoff, Ritchey, & Shaywitz, 1985). Neurological sequelae, most notably hemiparesis, headache, and seizures, are noted in sickle cell children who have suffered strokes (Trauner, 1998).

Neuropsychological consequences of stroke in sickle cell disease have been less well studied, although motor disturbances have been noted in cases with obvious neurological involvement. Early research on cognitive functioning in children with sickle cell anemia without neurological complications noted mixed results with regard to intellectual impairment, but a number of methodological concerns were present (Trauner, 1998). A more careful study by Swift and colleagues (1989) compared children with sickle cell anemia to sibling controls on a comprehensive neuropsychological test battery, including measures of constructional and motor skills. Subtle but widespread neuropsychological deficits were found to be associated with sickle cell anemia, with the sickle cell group performing more poorly on many measures. Findings for the Beery Developmental Test of Visual Motor Integration were in the predicted direction; however, they were not statistically significant. Hence, until more definitive research is conducted, it appears that children with sickle cell anemia (but without obvious cerebrovascular involvement) may not show specific motor disturbances.

ACUTE LYMPHOBLASTIC LEUKEMIA

Acute lymphoblastic leukemia (ALL), a malignancy most commonly found in children between the ages of 2 and 10, is responsible for 75–85% of the acute leukemias of childhood (Colby-Graham & Chordas, 2003). For a disease that was virtually always fatal in the past, modern-day intensive multiagent chemotherapy has resulted in survival rates approaching 80% (Veerman et al., 1996). However, prolonged survival has led to increased recognition of therapy-related morbidity. The treatment of childhood ALL has been found to be associated with neurotoxicity in both the central and peripheral nervous systems. It appears that central nervous system (CNS) toxicity is largely a result of CNS treatment that consists of chemotherapy, typically intrathecal and high-dose intravenous methotrexate and/or cranial radiotherapy. This CNS treatment can lead to structural alterations in the brain, including white matter changes, cortical atrophy, and calcifications (Ochs, 1989). Early studies noted that vincristine, an anticancer drug commonly used in treatment for ALL, was responsible for treatment-related peripheral neuropathy (Casey, Jellife, Le Quesne, & Millett, 1973). The earliest and most consistent clinical manifestations of peripheral neurotoxicity are depression of deep tendon reflexes, motor weakness and clumsiness, and sensory disturbances (Harila-Saari, Vainionpaa, Kovala, Tolonen, & Lanning, 1998; Sandler, Tobin, & Henderson, 1969).

In recent years, greater attention has been directed toward the wide spectrum of motor deficits manifest by children both during and after treatment for ALL. Survivors of childhood ALL frequently display both gross and fine motor impairments as a result of treatment. Indeed, in one study, gross motor difficulties were reported to be the most common (63%) abnormal finding on neurological examination; fine motor difficulties were less common (31%) (Harila-Saari, Huuskonen, Tolonen, Vainionpaa, & Lanning, 2001). Harila-Saari and colleagues (2001) also noted that 41% of the children had depressed deep tendon reflexes and 34% had dysdiadochokinesia, an impairment of the ability to make movements exhibiting a rapid change of motion, which is the result of cerebellar dysfunction. They suggested that the fine motor difficulties and depressed deep tendon reflexes were due to the peripheral neuropathy caused by vincristine, whereas the gross motor deficits and dysdiadochokinesia were likely a result of CNS toxicity, principally related to the CNS treatment. Importantly, a more recent study found that many of these neurologic signs were still evident 5 years after therapy for ALL (Lehtinen et al., 2002); 33% of the patients continued to have fine or gross motor difficulties and dysdiadochokinesia. Also, some children continued to exhibit depressed deep tendon reflexes. Consistent with these findings, Reinders-Messelink and colleagues (1996) reported problems with handwriting and fine motor skills 2 years after children completed treatment for ALL. These findings suggest that the majority of children treated for ALL have a favorable prognosis with regard to recovery of motor functioning once treatment for ALL is complete; however, some children do continue to show significant disability in multiple domains.

A recent study suggests that the motor problems of children treated for ALL may change over time. Reinders-Messelink and colleagues (1999) reported that problems in balance skills were most pronounced at the end of induction therapy, whereas half a year after induction therapy, these deficits had decreased. However, half a year after treatment the children exhibited a marked increase in fine motor problems. These authors suggested that vincristine neurotoxicity may be responsible for the increase in motor problems, particularly problems in balance, after induction therapy, and that methotrexate, another neurotoxic agent, may be responsible for the later appearance of fine motor problems. Indeed, the neurotoxic effects of methotrexate are known to appear 1 month to several years after treatment (Gilbert, Harding, & Grossman, 1989).

The findings of a study by Wright, Halton, Martin, and Barr (1998) that examined musculoskeletal and gross motor functioning following treatment for ALL lend support to the idea that the majority of observed motor problems do not lessen with increasing time off treatment. These investigators found that 12 months or more after treatment (median time off treatment, 40 months), children treated for ALL were able to perform most basic gross motor functions incorporated in the Gross Motor Function Measure, such as walking, running, and climbing stairs; however, they continued to score lower on these measures than did healthy same-age peers. Performance on the various gross motor skills measured by the BOTMP also revealed that relative to healthy controls, children treated for ALL continued to perform more poorly on tasks requiring strength, balance, and speed and agility. How these motor difficulties affect the child's daily functioning is not known. Thus, there is a need for long-term follow-up studies in this area.

The motor outcomes of children with ALL vary as a function of the treatment used. In general, children who received CNS irradiation show the most dramatic and consistent declines in visual–motor integration (Copeland et al., 1985; Espy et al., 2001) and fine motor skills (Copeland et al., 1985) compared to children with ALL who did not receive irradiation. This group of children also displays some declines in gross motor skills (Wright et al., 1998). ALL survivors who receive intrathecal and systemic methotrexate display motor deficits; however, these deficits tend to be less severe than those reported in children who receive CNS irradiation. Finally, for children who receive intrathecal methotrexate alone, no significant changes in motor skills are evident in most cases (Espy et al., 2001). It has been suggested that the effects of methotrexate on the CNS could be additive. Specifically, as methotrexate administered systemically easily crosses the blood–brain barrier (Balis & Poplack, 1989), it may potentiate the neurotoxic effects of the intrathecal methotrexate on the CNS, thereby having more detrimental effects on children who receive both as part of their treatment (Espy et al., 2001).

Sophisticated techniques for measuring neurological motor symptoms and signs have contributed greatly to our current knowledge of the motor deficits of children treated for ALL. One technique that is frequently used is the measurement of motor evoked potentials (MEPs). This allows investigators to evaluate the functioning of central and peripheral motor nervous pathways after treatment. Abnormal MEPs have been found within both the CNS and peripheral motor nervous tract at the end of therapy. Specifically, children treated for ALL display significantly prolonged MEP latencies within the entire motor pathway and significantly decreased MEP amplitudes in the peripheral motor nerves (Harila-Saari et al., 2001). Such findings suggest demyelination and loss of descending motor fibers or loss of muscle fibers (Harila-Saari et al., 2001). Lehtinen and colleagues (2002) reported that survivors of childhood ALL still demonstrated decreased motor nerve conduction in the peripheral nerves 5 years after treatment. These two studies indicate that the adverse effects of the ALL treatment on motor pathways are partially, but not totally, reversible, with conduction velocity remaining lower in ALL patients over time. Such alterations in the motor systems may consequently account for the persistent motoric deficits evident in many children following ALL treatment (Lehtinen et al., 2002).

PEDIATRIC HUMAN IMMUNODEFICIENCY VIRUS

Pediatric human immunodeficiency virus (HIV), the etiological agent of the acquired immune deficiency syndrome (AIDS), has reached epidemic proportions in recent years, affecting more than 1 million children worldwide (Belman, 1997). The virus has been found to adversely affect children's motor development, often resulting in delayed acquisition and performance of gross and/or fine motor skills. Furthermore, many infected children develop an HIV-associated encephalopathy, a condition characterized by a variety of movement disorders, such as ataxia, spasticity, and impaired muscle tone. A minority of children may also manifest motor deficits consistent with an extrapyramidal syndrome. All these effects are largely thought to be due to the action of the virus on the developing nervous system (Belman, 1997). As such, the earlier the child is infected (i.e., prenatally vs. postnatally), the more rapid the onset of motor symptoms and progression of the disease (Cohen et al., 1991).

Children who are infected with the HIV virus through vertical transmission (i.e., mother to child) have consistently been found to display delayed motor development compared to children unexposed to the virus, and to children born to HIV-infected mothers, but who do not acquire the disease themselves (known as seroreverters) (Chase, Vibbert, Pelton, Coulter, & Cabral, 1995; Chase et al., 2000; Gay et al., 1995). A study by Nozyce and colleagues (1994) confirmed that perinatally acquired HIV infection is associated with motor impairment in many infected children. In this study, all the children in the HIV-infected group showed delays on motor assessments. Similarly, a prospective study that assessed the outcomes of infants born to non-drug-using HIV-seropositive Haitian women found that as early as 3 months of age, the mean motor scores of HIV-infected infants on the Bayley Scales of Infant Development were significantly lower than those of uninfected infants (Gay et al., 1995). These early motor delays have been reported to persist over time in a large majority of infected children (Chase et al., 1995).

Other studies that have examined the outcomes of infants with perinatally acquired HIV suggest deficits in more specific domains of motor functioning. One prominent pattern seen in pediatric HIV infection is a decline in both gross and fine motor skills. This pattern of deterioration could be due to either a failure to acquire new motor skills or a loss of previously acquired milestones (Belman, 1990b; Chase et al., 1995). Msellati and colleagues (1993) reported gross motor retardation and deficits in fine motor skills to be far more common in their African sample of HIV-seropositive children at 6, 12, 18, and 24 months of age compared to a group of seroreverters and a group of children unexposed to the HIV virus. Boivin and colleagues (1995), using the Denver Developmental Screening Test, also observed that both gross and fine motor functioning distinguished between children in Zaire who were infected with HIV and their uninfected counterparts at follow-up periods from 3 to 18 months of age, with the infected children performing significantly worse.

Numerous studies have documented the relationship between neurological dysfunction and motor deficits in pediatric HIV patients (Knight, Mellins, Levenson, Arpadi, & Kairam, 2000; Msellati et al., 1993). Evidence for this association is highlighted in a study that reported that when HIV-positive children also had neurological deficits, these children exhibited significantly more motor problems than did HIV-positive children who did not have neurological deficits and seroreverters, with and without neurological diagnoses (Knight et al., 2000). These findings are in line with an earlier investigation, which found that both the child's HIV status and neurological diagnosis were important in predicting motor impairments (Mellins, Levenson, Zawadzki, Kairam, & Weston, 1994) and suggest that the CNS is the primary pathway through which HIV affects children's motor development.

One common manifestation of CNS disease in older infants infected with HIV is encephalopathy, with HIV-associated progressive encephalopathy often cited as the most severe and salient symptom of pediatric HIV infection (Wachsler-Felder & Golden, 2002). The age of onset is usually within the first year of life, although it may begin when the child is 2 or 3 years of age (Wachsler-Felder & Golden, 2002). In progressive encephalopathy, the young child frequently exhibits severe motor involvement. Specifically, infants and younger children have commonly been observed to display progressive corticospinal tract signs with concomitant loss of previously acquired milestones, muscle weakness, initial hypotonia with hyperreflexia, and eventual progression to spasticity, ataxia, tremor, and gait disturbances (Belman, 1990b; Belman et al., 1988). It has also been reported that some children with severe encephalopathy manifest extrapyramidal dysfunction, which is characterized by a host of motor symptoms, such as a loss of ambulatory abilities and bradykinesia, as well as rigidity and postural instability (Mintz et al., 1996).

Although these clinical features of HIV may be more pervasive and severe in children with HIV-related encephalopathy, a large proportion of pediatric HIV cases without encephalopathy demonstrate similar motor impairments. Indeed, the latter group of children, especially those younger in age (< 30 months), have consistently been reported to exhibit decreased strength, gait abnormalities, psychomotor retardation, poor head control, reflex abnormalities, poor motor coordination, and either increased or decreased motor tone (Englund et al., 1996; Pearson et al., 2000). Paucity of spontaneous movement has also been noted in these youngsters (Lord, Danoff, & Smith, 1995).

Studies with school-age children infected with the HIV virus perinatally, and who do not have an associated encephalopathy, have yielded less conclusive findings than studies of infants and younger children. Among school-age children infected through vertical transmission whose disease has not progressed to an advanced stage, there is a tendency to see more subtle disturbances in higher gross motor functions involving the lower extremities, such as running speed and agility (Parks, 1994). These children have also been found to display psychomotor slowing at 3–9 years of age (Cohen et al., 1991). As the disease progresses to an advanced stage, motor deficits become markedly more salient among this age group (Wachsler-Felder & Golden, 2002). Moreover, similar to the more pronounced motor deficits evident in children with HIV-related encephalopathy, many of the impairments observed in children without this condition are due to the effects of the virus on the corticospinal tract, including axonal and myelin degenerative changes (Belman, 1990a). Furthermore, basal ganglia calcification has frequently been documented in HIV-infected children (Belman, 1990a; Belman et al., 1988), suggesting that CNS motor centers are clearly being affected in children with HIV.

MENINGITIS

As a group, infections of the nervous system figure in the differential diagnosis of many neurological syndromes. Meningitis is a relatively common infectious disease process that is a major cause of acquired neurological disease in infancy and childhood. Viral and bacterial pathogens can cause meningitis, and although viral meningitis is more common than bacterial meningitis, bacterial disease is more likely to result in neuropsychological impairment and is the focus of discussion here. Bacterial meningitis is an inflammatory response to infection of the leptomeningeal cells and subarachnoid space, producing an acute clinical syndrome of fever, headache, neck stiffness, and altered mental status. After diagnosis is confirmed neurologically with clinical examination, laboratory tests, and imaging if required, treatment primarily consists of antibiotic treatment aimed at the infectious agent. In the past, high rates of mortality were associated with meningitis, but antibiotic treatment and vaccines have proven remarkably effective (see Solbrig, Healy, & Jay, 2000).

The most common bacterial pathogens include *Haemophilus influenzae*, *Streptococcus pneumoniae*, and *Neisseria meningitides*, and account for 75–80% of cases after the neonatal period. *N. meningitides* is now the predominant pathogen among children ages 2–18 years in the United States, group B *streptococci* are most commonly seen in neonates, *S. pneumoniae* is most frequent in adults, and *H. influenzae* is seen in children under age 5 and adults who test positive for HIV (Solbrig, Healy, & Jay, 2000). Bacterial meningitis causes profound disruption to the cerebrovascular and cerebral spinal fluid (CSF) dynamics, including inflammation and narrowing of cerebral blood vessels, and thrombosis in some cases. Raised intracranial pressure is also seen, with possible obstruction of CSF flow. Although treatment has been effective with regard to decreased mortality, there is continued concern regarding morbidity, with neurological sequelae seen in up to one-third of the children. Mental retardation, motor impairment, seizures, hemiparesis, and visual and hearing impairments have all been described (Snyder, 1994). Unfavorable outcomes have been associated with a young age, delay in initiation of treatment, focal neurological signs or coma upon admission, and a malignant clinical course.

Neuropsychological studies of children have focused on outcome following *H. influenzae* and group B streptococcal meningitis; a number of the studies include motor and perceptual–motor assessment, and these are emphasized here. A prospective cohort study of adverse outcomes from several types of bacterial meningitis was conducted by Grimwood and colleagues (1995). These authors noted increased abnormality in intellectual and neurological function in 158 children with meningitis compared to controls. Subtle neurological motor abnormalities were seen, and impaired visual–motor functioning was found in the affected versus control groups. Children with acute neurological complications had more adverse outcomes than did children with uncomplicated meningitis and control children.

Neurological, psychological, and academic capabilities of children following group B *Streptococcus* were evaluated by Wald and colleagues (1986) in a study of 34 children 3–18 years of age. Twenty-one siblings were used as controls. Of the total original population of 74 affected children (21 had died, two were institutionalized, 15 were assessed by phone, and two were lost to follow-up), nine children (12%) had major neurological sequelae including mental retardation, hemiparesis, deafness or blindness, so only 23 (32, depending on the task) children were able to complete the formal motor assessment measures. This group of affected children, including four of the nine children with severe sequelae, performed more poorly than did sibling controls on a perceptual motor task (Beery VMI), but the differences between groups disappeared when the children with severe sequelae were excluded from analysis. Therefore, the authors interpreted the results as indicating that children surviving group B streptococcal meningitis without major neurological sequelae appeared to be functioning normally or comparable to siblings in perceptual motor capabilities.

H. G. Taylor and associates have conducted a number of studies of *H. influenzae* meningitis in children (for more detailed summaries, see Anderson & Taylor, 2000; Taylor, Schatschneider, & Rich, 1992). An early study compared 97 school-age children who had been treated for *H. influenzae* type b meningitis to siblings with regard to neurological and developmental consequences (Taylor et al., 1990). Fourteen percent of the children had persisting neurological sequelae, but few other measurable differences appeared between the groups when methodological controls were applied. Neuropsychological performance was summarized by factor scores, with the attentional/motor factor showing no differences between the index and control groups. The authors concluded that there is a favorable prognosis for the majority of children treated for *H. influenzae* type b meningitis, and no obvious residual perceptual motor deficits are seen.

Several additional follow-up studies of children with *H. influenzae* meningitis are summarized by Anderson and Taylor (2000), including research completed in the United States, Canada, and Australia. Only general conclusions from these studies regarding the motor behavior of the affected children are presented here. Anderson and Taylor conclude that children with acute-phase neurological complications can show persisting impairments in perceptual/performance skills and response speed, as well as some evidence of "soft" neurological signs. Mild impairments in visuomotor coordination, gross motor skills, and executive functions are all documented in the postmeningitic children. However, the motor outcomes for the majority of affected children are generally good, with only subtle deficits apparent in the long term.

An additional study by Taylor's group (Taylor, Schatschneider, Petrill, Barry, & Owens, 1996) examined executive functioning in children at risk for sequelae from *H. influenzae* type b meningitis. Fifty-three affected school-age children were compared to 170 unaffected controls. A factor-analytic methodology was used for the analysis, with group differences seen in the factor related to response speed. Select weaknesses in executive motor functioning were therefore documented for the affected group.

Unfortunately, a number of inconsistencies and methodological concerns are noted when trying to understand the motor sequelae of bacterial meningitis in children (Anderson & Taylor, 2000). To summarize, research conducted to date suggests that it is likely that affected children who demonstrate more severe acute neurological complications will show residual motor impairment, but children who recover well initially may demonstrate only subtle motor changes affecting efficiency and speed of motor execution.

HYDROCEPHALUS

Motor deficits are commonly observed in children with hydrocephalus, a condition in which an excessive accumulation of CSF within the ventricular system of the CNS results in increased intracranial pressure (ICP). The accumulation of CSF may result from a blockage within the ventricular system, under absorption of CSF or excessive production of CSF (Del Bigio, 1993). The consequent increase in ICP causes expansion of the ventricles and displacement of adjacent brain structures. Hydrocephalus may be the result of congenital factors such as spina bifida and myelomeningocele or may be acquired by a variety of etiologies, the most common being intraventricular hemorrhage in premature infants, TBI, meningitis, tumor, and infectious diseases (Mataro, Junque, Poca, & Sahuquillo, 2001).

Motor deficit has been reported in up to 60% of children with hydrocephalus (Hoppe-Hirsch et al., 1998), with significant impairment in multiple motor domains. Children with early-onset hydrocephalus frequently display *gross motor* impairment (Wills, 1993). Impaired jumping ability, an indication of poor lower leg strength, and decreased handgrip strength, a marker of upper-limb gross motor function, have been observed in many school-age children with hydrocephalus (Hetherington & Dennis, 1999). Gait, posture, and balance have also been found to be impaired in children with hydrocephalus (Dennis & Barnes, 1994; Hetherington & Dennis, 1999).

Hydrocephalus often compromises the cerebellum (Anderson & Plewis, 1977), a neuroanatomical structure heavily involved in the regulation of balance, posture, and gait (Ghez, 1991). Ataxia, another consequence of cerebellar dysfunction, has been noted in children with hydrocephalus (Hetherington & Dennis, 1999). Furthermore, hydrocephalus can stretch, destroy, or interfere with the normal development of the corpus callosum (Fletcher et al., 1992), which may also contribute to balance or gait disturbances (Jinkins, 1991).

Spasticity and ambulatory status are two areas of gross motor functioning that can be impaired in children with acquired hydrocephalus, with more severe cases of hydrocephalus (i.e., progressive hydrocephalus) displaying greater disability (Fletcher et al., 1997). Fletcher and colleagues (1997) reported children with either progressive or arrested hydrocephalus as a result of intraventricular hemorrhage often presented with spastic hemiparesis. This impairment was significantly more common in children in the progressive group. Fletcher and colleagues also found that ambulation was impaired in some children with progressive hydrocephalus.

Significant research effort has been directed at characterizing the *fine motor* skills of children with hydrocephalus, largely due to the growing concern about the detrimental effects deficits in these skills can have on academic performance (Anderson, 1975; Brunt, 1980). Regardless of gross motor status, deficits in upper limb and hand function, including psychomotor speed and fine motor skills, are frequently reported in this population. Indeed, in an investigation of 187 children with hydrocephalus, Fletcher and colleagues (1995) observed abnormalities in fine motor coordination in 74% of children with shunted hydrocephalus and in 30% of children with arrested hydrocephalus. The finding that children with unshunted hydrocephalus had less severe fine motor deficits than those with shunted hydrocephalus was likely due to the less severe nature of their unshunted condition (see Fletcher et al., 1997). Consistent with the foregoing findings, Hetherington and Dennis (1999) reported that children with hydrocephalus scored significantly lower on measures of fine motor control, as well as on other upper-limb tests requiring dexterity and speed than did normally developing children.

In some cases of acquired hydrocephalus, *visuomotor and praxis* skills may be adversely affected (see Wills, 1993, for a review). Fletcher and colleagues (1997) found that tasks that require the effective integration of visual and motor skills were more severely impaired in children with shunted hydrocephalus relative to their unshunted counterparts. Anderson (1975) reported that children with hydrocephalus exhibited reduced writing speed and legibility and had difficulty controlling the force of handwriting movements. Difficulty with activities that require bilateral coordination, design copying, and tracing has also been reported in these children, as have impairments in sequential motor movements and problems in producing motor movements in response to verbal instructions (i.e., praxis deficits) (Brunt, 1980, 1984).

In addition to the notable movement abnormalities in children with hydrocephalus, it is clear that these children also demonstrate cognitive and neuropsychological characteristics that correlate with various aspects of cerebral dysfunction, particularly white matter pathology. Children with hydrocephalus often display reduced tactile–perceptual skills, reduced visuospatial skills, altered discourse characteristics affecting the usage of language, and possibly reduced attention affecting memory capabilities (Fletcher et al., 1992; Wills, 1993). Fletcher and colleagues (1995) consider these neuropsychological findings, particularly the impaired motor and visuospatial capabilities, as representative phenotypically of a prototypical nonverbal learning disability syndrome in children with hydrocephalus. Given the obvious white matter and callosal pathology frequently seen in hydrocephalus, impairments in nonverbal and motor functioning are consistent with such a diagnosis.

Although the literature is growing, many gaps in our knowledge still exist. One area in particular that needs clarification is the impact of hydrocephalus on different stages of development. Review of the research literature also reveals that it is dominated by studies focusing on children with hydrocephalus resulting from congenital factors such as spina bifida or myelomeningocele. Therefore, it is imperative that more attention be devoted to gaining a better understanding of the functioning of children with the acquired forms of this condition. Acquired hydrocephalus often arises from fundamentally different etiologies and these etiological differences likely contribute to the neurodevelopmental deficits observed in these youngsters.

EARLY EXPOSURE TO TOXINS

It has long been recognized that environmental factors have important effects on how children's brains develop and function. Extensive laboratory and clinical studies of several compounds, such as lead, mercury, and polychlorinated biphenyls, suggest that early exposure to these environmental chemicals can have detrimental effects on neurodevelopment. An important consequence of exposure to such toxins, both prenatally and/or postnatally, is significant impairment in children's motor development and functioning, with the degree of impairment often dependent on the extent of exposure.

The relationship between *lead* exposure prenatally and postnatally and cognitive deficits is well established in the research literature (Hammond & Dietrich, 1990). Until recently, however, motor performance has rarely been the focus of these investigations. Studies that have examined the effects of early lead exposure on children's motor development have consistently found that exposure affects visual–motor integration (Baghurst et al., 1995; Dietrich, Berger, & Succop, 1993). Both prenatal and postnatal blood lead concentrations have been shown to be adversely associated with scores on measures of visual–motor abilities in children 7 years of age (Baghurst et al., 1995). In a Cincinnati cohort, postnatal lead exposure was associated with poorer visual–motor functioning in 6-year-olds, and these findings remained even after adjusting for a range of covariates that may have influenced motor development, such as maternal IQ, socioeconomic status, and child sex (Dietrich et al., 1993). Consistent with these findings, a recent prospective study that compared a group of 4½-year-old children who grew up in a town in Yugoslavia with a lead smelter and another group of the same-age children from a non-lead-exposed town reported that children exposed to lead showed markedly more deviant performance on tasks requiring visual–motor integration (Wasserman et al., 2000).

Large-scale studies examining the impact of early exposure to relatively low levels of environmental lead have *not* been extensively documented in the research literature. The results of the Cincinnati Lead Study, in which exposure to lead was low to moderate (Dietrich et al., 1993), suggests, however, that even low levels of lead may have severe and pervasive effects on children's motor development. In this study, a comprehensive neuromotor assessment battery was administered to 245 6-year-old urban inner-city children. These children were followed from birth, with blood lead concentrations and neurobehavioral development assessed quarterly. Results indicated that neonatal blood lead levels were significantly associated with lower scores on the BOTMP subtest assessing upper-limb speed and dexterity and the composite score for fine motor performance. Postnatal blood lead levels were also associated with poorer performance on measures of bilateral coordination of the gross musculature and visual–motor control. Although the precise mechanisms involved in lead-associated developmental motor deficits at lower levels of exposure are not yet clear, the authors noted that the cerebellum is particularly sensitive to lead intoxication (Press, 1977), and that is it possible that cerebellar dysfunction may account for the motor problems present in these children.

Despite the evident relationship between exposure to lead at a young age and motor deficits, it has been questioned whether the adverse effects of lead exposure is related to motor development in general, or whether the association is confined to specific motor domains (i.e., fine motor skills). The study by Wasserman and colleagues (2000) found that there was a significant negative association between early lead exposure and fine motor and visual–motor functioning; however, exposure had no appreciable effects on gross motor skills assessed by the BOTMP. Similar results were also obtained using the McCarthy Scales of Children's Abilities (Wasserman et al., 1994). These findings suggest that the negative associations between lead exposure and motor development are not global but instead may be limited to specific areas of functioning. In contrast, however, at least two studies have demonstrated an association between blood lead concentration and one component of gross motor performance, impaired postural balance, as measured by postural sway on a microprocessor-based force platform (Bhattacharya, Shukla, Dietrich, Bornschein, & Berger, 1995; Bhattacharya et al., 1991). For a more detailed discussion of the balance and postural control problems of children exposed to lead, the reader is referred to Williams and Ho, Chapter 10, this volume.

A second environmental agent to which the developing brain is particularly sensitive is *methylmercury* (MeHg). Both prenatal and postnatal exposure to MeHg can adversely affect the CNS, but it appears to be most neurotoxic when the brain is developing rapidly (Myers & Davidson, 2000), thereby placing young children at heightened risk for developmental deficits. MeHg is a common environmental contaminant that is released into the environment from gold mining activities and slash-and-burn agricultural practices, which result in MeHg making its way into the water system where it is concentrated in fish and other sea life. As a result, populations that depend on fish as an important source of protein may achieve MeHg exposure levels that detrimentally affect brain development. Indeed, two of the most well documented outbreaks of poisoning from MeHg occurred in Minamata (1956) and Niigata (1965), Japan due to ingestion of contaminated fish (Kondo, 2000). These events provided unique opportunities for researchers to investigate the adverse effects associated with maternal consumption and fetal and neonatal affliction. Fetuses were affected with MeHg through umbilical circulation from their mothers who had eaten the contaminated fish and infants through breastfeeding (Kondo, 2000). Many of the infants who survived the high levels of MeHg exposure, were later found to exhibit cerebral-palsy-like motor symptoms (Kondo, 2000). Clinically, the symptoms were characterized by nonlocalized cerebral symptoms, with the children primarily presenting with primitive reflexes, ataxia, muscle weakness, and deformity of posture.

Although the detrimental consequences of high levels of MeHg exposure on motoric functioning may be particularly salient, as is the case with environmental lead, it is only recently that investigators have begun to examine the effects of lower mercury level exposure on child development. In a recent investigation conducted by Cordier and colleagues (2002), children 5–7 years of age residing in two Amerindian communities in French Guiana were compared. One community was deemed a high-MeHg-exposure area due to the environmental pollution from gold mining activities and the other a low-exposure community. Maternal hair MeHg concentrations obtained in December 1997 and June 1998 were used as a proxy for prenatal exposure. The results revealed an association between the mother's level of MeHg exposure and increased deep tendon reflexes and poorer coordination of the legs in their children. Importantly, this study illuminates a dose-dependent relationship between MeHg level exposure and motor impairment, with children showing diminished psychomotor performance with increasing maternal MeHg concentrations. Children with relatively low levels of exposure, however, still showed impairment in these domains. This position was supported in a recent report from the National Research Council (2000) that concluded that chronic low-dose prenatal exposure to MeHg (e.g., from maternal consumption of fish) is associated with developmental deficits. Poorer performance on tests requiring the use of fine motor skills was noted to be a particular area of vulnerability for children exposed to MeHg. Consistent with these findings, a case-control study of children with prenatal exposure to MeHg in the Faeroe Islands, where increased exposure to mercury is mainly due to consumption of whale meat, also revealed that tasks requiring speeded motor response were negatively affected by mercury exposure (Grandjean, Weihe, White, & Debes, 1998).

There is growing evidence that *polychlorinated biphenyls* (PCBs) are yet another environmental chemical that can interrupt neurodevelopmental processes during critical periods of development, resulting in negative effects on motor behavior. PCBs are complex mixtures of persistent contaminants that are ubiquitous in the environment, largely stemming from their use in electrical transformers, paper recycling, and other commercial processes. Although they have long been banned in Western countries, they continue to contaminate many water sources and soils. Moreover, similar to both lead and mercury, PCBs easily cross the placenta and may cause *in utero* injury to the developing brain (Patandin et al., 1999). The negative effects of prenatal exposure to environmental levels of PCBs on child development have been described in a number of prospective long-term follow-up studies, with the existing research suggesting that PCBs hinder neurodevelopment in children exposed early in life (Walkowiak et al., 2001).

The neonatal effects of PCBs on motor development are underscored in two well-known studies, one conducted in North Carolina and the other in Michigan. In North Carolina, the neonatal effects of transplacental exposure to PCBs at levels representative of the general population were examined in 912 infants using the Brazelton Neonatal Behavioral Assessment Scales (Rogan et al., 1986). The authors reported that higher PCB levels in maternal milk at birth were associated with less muscle tone (hyptonicity) and activity, as well as hyporeflexia. Lower psychomotor skills among those infants exposed to higher prenatal PCB levels were reported at follow-up, from

6–24 months of age (Gladen et al., 1988; Rogan & Gladen, 1991). In the Michigan study, maternal consumption of fish contaminated by PCBs was found to be predictive of newborn motor immaturity, with more abnormally hypoactive reflexes associated with higher maternal consumption (Jacobson, Jacobson, & Schwartz, 1984). The neurotoxic effects of prenatal PCB exposure on motor development have been found to persist into early school age with children at 4½ years of age manifesting subtle motor developmental delays (Vreugdenbil, Lanting, Mulder, Boersma, & Weisglas-Kuperus, 2002).

In addition to *in utero* exposure to PCBs, infants may also be exposed to relatively high PCB concentrations through human breast milk. However, unlike prenatal exposure to these compounds, a consistent association has not been found between postnatal exposures and adverse motor outcomes. In the North Carolina study mentioned previously, no deleterious effects on motor functioning were associated with breastfeeding (Gladen et al., 1988). In contrast, a study conducted in the Netherlands revealed that higher levels of PCB exposure via breastfeeding did in fact have a significant adverse effect on the psychomotor outcome among breast feeders (Koopman-Esseboom et al., 1996). The negative effect of postnatal PCB exposure via breastfeeding on psychomotor behavior was found to last up to at least 42 months of age (Walkowiak et al., 2001).

MALNUTRITION

The past few decades have seen several substantial advances in our understanding of the importance of micronutrients in child health and development. Accumulating data have underlined the important long-term adverse effects on motor functioning that may occur with iron deficiency anemia. Zinc and iodine are two other micronutrients whose significance in motor development is becoming increasingly appreciated. The roles of iron, zinc, and iodine on motor functioning are highlighted in observational studies of the characteristics of children deficient in these nutrients, as well as studies with treatment components that compare the developmental test performance of these children with that of healthy control groups.

Several consistent results have emerged from studies of the behavior and development of infants with *iron deficiency anemia*, a condition that affects 20–25% of infants worldwide (DeMaeyer & Adiels-Tegman, 1985; Florentino & Guirriec, 1984). These studies have reported that anemic infants scored significantly lower on tests of motor development relative to comparison groups without anemia (Lozoff et al., 1987; Walter, De Andraca, Chadud, & Perales, 1989). In a landmark study by Lozoff and colleagues (1987), it was found that Costa Rican infants 12–23 months of age with anemia, relative to both healthy controls and nonanemic iron-deficient infants, showed significantly lower scores on the psychomotor developmental index of the Bayley Scales of Infant Development. An examination of the specific motor functions that were impaired in the anemic group showed that many exhibited difficulties with walking up and down stairs, standing on one foot and balancing, and walking on a line. A second study conducted by Walter and colleagues (1989) confirmed the lower motor test scores among anemic infants reported by Lozoff and colleagues, especially on tasks requiring balance and coordination skills. Interestingly, there was no significant difference in performance between the control infants with normal iron status and nonanemic iron-deficient children. Motor–balance–coordination deficits were also described in an earlier study by Cantwell (1974), in which infants without anemia were compared with those who developed anemia at 6–18 months of age. The latter group was found to be far less proficient at tandem walking, balancing on one foot, and repetitive hand or foot movements. These three studies support the general observation by Oski and Honig (1978) that anemic children evidence poor fine and gross motor coordination.

More recently, investigators have extended their research on motor functioning in infants with iron deficiency anemia and have begun to investigate the physical activity levels of these children. Angulo-Kinzler, Peirano, Lin, Garrido, and Lozoff (2002) compared spontaneous motor activity in 6-month-old Chilean infants with or without iron deficiency anemia. They found that the anemic infants displayed reduced motor activity compared to their nonanemic counterparts, with the differences becoming even more pronounced at 12 and 18 months of age. Other studies on iron deficiency and motor activity have reported similar findings (Jahari, Saco-Pollitt, Husaini, & Pollitt, 2000; Lozoff et al., 1998). Sustained decreases in motor activity may have negative consequences for children's long-term motor development (Sameroff & McDonough, 1984), as children who are inactive and do not practice their existing capabilities may be less likely to acquire new or more complex skills (Neisser, 1997).

Studies examining the effect of treatment of iron deficiency in young children have produced conflicting results, with some showing improvements in motor skills while others showed lasting adverse effects. Stoltzfus and colleagues (2001) found significant improvements in motor development after 12 months of supplemental iron. Other studies have reported that following iron therapy, children who were previously anemic were found to accomplish motor milestones at a rate comparable to that of their healthy, same-age peers (Aukett, Parks, Scott, & Wharton, 1986) and to display improvements on measures of both gross and fine motor coordination (Oski & Honig, 1978). These studies suggest that replenishing iron levels may positively influence motor development in children. In contrast, a recent investigation suggested that some children, particularly those with more severe anemia resulting from iron deficiency, are at heightened risk for a long-lasting developmental disadvantage compared to their peers with better iron status. Indeed, in a follow-up to their 1987 study, Lozoff, Jimenez, Hagen, Mollen, and Wolf (2000) found that children who presented with severe, chronic iron deficiency in infancy still demonstrated markedly poorer performance on tests of motor functioning more than a decade later, even after controlling for background variables. The authors speculated that the long-lasting motor differences might be a direct consequence of delayed myelination during infancy as a result of insufficient iron. Alternatively, they proposed that indirect effects may result from lower levels of iron in the brain, such as altered neurotransmitter function and impaired myelination during the early years, which may disrupt the process of laying down the neural bases for some motor fundamentals. The findings of the foregoing studies suggest that the severity and chronicity of the iron deficiency may be factors in the motor outcomes of children with iron deficiency anemia. Future research is needed, however, to clarify these relationships.

In addition to poor iron consumption, malnourished children commonly consume diets with low *zinc* content or with constituents that reduce bioavailability. As a result, zinc deficiency is commonly found in populations where the diet is low in flesh foods and high in substances that inhibit zinc absorption, such as fiber, cows' milk, and the phytate found in foods of plant origin. Inadequate zinc intake may, in turn, adversely affect these children's motor functioning. Indeed, an examination of the relationship between maternal sources of zinc and infant development illuminates the negative effects that zinc deficiency may have on a child's developing motor skills (Kirksey et al., 1994). Kirksey and colleagues (1994) found that at 6 months of age, children of mothers with high intakes of plant zinc throughout the lactation period, which is lower in bioavailability than zinc from animal sources, were likely to exhibit low scores on measures of motor development. Furthermore, activity levels have been reported to be significantly lower in zinc-deprived children, compared to their counterparts with normal zinc status (Bentley et al., 1997).

Two recent studies have used zinc supplementation trials to examine the relation between zinc deprivation and activity in undernourished infants and toddlers (Bentley et al., 1997; Sazawal et al., 1996). In a trial conducted in India, children 6–35 months of age were randomly assigned to either a zinc-supplemented or a control group. Both groups received vitamins A, B1, B2, B6, D3, and E, and niacinamide as well. The authors found that children who received the zinc supplementation, given along with the selected vitamins, showed significantly greater activity levels compared to control participants. Interestingly, children in the zinc group spent 72% more time performing high-movement activities such as running, compared to children who did not receive zinc treatment. A similar study of Guatemalan infants ages 6–9 months also found an increase in play behavior and motor activity among infants who received the zinc supplement compared to the placebo control group. These differences became noticeable after 7 months of treatment when zinc-supplemented infants were more frequently observed to be sitting up and involved in play behaviors and less likely to be observed lying down than were the infants receiving the placebo. Thus, taken together, these studies suggest that zinc nutriture plays an important role in the development of motor skills, and that zinc deficiency may be a determinant of the lower activity levels associated with malnutrition in young children.

Like zinc, there is mounting evidence that *iodine* deficiency during intrauterine life, as well as early childhood, can greatly impair psychomotor development (DeLong, 1993). The most robust evidence of the role of iodine in motor development has come from randomized controlled trials of iodine supplementation of women of childbearing age in Papua New Guinea (Pharoah, Buttfield, & Hetzel, 1971). Results revealed that an injection of intramuscular iodine before conception eliminated endemic cretinism in the iodine-treated group, a condition marked by mental retardation, including significant motor impairment. Furthermore, among the noncretins, children whose mothers received iodized oil were found to exhibit better motor functioning 10 years later. Iodine deficiency during pregnancy has also been associated with cerebral palsy (DeLong, 1993).

Numerous observational studies have examined the motor outcome of children in iodine-deficient and/or iodine-sufficient areas, and nearly all have found poorer psychomotor development in children residing in areas characterized by iodine deficiency (Fernald, 1998). In a study of normal school children ages 6–16 years living in two iodine-deficient areas in Sicily, 19.3% of the children in one locality and 18.5% in the other were reported to display neuromuscular abnormalities, including increased tendon reflexes, clonus of the foot, Babinski sign, and minor disturbances in balance and gait, relative to children living in an iodine-sufficient area (Vermiglio et al., 1990). Similarly, an investigation of children residing in iodine-deficient areas in Iran found that 29% displayed crossed adductor reflex, and 39% presented with hyperreflexia (Azizi et al., 1995). Visuomotor coordination has also been reported to be particularly poor in iodine-deficient communities (Sankar et al., 1994). Therefore, there is conclusive evidence that iodine deficiency, both pre- and postnatally, may have detrimental effects on the child's motor functioning.

ACKNOWLEDGMENTS

Grants from the Alberta Children's Hospital Foundation and the Canadian Institutes of Health Research supported the preparation of this chapter.

REFERENCES

Alajouanine, T., & Lhermitte, F. (1965). Acquired aphasia in children. *Brain, 88,* 653–662.

Anderson, E. M. (1975). Cognitive deficits in children with spina bifida and hydrocephalus: A review of the literature. *British Journal of Educational Psychology, 45,* 257–268.

Anderson, E. M., & Plewis, I. (1977). Impairment of a motor skill with spina bifida cystica and hydrocephalus: An exploratory study. *British Journal of Psychology, 68,* 61–70.

Anderson, V. A., & Taylor, H. G. (2000). Meningitis. In K. O. Yeates, M. D. Ris, & H. G. Taylor (Eds.), *Pediatric neuropsychology: Research, theory, and practice* (pp. 117–148). New York: Guilford Press.

Angulo-Kinzler, R. M., Peirano, P., Lin, E., Garrido, M., & Lozoff, B. (2002). Spontaneous motor activity in human infants with iron-deficiency anemia. *Early Human Development, 66,* 67–79.

Aukett, M. A., Parks, Y. A., Scott, P. H., & Wharton, B. A. (1986). Treatment with iron increases weight gain and psychomotor development. *Archives of Disease in Childhood, 61,* 849–857.

Azizi, F., Kalani, H., Kimiagar, M., Ghazi, A., Sarshar, A., Nafarabadi, M., et al. (1995). Physical, neuromotor and intellectual impairment in non-cretinous schoolchildren with iodine deficiency. *International Journal for Vitamin and Nutrition Research, 65,* 199–205.

Baghurst, P. A., McMichael, A. J., Tong, S., Wigg, N. R., Vimpani, G. V., & Robertson, E. F. (1995). Exposure to environmental lead and visual–motor integration at age 7 years: The Port Pirie cohort study. *Epidemiology, 6,* 104–109.

Balis, F. M., & Poplack, D. G. (1989). Central nervous system pharmacology of antileukemic drugs. *Journal of Pediatric Hematology and Oncology, 10,* 74–86.

Bawden, H. N., Knights, R. M., & Winogron, H. W. (1985). Speeded performance following head injury in children. *Journal of Clinical and Experimental Neuropsychology, 7,* 39–54.

Belman, A. L. (1990a). AIDS and pediatric neurology. *Neurologic Clinics, 8,* 571–603.

Belman, A. L. (1990b). Neurologic syndromes associated with symptomatic human immunodeficiency virus infection in infants and children. In P. B. Kozlowski, D. A. Snider, P. M. Vietze, & H. M. Wisniewski (Eds.), *Brain in pediatric AIDS* (pp. 45–64). Basel, Switzerland: Karger.

Belman, A. L. (1997). Pediatric neuro-AIDS. *Neuroimaging Clinics of North America, 7,* 593–613.

Belman, A. L., Diamond, G., Dickson, D., Horoupian, D., Llena, J., Lantos, G., et al. (1988).

Pediatric acquired immunodeficiency syndrome. *American Journal of Diseases of Children, 142*, 29–35.

Bentley, M. E., Caulfield, L. E., Ram, M., Santizo, M. C., Hurtado, E., Rivera, J. A., et al. (1997). Zinc supplementation affects the activity patterns of rural Guatemalan infants. *Journal of Nutrition, 127*, 1333–1338.

Bhattacharya, A., Shukla, R., Dietrich, K. N., Bornschein, R. L., & Berger, O. (1995). Effect of early lead exposure on children's postural balance. *Developmental Medicine and Child Neurology, 37*, 861–878.

Bhattacharya, A., Shukla, R., Dietrich, K. N., Miller, J., Bagchee, A., & Bornschein, R. L. (1991). Functional implications of postural disequilibrium due to lead exposure. *Neurotoxicology, 14*, 179–190.

Boivin, M. J., Green, S. D. R., Davies, A. G., Giordani, B., Mokili, J. K. L., & Cutting, W. A. M. (1995). A preliminary evaluation of the cognitive and motor effects of pediatric HIV infection in Zairian children. *Health Psychology, 14*, 13–21.

Brink, J. D., Imbus, C., & Woo-Sam, J. (1980). Physical recovery after severe closed head trauma in children and adolescents. *Journal of Pediatrics, 97*, 721–727.

Brunt, D. (1980). Characteristics of upper limb movement in a sample of meningomyelocele children. *Perceptual and Motor Skills, 51*, 431–437.

Brunt, D. (1984). Apraxic tendencies in children with myelomeningocele. *Adapted Physical Activity Quarterly, 1*, 61–67.

Cantwell, R. J. (1974). The long-term neurological sequelae of anemia in infancy. *Pediatric Research, 8*, 342.

Carlin, T. M., & Chanmugam, A. (2002). Stroke in children. *Emergency Medicine Clinics of North America, 20*, 671–685.

Casey, E. B., Jellife, A. M., Le Quesne, P. M., & Millett, Y. L. (1973). Vincristine neuropathy. Clinical and electrophysiological observations. *Brain, 96*, 69–86.

Chaplin, D., Deitz, J., & Jaffe, K. M. (1993). Motor performance in children after traumatic brain injury. *Archives of Physical Medicine and Rehabilitation, 74*, 161–164.

Chase, C., Vibbert, M., Pelton, S., Coulter, D. L., & Cabral, H. (1995). Early neurodevelopmental growth in children with vertically transmitted human immunodeficiency virus infection. *Archives of Pediatrics and Adolescent Medicine, 149*, 850–855.

Chase, C., Ware, J., Hittelman, J., Blasini, I., Smith, R., Llorente, A., et al. (2000). Early cognitive and motor development among infants born to women infected with human immunodeficiency virus. *Pediatrics, 106*, E25.

Cohen, S. E., Mundy, T., Karassik, B., Lieb, L., Ludwig, D. D., & Ward, J. (1991). Neuropsychological functioning in human immunodeficiency virus type 1 seropositive children infected through neonatal blood transfusion. *Pediatrics, 88*, 58–68.

Colby-Graham, M. F., & Chordas, C. (2003). The childhood leukemias. *Journal of Pediatric Nursing, 18*, 87–95.

Copeland, D. R., Fletcher, J. M., Pfefferbaum-Levine, B., Jaffe, N., Ried, H., & Maor, M. (1985). Neuropsychological sequelae of childhood cancer in long-term survivors. *Pediatrics, 75*, 745–753.

Cordier, S., Garel, M., Mandereau, L., Morcel, H., Doineau, P., Gosme-Seguret, S., et al. (2002). Neurodevelopmental investigations among methylmercury-exposed children in French Guiana. *Environmental Research, 89*, 1–11.

Costeff, H., Groswasser, Z., & Goldstein, R. (1990). Long-term follow-up review of 31 children with severe closed head trauma. *Journal of Neurosurgery, 73*, 684–687.

Del Bigio, M. R. (1993). Neuropathological changes caused by hydrocephalus. *Acta Neuropathologica, 85*, 573–585.

DeLong, G. R. (1993). Effects of nutrition on brain development in humans. *American Journal of Clinical Nutrition, 57*, S286–S290.

DeMaeyer, E., & Adiels-Tegman, M. (1985). The prevalence of anaemia in the world. *World Health Statistics Quarterly, 38,* 302–316.

Demierre, B., & Rondot, P. (1983). Dystonia caused by putamino–capsulo–caudate vascular lesions. *Journal of Neurology, Neurosurgery, and Psychiatry, 46,* 404–409.

Denckla, M. B. (1994). Measurement of executive function. In G. R. Lyon (Ed.), *Frames of reference for the assessment of learning disabilities* (pp. 117–142). Baltimore: Brookes.

Dennis, M., & Barnes, M. A. (1994). Neuropsychologic function in same-sex twins discordant for perinatal brain damage. *Developmental and Behavioral Pediatrics, 15,* 124–130.

DePaepe, J. L., & Lange, E. K. (1994). Physical assessment. In R. C. Savage & G. F. Wolcott (Eds.), *Educational dimensions of acquired brain injury* (pp. 345–365). Austin, TX: Pro-Ed.

deVeber, G. (2002). Stroke and the child's brain: An overview of epidemiology, syndromes and risk factors. *Current Opinion in Neurology, 15,* 133–138.

deVeber, G. A., MacGregor, D., Curtis, R., & Mayank, S. (2000). Neurologic outcome in survivors of childhood arterial ischemic stroke and sinovenous thrombosis. *Journal of Child Neurology, 15,* 316–324.

Dietrich, K. N., Berger, O. G., & Succop, P. A. (1993). Lead exposure and the motor developmental status of urban six-year-old children in the Cincinnati Prospective Study. *Pediatrics, 91,* 301–307.

Dusser, A., Goutieres, F., & Aicardi, J. (1986). Ischemic strokes in children. *Journal of Child Neurology, 1,* 131–136.

Englund, J. A., Baker, C. J., Raskino, C., KcKinney, R. E., Lifschitz, M. H., Petrie, B., et al. (1996). Clinical and laboratory characteristics of a large cohort of symptomatic, human immunodeficiency virus-infected infants and children. *Pediatric Infectious Disease Journal, 15,* 1025–1036.

Espy, K. A., Moore, I. M., Kaufmann, P. M., Kramer, J. H., Matthay, K., & Hutter, J. J. (2001). Chemotherapeutic CNS prophylaxis and neuropsychologic change in children with acute lymphoblastic leukemia: A prospective study. *Journal of Pediatric Psychology, 26,* 1–9.

Ewing-Cobbs, L., Fletcher, J. M., & Levin, H. S. (1995). Traumatic brain injury. In B.P. Rourke (Ed.), *Syndrome of nonverbal learning disabilities: Neurodevelopmental manifestations* (pp. 433–459). New York: Guilford Press.

Ewing-Cobbs, L., Levin, H. S., & Fletcher, J. M. (1998). Neuropsychological sequelae after pediatric traumatic brain injury: Advances since 1985. In M. Ylvisaker (Ed.), *Traumatic brain injury rehabilitation: Children and adolescents* (2nd ed., pp. 11–26). Boston: Butterworth-Heinemann.

Fernald, L. C. (1998). Iodine deficiency and mental development in children. In S. M. Grantham-McGregor (Ed.), *Nutrition, health, and child development: Research advances and policy recommendations* (pp. 234–255). Washington, DC: Pan American Health Organisation, The World Bank, and Tropical Metabolism Research Unit of the West Indies.

Fletcher, J. M., Bohan, T. P., Brandt, M. E., Brookshire, B. L., Beaver, S. R., Francis, D. J., et al. (1992). Cerebral white matter and cognition in hydrocephalic children. *Archives of Neurology, 49,* 818–824.

Fletcher, J. M., Brookshire, B. L., Bohan, T. P., Brandt, M. E., & Davidson, K. C. (1995). Early hydrocephalus. In B. P. Rourke (Ed.), *Syndrome of nonverbal learning disabilities: Neurodevelopmental manifestations* (pp. 206–238). New York: Guilford Press.

Fletcher, J. M., Landry, S. H., Bohan, T. P., Davidson, K. C., Brookshire, B. L., Lachar, D., et al. (1997). Effects of intraventricular hemorrhage and hydrocephalus on the long-term neurobehavioral development of preterm very-low-birthweight infants. *Developmental Medicine and Child Neurology, 39,* 596–606.

Florentino, R. F., & Guirriec, R. M. (1984). Prevalence of nutritional anemia in infancy and childhood with emphasis on developing countries. In A. Stekel (Ed.), *Iron nutrition in infancy and childhood* (pp. 61–74). New York: Raven Press.

Gagnon, I., Forget, R., Sullivan, S. J., & Friedman, D. (1998). Motor performance following a mild traumatic brain injury in children: An exploratory study. *Brain Injury, 12*(10), 843–853.

Gay, C. L., Armstrong, D., Cohen, D., Lai, S., Hardy, M. D., Swales, T. P., et al. (1995). The effects of HIV on cognitive and motor development in children born to HIV-seropositive women with no reported drug use: Birth to 24 months. *Pediatrics, 96*, 1078–1082.

Ghez, C. (1991). The cerebellum. In E. R. Kandel, J. H. Schwartz, & T. M. Jessell (Eds.), *Principles of neural science* (3rd ed., pp. 853–868). New York: Elsevier.

Gilbert, M. R., Harding, B. L., & Grossman, S. A. (1989). Methotrexate neurotoxicity: In vitro studies using cerebellar explants from rats. *Cancer Research, 49*, 2502–2505.

Giroud, M., Lemesle, M., Madinier, G., Manceau, E., Osseby, G. V., & Dumas, R. (1997). Stroke in children under 16 years of age: Clinical and etiological difference with adults. *Acta Neurologica Scandinavica, 96*, 401–406.

Gladen, B. C., Rogan, W. J., Hardy, P., Thullen, J., Tingelstad, J., & Tully, M. (1988). Development after exposure to polychlorinated biphenyls and dichlorodiphenyl dichloroethene transplacentally and through human milk. *Journal of Pediatrics, 113*, 991–995.

Gordon, A. L., Ganesan, V., Towell, A., & Kirkham, F. J. (2002). Functional outcome following stroke in children. *Journal of Child Neurology, 17*, 429–434.

Grandjean, P., Weihe, P., White, R. F., & Debes, F. (1998). Cognitive performance of children prenatally exposed to "safe" levels of methylmercury. *Environmental Research, 77*, 165–172.

Grimwood, K., Anderson, V. A., Bond, L., Catroppa, C., Hore, R. L., Keir, E. H., et al. (1995). Adverse outcomes of bacterial meningitis in school-age survivors. *Pediatrics, 95*, 646–656.

Guthrie, E., Mast, J., Richards, P., McQuaid, M., & Pavlakis, S. (1999). Traumatic brain injury in children and adolescents. *Child and Adolescent Psychiatric Clinics of North America, 8*, 807–826.

Guttmann, E. (1942). Aphasia in children. *Brain, 65*, 205–219.

Hammond, P. B., & Dietrich, K. N. (1990). Lead exposure in early life: Health consequences. *Reviews of Environmental Contamination and Toxicology, 115*, 91–124.

Harila-Saari, A. H., Huuskonen, U. E. J., Tolonen, U., Vainionpaa, L. K., & Lanning, B. M. (2001). Motor nervous pathway function is impaired after treatment of childhood acute lymphoblastic leukemia: A study with motor evoked potentials. *Medical and Pediatric Oncology, 36*, 345–351.

Harila-Saari, A. H., Vainionpaa, L. K., Kovala, T. T., Tolonen, E. U., & Lanning, B. M. (1998). Nerve lesions after therapy for childhood acute lymphoblastic leukemia. *Cancer, 82*, 200–207.

Hetherington, R., & Dennis, M. (1999). Motor function profile in children with early onset hydrocephalus. *Developmental Neuropsychology, 15*, 25–51.

Hoppe-Hirsch, E., Laroussinie, F., Brunet, L., Sainte-Rose, C., Renier, D., Cinalli, G., et al. (1998). Late outcome of the surgical treatment of hydrocephalus. *Child's Nervous System, 14*, 97–99.

Jacobson, J. L., Jacobson, S. W., & Schwartz, P. M. (1984). Prenatal exposure to an environmental toxin: A test of the multiple effects model. *Developmental Psychology, 20*, 523–532.

Jaffe, K. M., Fay, G. C., Polissar, N. L., Martin, K. M., Shurtleff, H., Rivara, J. B., et al. (1992). Severity of pediatric traumatic brain injury and early neurobehavioral outcome: A cohort study. *Archives of Physical Medicine and Rehabilitation, 73*, 540–547.

Jahari, A. B., Saco-Pollitt, C., Husaini, M. A., & Pollitt, E. (2000). Effects of an energy and micronutrient supplement on motor development and motor activity in undernourished children in Indonesia. *European Journal of Clinical Nutrition, 54*, S60–S68.

Jinkins, J. R. (1991). Clinical manifestations of hydrocephalus caused by impingement of the corpus callosum on the falx: An MR study in 40 patients. *American Journal of Neuroradiology, 12*, 331–340.

Johnson, S. L. J., & Hall, D. M. B. (1992). Post-traumatic tremor in head injured children. *Archives of Disease in Childhood, 67*, 227–228.

Keidan, I., Shahar, E., Barzilay, Z., Passwell, J., & Brand, N. (1994). Predictors of outcome of stroke in infants and children based on clinical data and radiologic correlates. *Acta Paediatrica, 83*, 762–765.

Kirksey, A., Wachs, T. D., Yunis, F., Srinath, U., Rahmanifar, A., McCabe, G. P., et al. (1994). Relation of maternal zinc nutriture to pregnancy outcome and infant development in an Egyptian village. *American Journal of Clinical Nutrition, 60*, 782–792.

Klonoff, H., Clark, C., & Klonoff, P.S. (1993). Long-term outcome of head injuries: A 23 year follow up study of children with head injuries. *Journal of Neurology, Neurosurgery, and Psychiatry, 56*, 410–415.

Knight, W. G., Mellins, C. A., Levenson, R. L., Arpadi, S. M., & Kairam, R. (2000). Brief report: Effects of pediatric HIV infection on mental and psychomotor development. *Journal of Pediatric Psychology, 25*, 583–587.

Knights, R. M., Ivan, L. P., Ventureyra, E. C. G., Bentivoglio, C., Stoddart, C., Winogron, W., et al. (1991). The effects of head injury in children on neuropsychological and behavioural functioning. *Brain Injury, 5*, 339–351.

Kondo, K. (2000). Congenital Minamata disease: Warnings from Japan's experience. *Journal of Child Neurology, 15*, 458–464.

Koopman-Esseboom, C., Weisglas-Kuperus, N., de Ridder, M. A. J., Van der Paauws, C. G., Tuinstra, L. G. M., & Sauer, P. J. J. (1996). Effects of polychlorinated biphenyl/dioxin exposure and feeding type on infants' mental and psychomotor development. *Pediatrics, 97*, 700–706.

Kraus, J. F. (1995). Epidemiological features of brain injury in children: Occurrence, children at risk, causes and manner of injury, severity, and outcomes. In S. H. Broman & M. E. Michel (Eds.), *Traumatic head injury in children* (pp. 22–39). New York: Oxford University Press.

Krauss, J. K., Trankle, R., & Koop, K. H. (1996). Post-traumatic movement disorders in survivors of severe head injury. *Neurology, 47*, 1488–1492.

Lanska, M. J., Lanska, D. J., Horwitz, S. J., & Aram, D. M. (1991). Presentation, clinical course, and outcome of childhood stroke. *Pediatric Neurology, 7*, 333–341.

Lehtinen, S. S., Huuskonen, U. E., Harila-Saari, A. H., Tolonen, U., Vainionpaa, L. K., & Lanning, B. M. (2002). Motor nervous system impairment persists in long-term survivors of childhood acute lymphoblastic leukemia. *Cancer, 94*, 2466–2473.

Levin, H. S., & Chapman, S. B. (1998). Aphasia after traumatic brain injury. In M. T. Sarno (Ed.), *Acquired aphasia* (3rd ed., pp. 481–529). San Diego, CA: Academic Press.

Lord, D., Danoff, J. V., & Smith, M. R. (1995). Motor assessment of infants with human immunodeficiency virus infection: A retrospective review of multiple cases. *Pediatric Physical Therapy, 7*, 9–13.

Lozoff, B., Brittenham, G. M., Wolf, A. W., McClish, D. K., Kuhnert, P. M., Jimenez, E., et al. (1987). Iron deficiency anemia and iron therapy effects on infant developmental test performance. *Pediatrics, 79*, 981–995.

Lozoff, B., Jimenez, E., Hagen, J., Mollen, E., & Wolf, A. W. (2000). Poorer behavioral and developmental outcome more than 10 years after treatment for iron deficiency in infancy. *Pediatrics, 105*, E51.

Lozoff, B., Klein, N. K., Nelson, E. C., McClish, D. K., Manuel, M., & Chacon, M. E. (1998). Behavior of infants with iron-deficiency anemia. *Child Development, 69*, 24–36.

Mancini, J., Girard, N., Chabrol, B., Lamoureux, S., Livet, M., Thuret, I., et al. (1997). Ischemic cerebrovascular disease in children: Retrospective study of 35 patients. *Journal of Child Neurology, 12*, 193–199.

Mataro, M., Junque, C., Poca, M. A., & Sahuquillo, J. (2001). Neuropsychological findings in congenital and acquired childhood hydrocephalus. *Neuropsychology Review, 11*, 169–178.

Mellins, C. A., Levenson, R. L., Zawadzki, R., Kairam, R., & Weston, M. (1994). Effects of pediatric HIV infection and prenatal drug exposure on mental and psychomotor development. *Journal of Pediatric Psychology, 19*, 617–628.

Mintz, M., Tardieu, M., Hoyt, L., McSherry, G., Mendelson, J., & Oleske, J. (1996). Levodopa therapy improves motor function in HIV-infected children with extrapyramidal syndromes. *Neurology, 47*, 1583–1585.

Msellati, P., Lepage, P., Hitimana, D. G., van Goethem, C., van de Perre, P., & Dabis, F. (1993). Neurodevelopmental testing of children born to human immunodeficiency virus type 1 seropositive and seronegative mothers: A prospective cohort study in Kigali, Rwanda. *Pediatrics, 92*, 843–848.

Murdoch, B. E., Ozanne, A. E., & Cross, J. A. (1990). Acquired childhood speech disorders: Dysarthria and dyspraxia. In B. E. Murdoch (Ed.), *Acquired neurological speech/language disorders in childhood* (pp. 308–341). London: Taylor & Francis.

Myers, G. J., & Davidson, P. W. (2000). Does methylmercury have a role in causing developmental disabilities in children? *Environmental Health Perspectives, 108*, 413–420.

National Research Council. (2000). *Toxicological effects of methylmercury*. Washington, DC: National Academy of Science Research.

Neisser, U. (1997). Two perceptually given aspects of the self and their development. *Developmental Review, 11*, 197–209.

Nozyce, M., Hittelman, J., Muenz, L., Durako, S. J., Fischer, M. L., & Willoughby, A. (1994). Effect of perinatally acquired human immunodeficiency virus infection on neurodevelopment in children during the first two years of life. *Pediatrics, 94*, 883–891.

Obeso, J. A., & Narbona, J. (1983). Post-traumatic tremor and myoclonic jerking. *Journal of Neurology, Neurosurgery, and Psychiatry, 46*, 788.

Ochs, J. J. (1989). Neurotoxicity due to central nervous system therapy for childhood leukemia. *American Journal of Pediatric Hematology/Oncology, 11*, 93–105.

O'Flaherty, S., Chivers, A., Hannan, T., Kendrick, L., McCartney, L., Wallen, M., et al. (2000). The Westmed pediatric TBI multidisciplinary outcome study: Use of functional outcomes data to determine resource prioritization. *Archives of Physical Medicine and Rehabilitation, 81*, 723–729.

Oski, F. A., & Honig, A. S. (1978). The effects of therapy on the developmental scores of iron-deficient infants. *Journal of Pediatrics, 92*, 21–25.

Papero, P. H., Snyder, H. M., Gotschall, C. S., Johnson, D. L., & Eichelberger, M. R. (1997). Relationship of two measures of injury severity to pediatric psychological outcome 1–3 years after acute head injury. *Journal of Head Trauma Rehabilitation, 12*, 51–67.

Parks, R. A. (1994). Occupational therapy with children who are HIV positive. *Developmental Disabilities, 4*, 5–6.

Patandin, S., Lanting, C. I., Mulder, P. G., Boersma, E. R., Sauer, P. J., & Weisglas-Kuperus, N. (1999). Effects of environmental exposure to polychlorinated biphenyls and dioxins on cognitive abilities in Dutch children at 42 months of age. *Journal of Pediatrics, 134*, 33–41.

Pearson, D. A., McGrath, N. M., Nozyce, M., Nichols, S. L., Raskino, C., Brouwers, P., et al. (2000). Predicting HIV disease progression in children using measures of neuropsychological and neurological functioning. *Pediatrics, 106*, E76.

Pharoah, P. O., Buttfield, I. H., & Hetzel, B. A. (1971). Neurological damage to the fetus resulting from severe iodine deficiency during pregnancy. *Lancet, 13*, 308–310.

Press, M. F. (1977). Lead encephalopathy in neonatal Long-Evans rats: Morphologic studies. *Journal of Neuropathology, 36*, 169–195.

Reinders-Messelink, H. A., Schoemaker, M. M., Hofte, M., Goeken, L. N., Kingma, A., van den Briel, M. M., et al. (1996). Fine motor and handwriting problems after treatment for childhood acute lymphoblastic leukemia. *Medical and Pediatric Oncology, 27,* 551–555.

Reinders-Messelink, H., Schoemaker, M., Snijders, T., Goeken, L., van den Briel, M., Bokkerink, J., et al. (1999). Motor performance of children during treatment for acute lymphoblastic leukemia. *Medical and Pediatric Oncology, 33,* 545–550.

Rogan, W. J., & Gladen, B. C. (1991). PCBs, DDE, and child development at 18 and 24 months. *Annals of Epidemiology, 1,* 407–413.

Rogan, W. J., Gladen, B. C., McKinney, J. D., Carreras, N., Hardy, P., Thullen, J., et al. (1986). Neonatal effects of transplacental exposure to PCBs and DDE. *Journal of Pediatrics, 109,* 335–341.

Russell, M. L., Krouse, S. I., Lane, A. K., Leger, D., & Robson, C. A. (1998). Intervention for motor disorders. In M. Ylvisaker (Ed.), *Traumatic brain injury rehabilitation: Children and adolescents* (2nd ed., pp. 61–84). Boston: Butterworth-Heinemann.

Sameroff, A. J., & McDonough, S. C. (1984). The role of motor activity in human cognitive and social development. In E. Pollitt & P. Amante (Eds.), *Energy intake and activity: Current topics in nutrition and disease* (pp. 331–354). New York: Liss.

Sandler, S. G., Tobin, W., & Henderson, E. S. (1969). Vincristine-induced neuropathy. A clinical study of fifty leukemic patients. *Neurology, 19,* 367–374.

Sankar, R., Rai, B., Pulger, T., Sankar, G., Srinivasan, T., Srinivasan, L., et al. (1994). Intellectual and motor functions in school children from severely iodine deficient region in Sikkim. *Indian Journal of Pediatrics, 61,* 231–236.

Sazawal, S., Bentley, M., Black, R. E., Dhingra, P., George, S., & Bhan, M. K. (1996). Effect of zinc supplementation on observed activity in low socioeconomic Indian preschool children. *Pediatrics, 98,* 1132–1137.

Schoenberg, B. S., Mellinger, J. F., & Schoenberg, D. G. (1978). Cerebrovascular disease in infants and children: A study of incidence, clinical features, and survival. *Neurology, 28,* 763–768.

Snyder, R. D. (1994). Bacterial and spirochetal infections of the nervous system. In K. F. Swaiman (Ed.), *Pediatric neurology: Principles and practice* (2nd ed., Vol. 1, pp. 611–641). St. Louis, MO: Mosby.

Solbrig, M. V., Healy, J. F., & Jay, C. A. (2000). Bacterial infections. In W. G. Bradley, R. B. Daroff, G. M. Fenichel, & C. D. Marsden (Eds.), *Neurology in clinical practice: The neurological disorders* (3rd ed., Vol. II, pp. 1317–1351). Boston: Butterworth-Heinemann.

Spreen, O., Risser, A. H., & Edgell, D. (1995). *Developmental neuropsychology.* New York: Oxford University Press.

Stoltzfus, R. J., Kvalsvig, J. D., Chwaya, H. M., Montresor, A., Albonico, M., Tielsch, J. M., et al. (2001). Effects of iron supplementation and anthelmintic treatment on motor and language development of preschool children in Zanzibar: Double blind, placebo controlled study. *British Medical Journal, 323,* 1389–1393.

Swift, A. V., Cohen, M. J., Hynd, G. W., Wisenbaker, J. M., McKie, K. M., Makari, G., et al. (1989). Neuropsychologic impairment in children with sickle cell anemia. *Pediatrics, 84,* 1077–1085.

Taylor, H. G., Mills, E. L., Ciampi, A., duBerger, R., Watters, G. V., Gold, R., et al. (1990). The sequelae of *Haemophilus Influenzae* meningitis in school-age children. *New England Journal of Medicine, 323,* 1657–1663.

Taylor, H. G., Schatschneider, C., Petrill, S., Barry, C. T., & Owens, C. (1996). Executive dysfunction in children with early brain disease: Outcomes post-*Haemophilus Influenzae* meningitis. *Developmental Neuropsychology, 12,* 35–51.

Taylor, H. G., Schatschneider, C., & Rich, D. (1992). Sequelae of *Haemophilus Influenzae* meningitis: Implications for the study of brain disease and development. In M. G. Tramontana

& S. R. Hooper (Eds.), *Advances in child neuropsychology* (Vol. 1, pp. 50–108). New York: Springer-Verlag.

Trauner, D. A. (1998). Stroke in infants and children. In C. E. Coffey & R. A. Brumback (Eds.), *Textbook of pediatric neuropsychiatry* (pp. 839–852). Washington, DC: American Psychiatric Press.

Trauner, D. A., Chase, C., Walker, P., & Wulfeck, B. (1993). Neurologic profiles of infants and children after perinatal stroke. *Pediatric Neurology, 9*, 383–386.

VanHoff, J., Ritchey, A. K., & Shaywitz, B. A. (1985). Intracranial hemorrhage in children with sickle cell disease. *American Journal of Diseases of Childhood, 139*, 1120–1123.

Veerman, A. J., Hahlen, K., Kamps, W. A., VanLeeuwen, E. F., DeVaan, G. A., Solbu, G., et al. (1996). High cure rate with a moderately intensive treatment regimen in non-high risk childhood acute lymphoblastic leukemia: Results of protocol ALL VI from the Dutch Childhood Leukemia Study Group. *Journal of Clinical Oncology, 14*, 911–918.

Vermiglio, F., Sidoti, M., Finocchairo, M. D., Battiato, S., Lo Presti, V. P., Benvenga, S., et al (1990). Defective neuromotor and cognitive ability in iodine-deficient schoolchildren of an endemic goiter region in Sicily. *Journal of Clinical Endocrinology and Metabolism, 70*, 379–384.

Vreugdenbil, H. J. I., Lanting, C. I., Mulder, P. G. H., Boersma, E. R., & Weisglas-Kuperus, N. (2002). Effects of prenatal PCB and dioxin background exposure on cognitive and motor abilities in Dutch children at school age. *Journal of Pediatrics, 140*, 48–56.

Wachsler-Felder, J. L., & Golden, C. J. (2002). Neuropsychological consequences of HIV in children: A review of the literature. *Clinical Psychology Review, 22*, 441–462.

Wald, E. R., Bergman, I., Taylor, H. G., Chiponis, D., Porter, C., & Kubek, K. (1986). Long-term outcome of group B streptococcal meningitis. *Pediatrics, 77*, 217–221.

Walkowiak, J., Wiener, J. A., Fastabend, A., Heinzow, B., Kramer, U., Schmidt, E., et al. (2001). Environmental exposure to polychlorinated biphenyls and quality of the home environment: Effects on psychodevelopment in early childhood. *Lancet, 358*, 1602–1607.

Wallen, M. A., Mackay, S., Duff, S., McCartney, L. C., & O'Flaherty, S. J. (2001). Upper-limb function in Australian children with traumatic brain injury: A controlled, prospective study. *Archives of Physical Medicine and Rehabilitation, 82*, 642–649.

Walter, T., De Andraca, I., Chadud, P., & Perales, C. G. (1989). Iron deficiency anemia: Adverse effects on infant psychomotor development. *Pediatrics, 84*, 7–17.

Wasserman, G. A., Graziano, J. H., Factor-Litvak, P., Popovac, D., Morina, N., Musabegovic, A., et al. (1994). Consequences of lead exposure and iron supplementation on childhood development at age four years. *Neurotoxicology and Teratology, 16*, 233–240.

Wasserman, G. A., Musabegovic, A., Liu, X., Kline, J., Factor-Litvak, P., & Graziano, J. H. (2000). Lead exposure and motor functioning in 4½-year-old children: The Yugoslavia Prospective Study. *Journal of Pediatrics, 137*, 555–561.

Wills, K. E. (1993). Neuropsychological functioning in children with spina bifida and/or hydrocephalus. *Journal of Clinical Child Psychology, 22*, 247–265.

Wright, M. J., Halton, J. M., Martin, R. F., & Barr, R. D. (1998). Long-term gross motor performance following treatment for acute lymphoblastic leukemia. *Medical and Pediatric Oncology, 31*, 86–90.

Wulfeck, B. B., Trauner, D. A., & Tallal, P. A. (1991). Neurologic, cognitive, and linguistic features of infants after early stroke. *Pediatric Neurology, 7*, 266–269.

Yeates, K. O., Patterson, C. M., Waber, D. P., & Bernstein, J. H. (2003). Constructional and figural memory skills following pediatric closed-head injury: Evaluation using the ROCF. In J. A. Knight & E. Kaplan (Eds.), *The handbook of Rey–Osterrieth Complex Figure usage: Clinical and research applications* (pp. 383–392). Lutz, FL: Psychological Assessment Resources.

CHAPTER 9

Involuntary Motor Disorders in Childhood

DEBORAH DEWEY
DAVID E. TUPPER
SHAUNA BOTTOS

The study of childhood-onset involuntary motor disorders is an emerging area of interest for both neurologists and psychologists alike. Over the past two decades, we have witnessed great strides in our understanding of the neuropathophysiological mechanisms underlying pediatric movement disorders, largely due to the technological advances in neuroimaging that were previously unavailable. Delineation of the clinical features that distinguish one motor disorder from another has, as a consequence, become increasingly precise. In addition, advances in genetic technology have provided developmental neuroscience with an additional layer of biological understanding of a number of developmental disabilities.

While we may subsume a number of motor disturbances under the two broad categories of *hyperkinetic* (excessive) and *hypokinetic* (diminished) movement, these disorders of movement are not mutually exclusive because features of both may be evident as the disorder in question progresses over time. Although most motor disorders in the pediatric population are hyperkinetic in nature, such as tics and Tourette syndrome or Sydenham's chorea, there are pediatric conditions, including juvenile Huntington's disease, which may produce a hypokinetic state. The predominant focus of this chapter is on the types of motor deficits characteristic of children with Tourette syndrome and other tic disorders. The clinical and neuropsychological features of children with Sydenham's chorea and juvenile-onset Huntington's disease are also presented. After reviewing the broader symptoms of these disorders, we describe contemporary research on the basic pathophysiology, genetics, and treatment of each condition. The defining characteristic of disorders discussed in this chapter is that they all share unintended or involuntary movements as a primary symptom.

TICS AND TOURETTE SYNDROME

Epidemiological studies suggest that transient tics occur in 4–24% of schoolchildren (Shapiro & Shapiro, 1982), while the prevalence of Tourette syndrome (TS), a condition marked by multiple motor tics and at least one vocal tic, is approximately 1 to 8 per 1,000 in boys and 0.1 to 4 per 1,000 in girls (Leckman & Cohen, 1999). The onset of tics is typically during childhood between the ages of 5 and 10 (Arzimanoglou, 1998), with a tendency for tics to increase to a maximum severity during the prepubescent years then often to decline in frequency and severity by the beginning of adulthood (Leckman et al., 1998). Furthermore, children with TS and related disorders frequently display behaviors consistent with a number of behavioral and emotional disturbances, the most common being attention-deficit/hyperactivity disorder (ADHD) and obsessive–compulsive disorder (OCD) (Cohen & Leckman, 1994). Indeed, considerable controversy surrounds the etiological, and specifically the genetic, relationship among TS, ADHD, and OCD.

A tic is an involuntary, rapid, sudden, nonrhythmic, stereotyped motor movement or vocalization. There is often an associated prior sensation or irresistible "urge" to execute the tic, which is then followed by a transient relief (Jankovic, 1998). A distinction is often made between *simple* motor tics, in which discrete contractions in individual muscles or small groups of muscles occur, and *complex* motor tics, characterized by more muscles acting in a coordinated pattern to produce more complicated movements that may resemble purposeful voluntary movements (Bradshaw, 2001). Many children with TS display both simple and complex tics during the course of the disorder. However, the specific tic repertoire an individual with TS displays changes over time such that new motor or vocal tics may replace old ones over the course of months or years in a rather unpredictable fashion. Examples of common simple motor tics include head jerking, eye blinking, nose twitching, or a brief shrug of a shoulder. More complex tics may manifest as scratching, touching, rubbing, jumping, throwing, hitting, head or hand gestures, dystonic postures, adjustments for symmetry (Bradshaw, 2001), and complexities of gait, including retracing steps and twirling (Saunders-Pullman, Braun, & Bressman, 1999). Blocking tics, marked by a cessation of motor activity or speech, are also part of the tic spectrum (Saunders-Pullman et al., 1999). Tics may also be vocal or phonic and may manifest as sniffing, throat clearing, squealing, or snorting. Likewise, some children display more complex vocal tics, such as copropraxia (obscene gestures or behaviors), echolalia (repetition of others' speech), coprolalia (aggressive, obscene, or socially inappropriate words), echopraxia (imitation of others' behavior), and palilalia (repetition of one's own words or phrases) (Bradshaw, 2001). Most severe tics are associated with a large number of complex repetitive movements, including compulsions, stereotypies, and mannerisms (Lees & Tolosa, 1988). Compulsions are characterized by repetitive, intentional, and purposeful behaviors that are performed in response to intrusive impulses or thoughts (obsessions), whereas stereotypies are purposeless movements of entire body areas that are fragments of normal movements and are carried out in a uniformly repetitive fashion. Mannerisms are typically described as a bizarre mode of carrying out a purposeful act and are usually performed as a result of the incorporation of a stereotyped movement into goal-directed behavior (Arzimanoglou, 1998).

Motor tics have been reported to occur in many instances among children as isolated phenomena and therefore are considered acute transient tics. In contrast, tics that persist are deemed chronic. The fourth edition of *Diagnostic and Statistical Manual of Mental Disorders* (DSM-IV; American Psychiatric Association, 1994) recognizes three types of tic disorders on the basis of clinical criteria: transient tic disorder, chronic motor or vocal tic disorder, and Gilles de la Tourette syndrome. A diagnosis of transient tic disorder may be given when single or multiple motor and/or vocal tics are present, the tics occur many times a day, often in "bouts," and last at least 4 weeks but do not exceed 12 consecutive months, with an onset prior to 18 years of age (Arzimanoglou, 1998). The disorder cannot occur exclusively during substance intoxication or be due to known central nervous system disease, and the individual must display impaired functioning in social, academic, or occupational domains. Chronic tic disorder is similar to its transient counterpart in all the aforementioned factors, except that *either* vocal or motor tics (not both) must occur intermittently for a period of more than 1 year. TS is implicated when all the criteria for transient tic disorder are met; however, *both* vocal and motor tics must be present for more than 1 year, and the anatomic location, number, frequency, severity, and complexity of the tics change over time, in a waxing and waning manner.

Relative to other movement disorders, tics display the greatest range of phenomena resembling other forms of motor deficits. Indeed, children with tics often exhibit features similar to chorea (Saunders-Pullman et al., 1999), in which the child displays irregular, jerky, random, and brisk movements primarily affecting the limbs, face, jaw, and tongue. Similarly, the symptoms manifested by children with tic-related disorders often resemble myoclonus, a condition characterized by sudden, brief, jerky, and shock-like involuntary movements. Dystonia, a disordered tonicity of the muscles, is also not uncommon in children with TS (Saunders-Pullman et al., 1999).

Many children with TS and related disorders also show deficits in a vast array of motor skills. Sheppard, Bradshaw, Georgiou, Bradshaw, and Lee (2000) compared the movement sequencing performance of 12 children with TS and healthy age-matched control children. Performance was evaluated using a serial choice reaction time button-pressing procedure. Submovement execution times along the sequence were measured at two-way choice points. The authors manipulated the amount of advance information the child had regarding the next submovement in the sequence by illuminating a light-emitting diode under the next button to be pressed at particular stages of the sequence. They found that reducing the level of advance information resulted in a significant impairment in aspects of movement preparation for children with TS compared to the controls. More specifically, the time that each button was held down (i.e., movement preparation) became longer for children with TS as the amount of advance information decreased. Thus, children with TS appear to exhibit a disproportionate reliance on external visual cues to guide performance on tasks that require the sequencing of movements. The authors suggested that these findings were consistent with frontostriatal dysfunction involving the motor or dorsolateral prefrontal cortex circuitry. Dysfunction in these areas has been reported in neuroimaging studies of individuals with this disorder (discussed later).

In addition to difficulties with motor sequencing, recent studies that have focused on identifying the specific neuropsychological deficits associated with TS have reported that individuals with this disorder display specific impairments in visual–motor integration (Brookshire, Butler, Ewing-Cobbs, & Fletcher, 1994; Harris et al., 1995; Randolph, Hyde, Gold, Goldberg, & Weinberger, 1993; Schultz et al., 1998; Schultz, Carter, Scahill, & Leckman, 1999) and fine motor skills (Bornstein, 1990, 1991;

Bornstein, Baker, Bazylewich, & Douglas, 1991; Randolph et al., 1993; Schultz et al., 1998; Yeates & Bornstein, 1994). The studies by Bornstein and colleagues indicate that tasks that require simple motor speed (i.e., finger tapping) are not impaired in individuals with TS; however, fine motor tasks, which demand visual perceptual skills (i.e., Purdue Pegboard), are consistently impaired. Therefore, the motor skills deficits observed in individuals with TS do not appear to be the result of an impairment in basic motor skills but seem to be due to difficulties in the integration of visual information and motor outputs (Como, 2001; Schultz et al., 1998).

TS is also frequently associated with a wide array of neurological, behavioral, and cognitive difficulties, including problems in attention, disinhibition, and obsessive–compulsive symptoms (Barkley, 1997; Cohen, Deltor, Shaywitz, & Leckman, 1998; Como, 2001; Robertson, Trimble, & Lees, 1988; Schuerholz, Baumgartner, Singer, Reiss, & Denckla, 1996). There is debate as to whether or not there is a general deficit in the performance of executive function tasks that involve set and attention (Schultz et al., 1999). Schuerholz and colleagues (1996) conducted a study of children with TS with and without ADHD, and focused on identifying the psychoeducational and neuropsychological profiles of these disorders. Three groups of participants were recruited, a TS-only group, a TS-plus-ADHD group, and a group of children with TS and for whom ADHD was suspected but not confirmed. Unaffected siblings were used as controls. A comprehensive battery of neuropsychological and psychoeducational tests was administered. Learning disabilities were present in 23% of the total TS sample (all three groups) but not in the TS-only group. All TS subjects had significantly reduced scores on measures of choice reaction time consistent with prior research, but the TS-only group was also significantly poorer on a measure of executive functioning (letter word fluency). The authors interpreted this finding as suggestive of impairment in a left frontostriatal pathway subserving timed executive skills.

Pathogenesis of Tourette Syndrome

TS is considered a genetic disorder that is inherited in an autosomal dominant fashion (Pauls & Leckman, 1986). Support that genetic factors play an important role in the transmission and expression of TS and related disorders is evident in both twin and family studies. Hyde, Aaronson, Randolph, Rickler, and Weinberger (1992) in a study of monozygotic (MZ) twins found the concordance rate for TS to be 56% and the concordance rate for tic disorders to be 94%, which suggests a genetic basis for these conditions. Unfortunately, few studies have examined MZ twin pair's concordance rates for tic-related disorders compared to concordance rates for dizygotic (DZ) twins. An early study that compared MZ and DZ twins did find that MZ twins had a significantly higher concordance rate for TS than DZ twins (53% and 8%, respectively) (Price, Kidd, Cohen, Pauls, & Leckman, 1985). Moreover, when the presence of any type of tic disorder was examined among twin pairs, the concordance rate for the MZ twins (77%) was higher than the concordance rate for DZ twins (23%). Recently, there have also been case reports of families in which more than one relative met the criteria for TS or tics (Eidelberg et al., 1997). These findings provide compelling support for the role of genetics in the transmission of tic-related disorders.

Several lines of evidence suggest that dysfunction of basal ganglia circuits and their connections with frontocortical circuits may be of fundamental importance in the pathophysiology of TS. Recent magnetic resonance imaging (MRI) studies of boys with TS have revealed anatomical changes in the prefrontal, premotor, and orbito-frontal cortex (Peterson et al., 1993). Interestingly, functional imaging studies that have examined grip-force strength during unilateral or bimanual movements in adult patients with TS have found that the secondary motor areas were not activated during these tasks when compared with baseline conditions, indicating that the metabolic level in these areas was similar during rest and task performance (Serrien et al., 2002). The authors suggested that continuous activation of the secondary motor areas in movement preparation could be responsible for TS patients' involuntary urge to move. As mentioned previously, Sheppard and colleagues (2000) also observed abnormalities in movement preparation in children with TS and suggested that frontostriatal dysfunction may underlie such difficulties.

In vivo positron emission tomography (PET) and single-photon emission computed tomography (SPECT) studies have revealed reduced basal ganglia volume accompanied by decreased glucose metabolism and cerebral blood flow in adults with TS (Braun et al., 1993; Riddle, Rasmusson, Woods, & Hoffer, 1992). However, one must be cautious in extending these findings to children as long-term secondary effects of the disease and its treatment may be confounding factors. More research using neuroimaging techniques to study functional and anatomical changes in children with tic-related disorders is sorely needed.

Despite the recent advances in our understanding of the neuropathophysiology of TS, its neurobiochemical substrate remains unclear. Evidence is accumulating, however, to support the role of neurotransmitter dysfunction within the central nervous system in the pathogenesis of TS. In particular, the role of dopamine in the modulation of basal ganglia circuits has been emphasized in the neurobiology of tic disorders (Singer, 1994). Perhaps the most influential evidence for the dopamine hypothesis of TS comes from investigations of the effect of dopamine inhibiting and facilitating pharmacological agents. Such studies have found that the most effective treatment for symptoms of TS includes neuroleptics, such as haloperidol, which act as dopamine receptor antagonists (Shapiro & Shapiro, 1982). In contrast, dopamine agonists such as amphetamine and methylphenidate are reported to induce or exacerbate TS symptomatology (Castellanos et al., 1997). Further support for the importance of dopamine in TS is the body of evidence suggesting that different allelic forms of the D2 dopamine receptor may be related to the severity of tics (Comings et al., 1992). More recently, allelic variants at the dopamine D4 receptor have also been found to be associated with TS in some families (Grice et al., 1996). Thus, these findings suggest that TS is related to dopaminergic mechanisms.

In addition to dopamine, abnormal biochemical profiles of postmortem brains have implicated low serotonin levels, low glutamate levels in the globus pallidus, and low cortical cyclic AMP levels in the pathogenesis of TS (Singer, Hahn, & Moran, 1991). Some authors have attempted to reconcile these somewhat conflicting findings by suggesting that several neurotransmitter systems may operate in a cascading fashion in which different neurotransmitters may be involved in the different features characteristic of this disorder (Arzimanoglou, 1998). For example, it has been proposed that motor tics may be a consequence of overactivity of the dopaminergic system, whereas the attentional difficulties often characteristic of children with TS may be due to noradrenergic dysfunction (Arzimanoglou, 1998).

Given that no twin studies to date have yielded 100% concordance rates for the manifestation of TS and related disorders, environmental factors clearly play an important role in determining the presentation of this disorder. Factors such as adverse prenatal events, exposure to hormonal agents and central nervous system stimulants (Peterson, Leckman, & Cohen, 1995), and trauma (Jankovic, 2001) have all been implicated in the etiology of tic disorders. Postinfectious autoimmune mechanisms have also recently emerged as contributing factors for the pathogenesis of some cases of tics and TS (Church, Dale, Lees, Giovannoni, & Robertson, 2003). Indeed, clinical and systematic observations have revealed a subset of cases of acute-childhood-onset OCD and/or tic disorders immediately preceded by streptococcal infection (Kondo & Kabasawa, 1978). The term *pediatric autoimmune disorders associated with streptococcal infections* (PANDAS) has been applied to this subgroup of patients to indicate the hypothesized common etiopathogenesis. More specifically, it appears that in susceptible children, infection with group A beta-hemolytic streptococcus (GABHS) triggers the synthesis of antibodies against an epitope on the infectious agent, which cross-reacts with an epitope in the central nervous system (Snider & Swedo, 2003). When the cross-reactivity is directed toward an epitope in the basal ganglia and their associated circuits, movement disorders may ensue.

The clinical criteria for PANDAS have been described in detail by Swedo and colleagues (1998). For the current discussion, the neurological abnormalities characteristic of symptom exacerbation among this group of children are noteworthy and primarily include adventitious movements such as choreiform movements and tics. However, more subtle neurological signs may also be evident, such as motor hyperactivity or a deterioration in fine motor skills, the latter often manifesting as a worsening of the child's handwriting (Swedo et al., 1998).

Treatment

Nonpharmacological intervention has been deemed most appropriate for children with mild tics. Family counseling and education about the disorder are highly beneficial for optimal functioning of both the child and his or her caregivers. As mentioned earlier, the most effective and most common drug used with children with more severe tics or TS is the neuroleptic haloperidol (Kurlan, 1997). However, to avoid possible tardive dyskinesia, nonneuroleptic medications such as clonazepam and clonidine are often tried first. Botulinum toxin injections have also been used successfully to control either focal motor tics such as eye blinking or vocal tics (Scott, Jankovic, & Donovan, 1996), with the added benefits of lasting, on average, 3 to 4 months and having fewer serious complications.

SYDENHAM'S CHOREA

Sydenham's chorea (SC) is a well-recognized manifestation of rheumatic fever characterized by an array of neuropsychiatric symptoms. It affects children 5–15 years of age with a peak incidence at 8 years of age (Veasy et al., 1987). SC results from the development of antistreptococcal antibodies in reaction to the presence of GABHS, which by the process of molecular mimicry, cross-reacts with epitopes on the basal ganglia of susceptible hosts (Snider & Swedo, 2003). The course of SC is typically less than a year in duration, although there have been recent indications that remission may take longer for some patients (Cardosa, Vargas, Oliveira, Guerra, & Amaral, 1999).

In addition to the hallmark characteristic of frank chorea, the motor symptoms observed in patients with SC include gross fasciculations of the tongue, facial grimacing, loss of fine motor control, ballismus (abnormal swinging jerking movements), hypotonia, motor impersistence, gait disturbance, and speech abnormalities such as dysarthria (Aron, Freeman, & Carter, 1965). Children with SC also often display ataxia and clumsiness (Swedo, 1994). Moreover, any portion of the body may be affected, and the symptoms may be unilateral or bilateral. Thus, many of the clinical features are similar to those seen in children with tic-related disorders or PANDAS, which often poses diagnostic difficulties.

Pathogenesis of Sydenham's Chorea

Regional inflammation is thought to play a role in the specificity of the post-streptococcal neuropsychiatric symptomatology. In SC, recent functional imaging studies provide support for the involvement of basal ganglia and cortical structures, with increased basal ganglia blood flow and disruptions in the blood–brain barrier in the caudate nuclei evident during the acute symptomatic period (Goldman et al., 1993). These abnormalities resolve as the chorea remits, suggesting that they are etiologically related to the neuropsychiatric symptoms found in the patients. Increased volumes of the putamen, caudate, and globus pallidus in children with SC compared to healthy controls have also been reported by Giedd and colleagues (1995). Furthermore, similar abnormalities have recently been found in children with PANDAS (Giedd, Rapoport, Garvey, Perlmutter, & Swedo, 2000; Giedd, Rapoport, Leonard, Richter, & Swedo, 1996), which supports the similar neurobiology of these two disorders.

Several studies have demonstrated significantly higher concentrations of anti-neuronal antibodies in children with SC, OCD, and TS, compared with healthy controls (Kiessling, Marcotte, & Culpepper, 1993, 1994), thereby drawing attention to a potential common autoimmune response manifest in some individuals with these conditions. Additional evidence of a common autoimmune etiology in the pathogenesis of these disorders is the presence of a serologic marker, the D8/17 B lymphocyte antigen, which is present in increased expression among patients with these conditions (Murphy et al., 1997; Swedo et al., 1997). It appears that this marker is genetically determined and most likely inherited in an autosomal recessive fashion (Gibofosky, Khanna, Suh, & Zabriskie, 1991).

Treatment

For many children with SC, the disease is self-limited; therefore, bed rest and the avoidance of stress are the treatments of choice. However, for a subgroup of children whose disease is unrelenting, the focus of treatment may be prophylactic antibacterial therapy, and in severe cases steroids may also be used (Blunt, Brooks, & Kennard, 1994). Furthermore, for patients with moderate to severe movement disorders, the accompanying obsessive–compulsive symptoms and other psychological disturbances may interfere with the children's daily functioning, and, thus, other forms of pharmacotherapy may be required. In a recent study comparing the efficacy of haloperidol, carbamazepine, and valproic acid, drugs that have all demonstrated symptom relief for patients with SC, valproic acid emerged as the drug of choice for children with this disease (Pena, Mora, Cardozo, Molina, & Montiel, 2002). By the end of the first week of treatment with valproic acid, the number of patients who responded to this treatment was significantly higher than the number of those who responded to haloperidol or carbamazepine therapy. Furthermore, the time to improvement was significantly shorter for those children who received valproic acid. Thus, this drug appears to be both effective and safe because of its low effective dose and rapid response rate. More important, however, it may be a viable alternative to haloperidol and similar dopamine receptor blocking drugs, which are associated with such deleterious side effects as parkinsonism and dystonia.

JUVENILE-ONSET HUNTINGTON'S DISEASE

Huntington's disease (HD) is an autosomal dominant inherited neurodegenerative disorder involving the basal ganglia and cerebral cortex. The gene responsible was localized on the tip of chromosome 4 in the 4p16.3 region in 1983 and is now known to be identified by having an excessive number of trinucleotide (CAG) repeats (Gusella, MacDonald, Ambrose, & Duyao, 1993). Exon 1 of the HD gene contains a stretch of uninterrupted CAG trinucleotide repeats which encode a protein called huntingtin whose function is presently unknown.

The age of onset for HD is most commonly during midlife; however, it has been estimated that 3–10% of all HD cases may have a childhood onset of under 20 years of age (Harper et al., 1991). In addition, juvenile HD is inherited from the father in up to 90% of the cases (Martin & Gusella, 1986). Normal or asymptomatic individuals have 35 or fewer CAG repeats, whereas HD is caused by expansions of 36 or more CAG repeats. There is an inverse relationship between CAG repeat number and age of onset; a greatly expanded gene is associated with early onset of illness, as well as more rapid progression. Expansions of 50 or more CAG repeats often are associated with the juvenile form of HD.

Although the research examining the clinical features of juvenile-onset HD is sparse, it appears that children with this disease may manifest a number of features that distinguish them from adult-onset cases. Adult HD typically manifests as a triad of symptoms including a choreic movement disorder, cognitive disturbance, and psychiatric or behavioral disorder (Nance & Myers, 2001). Although the same triad of features may be present in childhood-onset cases, juvenile HD patients more often present with cerebellar symptoms, mental deterioration, seizure disorder (Markham & Knox, 1965; Nance & Myers, 2001), and oral motor dysfunction (dysarthria, dysphagia, or drooling) (Nance & Myers, 2001). Furthermore, chorea, a movement disorder characterized by brief, irregular, nonrhythmic movements, is far less common in children than in the adult population. Instead, children are more likely to display symptoms of rigidity (Bruyn, 1969; Nance & Myers, 2001). During the course of juvenile HD, rigidity and a pyramidal syndrome develops in approximately 80% of cases, convulsive seizures or myoclonus is evident in about 30% of cases, and cerebellar features such as ataxia develop in approximately 65% of cases (Katafuchi, Fuijimoto, Ono, & Kuda, 1984; Siesling, Vegter-van der Vlis, & Roos, 1997). Some authors have reported tremor and ataxia to be more commonly associated with the rigid type of juvenile HD than with the choreatic type (Katafuchi et al., 1984; Siesling et al., 1997). Severe dystonia has also been observed in some juvenile HD patients (Nance & Myers, 2001).

While adults with HD are more likely to have choreic symptomatology, and only develop rigidity and dystonia much later in the disease progression, children with HD are likely to have stiffness of the legs, walking on the toes, or scissoring of the gait as initial or early symptoms. Clumsiness of hand and arm movements, dysarthric speech, drooling and poor motor control are also likely, particularly in very young children. The earlier the symptoms begin, the less likely the child is to have chorea at any point in the disease course. On the other hand, the older the child, the more likely he or she is to have chorea as a presenting symptom (Nance, 2001).

Unlike adult HD, there is no empirical research available regarding the neuro-cognitive and neuropsychological characteristics of children with HD. Children with juvenile HD often demonstrate early development that is age-appropriate and only later show characteristics that suggest progressive dysfunction. Initially, diagnosis may be difficult, with children showing motor characteristics similar to children with nonprogressive cerebral palsy. In addition, other clinically similar conditions, such as benign hereditary chorea and progressive myoclonic epilepsy, need to be ruled out in the diagnosis (Gambardella et al., 2001; Gordon, 2003; O'Shea, 1991). Frequent falls, dysarthria, clumsiness, hyperreflexia, and oculomotor disturbances are noted in children with HD. Sometimes, moodiness, speech difficulty, learning difficulties, or non-specific behavioral problems can be seen as early signs of juvenile HD (Elliott, 1993; Kremer, 2002). Mental deterioration is likely first manifested by declining school per-formance, but the pattern of specific cognitive abnormalities is not known at this time.

In addition to the different clinical symptomatology characteristic of juvenile-onset HD, the clinical course of HD in children is often more progressive than in the adult population (Nance & Myers, 2001). Unfortunately, all HD children will eventu-ally lose their ability to walk, eat safely, and communicate orally as their disease evolves, ultimately becoming bed-ridden and fully dependent on their caregivers. There is no cure for HD, and death is the eventual outcome.

Pathogenesis of Juvenile-Onset Huntington's Disease

Neuropathologically, similar brain regions are affected in juvenile- and adult-onset HD. HD is characterized by diffuse and regional cerebral atrophy, which is most dra-matic in the caudate nuclei and, to a lesser extent, the putamen (Martin & Gusella, 1986). Loss of small, spiny GABA-ergic neurons in the dorsomedial aspects of the head of the caudate are noted early in disease progression, and later the putamen and complete caudate become involved. Postmortems have revealed that as many as 80% of HD brains display atrophy of the frontal lobes (Vonsattel, 2000). In addition, the cerebellum and the globus pallidus, areas not typically involved in adults with HD, may be implicated in the pathology of the disease in children (Jervis, 1963). The de-struction of the latter two regions has been suggested to account for the balance diffi-culties and rigidity more often seen in children with HD (Ho, Chuang, Rovira, & Koo,

1995). Postmortems of HD brains have also shown intraneuronal aggregates (inclusions) in nuclei and neuronal processes; these inclusions are composed of truncated derivatives of the mutant huntingtin protein.

Treatment

The main approach to treating juvenile HD is currently restricted to the relief of symptoms through pharmacotherapy. Dopamine-depleting or dopamine-blocking agents are occasionally used to reduce chorea; however, these may exacerbate the dystonia and rigidity that are commonly present in children with HD (Nance & Myers, 2001). Some children with severe rigidity may benefit from anti-parkinsonian or antispasticity medications, and botulinum toxin may be used to manage certain dystonic features (Nance & Myers, 2001).

Children with HD obviously have complex and special needs that change throughout the course of their illness. A comprehensive approach to managing neurological, psychological, and family symptoms is clearly required, and a chronic disease perspective is often required. A team of care providers ideally can work with the child, family, and school to optimize the child's health and functioning throughout the course of the disease. It is particularly beneficial to recognize that HD occurs in families, and there are often needs for care of parents and other family members beyond the specific child affected (O'Shea, 1991; Wolff, 1988).

CONCLUSION

This chapter has provided a broad overview of the motor symptoms and deficits commonly observed in children with tics and TS, SC, and juvenile-onset HD. Tremendous gains have been made in our understanding of the genetic and neurophysiological mechanisms that influence the presentation and course of these disorders, largely due to the functional neuroimaging procedures now in widespread use. A common unifying link among these diverse motor disturbances is the evident dysfunction of the basal ganglia and its associated circuits. In addition, twin, family, and molecular genetic studies have provided compelling evidence in support of a genetic susceptibility for such disturbances. However, these very studies have also drawn attention to the important influence environmental factors may have on both the onset and course of each disorder. Therefore, it appears that the pathogenesis of these movement disorders may best be conceptualized as involving critical interactions among genetic factors, neurobiological substrates, and environmental factors in the production of the clinical phenotypes. With the advent of more refined and novel means for studying pediatric motor disorders likely to come in the 21st century, we will undoubtedly gain a better understanding of the etiological and neuropsychological correlates of these conditions.

ACKNOWLEDGMENTS

Grants from the Alberta Children's Hospital Foundation and the Canadian Institutes of Health Research supported the preparation of this chapter.

REFERENCES

American Psychiatric Association. (1994). *Diagnostic and statistical manual of mental disorders* (4th ed.). Washington, DC: Author.

Aron, A. M., Freeman, J. M., & Carter, S. (1965). The natural history of Sydenham's chorea: Review of the literature and long-term evaluation with emphasis on cardiac sequelae. *American Journal of Medicine, 38,* 83–93.

Arzimanoglou, A. A. (1998). Gilles de la Tourette syndrome. *Journal of Neurology, 245,* 761–765.

Barkley, R. A. (1997). *ADHD and the nature of self-control.* New York: Guilford Press.

Blunt, S. B., Brooks, D. J., & Kennard, C. (1994). Steroid-responsive chorea in childhood following cardiac transplantation. *Movement Disorders, 9,* 112–114.

Bornstein, R. A. (1990). Neuropsychological performance in children with Tourette syndrome. *Psychiatric Research, 33,* 73–81.

Bornstein, R. A. (1991). Neuropsychological performance in adults with Tourette syndrome. *Psychiatric Research, 37,* 229–236.

Bornstein, R. A., Baker, G. B., Bazylewich, T., & Douglas, A. B. (1991). Tourette syndrome and neuropsychological performance. *Acta Psychiatrica Scandinavica, 84,* 212–216.

Bradshaw, J. L. (2001). *Developmental disorders of the frontostriatal system: Neuropsychological, neuropsychiatric, and evolutionary perspectives.* Philadelphia: Psychology Press.

Braun, A. R., Stoetter, B., Randolph, C., Hsiao, J. K., Vladar, K., Gernert, J., et al. (1993). The functional neuroanatomy of Tourette's syndrome: An FDG-PET study, I. Regional changes in cerebral glucose metabolism differentiating patients and controls. *Neuropsychopharmacology, 9,* 277–291.

Brookshire, B. L., Butler, I. J., Ewing-Cobbs, L., & Fletcher, J. M. (1994). Neuropsychological characteristics of children with Tourette syndrome: Evidence for a nonverbal learning disability. *Journal of Clinical and Experimental Neuropsychology, 16,* 289–302.

Bruyn, G. W. (1969). The Westphal variant and the juvenile type of Huntington chorea. In A. Barbeau & J. R. Brunette (Eds.), *Progress in neurogenetics* (pp. 666–673). Amsterdam: Excerpta Medica Foundation.

Cardosa, F., Vargas, A. P., Oliveira, L. D., Guerra, A. A., & Amaral, S. V. (1999). Persistent Sydenham's chorea. *Movement Disorders, 14,* 805–807.

Castellanos, F. X., Giedd, J. N., Elia, J., Marsh, W. L., Ritchie, G. F., Hamburger, S. D., et al. (1997). Controlled stimulant treatment of ADHD and comorbid Tourette's syndrome: Effects of stimulant and dose. *Journal of the American Academy of Child and Adolescent Psychiatry, 36,* 589–596.

Church, A. J., Dale, R. C., Lees, A. J., Giovannoni, G., & Robertson, M. M. (2003). Tourette's syndrome: A cross sectional study to examine the PANDAS hypothesis. *Journal of Neurology, Neurosurgery, and Psychiatry, 74,* 602–607.

Cohen, D. J., Deltor, J., Shaywitz, B. A., & Leckman, J. F. (1982). Interaction of biological and psychological factors in the natural history of Tourette's syndrome: A paradigm for childhood neuropsychiatric disorders. *Advances in Neurology, 35,* 31–40.

Cohen, D. J., & Leckman, J. F. (1994). Developmental psychopathology and neurobiology of Tourette's syndrome. *Journal of the American Academy of Child and Adolescent Psychiatry, 33,* 2–15.

Comings, D. E., Comings, B. J., Muhlemean, D., Dietz, G., Shahbahrami, B., Tast, D., et al. (1992). The dopamine D2 receptor locus as a modifying gene in neuropsychiatric disorders. *Journal of the American Medical Association, 266,* 1793–1800.

Como, P. G. (2001). Neuropsychological function in Tourette syndrome. In D. J. Cohen, C. G. Goetz, & J. Jankovic (Eds.), *Advances in neurology: Tourette syndrome* (pp. 103–111). Philadelphia: Lippincott, Williams & Wilkins.

Eidelberg, D., Moeller, J. R., Antonini, A., Kazumata, K., Dhawan, V., Budman, C., et al. (1997). The metabolic anatomy of Tourette's syndrome. *Neurology, 48,* 927–934.

Elliott, W. (Ed.). (1993). *Living with Juvenile Huntington's disease.* Cambridge, Ontario: Huntington Society of Canada.

Gambardella, A., Miglia, M., Labate, A., Magariello, A., Gabriele, A. L., Mazzei, R., et al. (2001). Juvenile Huntington's disease presenting as progressive myoclonic epilepsy. *Neurology, 57,* 708–711.

Gibofosky, A., Khanna, A., Suh, E., & Zabriskie, J. B. (1991). The genetics of rheumatic fever: Relationship to streptococcal infection and autoimmune disease. *Journal of Rheumatology, 30,* 1–5.

Giedd, J. N., Rapoport, J. L., Garvey, M. A., Perlmutter, S., & Swedo, S. E. (2000). MRI assessment of children with obsessive–compulsive disorder or tics associated with streptococcal infection. *American Journal of Psychiatry, 157,* 281–283.

Giedd, J. N., Rapoport, J. L., Kruesi, M. J. P., Parker, C., Schapiro, M. B., Allen, A. J., et al. (1995). Sydenham's chorea: Magnetic resonance imaging of the basal ganglia. *Neurology, 45,* 2199–2202.

Giedd, J. N., Rapoport, J. L., Leonard, H. L., Richter, D., & Swedo, S. E. (1996). Case study: Acute basal ganglia enlargement and obsessive–compulsive symptoms in an adolescent boy. *Journal of the American Academy of Child and Adolescent Psychiatry, 35,* 913–915.

Goldman, S., Amrom, D., Szliwowski, H. B., Detemmerman, D., Goldman, S., Bidaut, L. M., et al. (1993). Reversible striatal hypermetabolism in a case of Sydenham's chorea. *Movement Disorders, 8,* 355–358.

Gordon, N. (2003). Huntington's disease of early onset or juvenile Huntington's disease. *Hospital Medicine, 64,* 576–580.

Grice, D. E., Leckman, J. F., Pauls, D. L., Kurlan, R., Kidd, K. K., Pakstis, A., et al. (1996). Genetic association of alleles at the dopamine D_4 receptor locus with Tourette's syndrome. *American Journal of Human Genetics, 59,* 644–652.

Gusella, J. F., MacDonald, M. E., Ambrose, C. M., & Duyao, M. P. (1993). Molecular genetics of Huntington's disease. *Archives of Neurology, 50,* 1157–1163.

Harper, P. S., Morris, M. R., Quarrell, O. W. J., Shaw, D. J., Tyler, A. T., & Youngman, S. (1991). *Huntington's disease.* London: Saunders.

Harris, E. L., Schuerholz, L. J., Singer, H. S., Reader, M. J., Brown, J. E., Cox, C., et al. (1995). Executive function in children with Tourette syndrome and/or attention deficit hyperactivity disorder. *Journal of the International Neuropsychological Society, 1,* 511–516.

Ho, V. B., Chuang, S., Rovira, M. J., & Koo, B. (1995). Juvenile Huntington's disease: CT and MR features. *American Journal of Neuroradiology, 16,* 1405–1412.

Hyde, T. M., Aaronson, B. A., Randolph, C., Rickler, K. C., & Weinberger, D. R. (1992). Relationship of birth weight to the phenotypic expression of Gilles de la Tourette's syndrome in monozygotic twins. *Neurology, 42,* 652–658.

Jankovic, J. (1998). Tics and Tourette syndrome. In E. Tolosa, W. C. Koll, & O. S. Gershanik (Eds.), *Differential diagnosis and treatment of movement disorders* (pp. 99–107). Boston: Butterworth-Heinemann.

Jankovic, J. (2001). Tourette's syndrome. *New England Journal of Medicine, 345,* 1184–1192.

Jervis, G. A. (1963). Huntington's chorea in childhood. *Archives of Neurology, 9,* 244–257.

Katafuchi, Y., Fuijimoto, T., Ono, E., & Kuda, N. (1984). A childhood form of Huntington disease associated with marked pyramidal signs. *European Journal of Neurology, 23,* 296–299.

Kiessling, L. S., Marcotte, A. C., & Culpepper, L. (1993). Antineuronal antibodies in movement disorders. *Pediatrics, 92,* 39–43.

Kiessling, L. S., Marcotte, A. C., & Culpepper, L. (1994). Antineuronal antibodies: Tics and obsessive–compulsive symptoms. *Journal of Developmental and Behavioral Pediatrics, 15,* 421–425.

Kondo, K., & Kabasawa, T. (1978). Improvement in Gilles de la Tourette syndrome after corticosteriod therapy. *Annals of Neurology, 4*, 387–390.

Kremer, B. (2002). Clinical neurology of Huntington's disease: Diversity in unity, unity in diversity. In G. Bates, P. S. Harper, & L. Jones (Eds.), *Huntington's disease* (3rd ed., pp. 28–61). Oxford, UK: Oxford University Press.

Kurlan, R. (1997). Tourette syndrome: Treatment of tics. *Neurologic Clinics, 15*, 403–409.

Leckman, J. F., & Cohen, D. J. (Eds.). (1999). *Tourette's syndrome: Tics, obsessions, compulsions.* New York: Wiley.

Leckman, J., Zhang, H., Vitale, A., Lahnin, F., Lynch, K., Bondi, C., et al. (1998). Course of tic severity in Tourette syndrome: The first two decades. *Pediatrics, 102*, 14–19.

Lees, A. J., & Tolosa, E. (1988). Tics. In J. Jankovic & E. Tolosa (Eds.), *Parkinson's disease and movement disorders* (pp. 275–281). Baltimore: Urban & Schwarzenberg.

Markham, C. H., & Knox, J. W. (1965). Observations on Huntington's chorea in childhood. *Journal of Pediatrics, 67*, 46–57.

Martin, J. B., & Gusella, J. F. (1986). Huntington's disease: Pathogenesis and management. *New England Journal of Medicine, 315*, 1267–1276.

Murphy, T. K., Goodman, W. K., Fudge, M. W., Williams, R. C., Ayoub, E. M., Dalal, M., et al. (1997). B lymphocyte antigen D8/17: A peripheral marker for childhood onset obsessive–compulsive disorder and Tourette's syndrome? *American Journal of Psychiatry, 154*, 402–407.

Nance, M. (Ed.). (2001). *The juvenile HD handbook: A guide for physicians, neurologists, and other professionals.* New York: Huntington's Disease Society of America.

Nance, M. A., & Myers, R. H. (2001). Juvenile onset Huntington's disease—Clinical and research perspectives. *Mental Retardation and Developmental Disabilities, 7*, 153–157.

O'Shea, B. (1991). Juvenile Huntington's disease. *Irish Journal of Psychological Medicine, 8*, 149–153.

Pauls, D. L., & Leckman, J. F. (1986). The inheritance of Gille de la Tourette's syndrome and associated behavior: Evidence for autosomal dominant transmission. *New England Journal of Medicine, 315*, 993–997.

Pena, J., Mora, E., Cardozo, J., Molina, O., & Montiel, C. (2002). Comparison of the efficacy of carbamazepine, haloperidol and valproic acid in the treatment of children with Sydenham's chorea. *Arquivos de Neuro-Psiquiatria, 60*, 374–377.

Peterson, B., Riddle, M. A., Cohen, D. J., Katz, L. D., Smith, J. C., Hardin, M. T., et al. (1993). Reduced basal ganglia volumes in Tourette's syndrome using three-dimensional reconstruction techniques from magnetic resonance images. *Neurology, 43*, 941–949.

Peterson, B. S., Leckman, J. F., & Cohen, D. J. (1995). Tourette's syndrome: A genetically predisposed and an environmentally specified developmental psychopathology. In D. Cicchetti & D. J. Cohen (Eds.), *Manual of developmental psychopathology* (pp. 213–242). New York: Wiley.

Price, R. A., Kidd, K. K., Cohen, D. J., Pauls, D. L., & Leckman, J. F. (1985). A twin study of Tourette syndrome. *Archives of General Psychiatry, 42*, 815–820.

Randolph, C., Hyde, T. M., Gold, J. M., Goldberg, T. E., & Weinberger, D. R. (1993). Tourette's syndrome in monozygotic twins. Relationship of tic severity to neuropsychological function. *Archives of Neurology, 50*, 725–728.

Riddle, M. A., Rasmusson, A. M., Woods, S. W., & Hoffer, P. B. (1992). SPECT imaging of cerebral blood flow in Tourette syndrome. *Advances in Neurology, 58*, 207–211.

Robertson, M. M., Trimble, M. R., & Lees, A. J. (1988). The psychopathology of the Gilles de la Tourette syndrome. A phenomenological analysis. *British Journal of Psychiatry, 152*, 383–390.

Saunders-Pullman, R., Braun, I., & Bressman, S. (1999). Pediatric movement disorders. *Child and Adolescent Psychiatric Clinics of North America, 8*, 747–765.

Schuerholz, L. J., Baumgartner, T. L., Singer, H. S., Reiss, A. L., & Denckla, M. B. (1996). Neuropsychological status of children with Tourette's syndrome with and without attention deficit hyperactivity disorder. *Neurology, 46,958–965.*

Schultz, R. T., Carter, A. S., Gladstone, M., Scahill, L., Leckman, J. F., Peterson, et al. (1998). Visual–motor integration functioning in children with Tourette syndrome. *Neuropsychology, 12,* 134–145.

Schultz, R. T., Carter, A. S., Scahill, L., & Leckman, J. F. (1999). Neuropsychological findings. In J. F. Leckman & D. J. Cohen (Eds.), *Tourette's syndrome—Tics, obsessions, compulsion: Developmental psychopathology and clinical care* (pp. 80–103). New York: Wiley.

Scott, B. L., Jankovic, J., & Donovan, D. T. (1996). Botulinum toxin into vocal cord in the treatment of malignant coprolalia associated with Tourette's syndrome. *Movement Disorders, 11,* 431–433.

Serrien, D. J., Nirkko, A. D., Loher, T. J., Lovblad, K. O., Burgunder, J. M., & Wiesendanger, M. (2002). Movement control of manipulative tasks in patients with Gilles de la Tourette syndrome. *Brain, 125,* 290–300.

Shapiro, A., & Shapiro, E. (1982). Tardive dyskinesia and chronic neuroleptic treatment of Tourette patients. *Advances in Neurology, 35,* 413.

Sheppard, D. M., Bradshaw, J. L., Georgiou, N., Bradshaw, J. A., & Lee, P. (2000). Movement sequencing in children with Tourette syndrome and attention deficit hyperactivity disorder. *Movement Disorders, 15,* 1184–1193.

Siesling, S., Vegter-van der Vlis, M., & Roos, R. A. C. (1997). Juvenile Huntington disease in the Netherlands. *Pediatric Neurology, 17,* 37–43.

Singer, H. S. (1994). Neurobiological issues in Tourette syndrome. *Brain Development, 16,* 353–364.

Singer, H. S., Hahn, I. H., & Moran, T. H. (1991). Abnormal dopamine uptake sited in postmortem striatum from patients with Tourette's syndrome. *Annals of Neurology, 30,* 558–562.

Snider, L. A., & Swedo, S. E. (2003). Post-streptococcal autoimmune disorders of the central nervous system. *Current Opinion in Neurology, 16,* 359–365.

Swedo, S. E. (1994). Sydenham's chorea: A model for childhood autoimmune neuropsychiatric disorders. *Journal of the American Medical Association, 272,* 1788–1791.

Swedo, S. E., Leonard, H. L., Garvey, M., Mittleman, B., Allen, A. J., Perlmutter, S., et al. (1998). Pediatric autoimmune neuropsychiatric disorders associated with streptococcal infections: Clinical description of the first 50 cases. *American Journal of Psychiatry, 155,* 264–271.

Swedo, S. E., Leonard, H. L., Mittleman, B. B., Allen, A. J., Rapoport, J. L., Dow, S. P., et al. (1997). Identification of children with pediatric autoimmune neuropsychiatric disorders associated with streptococcal infections by a marker associated with rheumatic fever. *American Journal of Psychiatry, 154,* 110–112.

Veasy, L. G., Widemeier, S. E., Orsmond, G. S., Rhuttenberg, H. D., Boucek, M. M., Roth, S. J., et al. (1987). Resurgence of acute rheumatic fever in the intermountain area of the United States. *New England Journal of Medicine, 316,* 421–427.

Vonsattel, J. P. (2000). Neuropathology of Huntington's disease. *NeuroScience News, 3,* 45–53.

Wolff, G. (1988). Huntington disease carrier status and the problems involved for those affected: A psychotherapeutic experience. *Clinical Genetics, 34,* 172–175.

Yeates, K. O., & Bornstein, R. A. (1994). Attention deficit disorder and neuropsychological functioning in children with Tourette's syndrome. *Neuropsychology, 8,* 65–74.

CHAPTER 10

Balance and Postural Control across the Lifespan

HARRIET G. WILLIAMS
LAURA HO

The ability to regulate and maintain balance is often taken for granted; however, it provides the primary foundation for mobility, for use of the upper extremities, and for maintaining overall functional independence throughout life. The development of balance/postural control is a significant part of early development and changes in the capacity to maintain balance are a critical factor associated with aging and loss of functional ability. Children with poor balance/postural control often have difficulty with acquisition of both gross and fine motor skills and frequently show deficits in a variety of visuomotor or eye–hand coordination behaviors. Balance functions are also of concern to the aging individual; nearly one-third or more of elderly individuals 65+ fall each year. Frail elderly fall even more frequently and suffer serious injuries and hospitalizations as a result. For all ages, lack of appropriate control of balance and posture can have negative effects on both mental and physical health; these effects are manifested in a variety of ways and include loss of confidence in ability to perform physical tasks, loss of independence, withdrawal from social activities, and diminished self-image and self-esteem. The health care costs of falls and loss of independence for the elderly alone are estimated to reach some $132 billion by 2030. Add to this the increasingly greater health care costs of providing services to young children with a variety of developmental needs, and it is clear that it is important to understand the nature of balance/postural control, how it develops and declines, and what factors contribute to the development and maintenance of effective control of balance.

WHAT IS BALANCE?

Balance can be defined simply as the ability to maintain the center of gravity over the base of support (e.g., Nashner, 1997). The center of gravity in humans is located in the pelvic region; the exact location of the center of gravity at any given point in time is dependent on the position of the body (head, arms, legs, etc.). The base of support de-

fines the limits of stability and the limits of stability define the area within which the
center of gravity must be maintained to avoid disequilibrium, instability, or a fall (generally this is 12½ degrees in anterior–posterior and 16 degrees in medial–lateral directions).

   Balance is also frequently categorized as static or dynamic; static balance refers to
the ability to maintain the center of gravity over the base of support during quiet
standing or sitting (Woollacott & Tang, 1997). Dynamic balance is known as "moving balance" and involves maintaining balance when the center of gravity and base of
support are moving (as in reaching up for an object) or when the center of gravity is
moving outside the base of support (as in walking up a flight of steps). The processes
involved in maintaining balance are anticipatory, reactive, or a combination of the two
(e.g., Cordo & Nashner, 1982; Haas, Diener, Rapp & Dichgans, 1989; Inglin &
Woollacott, 1988; Nashner, 1977). Reactive control of balance occurs when perturbations or events that contribute to instability (e.g., a slip, push, or trip) are unexpected;
anticipatory control of balance occurs when instability is expected or can be predicted
and thereby is planned for (e.g., getting into or out of a car and walking down a flight
of stairs). Optimal balance functioning requires both effective reactive and anticipatory control applied appropriately to the demands made on the individual as he or she
is attempting to maintain stationary balance or stay in control while moving.

THE BALANCE/POSTURAL CONTROL SYSTEM

The current view of balance control is based on systems models (e.g., Shumway-Cook
& Woollacott, 2001; Woollacott & Shumway-Cook, 1990). This perspective of balance describes the body as a mechanical system with mass, which is subject to external
(e.g., gravity and inertia) and internal forces (e.g., muscular contraction). Balance is
also a multidimensional process, which involves the interaction and function of a number of physiological systems; these include among others, the peripheral nervous system (PNS) and central nervous system (CNS), the muscular system (e.g., strength and
muscular endurance), the skeletal system (joint range of motion, flexibility, bone
strength, etc.), and the visual, proprioceptive, and vestibular systems (e.g., Yim-Chiplis
& Talbot, 2000).

   The CNS is integral to maintenance of balance and postural control through its
systematic monitoring and integration of information from the three major sensory
systems and through organizing the appropriate motor output to activate the corrective responses needed to maintain balance. The former is referred to as sensory organization of posture/balance, the latter as the motor coordination component of posture/
balance.

   Input from the three primary sensory systems involved in balance/postural control
normally provide redundant information about the state of equilibrium of the body
and indicate whether or not a corrective response is needed and what the nature of
that response should be. The relative importance of different sources of sensory information to maintenance of balance appears to differ with age and the context in which
the perturbation to balance occurs. For example, young children who are just learning
to stand are more reliant on vision than are older children who have had considerable
experience in walking (e.g., Woollacott & Shumway-Cook, 1990). In contrast, regardless of age, when a person is standing on a narrow surface (e.g., a balance beam) and

balance becomes unstable, input from the ankle proprioceptors is more critical than vision to restoration of balance (Nashner, 1997). An individual's capacity for effective balance also depends on a number of other factors, such as attention, previous experience, use of medications, state of mind, and fatigue.

MOTOR COORDINATION ASPECTS OF POSTURE AND BALANCE CONTROL: AN OVERVIEW

The term *motor coordination* refers to the timing and sequence of activation of appropriate postural responses to correct for perturbations to balance. Motor coordination dimensions of postural/balance control provide information about the integrity of spinal and CNS functioning, as well as information important in interpreting sensory organization aspects of posture/balance. The timing, sequence, and control of postural responses represents the postural control system's plan of action for addressing instability, adapting to it, and bringing the body back into balance. Postural synergies are one form of response organized by the CNS to adjust to instability of the body. In general, evidence indicates that healthy, young individuals (children and adults) respond to external perturbations to balance by activating stereotyped muscle responses known as postural synergies. These responses involve activation of leg and trunk muscles and are specific to the direction of the induced sway. Muscles on the anterior surface of the body respond to posterior sway; muscles on the posterior surface to anterior sway. The most commonly studied postural synergy is the "ankle strategy" where responses are generally activated first in the stretched ankle muscles and radiate upward from the base of support in a distal–proximal sequence. Thus, in response to platform movement creating anterior sway, the stretched gastrocnemius muscle is activated first, followed by the hamstrings and then paraspinal muscles. Postural synergies are present in children as young as 15 months, undergo dramatic change from 4 to 6 years, and are generally adult-like by 7 to 10 years of age. Head control, head–trunk coordination, and development of anticipatory postural adjustments continue to develop to 8 years and beyond (see Nashner, 1977; Shumway-Cook & Woollacott, 2001; Woollacott, Shumway-Cook, & Williams, 1989). There is general consensus that for adults and most children 7 years or older, the timing and sequence of postural synergies are as follows (e.g., Peterka & Black, 1990a, 1990b; Woollacott & Jensen, 1996):

- 100 millisecond (msec): Center of pressure (COP) moves; passive properties of body biomechanics.
- 110 msec: Distal muscle contracts.
- 130–140 msec: Proximal muscle contracts (e.g., 20–30 msec later).
- 130 msec: Active torque generation occurs.
- 230 msec: COP reaches peak displacement.
- 260 msec: Peak sway is reached and body returns to upright position.

Although the foregoing is rather universally observed in the body's response to counteracting sway, other factors can and do affect these synergistic responses to perturbations of balance. These include support surface conditions, initial body position, stimulus velocity (e.g., the speed with which the platform, for example, is moved), displacement amplitude (e.g., the distance that the platform is moved), and problems with the vestibular system and/or the inner ear mechanism, as well as availability and accuracy of visual and proprioceptive information.

SENSORY ORGANIZATION OF POSTURE/BALANCE CONTROL

Integral to the maintenance and control of posture and balance is the capacity to detect disturbances to stability (Assaiante & Amblard, 1995). Detection of perturbations to balance is primarily a function of the visual, proprioceptive, and vestibular systems. Under typical circumstances, all three sources are available and provide accurate and redundant information about the state of equilibrium. This information is integrated and synthesized at higher levels of the nervous system. The nature and importance of each source of sensory input for balance control have been examined through use of an experimental paradigm that involves systematic removal and/or modification of inputs from the three sensory systems. The typical paradigm requires the individual to stand on a measurement platform under several of the following sensory conditions (Shumway-Cook & Horak, 1986; Shumway-Cook & Woollacott, 1985): (1) all relevant sources of sensory input are available; (2) proprioceptive and vestibular inputs are available (eyes are closed); (3) vision and vestibular information is available (ankle proprioception is removed or diminished); (4) proprioceptive and vestibular inputs are available along with conflicting visual information (e.g., sensory conflict employing the moving room condition: the walls and ceiling move, the floor does not); (5) vestibular information alone is available (eyes are closed and ankle proprioception is controlled for or dampened); and (6) vestibular information is available along with erroneous visual information (sensory conflict is present and ankle proprioception is reduced or controlled for).

The effect of these different sensory conditions on posture/balance control is typically assessed through examination of the change in amplitude or extent of sway. The universal outcome of studies using this paradigm is that balance control is best when all three sources of sensory information are accurate and available (e.g., redundant sensory conditions). In addition, most studies indicate that while there is some increase in sway when vision is removed, significantly greater increases in sway are observed when either ankle proprioception is eliminated or when conflicting visual information is present. The most dramatic effect on posture/balance (e.g., sway) occurs when vestibular information and/or vestibular information coupled with erroneous visual information are the only sources available for detecting sway. Thus, balance control is most effective when all three sources of sensory input are present and accurate, but control of balance is still possible and reasonably effective when at least two of the three sources of sensory information are available and accurate (e.g., Shumway-Cook & Woollacott, 2001).

DEVELOPMENT OF POSTURE/BALANCE CONTROL

For a growing child, good balance is important to a variety of aspects of development including psychosocial interactions with peers, participation in games and sport activities, and self-esteem. Factors that affect optimal development of posture and balance control may have long-reaching effects that are not immediately obvious but appear much later in development

Sensory Issues

Sensory organization of balance responses in children typically has been examined using a "moving platform" paradigm. The individual stands on a measurement platform embedded in the floor; unexpectedly, the platform is moved forward or backward (or rotated, etc.). This creates a disturbance to balance similar to the start or stop of a bus (or other moving surface) on which the individual is standing. In these circumstances, accurate visual cues derived from sway caused by movement of the platform are available and can be used to assess the nature and extent of the disturbance to equilibrium. Data from studies (e.g., Butterworth & Hicks, 1977; Foster, Sveistrup, & Woollacott, 1996; Woollacott, Debu, & Mowatt, 1987) using this approach have shown that visual input has little or no effect on the timing of postural synergies (latencies: 90–120 msec) in young children (as young as 2 years with some experience in standing/walking) or adults (Sundermier, Woollacott, Jensen, & Moore, 1996; Woollacott et al., 1987).

What effect does vision have on postural synergies in infants younger than 2 years of age? Sundermier and Woollacott (1998) categorized children by developmental levels: (1) "pull to stand" (7–9 months old who could pull the body with some assistance to a standing position) and (2) "newly walking" (13 months old with 4–8 weeks of walking experience) and tested them with "eyes open" and "eyes closed" on a moving platform. They examined both the latency of onset of gastrocnemius muscle activity and integrated electromyography (EMG). Data indicated that vision had little or no effect on the speed with which postural responses were activated. This suggests that during development, vision may be more involved with activation of slower acting pathways integral to maintaining posture/balance (e.g., those with latencies greater than 200 msec).

Results of this same study indicated that there were developmental differences in the effects of vision on amplitude of muscle activity (integrated EMG). Vision had no measurable effect on the amplitude or force of postural responses in 7–9-month-olds; in contrast for "newly walking" children, the amplitude of activity in the gastrocnemius muscle was significantly greater with vision than without. These data suggest that vision may play an important role in behavioral transitions that involve new challenges to balance associated with, for example, learning to sit, stand, and/or walk independently. Once the child gains experience and has acquired some mastery of these behaviors, the effect of vision seems to be minimized (e.g., Butterworth & Hicks, 1977; Woollacott & Sveistrup, 1992, 1994). Since the elevated activity observed in the gastrocnemius in "new walkers" when vision was present was greater than was functionally necessary to maintain balance, it may be that vision, under certain circumstances, acts to amplify proprioceptive-mediated responses that are necessary to adapt to new and different perturbations to balance.

Visual information seems not to significantly affect the speed of automatic postural responses (latency = 90–100 msec) in children or adults; however, the sway of infants just learning to stand and/or walk is strongly affected by the presence of erroneous visual cues. Typically, conflicting visual cues are created through the paradigm known as the "moving room" phenomenon. This environment creates erroneous visual information about sway (e.g., with regard to whether or not sway is occurring and the direction of sway). The individual, young or old, typically sways in concert with the room as visual input from the moving room indicates that the body is sway-ing in the direction opposite to the actual direction of sway. Most children and espe-cially older adults show increased sway under these conditions. In addition, the magni-tude and direction of this sway actually leads to falls in many individuals. This suggests that the young postural control system is reliant on vision and finds it difficult to ignore or suppress visual information even when it is inaccurate and may lead to in-creased instability. Once the child has some experience in walking the magnitude of the sway response to conflicting visual cues declines; however, this sway response is still present in adults (e.g., Sundermier et al., 1996).

Thus, the development of postural control in children is characterized by changes in the contribution of different sensory systems to balance and by enhanced integrative processes (e.g., Butterworth & Hicks, 1977; Forssberg & Nashner, 1982). Clearly, al-though vision is an important source of sensory input for postural control in young children, by 4 to 6 years proprioceptive inputs gain influence and integrative processes begin to emerge. With continued growth and development, children also display an in-creasingly greater capacity to substitute one source of sensory information for an-other (e.g., proprioceptive input for vision) (Shumway-Cook & Woollacott, 1985; Woollacott, Shumway-Cook, & Nashner, 1986) and to resolve "sensory conflict" (e.g., to suppress erroneous information when appropriate). In general, however, most children require more than vestibular input to control balance effectively (Woollacott et al., 1986)

Motor Coordination Components

Although postural synergies are present in children as young as 15 months, they are not refined until 7–10 years of age. During this time, important changes occur in vari-ous aspects of motor coordination and/or postural synergies. Although the appropriate distal–proximal sequence of muscle activation is present in children 1–3 years of age, latencies of postural synergies are longer than those of adults but shorter than those of 4–6-year-olds. Postural responses in children 1–3 years of age are also of longer dura-tion and more stretch reflex responses are present than in older children. There is a dramatic period of change in postural responses from 4–6 years. Latency of onset of postural responses is significantly slower and more variable during this time. This change is important to keep in mind since reduction in response variability may reflect important changes in the development of the young nervous system. The sequence of activation of muscles is appropriate and reflex responses typically seen in younger chil-dren are no longer present. By 7–10 years of age, latencies of postural responses are comparable to those of adults and the variability seen in 4–6-year-olds has decreased. Duration of muscle activity is now also more proportional to the magnitude of the per-turbation to balance than was true earlier in development. All of these changes allow children to adapt to various threats to balance more effectively (see Shumway-Cook & Woollacott, 1985, 2001).

Sundermier, Woollacott, Roncesvalles, and Jensen (2001) also provide evidence that with increasing age *and/or* developmental level, the muscle activity involved in re-sponses to perturbation of balance increases and is better coordinated. The improved timing of muscle activity is accompanied by both increased peak torque at the ankle and hip and decreased time to restabilize or recover balance. Both developmentally and chronologically younger children display less synergistic muscle activity, undergo greater sway, and take longer to stabilize. Overall, motor development level appears to be a better predictor of motor coordination aspects of balance control than does chronological age.

Balance control improves and is more robust as mastery of locomotor skills and regulatory abilities improve. Roncesvalles, Woollacott, and Jensen (2001) classified children as new, intermediate, and advanced walkers, runners–jumpers, gallopers, hoppers, and skippers. Overall, children with more advanced locomotor skills (hoppers, skippers) adjusted to increasing threats to stability without stepping or losing balance more effectively than did children with less mastery. They had faster recovery times and relatively larger muscle torques. In addition, responses of children with greater locomotor mastery were nearly similar to those of adults.

Development of Gait/Locomotion

Development of locomotion is a multidimensional phenomenon that involves a number of physiological and biomechanical systems and subsystems. Optimum posture/balance control is a critical component in the appropriate development of gait and all the locomotor skills (see Breniere & Bril, 1998; Bril & Breniere, 1993; Massion, 1992; Roncesvalles et al., 2001; Thelen, Kelso, & Fogel, 1987; Thelen, Ulrich, & Jensen, 1989). Some aspects of gait/locomotion that change during development include (1) *relative gait velocity* (speed of gait/height; low in children with less than 5 months of independent walking, increases and remains constant from 15–21 months of walking, approaches adult values at 3 years of independent walking); (2) *relative step length* (step length/height: follows a positive nonlinear pattern characterized by a dramatic increase in step length in the initial 6–8 months of independent walking followed by progressive but moderate increases thereafter); and (3) *center of mass (CM) acceleration* (negative prior to 5 years of independent walking and positive after; vertical acceleration of the CM results from hip acceleration and leg muscle capacity to control stability at foot contact) (Breniere & Bril, 1998). Data from Breniere, Bril, and Fontaine (1989) suggest that there are four phases of postural control integral to the development of efficient locomotion/gait. Phase 1 occurs at the onset of independent walking (vertical acceleration of the CM is negative, the swing phase very short, and duration of the double stance phase very long). This is the behavioral manifestation, in part, of a deficit in the muscular capacity required to counteract the effects of gravity. Phase 2 includes the period from 1–5 months of independent walking typically described as a period of "walking by falling" (gait velocity increases, stripe/step length increases). Phase 3 usually occurs between 5 and 8 months of independent walking and is a reflection of the system's attempt to control the "fall" aspect of locomotion. Because muscle strength at joints involved in locomotion is not yet sufficient to fully modify this "walking by falling" pattern, gait continues to be somewhat problematic. Phase 4 represents 4+ years experience in independent walking. The pattern of locomotion in this phase is similar to that of adults; the system now exhibits increased capacity to counteract the force of gravity and the inertia induced by movement. There are also accompanying changes in arm position and/or action as control of gait increases. During early weeks when newly walking children move with a wide base of support, the arms are held in fixed postures at high guard. As balance control improves (the base of support narrows), arm movement and arm–foot opposition become incorporated into the gait pattern. Arm action thus plays the dual role of stabilizing the body and also contributing to forward movement (Ledebt, 2000). Shortly after the child walks, he or she begins to explore other modes of locomotion and run, jump, gallop, hop, and skip patterns appear and are mastered in that order.

POSTURAL/BALANCE CONTROL AND AGING

Postural sway is a natural phenomenon and generally not significant in young healthy adults. With increasing age, however, sway becomes more obvious and of greater concern (Baloh, Jacobson, Enrietto, Corona, & Honrubia, 1998; Ring, Nayak, & Isaacs, 1989; Sheldon, 1963). There is evidence that increased postural sway is associated with increased risk of falling and fractures in the elderly. Baloh and colleagues (1998) have shown that older adults who have poor balance sway significantly more than those with good balance. Fernie, Gryfe, Holliday, and Llewellyn (1982) also report data that point to postural sway as an important indicator of increased risk of falling among institutionalized elderly and Lord and colleagues (1994) provide similar data on community-dwelling elderly. Although postural sway increases with age, the most dramatic increases in amount of sway occur after age 60 (Sheldon, 1963). Baloh and colleagues (1998) also report that the sway velocity of older individuals is higher than that of younger adults.

WHEN BALANCE FAILS: FALLS AMONG THE ELDERLY

Falling is a health hazard for the older adult. One in three older adults fall each year and falls have become the sixth leading cause of death among the elderly population. Ten percent of falls result in injuries serious enough to require hospitalization. Falls are also a significant factor in 40% of admissions to nursing homes and to premature institutionalization. Age-specific data indicate that the occurrence of injuries and deaths caused by falls increases with age, with the greatest increases among the oldest age groups (Kannus et al., 1999). Falls and their consequences inevitably lead to increased health care costs (e.g., costs of hospitalization, nursing home care, and other health care services). Health care costs have also been shown to increase monotonically with the frequency and severity of falls (Lord et al., 1994; Rizzo et al., 1998). Understanding who is at risk for falling and identifying risk factors for falls are important issues for scientists whose focus is on the elderly. Discriminating characteristics of fallers include problems with vision (decreased visual acuity, contrast sensitivity), reduced proprioception (decreased toe position sense, decreased sharp–dull sensations, and poor vibration sense), lower extremity disability (foot problems, reduced lower limb strength, arthritis, and reduced ankle strength), impaired cognitive function, and polypharmacy and gait/balance abnormalities. Tinetti, Speechley, and Ginter (1988) concluded that most of the factors that predispose individuals for falls are associated with impaired neurological and musculoskeletal functions integral to stability.

Sorock and Labiner (1992) examined the relationship between lower extremity sensory and motor function and first falls in community-dwelling older adults and reported that if two or three risk factors were present, the rate of falling increased 3.9 times. Increased numbers of risk factors are also associated with increased probability of recurrent falls. Graafmans and colleagues (1996) examined fall risk factors and found that if five risk factors were present, there was an 84% chance that individuals would experience additional falls. Tinetti and Williams (1998) also reported a strong relationship between incidence of falls and declines in activities of daily living (ADL) functioning over a 1–3-year interval; greater declines in ADL functions were associated with increased numbers of falls. Repetitive fallers also experienced a decline in social functioning at both 1- and 3-year follow-ups.

Risk factors for falls may be different for men and women. Campbell and colleagues (1990) reported that decreased levels of physical activity, having had a stroke, developing arthritis in the knees, impaired gait, and increased body sway were associated with increased risk for falls in men. In contrast, for women, total number of medications, postural hypotension, and muscle weakness were factors significantly associated with increased risk of falling. Generally, women are more likely than men to fall in the home; men are more likely to fall outside the home often during participation in physical activity (Campbell et al., 1990).

Sensory Organization of Posture/Balance and Aging

Most available evidence suggests that the increase in sway and accompanying decline in balance among elderly individuals is largely a result of multiple deficits in a number of physiological systems (e.g., Sinclair & Nayak, 1990). More specifically, sensory systems responsible for providing information to the postural control system for maintenance of balance deteriorate with age, as do central processes that organize, analyze, and integrate sensory information integral to balance. Changes that occur in the sensory organization of postural control with age often can and do have a dramatic effect on maintenance of balance. Because important changes occur with age in visual, vestibular, and proprioceptive systems and integration of information from all of these systems is critical to maintenance of balance, it seems logical that deficits in any one sensory system can lead to postural instability (Borger, Whitney, Redfern, & Furman, 1999). Vision clearly is important in maintaining effective postural control throughout life. After age 65, however, individuals tend to rely more on vision for regulating balance than is true at younger ages (Lord & Ward, 1994). Elderly individuals with poor functional balance also tend to show an overreliance on visual cues for maintaining stability (Sundermier et al., 1996). Declines in vision with advancing age can and often do lead to impaired postural stability and increased risk for falls. For example, Lord and Menz (2000) reported that postural sway (during standing on a compliant surface) was related to visual functions such as contrast sensitivity and stereopsis. Simoneau, Leibowitz, Ulbrecht, Tyrrell, and Cavanah (1992) also found that reduced visual acuity was associated with greater postural sway in the elderly and Lord, Clark, and Webster (1991) reported that increased postural sway in older adults was related to both poor visual acuity and contrast sensitivity. Because these functions typically decline with age, these data point to an important connection between impaired vision and increased incidence of falls among older adults.

Proprioceptive Function

Proprioceptive and somatosensory functions undergo marked declines with age (Kaplan, Nixon, Reitz, Rindfleish, & Tucker, 1985; Skinner, Barrack, & Cook, 1984). Still, it is clear that proprioceptive input is an important source of sensory input in maintenance of stability at all ages (Lord & Ward, 1994; Lord et al., 1991). Colledge and colleagues (1994) assessed sway in four age groups (20–40, 40–60, 60–70, and 70+ years) using posturography and found that at all ages individuals were more dependent on proprioceptive input than vision in maintaining balance. Similarly, Judge, King, Whipple, Clive, and Wolfson (1996) examined the relative importance of visual (amount of sway with eyes closed) and proprioceptive inputs (amount of sway on a compliant surface) to stability; they reported that in the elderly the effect of reduced proprioceptive input on balance was four times greater than the effect of reduced vision. The decline in proprioceptive function with age and the importance of proprioceptive input in maintenance of stability at all ages puts the older individual at increased risk for loss of balance and potentially for falling.

Vestibular

While it is clear that vestibular information plays an integral role in maintenance of balance, the relationship between vestibular function and the maintenance of stability as a function of age is less clear. Impairment of vestibular function is often present in elderly individuals and data indicate that the elderly have greater difficulty than young adults do in maintaining balance under conditions in which vestibular information is the primary source of sensory input available for detecting changes in stability (Peterka & Benolken, 1995). Under these conditions older individuals are clearly less stable and more likely to fall. Still other evidence indicates that variations in vestibular function seen in older adults are not significantly related to increased sway (Lord et al., 1991).

Intersensory Integration

Intersensory functions also appear to decline with age; the older individual becomes more reliant on the availability of accurate and redundant sensory inputs (e.g., visual, proprioceptive, and vestibular) for balance control. Peterka and Black (1990b) assessed postural sway in individuals 7 to 81 years old under a number of different sensory conditions. Results indicated that when vision was absent or conflicting, older adults fell more frequently than did younger individuals. When both visual and proprioceptive inputs were diminished or conflicting, sway and the likelihood of falls increased significantly more in older than in younger adults. This was especially true for individuals 55 years and older. Judge and colleagues (1996) report similar results and showed that risk of loss of balance increased some fivefold when both visual and proprioceptive inputs were diminished and sevenfold when there was conflicting visual and diminished proprioceptive inputs. In addition, repeated exposure to reduced or conflicting sensory inputs did not improve the capacity of older individuals to adapt to such conditions.

Borger and colleagues (1999) examined the effect of the "moving room" phenomenon on postural control of healthy older adults. Compared to younger individuals, older adults were more dramatically affected (e.g., showed significantly greater increases in sway) when there was conflicting visual information from the "moving room." In addition, when diminished proprioceptive inputs were coupled with erroneous visual cues from the moving room, age differences in sway and falls were even more dramatic. Together, all the foregoing data suggest the following: (1) that to maintain balance effectively, older adults require clear and redundant sensory input from both visual and proprioceptive systems; and (2) that the capacity of the older person to regulate balance when vestibular input is the primary source of sensory information available is at best problematic.

Motor Coordination and Balance Control in the Elderly

To effectively maintain balance, an individual must detect perturbations to balance and then organize an appropriate response to correct for loss of balance. Important changes take place in the organization and execution of postural responses with age.

Postural Synergies and Aging

Postural responses (e.g., synergies) undergo a number of changes with age (Nardone, Siliotto, Grasso, & Schieppati, 1995; Woollacott & Shumway-Cook, 1990; Woollacott et al., 1986). First, the speed with which postural synergies are activated is slower and more variable in the elderly than in young adults. This is particularly true of the distal muscles of the lower leg and is most evident in the tibialis muscle and more dramatic in individuals 55+ years (Peterka & Black, 1990a; Whipple, Wolfson, Derby, Singh, & Tobin, 1993). The slowing of the tibialis response is believed to contribute significantly to diminished ability to regulate backward sway. Weeks (1994) also reported that the elderly are less consistent in temporal scaling of postural synergies. Overall, older adults require more time to detect postural disturbances and to initiate responses to instability produced by that disturbance.

The typical sequencing of activation of muscles is also disrupted more frequently in older individuals. For example, older adults frequently employ a hip strategy (muscles are activated in a proximodistal sequence) in responding to perturbations to balance when the ankle strategy (distoproximal activation of muscles) is more efficient (Manchester, Woollacott, Zederbauer-Hylton, & Marin, 1989; Stelmach, Phillips, DiFabio, & Teasdale, 1989; Woollacott & Shumway-Cook, 1990). Sundermeir and colleagues (1996) compared postural control of older adults with and without balance problems and reported that older adults with poorer balance tended to employ the hip strategy more often than those with better balance. Other evidence indicates that some 25–40% of older individuals display temporal reversals of activation of muscles involved in postural responses (e.g., the quadriceps muscle is activated prior to the tibialis) (Peterka & Black, 1990a; Woollacott et al., 1986). Together with the data on the slowing of postural responses, these findings point to a widespread breakdown in the timing of muscle activity in elderly individuals.

There is also evidence that the variability of the relative amplitude of muscle activity involved in postural synergies increases with age (Daubney & Culhmam, 1999; Quoniam, Hay, Roll, & Harlay, 1995; Woollacott & Shumway-Cook, 1990; Woollacott et al., 1986). In general, older adults tend to over- or underestimate the amplitude and velocity of the postural response needed to correct for perturbations to balance than do younger adults. Thus, the available data indicate that older adults are less able to accurately scale muscle activity to the nature of the postural disturbance. This makes them more vulnerable to falling and the potential negative health consequences.

Older adults also frequently contract agonist and antagonist muscles simultaneously to reduce sway and maintain stability (e.g., Woollacott & Shumway-Cook, 1990). That is, they exhibit co-contraction of postural muscles, a condition that results in stiffening of joints. It has been suggested that this co-contraction of postural muscles is a kind of protective mechanism and may be a way that older adults compensate for their inability to fine tune postural responses (Woollacott, Inglin, & Manchester 1988).

Central Integrative Processes, Balance, and Aging

Three levels of control have been hypothesized to contribute to the regulation of balance: the stretch reflex, long-latency (e.g., long loop) postural synergies, and higher levels of integration involved in synthesizing vestibular, visual, and somatosensory information (Stelmach, Teasdale, DiFabio, & Phillips, 1989). Generally, data indicate that stretch reflex responses are maintained with age, while higher-level, central integrative control of posture declines dramatically (Colledge et al., 1994; Quoniam et al., 1995; Stelmach, Phillips, et al., 1989). This decline in central integrative processing is best illustrated in the change observed with age in the delicate timing of postural and voluntary responses.

Older individuals generally exhibit poor timing of postural responses and voluntary movement (e.g., Stelmach, Teasdale, et al., 1989). In young individuals, the postural framework needed to support voluntary action is set quickly and in advance of the onset of the voluntary response (e.g., appropriate stability is established prior to reaching for an object on a high shelf). This relationship is often disrupted and is slower and less consistent in elderly individuals. This can and often does result in loss of balance, accidental falls, and other injuries.

GAIT AND MOBILITY

Normal gait depends on adequate functioning and integration among a number of physiological systems (e.g., nervous, muscular, skeletal, circulatory, and respiratory). Injury to or disease in one or more of these systems frequently leads to impairment of gait, reduced mobility, and decreased independence (Imms & Edholm, 1981). Disturbances of gait are prevalent in the elderly (Imms & Edholm 1981). Older individuals perform more poorly than do young adults on clinical measures of gait and mobility; specific gait parameters including velocity, cadence, stride length, and single-stance duration all show age-related changes (Himann, Cunningham, Rechnitzer, & Paterson, 1988; Lord, Lloyd, & Li, 1996; Okuzumi et al., 1995).

Himann and colleagues (1988) described the relationship between age and self-selected speeds of walking. Persons younger than 62 showed a 1–2% decline per decade in normal walking speed. After 63 years of age, there was a 12% (females) to

16% (males) decrease in walking speed per decade. In general, older females walked at significantly slower speeds, had shorter strides, and took more steps than older males.

There is also evidence that older persons who perform poorly on clinical tests of gait and mobility tend to be at increased risk of falling (Lord et al., 1996). Gait characteristics such as decreased arm swing, increased trunk sway, slow walking speed, unequal or asymmetrical stepping, and broad-based gait are also more common in individuals who have fallen than in those who have not (Lord et al., 1996). Lord and colleagues (1996) reported that individuals who had had multiple falls had reduced and more variable cadence and increased stance duration than nonfallers.

PHYSICAL ACTIVITY, BALANCE, AND GAIT IN THE ELDERLY

It has been suggested that the decline that occurs in balance and gait in the elderly is not an inevitable consequence of aging and is therefore treatable (Wolfson et al., 1992). Results of research focused on the effect of physical activity on balance and gait have shown that physical activity is beneficial to individuals who are undergoing declines in balance and gait and that regular participation in physical activity can diminish the risk of falls in the elderly (Brown & Holloszy, 1991, 1993). For example, individuals 61–70 years old who participated in an exercise program 1 hour a day, 5 days a week for 3 months showed significant improvement in strength, range of motion, standing balance, and ADL. All these are important factors in maintaining stability and preventing falls. There were no changes in gait parameters (Brown & Holloszy, 1991).

In a follow-up study, Brown and Holloszy (1993) examined the effects of a moderate intensity endurance training program on the same elderly individuals who had completed the previous 3-month exercise program. Participants trained for 45 minutes a day, 4 days a week for 1 year. The training consisted of walking, brisk walking, uphill treadmill walking, stationary cycling, and jogging. The frequency, duration, and intensity of training were increased based on improvement in individual $VO_{2_{max}}$ values. Both gait and balance performance parameters showed significant improvement (single-limb stance, step, and stride length, etc.). The authors suggest that fast walking and jogging challenged both balance and gait and thus resulted in improvements in both.

Shumway-Cook, Gruber, Baldwin, and Liao (1997) examined the effects of a multidimensional exercise program on balance, mobility, and risk for falls in community-dwelling older adults who had a history of falling. An individualized exercise program was designed to focus on specific impairments and functional disabilities of individual participants. Data indicated that those persons involved in the individualized exercise program showed improvement in both balance and mobility and had a significant reduction in fall risk. The authors point out that adherence to the program was a critical factor in whether or not improvements were realized. Individuals who fully adhered to the exercise protocol had the greatest improvements in balance and mobility while those with low adherence showed less change. Other data (e.g., Rubenstein et al., 2000) indicate that low-to-moderate-intensity exercise (3 days/week for 12 weeks) can produce significant improvement in balance, gait, and hip and ankle strength. Participants also reported overall improved physical functioning and fewer falls per unit of activity. Overall then, current science indicates that participation in regular and systematic physical activity can and does help to improve balance and mobility in the elderly.

ABNORMAL POSTURAL CONTROL

Abnormal posture and balance control may result from impairments in a number of underlying physiological systems. A wide array of developmental disabilities and/or disease conditions are also accompanied by a diverse set of abnormal characteristics associated with balance and postural control. Some of the most common conditions characterized by or associated with balance dysfunction are discussed in the next section.

Developmental Coordination Disorder

Developmental coordination disorder (DCD) is a relatively new diagnosis. Problems with motor coordination associated with DCD affect a minimum of 5–8% of children and are not uncommon in children with a diagnosis of learning disabilities, attention-deficit/hyperactivity disorder, or other developmental disabilities (see Ahonen, Kooistra, Viholainen, & Cantell, Chapter 12, this volume, for a detailed discussion of DCD, and Dewey, Crawford, Wilson, & Kaplan, Chapter 18, this volume, for a discussion of the association between motor problems and other developmental disorders). A feature of children diagnosed with DCD is poor balance/postural control. Many point to the poor balance of these children as the underlying factor in the pervasive and diverse incoordination that characterizes DCD (Williams & Castro, 1997; Williams & Woollacott, 1997). Sway patterns of children with DCD indicate that the integrity of the postural control system may be compromised. Wann, Mon-Williams, and Rushton (1998) studied children with and without DCD who stood on a force platform with eyes open and closed. They reported that children with DCD swayed significantly more than did control children (children with DCD swayed 7.37 cm; age-matched control children 3.5 cm; younger nursery school children 4.89; and adults 4.86 cm; the latter three groups were not different in sway amplitudes). When these same children balanced without vision, mean sway amplitude increased significantly for children with DCD; in contrast there was no change in sway amplitude for control children. Wann and colleagues also reported that children with DCD display a significantly higher peak sway frequency under moving room conditions, a significant proportion of which was outside the frequency band of the room motion. These authors concluded that children with DCD rely more on vision in maintaining balance than do age-matched or younger control children and thus are more vulnerable to disruption of balance by optical flow. Vestibular and proprioceptive systems are known to be integral to eliciting rapid adjustments to postural instability and sway. Because visual information may contribute more to slower postural adjustments (Nashner & Berthoz, 1978), it may be that the tendency of DCD children to rely visual information to regulate balance places them at a disadvantage in responding to disturbances that require rapid immediate corrections.

Williams and Woollacott (1997) examined postural synergies in children with DCD. Children stood with eyes open and feet shoulder-width apart on a force platform. The platform was moved to perturb balance in either a forward or a backward direction. Although the latency of postural responses under these circumstances was similar for both groups, children with DCD were significantly more variable in activating such responses. The presence of this variability in onset latency in younger and older children with DCD places them at a disadvantage in responding to instability that may not necessarily improve with growth and development (Williams & Woollacott, 1997). These authors also provide evidence that children with DCD are significantly different from control children in the sequence in which muscles are activated in responding to disturbances of balance. Control children consistently exhibited a distoproximal pattern of leg muscle activation, whereas children with DCD often responded with a less efficient proximodistal pattern of activation (17–28% of trials). Some two-thirds of young and one-third of older children with DCD displayed a proximodistal pattern of muscle activation on 40% or more of perturbation trials. Children with DCD also exhibited different patterns of trunk and neck muscle activation. These data suggest that the inconsistent timing and sequencing of muscle activity are major factors in the balance and control problems of children with DCD (Williams & Woollacott, 1997).

Other work (Williams & Castro, 1997) indicates that children with DCD produce more force in proximal (trunk and thigh) than distal leg muscles in responding to instability in an upright stance. This suggests that children with DCD may rely more on proximal than distal muscle control in regulating balance and because proximal muscle control generally represents a cruder, less refined level of motor control, children with DCD may be faced with additional challenges when finely graded force generation is required.

Cerebral Palsy

Children diagnosed with cerebral palsy (CP) exhibit a wide range of abnormalities in posture and balance control (Crenna, 1998). Burtner, Qualls, and Woollacott (1998) studied characteristics of balance control during stance in children with spastic CP and concluded that factors affecting balance and gait in these children are a reflection of both CNS and mechanical factors. For example, restricted range of motion at the ankle, knee, and hip often results in dysfunctional postural responses in children with CP as do abnormalities of muscle tone associated with upper motor neuron syndromes. There is also evidence that when children with "typical or normal" development stand in a crouched position (similar to that of children with CP) or walk in that position, EMG activity in postural muscles resembles that of children with spastic diplegia. The organization of muscle activity in the crouched position is characterized by increased incidence of both proximodistal activation of muscle activity and coactivation of agonist/antagonist muscles. These data suggest then that position or configuration of the body (e.g., biomechanical factors) can and does affect the nature of muscle activity involved in postural control.

Abnormal timing of muscle activity is universally observed in postural responses of children with CP and includes (1) spasticity or a velocity dependent increase in tonic stretch reflexes, (2) muscular weakness, (3) excessive coactivation of antagonist muscle, and (4) increased stiffness around joints. Other timing difficulties observed in these children are significant delays in onset of postural synergies, problems with appropriate sequencing of muscle activity, and inappropriate timing of postural muscle activity in anticipation of and preparation for voluntary movements (Nashner, Shumway-Cook, & Marin, 1983).

Developmentally, for children without CP, distoproximal activation of muscle activity in response to disturbance of stability occurs around the time the child independently pulls to a stand and is complete at onset of independent walking. In contrast, children with CP exhibit numerous reversals of muscle activation even at the stage of independent walking (especially in the spastic leg) and numerous monosynaptic stretch reflexes are also present. These timing difficulties along with the delay in postural responses dramatically reduce the likelihood that corrective responses to instability will be effective (Burtner et al., 1998). Interestingly, older children with CP display muscle activation patterns that more closely resemble those of much younger "normal" children; both have increased reversals and more coactivation of muscles. For example, one 7-year-old with CP was reported to exhibit muscular activity similar to that of a "typical" 10-month-old; both were at the level of pull to stand, stood independently momentarily but could not walk independently. Children with "normal" development also tend to activate agonist muscles with little or no activity in antagonists and involve trunk muscles in responding to instability. In contrast, children with CP tend to activate both agonist and antagonist muscles with little or no involvement of trunk muscles (Burtner et al., 1998). Individuals with athetoid CP also have difficulty timing agonist and antagonist activity (antagonist activity is often activated prior to or simultaneous with agonist activity). This frequently results in decreased or inappropriate scaling of amplitude of postural responses, the outcome of which is an underestimation of the extent of the instability and an inadequate corrective response. In other words, the force output does not match the amplitude of the perturbation (Shumway-Cook & Woollacott, 2001). Individuals with CP are also characterized by an inability to adapt postural responses to changes in balance conditions and thus frequently respond with limited and fixed response patterns (Nashner et al., 1983).

Lead Exposure

Bhattacharya, Shukla, Dietrich, Bornschein, and Berger (1995) suggest that the ability of the child to maintain upright balance provides a window for examining the functional status of the central and peripheral nervous systems. Bhattacharya, Shukla, Bornschein, Dietrich, and Keith (1990) and Bhattacharya and colleagues together provide evidence that points to a strong association between postnatal exposure to lead and poor balance and postural instability in young children. They reported that total amount of sway (eyes open) was smaller for children with lower levels of lead exposure. Without vision, there was an even clearer dose–response relationship between sway area and level of lead exposure. Specifically, with greater levels of lead exposure, the center of pressure tended to move closer to the edges of the base of support resulting in greater instability on the part of the child.

When children's balance control was examined under conditions where vision was absent, proprioceptive input was dampened or there was a combination of the two, sway increased significantly. This suggests that as balance conditions became more demanding and there was a greater reliance on higher centers of the nervous system for integration of sensory information and control of balance, the effect of lead exposure was even more dramatic. The extreme increase in sway under conditions where proprioceptive input was dampened and/or vestibular information was the primary source of input for regulation of balance implies that lead exposure potentially may lead to functional impairment of these sensory systems. Shukla, Bhattacharya, Dietrich, and Bornschein (1991) have also shown that proprioceptive function is negatively affected by lead exposure.

Chronic Otitis Media

Otitis media is one of the most common diseases of infancy and early childhood. Many children develop recurrent and/or persistent otitis media; there is some suggestion that children with persistent inner-ear infections are at risk for vestibular, balance, and/or motor dysfunction (Casselbrandt et al., 2000; Hart, Nichols, Butler, & Barin, 1998; Orlin, Effgen, & Handler, 1997). Otitis media with effusion (OME) has been shown to affect the amount of postural sway (determined by dynamic posturography) (Casselbrant, Furman, Rubenstein, & Mandel, 1995). Children with OME display significantly greater sway and a higher sway velocity than do other children. The basis for this increased sway is not clear but could be a manifestation of impairment of the peripheral vestibular system (e.g., due to effects of toxic substances on or transmission of pressure to the labyrinth) (Golz, Angel-Yerger, & Parush, 1998). Integrity of the vestibular apparatus is considered to be integral to optimal motor development; infants with a hypoactive labyrinth are delayed in standing/walking and abnormalities of semicircular canals found in some children are also associated with delayed motor development (Crowe & Horak, 1988).

It may be that children with vestibular dysfunction (especially as a result of OME) are increasingly more dependent on visual and proprioceptive inputs for balance control in part because these senses provide more reliable inputs about posture/balance. Children with OME are in fact more sensitive to and affected by erroneous optical flow of the visual field than other children. They display significantly greater sway and are more variable than do "normal" children under these conditions (Casselbrandt, Redfern, Fall, Furman, & Mandel, 1998). This is especially true for higher-frequency visual stimulus conditions. We also know that children under 7 years and patients with vestibular impairments have difficulty adapting to conflicting sensory conditions (Jacob, Redfern, & Furman, 1995; Redfern & Furman, 1994). Older children with congenital and acquired vestibular deficits also have difficulty with balance when resolution of conflicting sensory information is involved (Golz et al., 1998). Thus, children with OME appear to show a heightened sensitivity to conflicting sensory input that resembles that of individuals with vestibular deficits who also tend to rely heavily on vision for stability.

Parkinson's Disease

Parkinson's disease is a slow, progressive disorder that results from degeneration of dopamine-producing cells in the brain. Symptoms of Parkinson's disease include limb tremor, stiffness and rigidity of muscles, slowness of movement (especially gait), and impaired balance. Mitchell, Collins, Deluca, Burrows, and Lipsitz (1995) also report that individuals with Parkinson's disease have slower gait speeds, smaller functional reach, higher scores on the Geriatric Depression Scale, and more reported falls over the past year. Parkinson's disease affects more than 500,000 people in the United States; most of these are over 50 years old. The average age of onset is 60 years; the incidence and prevalence of the disease increase dramatically in the 70s and 80s.

The effect of Parkinson's disease on balance has been examined in a number of studies. For example, Horak, Nutt, and Nashner (1992) studied selected characteristics of postural control in individuals with Parkinson's disease. Data indicated that total sway area for individuals with Parkinson's was significantly smaller than that for healthy older adults (it was not different from that of young adults). To counteract forward sway, individuals with Parkinson's exhibited a reversal of the typical sequence of activation of muscles (proximal muscles were activated prior to distal muscles), simultaneously activated trunk muscles, and coactivated quadriceps and hamstring muscles. To counteract backward sway, individuals with Parkinson's again displayed a proximal to distal sequence of muscle activation (paraspinal muscles were activated before hamstrings), reciprocal activation of paraspinal and abdominal muscles, and coactivation of hamstring and quadriceps muscles. These all reflect excessive antagonist activity. In addition, individuals with Parkinson's responded with less torque (force) than young adults and had a significantly slower rate of sway. When these Parkinson's patients were faced with dramatic changes in the support surface (e.g., horizontal displacement of a narrow beam on which they were standing), they were unable to modify postural responses appropriately and lost balance. Instead of adopting a hip strategy more appropriate to standing on a narrow surface, Parkinson's patients tended to employ a less effective ankle strategy with widespread coactivation of agonists and antagonists. The investigators concluded that postural instability observed in individuals with Parkinson's is not necessarily a result of either the inability to use sensory information or a delay in muscle response latencies. Rather, they suggest that poor balance control is more likely to be due to abnormal motor planning along with difficulty in executing appropriate sequencing of muscle activity and an inability to modify postural response patterns. Another factor that may affect postural control in Parkinson's patients is that of greater use of antidepressants to cope with depression (Mitchell et al., 1995). Antidepressants are known to have a negative effect on postural control mechanisms.

Data on displacement of the center of pressure (COP) of individuals with Parkinson's indicates that the COP tends to drift a greater distance in the medial–lateral direction than is true for the healthy elderly (Mitchell et al., 1995). In contrast, there is no difference in COP displacement between individuals with Parkinson's disease and healthy older adults in the anterior–posterior direction. The predominance of medial–lateral activity may be a strategy that individuals with Parkinson's adopt to help counteract the effect of restricted movement in the anterior–posterior plane.

Chong, Jones, and Horak (1999) examined the adaptation of leg muscle activity of Parkinson's patients in response to changes in support conditions. Leg muscle activity was evaluated under free stance, in supported stance, in a standing passive-toes-up condition (the platform surface was rotated), and in a voluntary rise to toes. Compared to healthy older adults, individuals with Parkinson's disease often failed to reduce activity in the tibialis muscle as would be expected when stance is supported.

Reductions of tibialis activity when it occurred were much slower in Parkinson's patients than in healthy adults; this was true both when stance was supported and during voluntary toe raises. A similar effect was also seen in soleus muscle activity. Thus, individuals with Parkinson's have difficulty in modifying postural responses to changes in support conditions. This lack of ability to adapt muscle activity occurred in all support conditions and suggests that the deficit is a general rather than a specific task dependent problem.

Peripheral Neuropathy

Van den Bosch, Gilsing, Lee, Richardson, and Aston-Miller (1995) studied the effect of peripheral neuropathy on sensitivity to ankle joint proprioception, an important source of information for optimum balance control. Results indicated that individuals with peripheral neuropathy had significantly higher thresholds for detecting movement at the ankle joint. Healthy older adults detected a 0.17-degree change in ankle-joint position with 75% accuracy; individuals with peripheral neuropathy detected ankle-joint movement only after a change of 1.74 degrees. When individuals with peripheral neuropathy stood with the feet inverted, the ankle-joint threshold was 6 times greater than that of healthy elderly; with the feet turned outward, the threshold was 6.6 times greater than that of healthy older adults. Clinical examination of toe position sense indicated that this threshold was also significantly higher for individuals with peripheral neuropathy. There was no difference in vibration thresholds. Given the diminished perception of ankle-joint movement and great toe position sense, this suggests the presence of a deficit in proprioceptive input from the feet and ankle joints, a condition that could have a serious destabilizing effect on stability (Richardson & Hurvitz, 1995).

SUMMARY AND CONCLUSION

The development of balance/postural control is a significant part of early development and changes in the capacity to maintain balance are critical factors associated with aging and loss of functional ability. Research has also found that a diverse set of abnormal characteristics associated with balance and postural control are characteristic of a number of developmental disabilities/disease conditions and adult disease conditions. Thus, balance and postural control are essential to motor functioning of children and adults

REFERENCES

Assaiante, C., & Amblard, B. (1995). An ontogenetic model for the sensori-motor organization of balance control in humans. *Human Movement Science, 14,* 13–43.

Baloh, R. W., Jacobson, K. M., Enrietto, J. A., Corona. S., & Honrubia, V. (1998). Balance disorders in older persons: Quantification with posturography. *Otolaryngology—Head and Neck Surgery, 119,* 89–92.

Bhattacharya, A., Shukla, R., Bornschein, R., Dietrich, K., & Keith, R. (1990). Lead effects on postural balance of children. *Environmental Health Perspectives, 89,* 35–42.

Bhattacharya, A., Shukla, R., Dietrich, K., Bornschein, R., & Berger, O. (1995). Effect of early lead exposure on children's postural balance. *Developmental Medicine and Child Neurology, 37,* 861–878.

Borger, L. L., Whitney, S. L., Redfern, M. S., & Furman, J. M. (1999). The influence of dynamic visual environments on postural sway in the elderly. *Journal of Vestibular Research, 9,* 197–205.

Breniere, Y., & Bril, B. (1998). Development of postural control of gravity forces in children during the first five years of walking. *Experimental Biological Research, 121,* 255–262.

Breniere Y., Bril, B., & Fontaine, R. (1989). Analysis of the transition from upright stance to steady state locomotion in children under 200 days of autonomous walking. *Journal of Motor Behavior, 21,* 20–37.

Bril, B., & Breniere, Y. (1993). Posture and independent locomotion in childhood: learning to walk or learning dynamic postural control? In G. Savelsbergh (Ed.), *The development of coordination in infancy* (pp. 337–358). Amsterdam: North-Holland.

Brogren, E., Hadders-Algra, M., & Forssberg, H. (1998). Postural control in sitting children with cerebral palsy. *Neuroscience and Biobehavioral Reviews, 22,* 591–596.

Brown, M., & Holloszy, J. O. (1991). Effects of a low intensity exercise program on selected physical performance characteristics of 60- to 71- year olds. *Aging, 3,* 129–139.

Brown, M., & Holloszy, J. O. (1993). Effects of walking, jogging and cycling on strength, flexibility, speed and balance in 60- to 72-year olds. *Aging Clinical Experimental Research, 5,* 427–434.

Burtner, P., Qualls, C., & Woollacott, M. (1998). Muscle activation characteristics of stance balance control in children with spastic cerebral palsy. *Gait and Posture, 8,* 163–174.

Butterworth, G., & Hicks, L. (1977). Visual proprioception and postural stability in infancy: a developmental study. *Perception, 6,* 255–262.

Campbell, A. J., Borrie, M. J., Spears, G. F, Jackson, S. L, Brown, J. S., & Fitzgerald, J. L (1990). Circumstances and consequences of falls experienced by a community population 70 years and over during a prospective study. *Age and Aging, 19,* 136–131.

Casselbrant, M., Furman, J., Mandel, E., Fall, P., Jurs-Lasky, M., & Rockette, H. (2000). Past history of otitis media and balance in four year old children. *Laryngoscope, 110,* 773–778.

Casselbrant, M., Furman, J., Rubenstein, E., & Mandel, E. (1995). Effect of otitis media on the vestibular system in children. *Annals of Otology, Rhinology, and Laryngology, 104,* 620–624.

Casselbrandt, M., Redfern, M., Fall, P., Furman, J., & Mandel, E. (1998). Visual-induced postural sway in children with and without otitis media. *Annals of Otology, Rhinology, and Laryngology, 107,* 401–405.

Chong, R. K., Jones, C. L., & Horak, F. B. (1999). Postural set for balance control in Alzheimer's but not in Parkinson's disease. *Journal of Gerontology, 54,* M129–135.

Colledge, N. R., Cantley, P., Peaston, I., Brash, H., Lewis, S., & Wilson, J. A. (1994). Ageing and balance: The measurement of spontaneous sway by posturography. *Gerontology, 40,* 273–278.

Cordo, P., & Nashner, L. (1982). Properties of postural adjustments associated with rapid arm movements. *Journal of Neurophysiology, 47,* 287–302.

Crenna, P. (1998). Spasticity and "spastic" gait in children with cerebral palsy. *Neuroscience and Biobehavioral Reviews, 22,* 571–578.

Crowe, T., & Horak, F. (1988). Motor proficiency associated with vestibular deficits in children with hearing impairments. *Physical Therapy, 68,* 1493–1499.

Daubney, M. E., & Culhmam, E. G. (1999). Lower-extremity muscle force and balance performance in adults aged 65 years and older. *Physical Therapy, 79,* 1177–1185.

Fernie, G. R., Gryfe, C. I., Holliday, P. J., & Llewellyn, A. (1982). The relationship of postural sway in standing to the incidence of falls in geriatric subjects. *Age and Aging, 11,* 11–16.

Forssberg, H., & Nashner, L. (1982). Ontogenetic development of postural control in man: Adaptation to altered support and visual conditions during stance. *Journal of Neuroscience, 2*, 545–552.

Foster, E., Sveistrup, H., & Woollacott, M. (1996). Transitions in visual proprioception: A cross-sectional developmental study of the effect of visual flow on postural control. *Journal of Motor Behavior, 28*, 101–112.

Golz, A., Angel-Yerger, B., & Parush, S. (1998). Evalution of balance disturbances in children with middle ear effusion. *International Journal of Pediatric Otorhinolaryngology, 43l*, 21–26.

Graafmans, W. C., Ooms, M. E., Hofstee, H. M., Bezemer, P. D., Bouter, L. M., & Lips, P. (1996). Falls in the elderly: A prospective study of risk factors and risk profiles. *American Journal of Epidemiology, 143*, 1129–1136.

Haas, G., Diener, H., Rapp, H., & Dichgans, J. (1989). Development of feedback and feedforward control of upright stance. *Developmental Medicine and Child Neurology, 31*, 481–488.

Hart, M., Nichols, D., Butler, E., & Barin, K. (1998). Childhood imbalance and chronic otitis media with effusion: Effect of tympanostomy tube insertion on standardized tests of balance and locomotion. *Laryngoscope, 198*, 665–670.

Himann, J. E., Cunningham, D. A., Rechnitzer, P. A., & Paterson, D. H. (1988). Age-related changes in speed of walking. *Medicine and Science in Sports and Exercise, 20*, 161–166.

Horak, F. B., Nutt, J. G., & Nashner, L. M. (1992). Postural inflexibility in parkinsonian subjects. *Journal of Neurological Science, 111*, 46–58.

Imms, F. J., & Edholm, O. G. (1981). Studies of gait and mobility in the elderly. *Age and Aging, 10*, 147–156.

Inglin, B., & Woollacott, M. (1988). Age-related changes in anticipatory postural adjustments associated with arm movements. *Journal Gerontology, 43*, M105–M113.

Jacob, R., Redfern, M., & Furman, J. (1995). Optic flow-induced sway in anxiety disorders associated with space and motion discomfort. *Journal of Anxiety Disorders, 9*, 411–425.

Judge, J. O., King, M. B., Whipple, R., Clive, J., & Wolfson, L. I. (1996). Dynamic balance in older persons: Effects of reduced visual and proprioceptive input. *Journal of Gerontology, 50*, M263–70.

Kannus, P., Parkkari, J., Koskinen, S., Niemi, S., Palvanen, M., Jarvinen, M., et al. (1999). Fall-induced injuries and deaths among older adults. *Journal of the American Medical Association, 281*, 1895–1899.

Kaplan, F. S., Nixon, J. E., Reitz, M., Rindfleish, L., & Tucker, J. (1985). Age-related changes in proprioception and sensation of joint position. *Acta Orhopedia Scandinavia, 56*, 72–74.

Ledebt, A. (2000). Changes in arm posture during the early acquisition of walking. *Infant Behavior and Development, 231*, 79–89.

Lord, S. R., Clark, R. D., & Webster, I. W. (1991). Physiological factors associated with falls in an elderly population. *Journal of the American Geriatrics Society, 39*, 1194–1200.

Lord, S. R., Lloyd, D. G., & Li, S. K. (1996). Sensori-motor function, gait patterns and falls in community-dwelling women. *Age and Aging, 25*, 292–299.

Lord, S. R., & Menz, H. B. (2000). Visual contributions to postural stability in older adults. *Gerontology, 46*, 306–310.

Lord, S. R., Sambrook, P. N., Gilbert, C., Kelly, P. J., Ngyun, T., Webster, I. W., et al. (1994). Postural stability falls and fractures in the elderly: Results from the Dubbo Osteoporosis Epidemiology Study. *Medical Journal of Australia, 160*, 684–691.

Lord, S. R., & Ward , J. A. (1994) . Age-associated differences in sensoi-motor function and balance in community dwelling women. *Age and Aging, 23*, 452–460.

Manchester, D., Woollacott, M., Zederbauer-Hylton, N., & Marin, O. (1989). Visual, vestibular and somatosensory contributions to balance control in the older adult. *Journal of Gerontology, 44*, M118–M127.

Massion, J. (1992). Movement, posture and equilibrium: Interaction and coordination. *Progress in Neurobiology, 38*, 35–56.

Mitchell, S. L, Collins, J. J., DeLuca, C. J., Burrows, A., & Lipsitz, L.A. (1995). Open-loop and closed-loop postural control mechanisms in Parkinson's disease: Increased mediolateral activity during quiet standing. *Neuroscience Letters, 97*, 133–136.

Nardone, A., Siliotto, R., Grasso, M., & Schieppati, M. (1995). Influences of aging on leg muscle reflex response to stance perturbation. *Archives of Physical Medicine and Rehabilitation, 76*, 158–165.

Nashner, L. (1977). Fixed patterns of rapid postural responses among leg muscles during stance. *Experimental Brain Research, 30*, 13–24.

Nashner, L. (1997). Practical biomechanics and physiology of balance. In G. Jacobson, C. Newman, & J. Kartush (Eds.), *Handbook of balance function testing* (pp. 261–279). San Diego, CA: Singular.

Nashner, L., & Berthoz, A. (1978). Visual contribution to rapid motor responses during postural control. *Brain Research, 150*, 403–407.

Nashner, L., Shumway-Cook, A., & Marin, O. (1983). Stance posture control in select groups of children with cerebral palsy: Deficits in sensory organization and muscular coordination. *Experimental Brain Research, 49*, 393–409.

Okuzumi, H., Tanaka, A., Haishi, K., Meguro, K. I., Yamazaki, H., & Nakamura, T. (1995). Age-related changes in postural control and locomotion. *Perceptual Motor Skills, 81*, 991–994.

Orlin, M., Effgen, S., & Handler, S. (1997). Effect of otitis media with effusion on gross motor ability in preschool-aged children: Preliminary findings. *Pediatrics, 99*, 334–337.

Peterka, R., & Benolken, M. (1995). Role of somatosensory and vestibular cues in attenuating visually induced human postural sway. *Experimental Brain Research, 105*, 101–110.

Peterka, R. J., & Black, F. O. (1990a). Age-related changes in human posture control: Motor coordination tests. *Journal of Vestibular Research, 1*, 87–96.

Peterka, R. J., & Black, F. O. (1990b). Age-related changes in human posture control: Sensory organization tests. *Journal of Vestibular Research, 1*, 73–85.

Quoniam, C., Hay, L., Roll, J. P., & Harlay, F. (1995). Age effects on reflex and postural responses to propriomuscular inputs generated by tendon vibration. *Journal of Gerontology, 50*, B155–B165.

Redfern, M., & Furman, J. (1994). Postrual sway in response to optic flow stimuli in vestibular patients. *Journal of Vestibular Research, 4*, 221–230.

Richardson, J. K., & Hurvitz, E. A. (1995). Peripheral neuropathy: A true risk factor for falls. *Journal of Gerontology, 50*, M211–M215.

Ring, C., Nayak, U. S., & Issacs, B. (1989). The effect of visual deprivation and proprioceptive changes on postural sway in healthy adults. *Journal of the American Geriatrics Society, 37*, 745–749.

Rizzo, J. A., Fiedkin, R., Williams, C. S., Nabors, J., Acampora, D., & Tenetti, M. E. (1998). Health care utilization and costs in Medicare population by fall status. *Medical Care, 36*, 1174–1188.

Roncesvalles, M., Woollacott, M., & Jensen, J. (2001). Development of lower extremity kinetics for balance control in infants and young children. *Journal of Motor Behavior, 33*, 189–192.

Rubenstein, L. Z., Josephson, K. R., Trueblood, P. R., Loy, S., Harker, J. O., Pietruszka, F. M., et al. (2000). Effects of a group exercise program on strength, mobility and falls among fall-prone elderly men. *Journal of Gerontology, 55A*, M317–M321.

Sheldon, J. H. (1963). The effect of age on the control of sway. *Gerontology Clinician, 5*, 129–138.

Shukla, R., Bhattacharya, A., Dietrich, K., & Bornschein, R. (1991). Effects of lead exposure on postural control pathways: An exploratory factor analysis. In J. G. Farmer (Ed.), *Proceedings of the 8th International Conference on Heavy Metals in the Environment* (pp. 16–20).

Shumway-Cook, A., Gruber, W., Baldwin, M., & Liao, S. (1997). The effect of multidimensional exercises on balance, mobility and fall risk in community-dwelling older adults. *Physical Therapy, 1,* 46–57.

Shumway-Cook, A., & Horak, F. (1986). Assessing influence of sensory interaction on balance. *Physical Therapy, 66,* 1548–1550.

Shumway-Cook, A., & Woollacott, M. (1985). The growth of stability: Postural control from a developmental perspective. *Journal of Motor Behavior, 17,* 131–147.

Shumway-Cook, A., & Woollacott, M. (2001). *Motor control: Theory and practical applications.* Philadelphia: Lippincott.

Simoneau, G. G., Leibowitz, H. W., Ulbrecht, J. S., Tyrell, R. A., & Cavanah, P. R. (1992). The effects of visual factors and head orientation on postural steadiness in women 55 to 70 years of age. *Journal of Gerontology, 47,* M151–M158.

Sinclair, A. J., & Nayak, U. S. L. (1990). Age-related changes in postural sway. *Comprehensive Therapy, 16U,* 44–48.

Skinner, H. B., Barrack, R. L., & Cook, S. D. (1984). Age-related decline in proprioception. *Clinical Orthopedics, 184,* 208–211.

Sorock, G. S., & Labiner, D. M. (1992). Peripheral neuromuscular dysfunction and falls in an elderly cohort. *American Journal Epidemiology, 136,* 584–591.

Stelmach, G. E., Phillips, J, DiFabio, R. P., & Teasdale, N. (1989). Age, functional postural reflexes, and voluntary sway. *Journal of Gerontology, 44,* B100–B106.

Stelmach, G. E., Teasdale, N., DiFabio, R. P., & Phillips, J. (1989). Age related decline in postural control mechanisms. *International Journal of Aging and Human Development, 29,* 205–223.

Sundermier, L., & Woollacott, M. (1998). The influence of vision on the automatic postural muscle responses of newly standing and newly walking infants. *Experimental Brain Research, 120,* 537–540.

Sundermier, L., Woollacott, M., Jensen, J., & Moore S. (1996). Postural sensitivity to visual flow in aging adults with and without balance problems. *Journal of Gerontology—Medical Sciences 51A,* m45–52.

Sundermier, L., Woollacott, M., Roncesvalles, N., & Jensen. J. (2001). The development of balance control in children: Comparisons of EMG and kinetic variables and chronological and developmental groupings. *Experimental Brain Research, 136,* 340–350.

Thelen, E., Kelso, J., & Fogel, A. (1987). Self-organizing systems and infant motor development. *Developmental Reviews, 7,* 39–65.

Thelen, E., Ulrich, B., & Jensen, J. (1989). The developmental origins of locomotion. In M. Woollacott & A. Shumway (Eds.), *Development of posture and gait across the lifespan* (pp. 25–47), Columbia: University of South Carolina Press.

Tinetti, M. E., Speechley, M., & Ginter, S. F. (1988). Risk factors for falls among elderly persons living in the community. *New England Journal of Medicine, 319,* 1701–1707.

Tinetti, M. E., & Williams, C. S. (1998). The effect of falls and fall injuries on functioning in community-dwelling older persons. *Journal of Gerontology, 53,* M112–M119.

Van den Bosch, C. G., Gilsing, M. G., Lee, S. G., Richardson, J. K., & Ashton-Miller, J. A. (1995). Peripheral neuropathy effect on ankle inversion and eversion detection thresholds. *Archives of Physical Medicine and Rehabilitation, 76,* 850–856.

Wann, J., Mon-Williams, M., & Rushton, K. (1998). Postural control and coordination disorders: The swinging room revisited. *Human Movement Science, 17,* 491–513.

Weeks, D. L. (1994). Age-related differences in temporal scaling of postural EMG activity. *Aging, 6,* 323–333.

Whipple, R., Wolfson, L., Derby, C., Singh, D., & Tobin, J. (1993). Altered sensory function and balance in older persons. *Journals of Gerontology, 48,* 71–76.

Williams, H., & Castro, A. (1997). Timing and force characteristics of muscle activity: Postural control in children with and without developmental coordination disorders. *Australian Educational and Developmental Psychologist, 14,* 43–54.

Williams, H., & Woollacott, M. (1997). Characteristics of neuromuscular responses underlying posture control in clumsy children. *Motor Development: Research and Reviews, 1,* 8–23.

Wolfson, L., Whipple, R., Derby, C. A., Amerman, P., Murphy, T., Tobin, J. N., et al. (1992). A dynamic posturography study of balance in healthy elderly. *Neurology, 42,* 2069–2075.

Woollacott, M., Burnter, P. Jensen, J., Jasiewicz, J., Roncesvalles, N., & Svesitrup, H. (1998). Development of postural responses during standing in healthy children and children with spastic diplegia. *Neuroscience and Biobehavioral Reviews, 22,* 583–589.

Woollacott, M., Debu, B., & Mowatt, M. (1987). Neuromuscular control of posture in the infant and child: is vision dominant? *Journal of Motor Behavior, 19,* 167–186.

Woollacott, M., Inglin, B., & Manchester, D. (1988). Response preparation and posture control. Neuromuscular changes in the older adult. *Annals of the New York Academy of Science, 515,* 42–53.

Woollacott, M., & Jensen, J. (1996). Posture and locomotion In J. Heuer & S. Keele (Eds.), *Handbook of perception and action* (2nd ed., pp. 333–403). New York: Academic Press.

Woollacott, M., & Shumway-Cook, A. (1990). Changes in posture control across the lifespan. *Physical Therapy, 70,* 53–61.

Woollacott, M. H., Shumway-Cook, A., & Nashner, L.M. (1986). Aging and posture control: changes in sensory organization and muscular coordination. *International Journal of Aging and Human Development, 23,* 97–114.

Woollacott, M., Shumway-Cook, A., & Williams, H. (1989). Development of posture and balance control. In M. Woollacott & A. Shumway-Cook (Eds.), *Development of posture and gait across the lifespan* (pp. 77–96). Columbia: University of South Carolina Press.

Woollacott, M., & Sveistrup, H. (1992). Changes in the sequencing and timing of muscle response coordination association with developmental transitions in balance abilities. *Human Movement Science, 11,* 23–36.

Woollacott, M., & Sveistrup, H. (1994). The development of sensorimotor integration underlying posture control in infants during the transition to independent stance. In S. Swinnen, H. Heuer, J. Massion, & P. Casaer (Eds.), *Interlimb coordination: Neural, dynamical and cognitive constraints* (pp. 371–389). San Diego, CA: Academic Press.

Woollacott, M., & Tang, P. (1997). Balance control during walking in the older adult: Research and its implications. *Physical Therapy, 77,* 646–660.

Yim-Chiplis, P., & Talbot, L. (2000). Defining and measuring balance in adults. *Biological Research for Nursing, 1,* 321–331.

PART III

NEUROPSYCHOLOGICAL MANIFESTATIONS

CHAPTER 11

Developmental Phonological Disorder

MEGAN HODGE

LESLIE WELLMAN

The focus of this chapter is children with phonological disorder of unknown origin (i.e., developmental phonological disorder, or DPD; American Psychiatric Association, 1994). Children whose speech is difficult to understand because they make many pronunciation errors have been labeled as articulation disordered, speech disordered, and, more recently, phonologically disordered. Understanding what is meant by phonological disorder requires examination of language, with emphasis on speech perception and production processes. The next section provides a brief overview of mental processes hypothesized to underlie spoken language. Following this, DPD is defined within the context of childhood speech disorders. Two classification systems based on hypothesized etiology and underlying deficits in DPD are then described. Next, information about DPD from a neuropsychological perspective is summarized, followed by a discussion of the hypothesized neurological bases of DPD. Final sections examine the relationship between DPD and other childhood motor disorders and the assessment and treatment implications of applying a neuropsychological perspective to subtypes of DPD.

THE SPEECH–LANGUAGE CONNECTION

Speaking involves transforming a mental representation of an intention into a sequence of rapid, coordinated movements of muscles in the trunk, neck, and upper airway to generate the sounds of language (Levelt, 1989). Speech is an acoustic representation of language that is the product of a chain of overlapping cognitive, linguistic, and sensorimotor processes. Speech sounds are produced in sequences that conform to the permissible syllable and word structure, as well as the stress and intonation patterns, of a particular language. Together, these aspects constitute the sound system or *phonology* of a language. Speech refers to the motor aspects of language as characterized by articulation, speaking rate, loudness, and prosody (Mapou, 1995).

Language is a code that links a set of linguistic forms (i.e., phonological forms, words, and grammatical structure) to a number of aspects of meaning (Mapou, 1995). Linguistic aspects of speaking include accessing the appropriate words within the mental lexicon (concepts, categories, actions, properties, relationships), retrieving the abstract phonological representations of these words (specification of their component consonant and vowel sound types, i.e., phonemes, and how these are organized into structures such as syllables), and coding appropriate grammatical structures. Transformation from the abstract phonological representation of the sequence of words in an intended utterance to the physical sound signal that is perceived as speech involves a series of mental processes: sensory, perceptual (which links sensory to cognitive–linguistic), cognitive, linguistic, and speech motor control (which links linguistic to sensorimotor) (Dodd, 1995; Van der Merwe, 1997). These are shown in Figure 11.1, which is adapted from Dodd and McCormack (1995), Duffy (1995), Stackhouse and Wells (1997), and Van der Merwe (1997). Although not shown specifically in Figure 11.1, working memory is critical to and underlies all speech processes. It is the system that enables us to form intentions, hold information in consciousness, rehearse received input, access and activate long-term knowledge, make judgments about incoming information, decide on a plan of action, and monitor expression of information. Figure 11.1 is intended to identify component processes in speaking rather than present a model of how these processes occur and interact during speech development. The

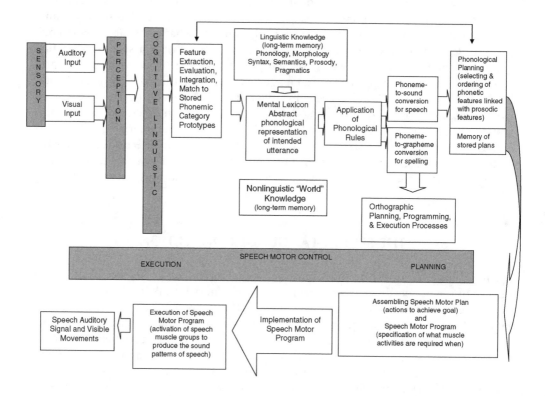

FIGURE 11.1. Spoken language processes.

reader is referred to Baker, Croot, McLeod, and Paul (2001) for a review of psycholinguistic models of speech development and their application to clinical practice.

As shown in Figure 11.1, a set of phonological rules transforms the lexical phonological specification of the words selected to express one's intended meaning to a phonological plan for speaking (phoneme to sound conversion). The phonological plan includes specifications for individual consonant and vowel segments, as well as for prosodic features such as intonation and syllable stress. This phonological plan can be assembled on line or, alternatively, accessed as a whole from routines stored in memory. The mental processes that derive precise instructions from the phonological plan for articulation of individual sounds and how these are modified when combined in sequences are referred to as *speech motor planning and programming*. Van der Merwe (1997) proposed that in the speech motor planning stage, motor goals are specified to formulate action strategies (e.g., close lips and raise soft palate for /b/ in "boy"). Then these actions are translated into speech motor programs that specify what particular muscles will act, with what force, and at what time to achieve the speech target, in view of current phonetic contextual conditions. Once the motor program is constructed, it is implemented by sending neural signals from the brain to muscles of the speech mechanism. These muscles act in concert at appropriate times and with appropriate forces to generate the necessary air pressures, air flows, and airway resistances to make sound energy, and to shape the oral and pharyngeal cavities to filter the sound energy into the intended consonant and vowel sequences in the speech signal (Minifie, Hixon, & Williams, 1973). Abnormalities in muscle function (e.g., tongue paralysis) or in peripheral anatomical structures (e.g., cleft palate), which affect the timing or accuracy of movements of the articulators, will result in speech production errors even if the abstract phonological representation, phonological plan, speech motor plan, and program are formulated accurately (Dodd & McCormack, 1995; Duffy, 1995; Hodge & Wellman, 1999).

When do children start to develop mental lexicons and abstract phonological (sound) representations for the words of a language and the grammatical and syntactic rules and associated prosodic patterns for combining these words into understandable, meaningful utterances? Kent (1992) reported that at some point between 6 and 8 months of age, infants begin to focus their attention on the characteristic features of the sound patterns of their native language. He reported that productive preference for the sound patterns of the ambient language is evident in infants' prespeech vocalizations by 8–10 months. For children, exposure to spoken language and opportunities to practice using spoken language are necessary to develop speech skills. Thus, a spoken language processing system must include input components, as shown in the left side of Figure 11.1, as well as output components.

According to the Fuzzy Logic Model of Perception (Massaro, 1994), auditory and, if available, visual speech signals are received via their respective sensory system. Then, through auditory (and visual) perceptual phonological processing, acoustic and visual features are evaluated, integrated, and matched to phonetic features for a syllable or other units (e.g., phoneme and allophone). This phonological input retrieves the phonological form of the word by activating the lexical item in long-term memory. The phonological form activates the semantic feature of the word and we get word meaning (Caplan, 1995). To say the word, the auditory–perceptual feature-based representation of the word in the phonological lexicon activates speech motor planning and the programming processes that generate movements to produce the sound patterns of the physical speech signal.

Speaking is a complex, skilled behavior that develops from birth and reaches adult-like proficiency in later childhood. According to Shriberg, Tomblin, and McSweeny. (1999), the sociobiological period for speech acquisition is 0–8 years, 11 months. That is, children age 9 years and older who have persisting speech sound errors have passed the period where "normalization" of speech delay occurs. The Verbal Motor Production Assessment for Children (VMPAC; Hayden & Square, 1999) was designed to identify the presence and determine the nature of motor impairments in children with speech disorders. In the normative information for the VMPAC, the range between 7 and 12 years is collapsed into one group for perceptual–behavioral measures of global motor control, focal oromotor control, sequencing (nonspeech and speech movements), and motor control in connected speech. This suggests that no significant differences in performance on these VMPAC tasks were observed across this age span. However, Walsh and Smith (2002) reported that significant changes in speech motor control processes occur during adolescence, based on a kinematic study of lip and jaw movements. These more sensitive measures suggest that refinement of speech motor skill continues into adolescence.

WHAT IS DEVELOPMENTAL PHONOLOGICAL DISORDER?

According to the fourth edition of the *Diagnostic and Statistical Manual of Mental Disorders* (DSM-IV; American Psychiatric Association, 1994), phonological disorder is a failure to use developmentally expected speech sounds that are appropriate for the child's age and dialect such that the resulting speech difficulties interfere with academic or occupational achievement and/or social communication. Errors in sound production, use, representation (e.g., difficulty sorting out which sounds in a language make a difference in meaning) and organization (e.g., errors of selection and ordering of sounds within syllables and words) may occur. When production of isolated sounds is impaired, these are referred to as errors in articulation and reflect a breakdown at a relatively peripheral level of the speech production process. When linguistic factors result in speech production errors, these are referred to as phonological impairments and are thought to reflect higher-level deficits in the knowledge of how sounds are combined to convey meaning (Dodd, 1995; Fey, 1992). Severity may range from mild to so severe that the child's speech is unintelligible even to familiar listeners.

Phonological disorders may have known or unknown origins. They can be associated with clear causal factors such as hearing loss, structural deficits of the speech mechanism (e.g., craniofacial conditions such as cleft palate), neuromuscular conditions (e.g., cerebral palsy and muscular dystrophy), cognitive limitations, or psychosocial problems. According to DSM-IV when mental retardation, a speech motor or sensory deficit, or environmental deprivation are present, a diagnosis of phonological disorder can only be made if the speech difficulties are in excess of those usually associated with these problems. The number of children with phonological disorders associated with known causal factors is small in comparison to the number of preschool children who present with phonological disorders of unknown origin. The phonological disorders of these latter children are often referred to as developmental (i.e., DPD) and may be accompanied by delayed speech onset. Estimated prevalence of DPD in the general population of children of late preschool to early school age is approximately 3% (Shriberg et al., 1999) to 10% (Geirut, 1998).

The heterogeneity of children with DPD is widely acknowledged. Two current classification systems for children with speech delays of unknown origin (DPD) also include children with speech praxis problems (i.e., diagnosed with developmental verbal dyspraxia, or DVD; Dodd, 1995) or suspected developmental apraxia of speech (DAS; Shriberg, Austin, Lewis, McSweeny, & Wilson 1997). Authors who use the term *DVD* view children with this diagnosis as having speech praxis problems that are part of a larger language deficit (hence "verbal" dyspraxia). DVD has its origins in the British literature. Authors who use the term *DAS* view these children as having speech praxis problems that can occur in isolation from other language deficits. DAS is used more commonly in the North American literature. Controversy and confusion over the use of these terms is long standing. Even when acknowledged "experts" make the diagnosis of DAS, the children identified are heterogeneous and experience a range of speech, language, social interaction, behavioral, and academic delays and disabilities (Ball, Bernthal, & Beukelman, 2002). In this chapter, DVD and DAS are used to refer to the same population of children.

Both the Shriberg and the Dodd research groups have conducted systematic research to develop classification systems of speech disorders based on underlying deficits and etiological factors. These two research groups have taken somewhat different but complementary approaches to this challenge. Their contributions to understanding the underlying mechanisms of DPD are described in the following two sections.

Developmental Phonological Disorder within the Context of Childhood Speech Disorders

Shriberg's Speech Disorders Classification System

The Speech Disorders Classification System (SDCS; Shriberg, Austin, et al., 1997; Shriberg et al., 1999) uses *child speech disorders* as a cover term to unify theoretical and applied aspects of speech disorders specific to both developmental and nondevelopmental issues. There are two primary divisions under this cover term. Developmental speech disorders are those with onsets during the developmental period (birth to 8 years, 11 months). Nondevelopmental speech disorders have their onset after 9 years. Developmental speech disorders are divided into those with known (e.g., cerebral palsy, cleft palate, and mental retardation) versus unknown origin. Using the definition introduced previously, children in this latter group (i.e., children with developmental speech disorders of unknown origin), would be considered to have DPD. This group of children is subdivided into two further classifications: *speech delay* (3 years to 8 years, 11 months) and *questionable residual errors* (6 years to 8 years, 11 months). Age-inappropriate speech sound deletions and substitutions that reduce speech intelligibility characterize *speech delay* (SD). Shriberg and Kwiatkowski (1994) noted that children with such patterns often have concurrent deficits in language and some have later deficits in reading and/or spelling. The second classification under developmental speech disorder of unknown origin is *questionable residual errors* (QRE).

QRE are characterized by speech errors limited to clinical distortions of fricative (e.g., /s/), affricate (e.g., "ch" as in *chair*), and/or liquid sounds (/r/ and /l/). According to Shriberg, Austin, and colleagues (1997) these errors do not affect a child's speech intelligibility and these children do not appear to be at higher risk for language deficits. The authors reported that some children with SD and QRE normalize by age 9 years. After the age of 9, children with SD who do not normalize are classified as RE-A (i.e., remaining errors are residuals of the developmental period). At age 9, children who had QRE who retain one or more clinical distortions are classified as RE-B. This distinction is made for genetic studies so that when the speech of family members of an affected child is assessed, speakers with residual errors who formerly had SD can be differentiated from those with residual errors who formerly had only QRE. According to Shriberg and colleagues (1999), "the hypothesis of two primary forms of child speech disorders of currently unknown origin, SD and QRE (or, if these persist after 9 years, RE-A and RE-B), is central to the interpretation of prevalence and comorbidity data for speech genetics studies" (p. 1463). Shriberg (1994) hypothesized that only SD is genetically transmitted while QRE (RE-B) arises from environmental variables.

Shriberg, Austin, and colleagues (1997) identified four putative etiological classifications under the umbrella of SD. These include (1) speech delay, unknown origin, possible genetic; (2) speech delay—otitis media with effusion; (3) speech delay—DAS; and (4) speech delay—developmental psychosocial involvement. In a series of three related papers, Shriberg, Aram, and Kwiatkowski (1997a, 1997b, 1997c) described their search for a DAS phenotype based on surface descriptions of speech errors and related behaviors. They concluded that children who have one or a combination of characteristics such as late speech onset, greatly reduced phonetic inventories, very low percent consonants correct scores, inconsistent errors, and atypical errors do not warrant the term *suspected DAS* because they are not descriptively different from other children who have been labeled late talkers or with speech delay of unknown origin. Shriberg and colleagues (1997c) proposed that only children who show impaired speech movement patterns (subtype 1) and/ or disturbed syllable stress patterns (subtype 2), regardless of other characteristics, warrant the diagnostic term *suspected DAS*. The first subtype is characterized by obvious difficulties in several areas common to acquired apraxia of speech (AOS) in adults. These include clearly documented nonspeech oral apraxia, observed groping of the articulators (e.g., tongue and lips) or other difficulties in speech onsets, and marked token-to-token inconsistencies (substitutions, deletions, distortions) with both phonetically simple and complex words. The second subtype of suspected DAS is characterized by inappropriate stress on multisyllabic utterances. For example, the word *banana* has three syllables and the primary stress is on the second syllable (*ba NA na*). An inappropriate stress pattern would put primary stress on all three syllables (i.e., *BA NA NA*). Shriberg and colleagues concluded that use of inappropriate stress was the only linguistic domain that differentiated some children with suspected DAS from those with other subtypes of SD. From a convergence of psycholinguistic, neurolinguistic, and developmental biolinguistic perspectives, Shriberg and colleagues developed the following five hypotheses about DAS: (1) inappropriate stress is a diagnostic marker for at least one subtype of DAS, (2) the psycholinguistic loci of inappropriate stress in this subtype of DAS are in phonological representational processes, (3) the proximal origin of this subtype of DAS is a neurogenically specific deficit, (4) the distal origin of this subtype of DAS is inherited genetic polymorphism, and (5) significant differences between AOS in adults and findings for this subtype of DAS call into question the inference that the latter is an apractic, motor speech disorder.

Dodd's Subtypes of Childhood Speech Disorders

Dodd (1995) described procedures for classifying childhood speech disorders into five subgroups: (1) articulation disorder, (2) delayed phonological acquisition, (3) consistent deviant disorder, (4) inconsistent deviant disorder, and (5) other (including DVD). She acknowledged that functional articulation and phonological disorder could co-occur but emphasized the importance of distinguishing between articulation and phonological errors as the treatment for each differs markedly. The following descriptions of these five subgroups are summarized from Dodd and Bradford and Dodd (1996).

Articulation Disorder. Articulation disorder is defined as lack of ability to produce a perceptually acceptable version of one or more sounds. In the majority of cases of functional articulation disorder (i.e., no known cause), the most common sounds affected are /s/, /r/ and the voiceless and voiced cognates of interdental fricative "th" as in *think* and *that*. A child's age needs to be taken into account as some studies suggest that fricatives and affricates may not be acquired up to 7 years. Dodd (1995) noted that the range of sounds affected is much greater when articulation disorders result from known causes such as neuromuscular impairment or anatomical abnormalities of the speech production mechanism.

Delayed Phonological Acquisition. Some children have phonological and articulation skills that follow the normal course of development but at a noticeably slower rate and thus are typical of a younger chronological age. When diagnosing delayed phonological acquisition, it is important to consider whether the child's phonological system is continuing to change spontaneously, if it is following a normal course of development, and how co-occurring error patterns cluster. In some cases the cluster of error patterns reflects a phonological system that is typical of a younger age group. In other cases earlier developmental error patterns may co-occur with those typical of older children.

Consistent Deviant Disorder. This classification is used for children who use non-developmental phonological rules (e.g., delete all initial stops) in addition to error patterns that may or may not be age appropriate.

Inconsistent Deviant Disorder. This is defined by the extent of variability of speech errors after excluding errors that could be explained by (1) context-specific influences, (2) in transition from incorrect to correct production, (3) linguistic load, or (4) a set of complex phonological rules. Dodd (1995) developed a 25-word test to calculate an index of consistency. She suggested that children producing 10 or more of the words differently on at least two of three "elicited" occasions should be classified as having inconsistent deviant disorder.

Other. Dysfluency, dyspraxia, and dysarthria are grouped under this subtype. Bradford and Dodd (1996) observed that DVD has been described as an articulation disorder, a phonological disorder, and a combination of these. Etiological hypotheses include motor planning or programming difficulties versus a breakdown in linguistic as well as motor processes. It has been hypothesized that some children with DVD have a general motor problem because of the co-occurrence of oral apraxia, limb apraxia, and occulomotor apraxia. Ozanne (1995) described DVD as a multideficit disorder comprising both a motor disturbance and associated language deficits. Bradford and Dodd observed that while the diagnosis of DVD has relied on a cluster of symptoms, these clusters have not been organized in a way to allow systematic evaluation. Ozanne proposed that to be diagnosed with DVD, a child had to evidence difficulties at three levels of speech production: phonological planning, phonetic programming, and orospeech motor control. She described characteristics of breakdowns at each level. Inconsistent articulation was hypothesized to reflect a phonological planning deficit; articulatory groping and differences between voluntary and involuntary phoneme production were thought to reflect breakdowns at the phonetic programming level; and impaired performance on diadochokinetic and oromotor tasks (e.g., nonspeech tongue movements) was thought to reflect a reduction in orospeech motor programming integrity.

Support for Dodd's Hypothesized Deficits
Underlying Developmental Phonological Disorder

Bradford and Dodd (1996) conducted a series of experiments to identify the impairments underlying speech disorders of unknown origin in children (i.e., DPD) who presented with differing patterns of delayed or deviant phonological processes. Subjects were assigned to one of four groups based on measures of language comprehension, oral and speech motor control, speech production patterns, and the consistency of these patterns at the word and conversational levels. The four groups included articulation and phonological delay (PD), consistent deviant (CD), inconsistent deviant (ID) and developmental verbal dyspraxia (DVD). Each subject was assessed on experimental tasks that included oromotor tasks (single and sequenced movements), fine motor tasks (upper limb speed and dexterity), visuomotor integration tasks (cutting, tracing, copying), and novel-word-learning tasks (recognition, imitation, and elicited speech). Based on their findings, Bradford and Dodd proposed specific underlying deficits for each classification.

Children assigned to the *delayed group* (articulation and phonological delay) (PD) were less severe than the other groups on measures of consonants correct, similar to the CD group on measures of consistency and did not have significant difficulty on the oral tasks. Errors produced on the diadochokinetic tasks were attributed to phonological patterns and not speech motor planning. On the experimental tasks, the PD group performed like the control group on oromotor, fine motor, and novel-word-learning (recognition and imitation) tasks. However, the children in the control group improved speech accuracy across trials, while the children with PD did not. Bradford and Dodd (1996) hypothesized that the PD children have no specific underlying deficit. Rather, their speech impairment may be attributed to delayed neurological maturation or an impoverished environment.

Children assigned to the CD group made fewer consonant errors than did the ID and DVD groups, had consistent error patterns, and were similar to the PD group in terms of oromotor function and diadochokinetic tasks. They performed like the control group on oromotor proficiency, fine motor tasks (dexterity and coordination), and learning to recognize and say new words. Therefore, these children did not appear to have deficits in oromotor skills, fine motor planning, integration of perceptual and motor information, or speech motor planning. It was hypothesized that the underlying impairment resulting in consistent nondevelopmental error patterns was a cognitive linguistic deficit (i.e., difficulty abstracting appropriate rules for internal representations of lexical output).

Children assigned to the ID group had more consonants incorrect and less consistency in error patterns than those in the PD or CD groups. The ID group performed in a similar fashion to the DVD group but to a lesser degree. On the experimental tasks, the ID group performed similarly to the control group on measures of oromotor function, visuomotor integration (untimed), and novel word learning. Performance on fine motor (speed and dexterity) tasks was significantly poorer than that of the control group, suggesting that organizing complex sequences of movements became more difficult when time was a performance factor. It was hypothesized that ID phonology was suggestive of a breakdown at the level of constructing or storing and retrieving plans for action (phonological planning), which is exacerbated when time limits are placed on the performance of complex actions.

Children assigned to the DVD group were similar to those in the ID group on most measures but had more difficulty on the oral function tasks involving the tongue and had the greatest proportion of prosodic deviations. On the experimental tasks, the children in the DVD group had more difficulty with oromotor sequences, visuomotor integration, fine motor speed and dexterity and novel word learning (imitative and elicited, accuracy across trials). Like the ID group, the DVD group showed deficits in organizing and implementing speech motor plans. Their poor performance on imitation suggested poor oromotor/fine motor planning deficits, (i.e., deficits in extracting information from a model, formulating an appropriate plan from a model, or implementing the plan). Further, their difficulty on fine motor tasks suggested more general deficits at the level of organizing and integrating sensory information into a plan of action. Ozanne (1995) also reported that, as a group, children with DVD performed poorly in comparison to control children on repetition of simple and complex sequences of hand movements. Their performance on fine motor tasks mirrored that for speech motor tasks. They were far less accurate than children in the CD and ID phonology groups in their ability to formulate place, timing, and sequencing of sounds in speech despite their ability to articulate isolated sounds. Based on these results, it was proposed that children with DVD exhibit deficits at the levels of phonological planning, phonetic programming, and oro/speech motor control.

NEUROPSYCHOLOGICAL PROFILES OF CHILDREN WITH DEVELOPMENTAL PHONOLOGICAL DISORDER

Children with DPD are usually diagnosed in the preschool years by speech–language pathologists (SLPs) on referral by public health nurses, preschool teachers, pediatricians, or parents. Neuropsychological test batteries are not typically administered to these children because of their young age and the discipline-specific perspective of SLPs. No established precedent for profiling the neuropsychological characteristics of children with DPD was located in the literature. According to Luria (cited in Lehr,

1990), the three hierarchical functional units of the cortical system are arousal (regulates cortical tone), sensory input (receives, analyzes, and stores information), and organizational and planning units (programming, regulation, verification of activity). Each unit has a primary area (receives impulses from and sends impulses to the periphery), a secondary area (information processing), and a tertiary area (receives input from two or more secondary areas and integrates information). Such hierarchical frameworks, which propose that skills at higher levels are dependent on skills at lower levels for full expression, are the basis for models of neuropsychological assessment.

Mapou's (1995) cognitive framework for neuropsychological assessment was selected to organize this discussion of neuropsychological characteristics of children with DPD because of its clinical emphasis and inclusion of cognitive and motor functioning. This hierarchical framework has four levels. At the base of the framework is "global functioning," as assessed by measures of general intellectual achievement abilities. The level above is labeled "foundational skills," which include arousal and attention; sensory (visual, auditory, somatosensory) and motor functions (lateral dominance, fine motor, sensorimotor integration, and praxis); and executive, problem-solving, and reasoning abilities. These foundational skills are fundamental to the effective expression of skills at higher levels in the framework. The next level is labeled "modality-specific skills," which include language (spoken and written) and visuospatial (nonverbal intellectual) functions. "Integrated skills" are at the highest level of the framework and include learning and memory, which require interaction, integration, and coordinated functioning of skills at lower levels. Personality style and emotional functioning are not included in the framework per se, but Mapou noted that these could mediate performance on neuropsychological measures.

Because by definition the cause of DPD is unknown, it is assumed that for children with a diagnosis of DPD, skills at the lowest level of Mapou's (1995) framework (i.e., general intellectual function) are intact. Similarly, it is assumed that at the second level (i.e., "foundational" skills), primary sensory and motor impairments have been excluded as causal factors for children with DPD. The remaining skills at levels two and three of Mapou's framework were used to organize a review of neuropsychological characteristics of children with DPD in the following sections. Characteristics at the level of foundational skills are described first, followed by a summary of characteristics relevant to modality specific skills (i.e., language and nonverbal intellectual functions). Little information has been published about the reasoning and problem-solving skills or general learning abilities of children with DPD. However, the academic outcomes of children with DPD have been studied and are summarized at the end of the review.

Attention

Little information has been published about the attentional abilities of children with DPD. However, when one looks at the population of children diagnosed with attention-deficit/hyperactivity disorder (ADHD), these children are at higher risk for a DPD than are children without ADHD (American Psychiatric Association, 1994).

The issue of how attentional abilities may affect outcome in children with DPD is one of interest. Kwiatkowski and Shriberg (1998) developed a two-parameter framework that attempted to subsume all elements relevant to intervention with children with speech delay under two domains termed *capability* and *focus*. A child's capability is assessed by measures of linguistic status and is constrained by risk factors (mechanism, cognitive, linguistic, and psychosocial constraints). The construct of focus reflects the attention–motivational constraints on a child's learning and is operationally defined as the amount of motivational support that a child needs to persist on a difficult task. Based on both retrospective and prospective studies, Kwiatkowski and Shriberg found that pretreatment capability is the most important predictor of speech normalization rate but pretreatment measures of focus added significantly to the predictive variance. These authors suggested that regardless of how well-developed linguistic analyses and specific treatment procedures are for children with DPD, individual differences in these children's attention and motivation play a central role in their learning and generalization and therefore in speech normalization outcomes.

Sensory Function

Dodd (1995) concluded that fluctuating hearing loss may be a contributing factor to phonological disorder but it is rarely a sole cause. She also stated that there is little evidence for central auditory processing deficits being a cause of phonological disorder in the absence of a more general learning disability. Information about the auditory processing skills of children diagnosed with DPD or with DAS specifically is scarce. A review by Hall, Jordan, and Robin (1993) revealed a range of severity levels on measures of auditory discrimination, sound recognition, auditory memory, and auditory sequencing abilities, with below-normal functioning reported in all but one of five studies for children with DAS. These results are congruent with reports of poorer performance on measures of phonological awareness in children with DVD/DAS (Stackhouse & Snowling, 1992).

Motor Skills

Bradford and Dodd (1994, 1996) examined oromotor (nonspeech) tasks and fine motor tasks for four groups of children with speech disorder of unknown origin. Oromotor tasks involved movements of the lips and tongue in a nonspeech context and sequences of two oral movements. Fine motor skills were assessed with two subtests of the Bruininks–Oseretsky Test of Motor Proficiency (i.e., upper limb speed and dexterity; visuomotor integration) (Bruininks, 1978). Children with delayed phonological and/or articulation skills performed as well as the normal control group on visuomotor integration tasks. Children with consistent deviant phonology also did not differ from normal controls on the oromotor tasks and the tasks that assessed speed, dexterity, and coordination of fine motor movements. Children with inconsistent deviant phonology performed like normal peers on oromotor single movements and in sequencing two nonspeech movements or postures. They were able to complete untimed motor tasks that required integration of visual information (e.g., tracing and copying cutting) like the normal controls. However, their performance was significantly poorer than that of their normal peers on tasks that required speed and dexterity of fine motor movements. Bradford and Dodd (1994, 1996) also found that these children had more difficulty organizing complex sequences of movement when time was included as a performance factor.

A greater proportion of children diagnosed with DVD had difficulty with tongue movements in nonspeech contexts. This aside, the children with DVD performed as well as controls in producing single oral movements in context, but their ability to organize the production of two oral movements following a model was significantly impaired. Children diagnosed as having DVD also had difficulty with both of the fine motor subtests (speed and dexterity and visuomotor integration) pointing to deficits in integrating sensory information into a plan of action and coordinating speed and dexterity of complex hand movements. Davis, Jakeilski, and Marquardt (1998) included fine and gross motor difficulties in the list of characteristics associated with DAS. Dewey, Roy, Square-Storer, and Hayden (1988) also reported that children with poor sequential motor performance for speech had lower scores on measures of limb praxis than did children with normal speech or speech disorder without impairments in speech sequential motion abilities.

Stark and Blackwell (1997) compared isolated oral movements (Iso-VOM), repeated oral movements (Rep-VOM), and a series of different movements (Seq-VOM) in children with normal language (LN), children with language impairment only (LI-O), and children with both language impairment and speech errors (LI-A). The mean age of the subjects was 8 years with standard deviations of less than or equal to 1 year. Accuracy and coordination of movement measures were also correlated with scores on a nonword repetition task and a phoneme identification task. The children with LI-O did not differ from normal children on measures of isolated and repeated oral movements, whereas the children with LI-A had significantly lower scores on these tasks. The children with LI-A did not differ from the normal group on Seq-VOM, whereas the LI-O groups' scores were significantly lower. While performance on the Iso-VOM was correlated significantly with nonword repetition in both LI groups, performance on Seq-VOM was correlated significantly with phoneme identification in the LI-O group only. On the basis of these results, the authors speculated that children with language impairment and persisting speech errors have developmental anomalies affecting the final cortical pathways for speech motor control. The children with language impairment who do not show persisting speech errors instead may have anomalies affecting the supplementary motor cortex and the widespread sequential motor–phoneme identification system proposed by Ojemann and Mateer (1977).

The findings reported by Stark and Blackwell (1997) are congruent with the *motolinguistic* model of cortical motor speech disorders proposed by Crary (1993). In his model, overlapping motor and speech–language functions exist within the left-hemisphere language areas. There are various steps or levels of information processing that pertain to both motor and speech–language functions along an anterior to posterior continuum. Frontal areas are important for volitional execution of speech or other oral movements. Disturbances here would result in movement execution difficulties such as articulation (i.e., performing the motor actions for the sounds of speech) at the level of single movements as seen in children with dysarthria. The posterior areas (temporoparietal) are important for linguistic formulation and for selecting and ordering complex serial movements for both motor and speech–language functions. Disturbances here would result in specific language impairment and difficulty selecting and ordering targets within a sequence. Between the ends of the continuum, motor and speech–language functions overlap. Disturbances here may permit correct sequential ordering but impair ability to perform sequences. Implications of Crary's model are that motor, speech, and language dysfunctions may occur independently. However, they may also co-occur and when this happens these dysfunctions are interrelated. Crary's model offers a valuable but as yet largely untested framework for understanding the relationships among speech, language, and motor function and dysfunction in children.

Language Functions

Spoken Language

Spoken language encompasses knowledge of the meaning of words, how words relate to each other, word order and grammar, and the ability to listen and organize ideas into words and then express these using speech. DSM-IV (American Psychiatric Association, 1994) identifies expressive language disorder, mixed receptive–expressive language disorder, and phonological disorder as three different diagnoses under the broader heading of communication disorders. Phonological disorder can be present without an associated language disorder. However, according to DSM-IV (American Psychiatric Association, 1994), the most common associated feature of expressive language disorder is phonological disorder and phonological disorder is also often present in children with mixed receptive–expressive language disorder.

In expressive language disorder, the child's scores on standardized, individually administered measures of expressive language development are substantially below those obtained from standardized measures of both nonverbal intellectual capacity and receptive language development. The disorder may be manifested clinically by a markedly limited vocabulary, verb-tense errors, difficulty recalling words, or difficulty producing sentences of developmentally appropriate length or complexity. Mixed receptive and expressive language disorder differs only in that the child's scores on standardized, individually administered measures of both receptive and expressive language development are substantially below those obtained from standardized measures of nonverbal intellectual capacity. Symptoms include those for expressive language disorder, as well as difficulty understanding words, sentences, or specific types of words such as spatial terms. The terms *developmental language impairment* and *specific language impairment* (SLI) are used interchangeably in the literature and refer to children who have expressive or receptive–expressive language disorders of unknown origin.

Controversy exists about the etiology of SLI. It is diagnosed in children who fail to develop spoken language in the normal fashion for no apparent reason (i.e., with no concomitants such as mental retardation, sensory disorders, frank neurological damage, serious emotional problems, or environmental deprivation) (Nelson, 1998). Children diagnosed with SLI exhibit a heterogeneous distribution of linguistic profiles at the level of information decoding and encoding. Recent studies of SLI suggest that it arises from limited linguistic processing capacity with possible compromises in the development of higher-level cognitive skills such as complex linguistic structures, mature lexical development, problem solving, and literacy (Ahmed, Lombardino, & Leonard, 2001). In these authors' review of taxonomies for subtyping child language disorders, children with articulation and phonological disorders in combination with other language difficulties appear repeatedly.

Shriberg and colleagues (1999) studied the prevalence of DPD and its comorbidity with SLI in the United States in a demographically representative sample of 1,328 monolingual, English-speaking, 6-year-old children. Their primary findings were as follows: a prevalence of DPD of 3.8%, with a higher (approximately 1½ times) prevalence in boys (4.5%) than in girls (3.1%); of those children with DPD, approximately 11–15% also had SLI. The diagnosis of SLI was made if a child scored at the 10th percentile or lower on two or more of five composite scores developed from seven language measures (Tomblin, Records, & Zhang, 1996). This sample was then categorized by language status (normal or SLI) and cognition (normal or impaired). Normal cognition was defined as having an IQ greater than 87 on the Block Design and Picture Completion tests of the Wechsler Preschool and Primary Scale of Intelligence—Revised (WPSI-R; Wechsler, 1989). This categorization resulted in 3.8% of boys and 1.5% of girls with normal cognition and normal language having speech delay, while 7.6% of boys and 4.8% of girls with normal cognition and SLI had speech delay. The sex pattern was reversed for children with low cognition. For children with low cognition and normal language, 2.5% of boys and 6.1% of girls had speech delay, whereas for children with low cognition and language impairment, 13.7% of boys and 17.9% of girls had speech delay. Based on these findings, children with DPD have a greater probability of also having SLI than do children without DPD.

Written Language (Reading and Spelling)

Larrive and Catts (1999) compared children with DPD and children with normally developing phonological and language abilities on measures of expressive phonology, phonological awareness, and language ability at the end of kindergarten and then on a reading achievement test a year later. Overall, children with expressive phonological disorders performed more poorly on the reading test than did children in the control group, but there was a great deal of variability in the children with phonological disorders. The authors then used the measures taken in kindergarten to predict which children in the phonological disorders group would have good versus poor reading outcomes. Greater severity of phonological disorder, poorer phonological awareness, and poorer language skills characterized children with poor reading outcomes. Expressive phonology and phonological awareness measures accounted for a significant amount of the variance in first-grade reading achievement.

Dodd and colleagues (1995) investigated the acquisition of literacy skills (spelling and reading) in children with phonological *delay* and disorder (*consistent deviant* and *inconsistent deviant*). In the first experiment, they looked at spelling skills assessed by measures of word spelling (real and nonsense words), phoneme segmentation and rule derivation. The *delayed* group spelled real words as well as the control group but qualitative differences were noted in that half of the children in the *delayed* group spelled at a level six months below chronological age and the group as a whole had fewer plausible errors. Errors for the *delayed* group were more suggestive of visual processing and not phonological processing difficulties. The *delayed* group had more difficulty with nonsense spelling, phoneme segmentation and rule derivation. The *consistent deviant* group performed poorly on all measures. Spelling was often non-phonetic (i.e., strings of unrelated letters). The *inconsistent deviant* group was not significantly different from the other disorder groups but the number of subjects was small (*n* = 5).

In the second experiment, Dodd and colleagues (1995) assessed reading accuracy (real and nonsense words) and comprehension with the same population. The *delayed* group was similar to the control group in their ability to read words (real and nonsense words) and reading comprehension. There were qualitative differences in that the *delayed* group appeared to use more of a visual route for word recognition. The CD group differed significantly on all measures, while the ID group differed primarily on measures of reading accuracy but not reading comprehension.

In a third experiment, Dodd and colleagues (1995) looked at a group of children who had received treatment for a speech disorder between the ages of 3 and 6 years but had been discharged from active treatment for at least 12 months and whose current ages were between 6 and 10 years. These children were assessed on measures of reading and spelling. They found that children with a history of phonological disorder performed more poorly on reading and spelling tasks than did children without a history of phonological disorder. However, those children with a history of articulation disorder or *delayed* phonological development were less likely to have reading and spelling difficulties than children with a history of *consistent* or *inconsistent* phonological disorder. They hypothesized that there was a common phonological deficit at the cognitive–linguistic level underlying difficulties with speaking, reading, and spelling because there were impairments at the level of input processing (auditory, visual) and output processing (speech, writing). The authors observed that the residual nature of the deficit, despite improvements in spoken output, has implications for intervention.

Lewis and Freebairn (1992) conducted a cross-sectional study at preschool age, grade-school age, adolescence, and adulthood to examine the performance of people with a history of preschool phonological disorder on measures of phonology, reading, and spelling. At each age, subjects with a history of disorder performed more poorly than did matched control subjects. When successive age groups were compared, a steady improvement on all measures was found as age increased. The greatest amount of change occurred between preschool and grade school. Subjects with a history of other language problems in addition to phonological disorder performed more poorly on reading and spelling measures than did those with only a history of phonological disorder. The authors concluded that the remnants of a preschool phonological disorder are detectable on literacy measures past grade school and into adulthood.

Raitano, Pennington, Tunick, Boada, and Shriberg (2004) examined how comorbid language impairment (LI) and the persistence of a speech sound disorder (SSD) related to preliteracy skills in a sample of 101 5- to 6-year-old children with a history of SSD. Their criteria for SSD were similar to that for DPD, as described in this chapter. The sample included 49 children whose SSD had normalized and did not have comorbid LI, 29 children who had persisting SSD and without comorbid LI, 13 children with persisting SSD and normalized LI, and 10 children with persisting SSD and LI. The investigators also compared these children's preliteracy measures with those obtained from a control group. Results revealed that the entire group of children with SSD performed less well than control participants on tasks assessing phonological awareness and letter-knowledge skills, even after the effects of nonverbal IQ and socioeconomic status were controlled. Robust main effects for SSD persistence and LI status on phonological awareness skills were found and appeared additive (no significant interaction). Children with normalized SSD and no concurrent LI performed less well on phonological awareness tasks than control participants without a history of speech or language disorder, even when nonverbal IQ was statistically controlled. The authors concluded that children with a history of SSD, whether or not it has normalized or is accompanied by language impairment, are at risk for deficits on preliteracy tasks that are predictive of later reading difficulties. In agreement with previous literature, children with persisting SSD and comorbid language impairment appeared at greatest risk.

Nonverbal Intellectual Functioning

Based on the definition of DPD, one might assume that compared to their verbal skills, nonverbal skills are a relative strength for children with DPD. Shriberg and colleagues (1999) provided the most comprehensive information to date about the nonverbal skills of children with DPD. Children in their sample were assessed on the Block Design and Picture Completion subtests of the WPPSI-R (Weschler, 1989). Of the boys in their sample with DPD, 63.4% had normal language and normal cognition, 15.2% had normal cognition and language impairment, 15.2% had low cognition and language impairment, and 6.1% had low cognition and normal language. In the girls identified with DPD, 38.9% had normal cognition and normal language, 11.1% had normal cognition and language impairment, 27.8% had low cognition and language impairment, and 22.2% had low cognition and normal language.

Hall and colleagues (1993) reviewed available literature that described intellectual abilities of the subgroup of children with DPD diagnosed with DAS. They found that some authors have reported that a diagnosis of DAS excludes children with decreased intellectual functioning (Davis et al., 1998; Marquardt & Sussman, 1991). They also noted that authors varied in terms of how normal intelligence was defined (e.g., a nonverbal IQ of 90 and above vs. 80 and above) and that some studies reported the occurrence of DAS in populations of children who functioned within the mentally retarded range of intellectual potential (Ferry, Hall, & Hicks, 1975). Thus, given the state of the literature, no conclusive statement about nonverbal intellectual functioning in children with DAS can be made at this time. What can be said, however, is that children with a diagnosis of DAS have a greater likelihood of having comorbid conditions that are associated with decreased performance on verbal and nonverbal measures of intellectual potential.

Academic Outcomes of Children with Developmental Phonological Disorder

Geirut (1998) stated that children with phonological disorders often require other types of remedial services in addition to speech–language therapy, with 50–70% exhibiting general academic difficulty through grade 12. Based on a review of the literature, she concluded that retrospective studies have shown that adults who were diagnosed and treated for phonological disorders in childhood continued to have difficulty processing information about language in general and the sound system in particular. While these adults did not have trouble producing speech sounds, they consistently made more errors in retrieval, manipulation, and comprehension of linguistic information and were slower to interpret language than were adults without a history of phonological disorders. Gierut observed that while the literature suggests that individuals with phonological disorders may be disadvantaged in situations that require the comprehension and production of language, this does not mean that DPD was the cause of their lower educational achievement. However, based on her literature review, she stated that children who receive some type of treatment for their phonological disorder have better long-term social, academic, and communication prognoses than do those who do not.

Considering the classification systems for children with DPD proposed by Dodd and Shriberg, it might be expected that those children with only articulation disorder or QRE would not show specific deficits in language. Children with phonological delay would also not be expected to show difficulties beyond those associated with immaturity. In Dodd's classification, children with CD phonology and ID phonology were identified as having difficulty in learning rules about the ambient phonological system and generating phonological plans. Whether these specific learning problems are reflected in other realms or reflect more general deficits in processing is unknown. However, these children are certainly at higher risk for persisting spoken language problems as well as written language difficulties, which puts them at greater risk for lower academic achievement.

Children with DVD or suspected DAS appear to be at greatest academic risk as they have a much higher probability of co-occurring expressive language disorders and fine motor and gross motor coordination and integration difficulties (Hall et al., 1993; Portwood, 2000). Hall and colleagues (1993) observed that most children exhibiting DAS required special educational programs, in addition to speech and language services, to prosper in their school setting. These authors acknowledged that their sample of children consisted of more severely involved individuals because of the nature of their clinic. Of note are the results of a preliminary, controlled follow-up study of 10 children who were identified by age 4 years as having DAS and average cognitive and receptive language function (Lewis, Freebairn, Hansen, & Taylor, 2002). At school age, eight children demonstrated improvement in articulation scores, but their syllable sequencing, nonsense word repetition, and language abilities remained poor. Comorbid disorders of reading and spelling were observed. The authors suggested that the phenotype for DAS changes with age as the children showed a broader spectrum of language and learning difficulties at school age than at age 4 years.

NEUROLOGICAL BASES
OF DEVELOPMENTAL PHONOLOGICAL DISORDER

The identification of subtypes of developmental phonological disorder (Dodd, 1995; Shriberg & Kwiatkowski, 1994; Shriberg et al., 1997a, 1997b, 1997c, 1999) suggests that there is more than one underlying mechanism for DPD. For children classified as having articulation disorder only or phonological delay, Dodd (1995) hypothesized that the underlying mechanism was one of overall neurological immaturity with no specific site implicated. Shriberg (1994) hypothesized that the subgroup of children with questionable residual errors (similar to Dodd's articulation disorder classification) did not have any neurological delay or difference but, rather, that their errors resulted from environmental variables.

Dodd (1995) summarized her perspectives on plausible causal and maintaining factors for developmental speech disorders of unknown origin. In regard to organic causes, she identified conditions that can result in poor gross and fine motor coordination, hyperactivity, and severe distractibility, such as undiagnosed neurological conditions (e.g., seizures) or genetic predispositions, and health issues (e.g., malnourishment and living conditions promoting upper respiratory infections). Nonorganic causes of childhood speech disorders of unknown origin were associated with the language-learning environment, which must provide adequate exposure to the language with opportunities for adult–child interaction around shared activities of interest to the child. Possible reasons for inadequate exposure to language that she identified included disordered language models provided by caregivers, multiple births, and stressful communicative environments.

There is clear evidence of a familial basis for DPD. Felsenfeld, McGue, and Broen (1995) conducted a 28-year follow-up study investigating familial aggregation in DPD. They compared the children of a group of 24 adults with a documented history of DPD, which persisted through at least the end of the first grade (probands), with a control group of 28 adults who were known to have normal articulation abilities as children. The results of their study demonstrated that children of the proband subjects performed significantly more poorly on all measures of articulation and expressive language and were more likely to have received articulation treatment. A correspondence between affected parent and children for specific articulatory error patterns or phonological processes was not evident in the proband families. Felsenfeld and colleagues (1995) concluded that their results agreed with most previous family studies (e.g., Lewis & Freebairn, 1992) that have demonstrated an increased rate of occurrence of speech–language disorders of unknown origin in families who have a first-degree relative who is similarly affected. Lai, Fisher, Hurst, Varga-Khadem, and Monaco (2001) identified the first gene linked to speech (FOXP2 gene located on chromosome 7q31) by studying a British family (the KE family), half the members of which are affected by a severe disorder of speech and language, described by the authors as DVD. The finding of an isolated gene was not expected as a multigenic mechanism with variable expression has been hypothesized to underlie familial speech disorders (e.g., Lewis & Freebairn, 1992). However, the identification of this gene provides the groundwork for future research in developing the genetic map underlying transmission of spoken language behaviors. More recently, Lewis, Shriberg, and colleagues (2002) showed genetic linkage to a region of chromosome 7q31 for 10 families ascertained through a preschool child with a phonological disorder.

Based on these findings, it is hypothesized that children with DPD have associated brain-related abnormalities when the underlying deficit appears to be one of difficulty in abstracting cognitive–linguistic rules for the ambient phonological system, applying these rules to generate phonological plans, or translating these phonological plans to speech motor plans and programs that direct the movements of the articulators for speech. These neural abnormalities could be the result of a genetic predisposition that results in an impoverished neural substrate for developing sufficient and efficient neuronal connections for phonological processing and speech planning and programming, or of damage to the developing brain *in utero* or during the early postnatal period, that inhibits establishment of these neural networks.

Areas of the brain that are hypothesized to be involved in processing phonological information and in translating abstract phonological representations to motor plans for speech include peri-Sylvian areas in the temporal, parietal, and inferior frontal lobes in the dominant hemisphere (Duffy, 1995). The supplemental motor area in the superior medial frontal cortex and links between cortical areas to subcortical components of the motor system (e.g., basal ganglia, thalamus, and cerebellum) are also involved in speech motor programming. Integrity of the upper and lower motor neuron pathways is also necessary for execution of speech movements (Duffy, 1995).

Bennett and Netsell (1999) described the insula's potential involvement in all aspects of speech and language processing. They argued, like Habib and colleagues (1995), that the insular cortex, with its massive afferent and efferent connections, provides an extensive network for receptive and expressive speech–language processing and is a crucial element in several distinct networks involving verbal and nonverbal communication. Bennett and Netsell state, "The insula is contiguous with Broca's area, Wernicke's area, the supramarginal gyrus and the angular gyrus. The insula spans essentially the entire length of the 'language zone' and is medial to these language regions above and below the Sylvian fissure" (p. 262). Paulesu and colleagues (1996) stated that the insula might normally act as an anatomical bridge between Broca's area, superior temporal cortex, and inferior parietal cortex. On the basis of positron emission tomography (PET) scan results that showed abnormal activity in the left insula for five adults whose only cognitive difficulty was phonological processing, these authors proposed that a dysfunctional left insula would weaken the connectivity between anterior and posterior language areas resulting in phonological processing deficits. Bennett and Netsell referred to Dronkers' area as a small region, approximately 5 mm in diameter, located on the superior aspect of the left insular precentral gyrus. Dronkers (1996) identified this as a region necessary for the planning of speech articulation based on her findings from a double dissociation study of brain lesions in adult patients with and without acquired apraxia of speech. Bennett and Netsell also described a series of studies with patients with oral apraxia that implicated damage to the insula. They speculated that lesions to other discrete regions of the insula are responsible for disorders in planning nonverbal oral movements and similarly that limb apraxia might result from lesions to yet another insular region.

Some type of brain difference, either inherited or the result of a pre- or perinatal event, is a widely supported hypothesis for the etiology of suspected DAS (Crary, 1993; Hall et al., 1993; Shriberg et al., 1997c.) Bennett and Netsell (1999) hypothesized that DAS results from damage or delayed development of Dronkers' area (site of lesion for acquired apraxia of speech in adults) and/or its neuronal connections. The coexistence of language problems could result from damage to other insular regions and their neuronal connections. Bennett and Netsell hypothesized that damage *in utero* or an acquired insult to the insula at various points in the development of speech and language could delay or disrupt emerging inter- and intrainsular connections. A child could show various degrees of speech and language disturbances depending on the locus, timing, and extent of these disruptions. These authors suggested that children who demonstrate early signs of DAS only, or speech and language problems that eventually remit, might be associated with eventual *normalized* function of the insula.

According to Portwood (2000), developmental disorders have their origins in the dysfunctional transmission and interpretation of messages within the systems of the brain. "Specific learning difficulties such as dyspraxia and dyslexia occur when the cortex persists in a state of immaturity. There has been insufficient 'pruning' and information takes longer to process. Dyspraxia is a result of such immaturity in the right hemisphere, dyslexia on the left" (p. 18). The left hemisphere is specialized in process-ing information sequentially, while the right hemisphere specializes in combining parts to make a whole (Portwood, 2000). She noted that while the left hemisphere is more efficient at processing verbal information, language should not be considered to be in the left hemisphere. However, speech perception and subsequent generation of lan-guage require sequential analytic processing for which the left hemisphere is special-ized. The purpose of hemisphere specialization is to improve the efficiency of the brain, and research has shown that it is necessary to have effective processing on both sides of the brain for optimum efficiency. The specialization of the left hemisphere for language processing appears to follow a developmental progression. Children up to the age of 3 appear to have no hemispheric preference in visual and auditory process-ing, but evidence suggests that a preference is well established by age 6 years. By age 12 years, the process of specialization appears virtually complete. Using functional magnetic resonance imaging techniques, Shaywitz and colleagues (1995) demonstrated that when male subjects performed phonological processing tasks, activity was almost exclusively present in the left hemisphere, whereas for female subjects, centers were ac-tivated in both hemispheres. This male–female difference has also been observed in tasks of visual imagery and spatial ability that show boys using the right hemisphere and girls using both (Portwood, 2000). Based on these types of studies, Portwood con-cluded that females have the capacity to analyze information using both hemispheres simultaneously, while males have evolved so that the left hemisphere processes lan-guage and the right hemisphere processes visuospatial stimuli. Therefore, females have systems that can be used in the right hemisphere if the left hemisphere has processing difficulties. However, this is not the case in males. These male–female differences in hemispheric processing of information provide one explanation for the higher rates of language and speech-related problems in boys compared with girls (Portwood, 2000). They may also partially account for the finding of the reversal of this trend in children with low cognitive function (Shriberg et al., 1999) where a greater proportion of fe-males than males had speech delay. While girls with unilateral hemisphere damage would not be at as great risk for language and visuospatial problems as boys, girls with bilateral hemispheric involvement would be at risk for both speech–language and visuospatial deficits and lowered cognitive function.

Conclusive evidence for brain differences in at least some individuals diagnosed with DVD comes from magnetic resonance imaging analyses of affected and unaf-fected members of the KE family and a group of age-matched controls (Watkins et al., 2002). These authors found a number of motor- and speech-related brain regions in which the affected family members had significantly different amounts of gray matter compared with the unaffected and control groups, which did not differ from each other. The caudate nucleus was one of several regions that were abnormal bilaterally. It also showed functional abnormality in a related PET study. Furthermore, the vol-ume of the caudate nucleus correlated significantly with performance of affected fam-ily members on a test of oral praxis, a test of nonword repetition, and the Wechsler in-telligence scales. Compared to unaffected family members and the control group, the affected family members were also found to have increased amounts of gray matter bi-laterally in the putamen, abnormally large amounts of gray matter in the left frontal opercular regions (pars triangularis and anterior insular cortex), significantly less gray matter in the left supplementary motor area, abnormal amounts of gray matter in re-gions of the posterior lobe of the cerebellum, and significantly more gray matter in the planum temporale bilaterally. Based on their findings, the authors observed that the relationship between size and function is not straightforward and that a larger volume in a particular brain structure does not necessarily impart an advantage to an individual. It is expected that well-designed neuroimaging studies will continue to elucidate brain–behavior relationships for children identified with various subtypes of DPD.

RELATIONSHIP OF DEVELOPMENTAL PHONOLOGICAL DISORDER TO OTHER DEVELOPMENTAL MOTOR DISORDERS

For children with phonological disorders of known origin where the cause is neuromuscular (e.g., cerebral palsy and muscular dystrophy) and the effect is to disturb normal development of speech motor control, other motor systems of the limbs and trunk are often also affected, resulting in movement disturbances in posture and gross and fine motor behaviors. Even in cases in which the predominant early signs involve impaired control of muscles used in speech and swallowing (e.g., congenital suprabulbar paresis), associated disturbances in gross and fine motor abilities and delays in motor milestones are common (Clarke, Carr, Reilly, & Neville, 2000).

The co-occurrence of fine and gross motor problems in at least some children diagnosed with DAS is well established (Bradford & Dodd, 1994, 1996; Crary, 1993; Davis et al., 1998). Portwood (2000) used the term *dyspraxia* synonymously with developmental coordination disorder (DCD). She subsumes children with DVD under this larger diagnosis. Hodge (1998) also argued that the definition of DCD should be broadened to include children who have a DCD specifically affecting movement control for speech.

Portwood (2000) reported that 50% of children diagnosed with isolated DCD show evidence of late acquisition of a single word vocabulary with significant articulation problems until the age of 8 or 9 years. She noted these children's speech and language skills are delayed (i.e., they appear to follow a normal progression but at a slower rate). Portwood differentiated these children with isolated DCD from those children with disordered language expression and comprehension that occurs comorbidly with DCD. The comorbidity of motor delay (falling within the criteria for DCD) and SLI has also been reported in recent neurological and neuropsychological investigations of children with developmental language impairment of unknown origin (Ahmed et al., 2001; Trauner, Wulfeck, Tallal, & Hesselink, 2000). Hill (1998) compared children diagnosed with SLI, DCD, age-matched control children, and younger children matched on language age on three tasks using familiar and unfamiliar actions to identify rate of dyspraxic deficits in these four groups. Of the 19 children who met criteria for SLI, subsequent testing identified 11 of these children as falling with the range for those with DCD on a measure of motor development.

IMPLICATIONS FOR ASSESSMENT AND TREATMENT OF CHILDREN WITH DEVELOPMENTAL PHONOLOGICAL DISORDER

Children with DPD can exhibit a range of surface level speech errors. Assessment strategies that can classify children with DPD into more homogeneous subgroups should result in selection of more appropriate treatments with better prediction of outcomes.

Classification systems that are based on the assumption that there are several subtypes of DPD that have different underlying deficits (Bradford & Dodd, 1994, 1996; Dodd, 1995; Shriberg, Austin, et al., 1997) provide a framework for selecting assessment strategies, interpreting results, and planning intervention. Models such as those proposed by Crary (1993) provide a basis for increasing our understanding of the relationships among observed speech, language and motor dysfunction, and underlying neural processes and substrates. Based on the information reviewed in this chapter, children with isolated articulation disorders or residual speech sound errors and no language difficulties are likely to have more positive academic outcomes than children with a cognitive–linguistic basis to their speech disorder (i.e., CD, ID, and DVD) (Dodd, 1995). However, even children who demonstrate a "normalized" speech sound disorder by age 6 and do not have a concurrent language impairment appear at some risk for later reading difficulties (Raitano et al., 2004). Of all the children with phonological disorders of unknown origin, children diagnosed with DVD/DAS appear to be at greatest risk for later academic difficulties.

Geirut (1998) addressed the efficacy of treatment for DPD. She observed that there is consensus in the literature that the primary goal of treatment is to improve the child's speech intelligibility and thereby increase communicative effectiveness. She describes this as a two-pronged task that involves teaching accurate articulation of speech sounds and facilitating the conceptual organization, lexical representation, and storage of speech sound information in memory. There is a range of available treatment methods that are classified broadly as those that adopt a sensorimotor approach as opposed to those that use a cognitive–linguistic approach to intervention. Dodd (1995) cautioned that remediating surface speech sound errors without addressing an underlying impairment in deriving and applying phonological rules will likely result in persisting deficits in reading and spelling.

McCauley and Strand (1999) addressed the nature of treatment for children who have phonological delay, as well as speech motor planning difficulties. They argued that cognitive–linguistic treatment approaches and traditional articulation treatment approaches, by themselves, do not meet the needs of children with speech motor planning and programming deficits. They recommended that treatment procedures that help these children to focus on learning the movement patterns and sequence of movement patterns used to produce words and word combinations be included in intervention. Examples of such procedures are provided in McCauley and Strand (1999), Square (1999), Strand and McCauley (1999), and Strand and Skinder (1999).

With increasing knowledge of the positive relationship between DPD in preschool and persisting poor performance on measures of spelling and reading, there is increasing focus on teaching phonological awareness directly to preschool children with developmental phonological delay to facilitate development of their early literacy skills. In light of the higher prevalence of SLI in children with DPD compared to the general population of kindergarten-age children, assessment procedures should include determination of the adequacy of these children's language skills. For example, Tomblin and colleagues (1997) indicated that the presence of a speech disorder significantly increases the probability of girls with language disorder being identified and enrolled for treatment.

Finally, as identified by Bradford and Dodd (1996), children with different types of phonological disorder differ in nonspeech gross and fine motor abilities as well as in their speech motor control abilities. Recent neuropsychological studies of children with SLI also suggest that that these children are at higher risk for motor delays than are children without SLI (Trauner et al., 2000). Based on these findings, it is recommended that preschool children who are referred for specific concerns about their speech and language deficits should also be screened for gross and fine motor delays as they are at higher risk than children without speech–language disorders. Potentially this will lead to earlier identification of and consequently earlier intervention for gross and fine motor deficits (i.e., prior to school entry), as well as a fuller picture of the nature of these children's developmental disorders (Hodge, 1998). Portwood (2000) reported that in her experience, speech–language pathologists are the primary route of referral for children suspected of having fine and gross motor coordination difficulties. Missiuna, Gaines, and Pollock (2002) outlined the role of the speech–language pathologist in recognizing and referring preschool children at risk for DCD and provided practical guidelines to support speech–language pathologists in this role. Clearly, applying a transdisciplinary perspective to children with developmental motor disorders (Hodge, 2003), whether these disorders are manifested first or primarily in goal-directed motor behavior that generates speech or in fine and gross motor skill development, appears essential to better understand the nature of the underlying impairment and maximize the motor, academic and social outcomes for these children.

CASE STUDY

J was assessed and diagnosed with a severe phonological delay at 3 years of age. Expressive language (grammar and syntax) was also delayed. Prenatal history was marked by maternal complications (flu, chicken pox), but subsequent health history was unremarkable. Familial history was significant for dyslexia, speech difficulties, and hyperactivity (paternal uncle). The parents reported no concerns regarding feeding and gross or fine motor skills.

J was seen for treatment once a week for the next year. Treatment focused on developing accurate articulation for a variety of sound types made with the tongue: stridents (s, f, sh, ch), velars (k, g) and liquids (l, r). Improvements were noted for production of target sounds in structured tasks with some generalization of "s", "f," and "k" to spontaneous conversation. Despite improvement at the word level, the parents reported that J was unintelligible to most people.

Reassessment at the beginning of kindergarten revealed normal hearing bilaterally, normal middle-ear function, speech recognition thresholds consistent with pure-tone results, and excellent word recognition scores. Both receptive vocabulary and expressive language scores were above the mean on standardized tests. However, mean length of utterance was not assessed because speech intelligibility was poor. In conversation, grammatical markers were deleted, particularly /s/ endings (e.g., possessive /-s/, regular third-person-singular verb tense). On single word articulation testing, errors were predominantly on consonant sequences, stridents, velars, and liquids. In conversation many more speech errors were noted, including sound and syllable deletions and sound prolongations. The Screening Test for Developmental Apraxia of Speech (Blakeley, 1980) was administered. According to this test, J's performance indicated that he had a 99% probability of DAS. The following behaviors were observed: oral articulatory groping for nonspeech movements, reduced verbal sequencing for consonant–vowel combinations, multiple distinctive feature errors per misarticulated sound, and slow speaking rate. Some hypernasality was noted. Examination of the oral mechanism revealed a bifid uvula but an intact hard palate. Follow-up of J's soft palate function via acoustical and aeromechanical examinations of resonance balance and velopharyngeal competency indicated that it was within normal limits. Further intensive speech treatment was recommended. Individual treatment was scheduled 4 months later. J was seen on a weekly basis over the subsequent 9 months. Treatment goals and outcomes were as follows:

- *Goal 1.* Consistent production of s, z, f, sh, ch, ing, th (voiced and voiceless), s blends and l blends in conversation. This goal was attained with the exception of target sounds in multisyllabic words. J achieved accuracy on complex combinations by slowing the rate of speech but articulatory groping was noted.
- *Goal 2.* Appropriate breath support and timing of inhalations in conversation. This was achieved as evidenced by a marked decrease in audible inhalations at inappropriate times. It was noted that J used short breath groups and increased his loudness level when excited. These behaviors could be altered with verbal cueing.
- *Goal 3.* Appropriate rate of speech to improve articulatory precision. J significantly reduced the rate of speech but needed verbal reminders to maintain a slowed rate in conversation.

Pre- and posttreatment intelligibility at the single word and sentence level was measured using the Test of Children's Speech (Hodge & Wellman, 1999). Comparison of the pre- and posttreatment results indicated that J made a 22% gain (63–85) in single word intelligibility and a 25% (70–95) gain in sentence intelligibility, and decreased his speaking rate from 170 to 125 in words per minute. Conversational speech was judged to be intelligible with careful listening. Unusual prosody, minimal oral opening during speech production, articulatory groping behaviors, intermittent hypernasality, and decreased articulatory precision on multisyllabic combinations continued to be present.

J was seen for eight additional treatment sessions to monitor rate control and improve multisyllabic word articulation. A finger-tapping strategy was introduced to facilitate a slower speaking rate. During telephone follow-up at 6-month intervals over the next 2 years the parents reported that J was more intelligible to unfamiliar listeners and was using conversational repair strategies effectively (e.g., repeating with greater oral opening, reducing rate, and tapping to cue syllables). At the end of the follow-up period, the parents reported that J was still making gains sequencing multisyllabic words but that speech prosody and rate continued to be unusual. They also mentioned that the grade 3 curriculum was difficult for J, necessitating extra practice at home on reading comprehension and written language skills. Information about J's fine motor skills and preferred social activities was not reported.

ACKNOWLEDGMENTS

We wish to thank Deborah Dewey, Robin Gaines, and Susan Rvachew for their very helpful suggestions in the preparation of this chapter and acknowledge support from the Canadian Language and Literacy Research Network in manuscript preparation.

REFERENCES

Ahmed, S., Lombardino, L., & Leonard, C. (2001). Specific language impairment: Definitions, causal mechanisms and neurobiological factors. *Journal of Medical Speech–Language Pathology, 9,* 1–15.

American Psychiatric Association. (1994). *Diagnostic and statistical manual of mental disorders* (4th ed.). Washington, DC: Author.

Baker, E., Croot, K., McLeod, S., & Paul, R. (2001). Psycholinguistic models of speech development and their application to clinical practice. *Journal of Speech, Language and Hearing Research, 44,* 685–702.

Ball, L., Bernthal, J., & Beukelman, D. (2002). Profiling communication characteristics of children with developmental apraxia of speech. *Journal of Medical Speech–Language Pathology, 10,* 221–229.

Bennett, S., & Netsell, R. (1999). Possible roles of the insula in speech and language processing: Directions for research. *Journal of Medical Speech–Language Pathology, 7,* 255–272.

Blakeley, R. W. (1980). *Screening test for developmental apraxia of speech.* Tigard, OR: C. C. Publications.

Bradford, A., & Dodd, B. (1994). The motor planning abilities of phonologically disordered children. *European Journal of Disorders of Communication, 29,* 349–369.

Bradford, A., & Dodd, B. (1996). Do all speech-disordered children have motor deficits? *Clinical Linguistics and Phonetics, 10,* 77–101.

Bruininks, R. H. (1978). *Bruininks–Oseretsky test of motor proficiency examiner's manual.* Circle Pines, MN: American Guidance Service.

Caplan, D. (1995). Language disorders. In R. Mapou & J. Spector (Eds.), *Clinical neuropsychological assessment: A cognitive approach (pp. 83–111).* New York: Plenum Press.

Clarke, M., Carr, L., Reilly, S., & Neville, B. (2000). Worster-Drought syndrome, a mild tetraplegic perisylvian cerebral palsy: Review of 47 cases. *Brain, 123,* 2160–2170.

Crary, M. (1993). *Developmental motor speech disorders.* San Diego, CA: Singular.

Davis, B., Jakeilski, K., & Marquardt, T. (1998). Developmental apraxia of speech: Determiners of differential diagnosis. *Clinical Linguistics and Phonetics, 12,* 25–45.

Dewey, D., Roy, E. A., Square-Storer, P., & Hayden, D. (1988). Limb and oral praxic abilities in children with verbal sequencing deficits. *Developmental Medicine and Child Neurology, 30,* 743–751.

Dodd, B. (1995). Procedures for classification of subgroups of speech disorder. In B. Dodd (Ed.), *The differential diagnoses and treatment of children with speech disorder* (pp. 49–64). San Diego, CA: Singular.

Dodd, B., Gillon, G., Oerlemans, M., Russell, T., Syrmis, M., & Wilson, H. (1995). Phonological disorder and the acquisition of literacy. In B. Dodd (Ed.), *The differential diagnoses and treatment of children with speech disorder* (pp. 125–146). San Diego, CA: Singular.

Dodd, B., & McCormack, P. (1995). A model of speech processing for differential diagnosis of phonological disorders. In B. Dodd (Ed.), *The differential diagnoses and treatment of children with speech disorder* (pp. 65–90). San Diego, CA: Singular.

Dronkers, N. (1996). A new brain region for coordinating speech articulation, *Nature, 383,* 159–161.

Duffy, J. (1995). *Motor speech disorders: Substrates, differential diagnosis and management.* St. Louis, MO: Mosby.

Felsenfeld, S., McGue, M., & Broen, P. (1995). Familial aggregation of phonological disorders: Results from a 28-year follow-up. *Journal of Speech and Hearing Research, 38,* 1091–1107.

Ferry, P., Hall, S., & Hicks, J. (1975). "Dilapidated" speech: Developmental verbal dyspraxia. *Developmental Medicine and Child Neurology, 17,* 749–756.

Fey, M. (1992). Articulation and phonology: Inextricable constructs in speech pathology. *Language Speech and Hearing Services in the Schools, 23,* 225–232.

Geirut, J. (1998). Treatment efficacy: Functional phonological disorders in children. *Journal of Speech, Language, and Hearing Research, 41,* S85–S100.

Habib, M., Daquin, G., Milandre, L., Royere, M., Rey, M., Lanteri, A., et al. (1995). Mutism and auditory agnosia due to bilateral insula damage-role of the insula in human communication. *Neuropsychologica, 33,* 327–339.

Hall, P., Jordan, L., & Robin, D. (1993). *Developmental apraxia of speech: Theory and clinical practice.* Austin, TX: Pro-Ed.

Hayden, D., & Square, P. (1999). *Verbal motor production assessment for children.* New York: The Psychological Corporation.

Hill, E. L. (1998). A dyspraxic deficit in specific language impairment and developmental coordination disorder? Evidence from hand and arm movements. *Developmental Medicine and Child Neurology, 40,* 388–395.

Hodge, M. (1998). Developmental coordination disorder: A diagnosis with theoretical and clinical implications for developmental apraxia of speech. *American Speech–Language–Hearing Association Special Interest Division 1 Newsletter: Language Learning and Education, 5,* 8–12.

Hodge, M. (2003). Clinical classification of children with developmental speech disorders: A transdisciplinary perspective. In L. Shriberg & T. Campbell (Eds.), *Proceedings of the 2002 Childhood Apraxia of Speech Research Symposium* (pp. 215–221). Carlsbad, CA: Hendrix Foundation.

Hodge, M., & Wellman, L. (1999). Management of children with dysarthria. In A. Caruso & E. Strand (Eds.), *Clinical management of motor speech disorders in children* (pp. 209–280). New York: Thieme.

Kent, R. (1992). Phonological development as biology and behavior. In R. Chapman (Ed.), *Processes in language acquisition and disorders* (pp. 67–85). St. Louis, MO: Mosby.

Kwiatkowski, J., & Shriberg, L. (1998). The capability–focus framework for child speech disorders. *American Journal of Speech–Language Pathology, 7,* 27–38.

Lai, C., Fisher, S., Hurst, J., Varga-Khadem, F., & Monaco, A. (2001). A forkhead-domain gene is mutated in a severe speech and language disorder. *Nature, 413,* 519–523.

Larrivee, L., & Catts, H. (1999). Early reading achievement in children with expressive phonological disorders. *American Journal of Speech–Language Pathology, 8,* 118–128.

Lehr, E. (1990). *Psychological management of traumatic brain injuries in children and adolescents.* Rockland, MD: Aspen.

Levelt, W. J. M. (1989). *Speaking: From intention to articulation.* Cambridge, MA: MIT Press.

Lewis, B., & Freebairn, L. (1992). Residual effects of preschool phonology disorders in grade school, adolescence and adulthood. *Journal of Speech and Hearing Research, 35,* 819–831.

Lewis, B., Freebairn, L., Hansen, A., & Taylor, H. (2002). School-age follow-up of children with apraxia of speech. *The ASHA Leader, 15,* 162.

Lewis, B., Shriberg, L., Freebairn, L., Hansen, A., Schick, J., & Iyengar, S. (2002). Phenotypes of families showing genetic linkage to chromosome 7. *The ASHA Leader, 15,* 162.

Mapou, R. (1995). A cognitive framework for neuropsychological assessment. In R. Mapou & J. Spector (Eds.), *Clinical neuropsychological assessment: A cognitive approach* (pp. 295–237). New York: Plenum Press.

Marquardt, T., & Sussman, H. (1991). Developmental apraxia of speech: Theory and practice. In D. Vogel & M. Cannito (Eds.), *Treating disordered speech motor control: For clinicians by clinicians* (pp. 341–390). Austin, TX: Pro-Ed.

Massaro, D. W. (1994). Psychological aspects of speech perception. In B. Dodd & R. Campbell (Eds.), *Hearing by eye: The psychology of lip reading* (pp. 53–83). Hillsdale, NJ: Erlbaum.

McCauley, R., & Strand, E. (1999). Treatment of children exhibiting phonological disorder with motor speech involvement. In A. Caruso & E. Strand (Eds.), *Clinical management of motor speech disorders in children* (pp. 187–208). New York: Thieme.

Minifie, F., Hixon, T. J., & Williams, F. (1973). *Normal aspects of speech, hearing and language*. Englewood Cliffs, NJ: Prentice-Hall.

Missiuna, C., Gaines, B., & Pollock, N. (2002). Recognizing and referring children at risk for developmental coordination disorders: Role of the speech-language pathologist. *Journal of Speech–Language Pathology and Audiology, 26,* 172–179.

Nelson, N. W. (1998). *Childhood language disorders in context: Infancy through adolescence* (2nd ed.). Boston: Allyn & Bacon.

Ojemann, G., & Mateer, C. (1977). Human language cortex: Location of memory, syntax and sequential motor–phoneme identification systems. *Science, 205,* 1401–1403.

Ozanne, A. (1995). The search for developmental verbal dyspraxia. In B. Dodd (Ed.), *The differential diagnoses and treatment of children with speech disorder* (pp. 91–109). San Diego, CA: Singular.

Paulesu, E., Frith, U., Snowling, M., Gallagher, A., Morton, J., Frackowiak, R., et al. (1996). Is developmental dyslexia a disconnection syndrome? *Brain, 119,* 143–157.

Portwood, M. (2000). *Understanding developmental dyspraxia.* London, UK: Fulton.

Raitano, N., Pennington, B., Tunick, R., Boada, R., & Shriberg, L. (2004). Pre-literacy skills of subgroups of children with speech sound disorders. *Journal of Child Psychology and Psychiatry, 45,* 821–835.

Shaywitz, B. A., Shaywitz, S. E., Pugh, K. R., Constable, R. T., Skudlarski, P., Fulbright, R. K., et al. (1995). Sex differences in the functional organization of the brain for language. *Nature, 373,* 607–609.

Shriberg, L. (1994). Five subtypes of developmental phonological disorders. *Clinics in Communication Disorders, 4,* 38–53.

Shriberg, L., Aram, D., & Kwiatkowski, J. (1997a). Developmental apraxia of speech: I. Descriptive and theoretical perspectives. *Journal of Speech, Language, and Hearing Research, 40,* 273–285.

Shriberg, L., Aram, D., & Kwiatkowski, J. (1997b). Developmental apraxia of speech: II. Toward a diagnostic marker. *Journal of Speech, Language and Hearing Research, 40,* 286–312.

Shriberg, L., Aram, D., & Kwiatkowski, J. (1997c). Developmental apraxia of speech: III. A subtype marked by inappropriate stress. *Journal of Speech, Language and Hearing Research, 40,* 313–337.

Shriberg, L., Austin, D., Lewis, B., McSweeny, J., & Wilson, D. (1997). The speech disorders classification system (SDCS): Extensions and lifespan reference data. *Journal of Speech, Language, Hearing Research, 40,* 723–740.

Shriberg, L., & Kwiatkowski, J. (1994). Developmental phonological disorders I: A clinical profile. *Journal of Speech, Language and Hearing Research, 37,* 1100–1126.

Shriberg, L., Tomblin, B., & McSweeny, J. (1999). Prevalence of speech delay in 6-year-old children with speech delay and comorbidity with language impairment. *Journal of Speech–Language–Hearing Research, 42,* 1461–1481.

Square, P. (1999). Treatment of developmental apraxia of speech: Tactile-kinesthetic, rhythmic, and gestural approaches. In A. Caruso & E. Strand (Eds.), *Clinical management of motor speech disorders in children* (pp. 149–185). New York: Thieme.

Stackhouse, J., & Snowling, M. (1992). Developmental verbal dyspraxia II: A developmental perspective on two case studies. *European Journal of Disorders of Communication, 27,* 35–54.

Stackhouse, J., & Wells, B. (1997). *Children's speech and literacy difficulties: A psycholinguistic framework.* San Diego, CA: Singular.

Stark, R., & Blackwell, P. (1997). Oral–volitional movements in children with language impairments. *Child Neuropsychology, 3,* 81–97.

Strand, E., & McCauley, R. (1999). Assessment procedures for treatment planning in children with phonologic and motor speech disorders. In A. Caruso & E. Strand (Eds.), *Clinical management of motor speech disorders in children* (pp. 73–107). New York: Thieme.

Strand, E., & Skinder, A. (1999). Treatment of developmental apraxia of speech: Integral stimulation methods. In A. Caruso & E. Strand (Eds.), *Clinical management of motor speech disorders in children* (pp. 109–148). New York: Thieme.

Tomblin, J. B., Records, N. L., Buckwalter, P. R., Zhang, X., Smith, E., & O'Brien, M. (1997). Prevalence of specific language impairment in kindergarten children. *Journal of Speech, Language, and Hearing Research, 40,* 1245–1260.

Tomblin, J. B., Records, N. L., & Zhang, X. (1996). A system for the diagnosis of specific language impairment in kindergarten children. *Journal of Speech, Language, and Hearing Research, 39,* 1284–1294.

Trauner, D., Wulfeck, B., Tallal, P., & Hesselink, J. (2000). Neurological and MRI profiles of children with developmental language impairment. *Developmental Medicine and Child Neurology, 42,* 470–475.

Van der Merwe, A. (1997). A theoretical framework of the characterization of pathological speech sensorimotor control. In M. McNeil (Ed.), *Clinical management of sensorimotor speech disorders* (pp. 1–25). New York: Thieme.

Walsh, B., & Smith, A. (2002). Articulatory movements in adolescence: Evidence for protracted development of speech motor control processes. *Journal of Speech, Language and Hearing Research, 45,* 1119–1133.

Watkins, K. E., Vargha-Khadem, F., Ashburner, J., Passingham, R. E., Connelly, A., Friston, K. J., et al. (2002). MRI analysis of an inherited speech and language disorder: Structural brain abnormalities. *Brain, 125,* 465–478.

Weschler, D. (1989). *WPPSI-R manual: Weschler Preschool and Primary Scale of Intelligence—Revised.* New York: Psychological Corporation.

CHAPTER 12

Developmental Motor Learning Disability

A NEUROPSYCHOLOGICAL APPROACH

TIMO AHONEN
LIBBE KOOISTRA
HELENA VIHOLAINEN
MARJA CANTELL

What are the motor problems associated with developmental coordination disorder, specific developmental disorder of motor function, and developmental dyspraxia? Are the motor problems associated with these disorders the same or different? Is there a better way of conceptualizing and describing these problems in children? The aim of this chapter is to present findings from studies that have examined these questions. We begin with a discussion of the various definitions and descriptions of developmental motor problems that have appeared in the research literature. We then discuss the current thinking on developmental motor disorders and the results of recent research that has investigated the long-term outcomes of children with these problems. Finally, we present a recently advanced neuropsychological theory of motor skills learning that could assist us in developing a better understanding of the motor learning disability experienced by these children.

FROM DYSPRAXIA AND DEVELOPMENTAL COORDINATION DISORDER TO MOTOR LEARNING DISABILITY

Many different terms have been applied to children who appear physically and intellectually normal yet lack the motor competence needed to cope with the demands of everyday living. Developmental clumsiness was first mentioned in the beginning of the century when Dupré (cited in Ford, 1966) described children with familial motor problems. The problems noted were atypical reflexes, associated movements, awkward voluntary movements, and diffuse mild hypotonia. Dupré called this a "motor deficiency." Collier, a contemporary, used a term *congenitally maladroit* and distinguished developmental clumsiness from cerebral palsy (cited in Ford, 1966).

In the 1930s, Orton suggested that atypical clumsiness, which he labeled "dyspraxia," was one of the developmental disorders typically found in children with dyslexia. He advanced the idea that the nature of the motor disorder was similar to other specific developmental difficulties in childhood. Moreover, he thought dyspraxia could not be explained by any neurological hard signs in the pyramidal or extrapyramidal systems, or in the cerebellum. He believed that dyspraxia was related to problems in voluntary movement planning (praxis) or visuospatial recognition (gnosia). He reported that children with these problems were not only delayed in learning the most simple movements, such as walking and running, but also delayed in manual and visuomotor tasks (Orton, 1937). Orton was among the first to suggest that clumsy children might have a specific motor learning problem (i.e., learning complex body movements and movements necessary for speech and writing). A decade later, Annell (1949) noted that although these children had normal or above-normal IQ, they had an obvious delay in learning everyday motor skills such as dressing, riding a bike, or fastening buttons.

In the 1960s, the term *developmental clumsiness* appeared in several publications (Gubbay, Ellis, Walton, & Court, 1965; Walton, Ellis, & Court, 1962), and in the 1970s, Gubbay (1975a, 1975b) defined clumsiness as developmental apraxia and agnosic ataxia. He considered clumsiness to be an expressive (apraxic) problem, a receptive (agnosic) problem, or an ataxic problem (seen as unsteady or uncoordinated movement)—or a combination of these three. Thus, overt manifestations of clumsiness were thought to vary considerably across individuals (Sugden & Sugden, 1990).

Into the 1980s, researchers such as Henderson and Hall (1982) continued to use Gubbay's (1975a) definition of clumsiness: "children whose level of competence in motor skills is significantly below the norm but who show no evidence of disease of the nervous system" (p. 39). Haubenstricker (1982) also identified a group of children "whose learning disability is manifested primarily in inadequate or inappropriate motor behaviour" (p. 41). By the end of the 1980s, the third revised edition of the *Diagnostic and Statistical Manual of Mental Disorders* (DSM-III-R; American Psychiatric Association, 1987) had labeled "clumsiness" as developmental coordination disorder (DCD). This diagnosis was developed to set developmental disorders of motor performance apart from other specific developmental disorders. Shortly after that, the World Health Organization (WHO; 1989, 1992) added the diagnosis "specific developmental disorder of motor function" (SDDMF) to ICD-10, under disorders of psychological development. The definition of DCD was further refined in DSM-IV (American Psychiatric Association, 1994). Table 12.1 provides the DSM-IV and ICD-10 definitions for DCD and SDDMF.

In the motor development area, and particularly among clinicians, the terms *developmental coordination disorder* and *developmental dyspraxia* are often used interchangeably. Among researchers in the field, however, they are rarely used synonymously, and there is much debate about their exact definitions. For some, the term *dyspraxia* has a much more specific meaning in that a clear line is drawn between deficits of movement planning or praxis and deficits of movement execution with disorders of execution not being included in the developmental classification rooted in the

TABLE 12.1. Definition of DCD and SDDMF

Developmental coordination disorder (DSM-IV, American Psychiatric Association, 1994)	Specific developmental disorder of motor function (ICD-10; World Health Organization, 1992)
Performance of daily activities that require motor coordination is substantially below that expected given the person's chronological age and measured intelligence (criterion A).	The child's motor coordination, on fine or gross motor tasks, should be significantly below the level expected on the basis of his or her age and general intelligence. This is best assessed on the basis of an individually administered, standardized test of fine and gross motor coordination. The difficulties in coordination should have been present since early in development (i.e., they should not constitute an acquired deficit). It is usual for the motor clumsiness to be associated with some degree of impaired performance on visuospatial cognitive tasks.
The disturbance in Criterion A significantly interferes with academic achievement or activities of daily living (criterion B).	
The diagnosis is made if the coordination difficulties are not due to a general medical condition (e.g., cerebral palsy, hemiplegia, or muscular dystrophy) and the criteria are not met for pervasive developmental disorder (criterion C).	
If mental retardation is present, the motor difficulties are in excess of those usually associated with it (criterion D).	

term *dypraxia* (Sugden & Keogh, 1990). Even more specific is the definition of dyspraxia proposed by Denckla and Roeltgen (1992) and Dewey (1995), who reserve the term *dyspraxia* for a disorder of gesture. According to their definition, the core deficit in developmental dyspraxia is a deficit in the performance of representational gestures (gestures relating to meaningful acts), nonrepresentational gestures (gestures relating to meaningless acts) and gesture sequences. This definition is more specific than the one proposed by Ayres (1972, 1985). She defined developmental dyspraxia as a disorder in planning and carrying out skilled, nonhabitual motor acts in the correct sequence. Some new research, which has attempted to bridge this definitional issue, suggests that it is possible to conceptualize DCD as either a planning disorder or a co-ordination/execution disorder. Planning disorders would be characterized by problems in knowing what to do and how to move, while coordination/execution disorders would be characterized by poorly coordinated performance in children who know what to do (Dewey, 2002).

PROBLEMS WITH THE PRESENT DEFINITIONS OF DEVELOPMENTAL COORDINATION DISORDER, SPECIFIC DEVELOPMENTAL DISORDER OF MOTOR FUNCTION, AND DEVELOPMENTAL DYSPRAXIA

Because of the difference definitions and diagnostic criteria proposed for DCD, SDDMF, and developmental dyspraxia, a fundamental question that must be addressed is whether these disorders constitute a unitary syndrome in terms of symptoms, etiology, treatment response, and outcome (Cantell, Kooistra, & Larkin, 2001).

The descriptions of the specific motor problems that are experienced by children with DCD, SDDMF, and developmental dyspraxia are often very similar. Both DSM-IV (i.e., DCD) and ICD-10 (i.e., SDDMF) diagnostic manuals describe movement at a functional level—that is, they refer to everyday goal-directed actions and acknowledge that the pattern of motor difficulties varies with age (Henderson & Barnett, 1998a). Definitions of dyspraxia also refer to everyday actions and indicate that the motor performance of children with dyspraxia can change with practice but that competent motor skills in one area do not generalize to other similar activities (Ayres, 1972, 1985). Of note is the fact that ICD-10 specifically mentions that children with dyspraxic deficits would be included in the diagnostic category of SDDMF. No mention of dyspraxia is made, however, within DSM-IV.

DSM-IV and ICD-10 use some of the same diagnostic criteria for inclusion; however, there are some clear differences, the most notable being that DSM-IV allows for the inclusion of children with mental retardation (MR) if the motor problems exceed those usually associated with MR, whereas, ICD-10 mandates that children must display normal IQ to be diagnosed with SDDMF. In terms of developmental dyspraxia, Gubbay (1975a) stated that children with developmental dyspraxia display normal intelligence and suggested that children with MR could not be diagnosed as dyspraxic. However, Dawdy (1981) questioned the idea that children needed to demonstrate normal intelligence before being diagnosed as developmentally dyspraxic. He suggested that children's motor skills should be compared to their level of cognitive development. If their motor skills were significantly poorer then one would expect based on intellectual level that dyspraxia was a possible diagnosis.

The inclusion of children with MR is a complicated one. Little attention has been paid to the IQ–motor ability discrepancy notion in the movement disorders literature. Further, "no attempt has been made to find out whether the motor difficulties experienced by intelligent children differ in any way from those experienced by less intellectually able children" (Henderson & Barnett, 1998b, p. 223). Finally, no normative data for the entire spectrum of movement difficulties are available and the research literature does not provide any indication of the appropriate discrepancy between motor and intellectual ability.

It is clear that children with motor problems display a wide range of cognitive ability. It has been suggested that there is a relationship between IQ and motor skills, with children with developmental motor problems obtaining higher scores on the Verbal IQ than Performance IQ on the Wechsler scales (Henderson & Barnett, 1998a). In contrast, Laszlo and Sainsbury (1994) claimed that motor problems do not appear to be correlated with IQ. Further, Knuckey and Gubbay (1983) failed to find an IQ difference between control children and children with motor problems.

Both DSM-IV and ICD-10 diagnostic criteria exclude children with medical conditions (e.g., cerebral palsy and muscular dystrophy) and identifiable neurological disorders (i.e., seizure disorders). The definition of SDDMF allows, however, for the inclusion of children with some neurodevelopmental immaturities (i.e., premature children). Similarly, Gubbay (1975a) stated that children with dyspraxia display normal findings on conventional neurological exams. Therefore, children with disorders such as cerebral palsy and neuromotor disorders such as muscular dystrophy would be excluded from this diagnosis. The line between these identifiable medical and neurological conditions and lesser disabilities of motor function and control is difficult.

It has been suggested that the presence of "soft" neurological signs may provide some indication of a neurological impairment and that children who display these signs should be excluded from a diagnosis of DCD, SDDMF, or developmental dyspraxia. However, there are few normative data on the occurrence of these signs, as our knowledge about the evolution of these signs is incomplete, and we know very little about their presence or absence and neurological development. It is possible that technological developments such as functional magnetic resonance imaging (fMRI) and positron emission tomography (PET) could enable the detection of heterogeneous neuropathological and pathophysiological lesions in the brains of children with various conditions which have associated motor impairments (Jongmans, Mercuri, Dubowitz, & Henderson, 1998). However, even if lesions or developmental abnormalities are detected, they may not always be associated with motor clumsiness. Therefore, the question remains as to where the line should be drawn between identifiable medical and neurological conditions and lesser disabilities which result in impairments of motor function and control.

Different requirements concerning assessment are also noted for these three diagnoses. In ICD-10, standardized tests of fine and gross motor coordination are advocated, while DSM-IV does not give any specific details on assessment. Although no specific requirements for the assessment of dyspraxia have been noted, recent definitions state that children with dyspraxia display a deficit in gestural performance (Dewey, 1995). Therefore, some measure of gestural performance is needed to confirm this diagnosis. At present, there are no generally accepted criteria that identify children with these disorders of motor function.

DSM-IV includes a specific prevalence of 6% in the age range of 5–11 years. Early studies of children with developmental dyspraxia reported a prevalence of between 4 and 8% in school-age children (Gubbay, 1975a; Henderson & Hall, 1982). ICD-10 does not provide prevalence rates. The developmental course of motor disabilities is described to vary with age in DSM-IV, ICD-10, and studies of children with developmental dyspraxia. DSM-IV suggests that in some cases, lack of coordination continues throughout adolescence into adulthood (see more details on developmental course below); ICD-10 does not provide any details regarding the developmental course. Studies of children with developmental dyspraxia have suggested that some of these children outgrow their problems in adolescence, whereas others continue to evidence difficulties into adulthood (Knuckey & Gubbay, 1983).

As indicated by the foregoing discussion, the diverse terminology used to label motor problems and the different definitions of the disorder still beg the question of whether we are referring to one disorder or many. In an attempt to address this issue, an international consensus meeting was organized in 1994 at the University of Western Ontario, London, Canada. In a consensus statement developed from the meeting, participants agreed to use the term *developmental coordination disorder* when referring to children with developmental motor problems. The London Consensus also described DCD as a chronic and usually permanent condition characterized by impairment of motor performance that was sufficient to produce functional motor performance deficits that were not explicable by the child's age or intellect, or by other diagnosable neurological or spatial–temporal organizational problems (Polatajko, Fox, & Missiuna, 1995). Despite this consensus, however, a number of terms continue to be used to describe and diagnose children with developmental motor deficits. Further, no universally agreed-on set of characteristics has been identified for these children. The field, however, does seem to agree on the fact that these problems are not due to general intellectual or gross sensory, motor, or neurological impairments (Smyth, 1992).

Recently several researchers, especially those involved in DCD intervention studies, are suggesting a new perspective, based on motor learning theory, that may better explain the specific difficulties that children with DCD have in learning motor skills (Hands & Larkin, 2001; Larkin & Parker, 2002; Missiuna & Mandich, 2002). Specifically, they have proposed that children with DCD, SDDMF, or developmental dyspraxia, may all be seen as having a "motor learning disability" (MLD). Therefore, in the remainder of this text, we use the term MLD, as we try to make our point that it is motor learning problems that all these children have in common.

THE PROBLEMS OF CHILDREN
WITH MOTOR LEARNING DISABILITIES

As described in the previous sections, children with MLD have typically been identified as having a general delay in motor development (i.e., late achievement of age-relevant milestones, such as walking, self-care, and handwriting). Further, it has been suggested that the movement difficulties of these children simply reflect performance at the lower end of the normal distribution (Ingram, 1963). In their review of 33 studies on developmental motor problems, Wall, Reid, and Paton (1990) concluded that the most typical features in these children were delayed motor development, slowness to dress, writing problems, poor balance, difficulties in ball skills, and gait problems.

Other investigators have suggested that MLD may be part of the spectrum of cerebral palsy (Dare & Gordon, 1970). Blondis, Snow, Roizen, Opacich, and Accordo (1993) used the term *minimal/mild cerebral palsy* to describe MLD and suggested that it forms a subtype of the "clumsy child syndrome." It is possible that mild impairment of perceptual motor abilities is consistent with a very mild degree of cerebral palsy, which may result in ungainly motor activity. However, the issue of the distinction between mild cerebral palsy and clumsiness is still unclear (Denckla & Roeltgen, 1992). The specific problems experienced by children with MLD are often not understood by others and can result in low motivation and poor self-perception and interfere profoundly with learning and performance (Neumann & Walker, 1996).

Although there is a broad agreement that the motor behaviors of children with MLD are qualitatively inferior to those of typically developing children, a clear understanding of the specific motor difficulties these children experience is still lacking (Cermak, Gubbay, & Larkin, 2002). One way to examine the motor performance of these children is to investigate the quality of their performance of motor skills. Research that has done this has reported that children with MLD display inconsistency, large trial-to-trial variation (Haubenstricker, 1982), perseveration, rhythmical difficulties (Denckla, 1984), inadequate use of force and tempo (Lundy-Ekman, Ivry, Keele, & Woollacott, 1991), and variable patterns of movement execution (Hoare, 1994) .

It appears then that children with MLD experience many different types of motor problems. Williams (2002) recognized the extensive heterogeneity of these motor control problems. She stated that in the research literature, 11 different types of motor problems were frequently reported. Like Wall and colleagues (1990), she found that slow reaction and movement times, as well as problems in balance and postural control, were consistently reported. She also stated that there is some evidence in the research literature that children with MLD have central nervous system involvement in their motor control difficulties. For example, Williams and Burke (1995) reported that the force of the conditioned patellar tendon reflex was greater in children with MLD than in children without MLD, which suggested that MLD may be linked to an increased sensitivity of the peripheral reflex loop.

SUBGROUPING EFFORTS OF MOTOR LEARNING DISABILITIES

Among the children with MLD, there are those who have MLD as an isolated disorder, but many of them are faced with additional problems. Poor coordination can affect a range of skills from self-care to athletic competence (Denckla & Roeltgen, 1992). The existence of additional or "comorbid" problems can either highlight or disguise MLD and therefore may have an effect on its diagnosis (see Piek & Pitcher, Chapter 14, and Dewey, Crawford, Wilson, & Kaplan, Chapter 18, this volume, for a more detailed discussion of this issue). Henderson and Hall (1982) identified three distinct subgroups of clumsy children. The children in the first group had above-average intelligence and no academic problems. Their motor impairments seemed to be an isolated problem. The second group was characterized by low academic achievement and their IQs were at the lower end of the normal range. The children in this group also had social and behavioral problems. In a third group, children were of mixed ability and could not readily be classified in either of the preceding groups. Henderson (1987, 1993) noted that classifying MLD as a "pure" disorder (i.e., not associated with any other developmental disorders) would result in including only children with high IQ. Children who displayed other problems in addition to MLD would be excluded from the diagnosis.

Many others acknowledge the existence of specific subtypes of motor performance deficits (Ahonen, 1990; Cermak, 1985; Deuel & Doar, 1992; Miyahara, 1994). Some studies have emphasized a distinction between motor planning and motor execution (David et al., 1981; Dewey & Kaplan, 1992), whereas others have sought to describe subgroup differences in terms of underlying deficits in sensory processing (Hulme, Smart, & Moran, 1982; Laszlo, Bairstow, Bartrip, & Rolfe, 1988; Mon-Williams, Pascal, & Wann, 1994). In an attempt to refine the search for subtypes, some researchers have turned to statistical clustering approaches (Ahonen, 1990; Dewey & Kaplan, 1994; Dewey, Kaplan, Wilson, & Crawford, 1999; Hoare, 1994; Miyahara, 1994). For example, Hoare (1994) tried to identify homogeneous groups within a pool of children with perceptual motor problems. She based her cluster analysis on five factors of movement dysfunction (i.e., manual dexterity, gross body coordination, vision, balance/hop, and active kinesthesis). Five subtypes were found: gross motor problems, good visual perception, perceptual dysfunction, good kinesthetic processing, and execution problems. Additional information related to the existence of distinct motor profiles has come from studies that have included children with learning disabilities. Miyahara (1994) identified four subtypes of children: a subtype with gross motor problems, another one with poor balance, a group with no motor problems, and a fourth group with good balance but poor running speed.

A key problem with the studies using statistical clustering techniques is that their outcomes are entirely dependent on the measures used (Aldenderfer & Blashfield, 1984; MacNab, Miller, & Polatajko, 2001; Morris, Blashfield, & Satz, 1981), which seriously limits the validity of these studies and thus undermines their attempts to generate specific information concerning etiology and treatment of MLD. In view of the limitations of these studies, Kaplan, Wilson, Dewey, and Crawford (1998) argued that the usefulness of subtyping is questionable, although some broad subgroups of developmental disorders might exist. They concluded that because there is such a large degree of overlap between different childhood disorders, comorbidity was the rule rather than the exception. Dewey (2002) suggested that instead of investigating subtypes of MLD, it may be useful to investigate the combinations of problems (i.e., motor, attention, and learning) displayed by children with developmental disorders as this would provide a clearer picture of the child's overall disability.

POSSIBLE CAUSES OF MOTOR LEARNING DISABILITIES

About 6% of all children display MLDs. Some studies report slightly different prevalence rates, but the range is between 4 and 13%, depending on the cutoff system and tests used (Kadesjo & Gillberg, 1999; Wright & Sugden, 1996). The severity of the problems varies with about 5% of children having a clearly notable MLD and 2% of children having a more serious form of MLD that profoundly interferes with daily life activities (Ahonen, 1990; Knuckey & Gubbay, 1983; van Dellen, Vassen, & Schoemaker, 1990). MLD is nearly without exception reported to occur three times more often in boys than in girls (Henderson & Hall, 1982; Keogh, Sugden, Reynard, & Calkins, 1979; Schoemaker, Hijlkema, & Kalverboer, 1994). Brenner and Gillman (1966), Gubbay (1975a), and Iloeje (1987), however, failed to find this male preponderance.

There is no single factor that causes MLD and its etiology remains unclear (Wall et al., 1990). Various causes of MLD have been postulated. Pre- or perinatal incidents affecting early brain development are thought to play a critical role. Affected children with motor dysfunctions, therefore, were once considered to be suffering from "minimal brain damage" (Blondis eta l., 1993; Gubbay, 1985; Kalverboer, de Vries, & van Dellen, 1990; Walton et al., 1962). (It is important to note that the view that "brain damage" is the primary aspect of MLD has been completely abandoned.) Although some studies have found a higher occurrence of pre- or perinatal incidents, others have not. Therefore, no definite conclusion with respect to the causal role of such incidents can be made (Cermak et al. , 2002). More neurologically oriented researchers, using electroencephalograms (EEGs) and other brain mapping techniques, have not been able to demonstrate causal relationships between MLD and factors such as metabolic problems, maternal drug use, or vitamin deficiencies (Gubbay, 1975a; Knuckey & Gubbay, 1983).

In the absence of a clear neurological basis for MLD, many researchers have focused on neurological soft signs, such as hypotonia and associated, mirror, or choreiform movements. These signs appear as a form of deviant performance on subtests in neurological examinations but cannot be linked to concrete neurological abnormalities (Neumann & Walker, 1996). Although more soft signs are found in children with MLD than in controls (Henderson & Hall, 1982; Iloeje, 1987; Losse et al., 1991) their etiological significance for MLD is still disputed (Touwen, 1993).

Parts of the central nervous system, which have a predominant role in motor control, are the basal ganglia, the cerebellum, and the motor cortex. Dysfunction of these structures could result in movement difficulties such as coordination and timing problems, hypotonia, and dysmetria (Greer, 1984). Although these signs are sometimes present in children with MLD, they do not offer a satisfactory explanation for all the problems experienced by these children (Henderson, 1993). Recently, Wilson, Thomas, and Maruff (2002) studied procedural learning in children with MLD. Their findings suggested that MLD is an impairment in the ability to automatize motor skills. Furthermore, reduced automatization was linked to immaturity in the development of neural pathways from the motor centers of the cortex to the basal ganglia.

At a psychological level, researchers have examined whether MLD is due to processing deficits. Most of this research has concentrated on deficits in perceptual processes that involve the input of information such as visual (Hulme, Biggerstaff, Moran, & McKinlay, 1982; Lord & Hulme, 1987b) or kinesthetic (Laszlo & Bairstow, 1985; Lord & Hulme, 1987a) processes (see Wilson, Chapter 13, this volume, for a more detailed discussion). Other studies have focused on the central decision processes of motor preparation (Smyth & Glencross, 1986; van Dellen & Geuze, 1988). Although the findings of these two studies were not identical, results indicated that children with MLD had problems in selecting the right response, particularly in situations in which they have to process a large amount of information. Some studies have also investigated output related processes; Bairstow and Laszlo (1989) concluded that children with MLD had difficulties in converting current movement information into the appropriate motor commands.

The foregoing discussion clearly shows that the problems of children with MLD are multidimensional and that no single factor has been identified as the direct cause of MLD (Kalverboer, 1988). MLD has often cumulative long-term effects on cognitive and social emotional development (see the following section). Therefore, there is a need for exploration of multicausative models in order to understand the interplay between genetic predisposition, brain structure and pre- and postnatal experience in MLD (Cermak et al., 2002; Hadders-Algra, 2002).

PERSISTENCY OF MOTOR LEARNING DISABILITY AND LONG-TERM OUTCOMES

The literature on MLD in later childhood and adolescence offers two different and sometimes contradictory views on how persistent the problems are (Cantell & Kooistra, 2002; Cantell, Smyth, & Ahonen, 1994, 2003). There is an optimistic view of MLD that states that it is mostly confined to childhood and it decreases with age. This is supported by Erhardt, McKinlay, and Bradley (1987), who showed that it took uncoordinated adolescents longer to reach a ceiling in terms of their motor performance. Hall (1988) claimed that this finding showed that motor problems disappear by adolescence and that, therefore, they could not be called a long-term disability. The results of Knuckey and Gubbay (1983) could also be interpreted as falling into this optimistic category. They found that children with mild to moderate MLD improved to normality by age 16–20 years and concluded that MLD is a problem that is largely confined to childhood rather than a long-term disability. However, they also showed that a particular category of children with severe MLD had a less favorable outcome. Knuckey and Gubbay suggested that a maturational lag might be the etiology in mild MLD, whereas, structural lesions involving the cerebral cortex might be present in the more severely afflicted children.

The more pessimistic view is that MLD does not disappear as a function of age. In at least four different follow-up studies (Ahonen, 1990; Geuze & Borger, 1993; Gillberg & Gillberg, 1989; Losse et al., 1991), the results have shown that more than half of the children with MLD continue to display poorer motor performance into adolescence. Losse and colleagues (1991) followed a group of 16 children with MLD into adolescence and found that the prognosis for these children was not favorable. At the age of 16, a majority of the adolescents had motor difficulties in addition to a range of educational, social, and emotional problems. Likewise, Geuze and Borger (1993), in a 5-year follow-up of 19 children with MLD found that half of the population still experienced serious motor problems between the ages of 11 and 17 years. The same results with respect to persistency of MLD into adolescence were found by Ahonen (1990) and Cantell and colleagues (1994, 2003) who followed 65 children until the age of 17. Gillberg and Gillberg (1989) discussed movement problems in the wider context of motor/perceptual dysfunction (MPD) and deficits in attention, motor control, and perception (DAMP). They have reported that half of the children with DAMP stayed persistently clumsy between ages 7 and 13, while the other half of their population improved and displayed motor performance similar to the control children by 13 years of age. Interestingly, however, a different picture emerged with respect to academic and behavioral outcome; most of the children with DAMP had persistent academic or behavioral problems up to 13 years of age. It was concluded that catching up with motor development did not always result in the disappearance of academic and social problems.

An important reason for investigating the long-term outcome of MLD is the disproportionate incidence of academic, behavioral, and social problems that these children have (Ahonen, 1990; Cantell et al., 1994, 2003; Deuel, 1992; Geuze & Borger, 1993; Henderson, 1987; Losse et al., 1991; Smyth, 1992). For example, Cantell and colleagues (2003) found that at the age of 17, only 29% of the adolescents with MLD were attending high school and 10% did not attend any education at all and were unemployed. Teachers also reported other problems, such as a lack of friendships in these adolescents. The reasons for these problems are not entirely clear, although it has been hypothesized that poor motor coordination has wide-reaching effects on children's learning skills and interaction with others.

The conclusion that can be drawn from these studies is that MLD does not disappear as a function of age. An alternative way to consider these findings would be to say that while some children with MLD do "grow out of it," some do not. Unfortunately, none of the follow-up studies have reported what has happened to those children who were originally judged to be lacking in coordination but who had caught up with their control groups in terms of their motor development during adolescence. Recently, some retrospective studies have suggested that several pathways for MLD exist (Cousins & Smyth, 2003; Fitzpatrick, 2003) and that mechanisms such as adaptation and compensation would be worth studying (Cantell & Kooistra, 2002; May-Benson, Ingolia, & Koomar, 2002).

The same controversy on positive and negative outcomes can be found in studies that have focused on the slightly different but related research areas of minimal brain dysfunction (MBD) or minor neurological dysfunction (MND). Soorani-Lunsing, Hadders-Algra, Huisjes, and Touwen (1994) and Hadders-Algra (2002), differentiated between two types of MND, "complex MND," which is a persistent type and "simple MND," which is a transient type. The persistent one was related to a negative academic and behavioral outcome, whereas the transient type had a positive long-term outcome resulting in the normalization of both the neurological functions and other functions, like motor, behavioral, and cognitive functions.

Overall, the findings of studies that have investigated long-term outcomes suggest that problems in perceptual motor development early in the school years may have a disadvantageous effect on educational and social development, although it may only be the case for the most severely affected children (Cantell et al., 1994, 2003; Hadders-Algra, 2002; Soorani-Lunsing et al., 1994; Touwen, 1993). The resolution of the MLD itself may not be the most important factor in determining a successful outcome for children in social and educational terms. Children who are initially categorized as having impaired motor development may remain in a group of "difficult" children in school even if their motor performance improves to the level of their peers in adolescence (Norwich, 1997). Obviously, an important question for future research is how lack of basic motor competence, lack of practice, and lack of motivation interact to affect long-term outcomes in children with MLD.

MODELS OF MOTOR LEARNING

It has been suggested that the motor problems of children with DCD can be explained using four key components of motor learning theory (i.e., the stage of the learner, the type of task, the scheduling of practice, and the type of feedback) (Missiuna & Mandich, 2002). Fitts and Posner (1967) described three stages of skill acquisition (i.e., cognitive, associative, and autonomous), which have been used in designing recent intervention efforts in children with MLD (Miller, Polatajko, Missiuna, Mandich, & Macnab, 2001; Wright, 1998). From a motor learning perspective, the motor problems seen in these children typically reflect basic difficulty in learning and executing novel motor tasks, as well as generalizing these newly acquired skills to new situations (Goodgold-Edwards & Cermak, 1990; Missiuna, 1994). In other words, children with MLD do not appear to have the basic skills required to analyze task demands, interpret appropriate cues from the environment, and use knowledge of their performance to prepare for upcoming actions (Lefebvre & Reid, 1998). (It is important to note that some of these learning problems have also been described in children with dyspraxia, which, once again, shows the overlap of the terminology used for identifying problems in motor skills.) Motor learning theory can also be viewed from an ecological or dynamic systems perspective as suggested by Missiuna and Mandich (2002) and Larkin and Parker (2002). These perspectives imply that factors related to the learner's attributes, physique, fitness, cognition, and motivation are important to consider when selecting learning tasks and instructional designs. It is assumed that learning occurs when the multiple systems within the child interact cooperatively with the functional task demands and with the environmental context. As a consequence, the role of the teacher or therapist is to analyze the movement problems or action goals, thereby taking into account the variable features of the task, the child, and the environment. These are seen as "constraints," related to the learner, the task, and the environment (Newell, 1986).

Recently, several researchers in the field, especially those involved in intervention, have proposed an alternative perspective that may assist us in better understanding of the specific difficulties children with MLD experience in learning motor skills (Hands & Larkin, 2001; Larkin & Parker, 2002; Missiuna & Mandich, 2002). This view, based on Gentile's (1998) theory of motor learning, proposes that there are two types of motor learning processes, that is, explicit and implicit. Explicit processes involve the conscious mapping of a set of correspondences between the child and the environmental conditions in order to achieve the action goal. Implicit processes include the unconscious organization of components such as the positioning of the joints and response to gravity. These processes are at first only crudely organized, but with continued practice they become more controlled and finely tuned. As a result, the performance efficiency increases. Gentile's concepts of explicit and implicit learning processes are consistent with the neuropsychological approach, which we describe in the next section.

A NEUROPSYCHOLOGICAL APPROACH TO MOTOR LEARNING

As the foregoing review has shown, we know much about the clinical features of children with MLD. We also know that these children may have a variety of difficulties in motor control. Therefore, it is possible that within the MLD population there are different subgroups of children with different core deficits underlying their motor problems. We can also assume that behind these core deficits there may be individual differences in brain development and functioning. What is lacking though is a consistent theory that takes into account these various research findings.

Recently, Willingham (1998) formulated a detailed neuropsychological theory of motor skill learning, the "control-based learning theory" (COBALT), which may assist in integrating the research findings concerning developmental motor problems. Its key assumption is that learning new motor skills evolves directly from motor control processes. The theory uses three principles of motor control to further our understanding of motor skill learning: (1) the neural separability principle, (2) the disparate representation principle, and (3) the dual-mode principle (see the conceptual framework in Figure 12.1.). *The neural separability principle* proposes that different cognitive components of motor control (i.e., strategic processes, perceptual–motor processes, sequencing processes, and dynamic processes) are associated with anatomically distinct parts of the brain. This principle is very similar to the theory of dynamic localization proposed by Luria (1973) and suggests that groups of simultaneously working zones of the brain are responsible for the performance of complex mental activity. *The disparate representation principle* proposes that the different cognitive components of complex activity utilize different forms of representation. *The dual-mode principle* proposes that motor acts can be executed in either a conscious, effortful or an unconscious, automatic mode.

It is important to note here that Willingham's (1998) theory was originally devised to account for the development of spatial accuracy in normal motor behavior. For the purpose of this chapter, therefore, it is used as a conceptual framework with

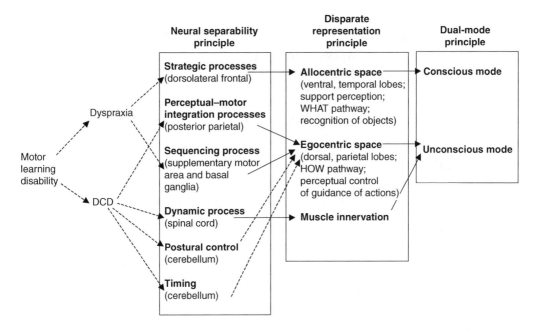

FIGURE 12.1. A schematic diagram of the process contributing to motor learning disability derived from the theory of Willingham (1998). Solid lines show connections suggested by Willingham, the dashed lines show hypothetical connections suggested by the authors.

some modifications added to it, to account for the typical motor difficulties seen in children with MLD (i.e., difficulties in temporal accuracy and postural control). In the following sections, we summarize the main points of the COBALT theory, and then we try to align the findings of the research on MLD and the theory's main concepts.

Neural Separability Principle

The COBALT theory identifies four separate processes with distinct neural bases that underlie motor control: strategic, perceptual–motor integration, motor sequencing, and dynamic processes. The *strategic processes* identify the *goal* of motor activities. The dorsolateral frontal cortex is the main structure responsible for these high-level planning processes of motor activity (Willingham, 1998). According to Fuster (2000), the entire cortex of the primate's frontal lobe seems to be dedicated to organismic action. It can be considered as a whole motor or executive cortex. The executive functions can be conceptualized as a hierarchical system of action control comprising volition, planning, selection, programming, and performance of movement (Seitz, Stephan, & Binkofski, 2000). Frontal executive networks are hierarchically organized, similar to posterior perceptual networks. At the top is the prefrontal cortex, which represents the broad schemas of action in skeletal and speech domains. One of the most consistent components of the prefrontal lesion syndrome is the difficulty in formulating and enacting plans of behavioral, linguistic, or cognitive action (Fuster, 2000).

When trying to understand acquired or developmental disorders of voluntary motor actions the concept of planning is very central. In the typology of apraxia in adults, Roy (1978) identified three types of apraxia: (1) planning apraxia with two subcategories (i.e., *primary* and *secondary* planning apraxia), (2) execution apraxia, and (3) unit apraxia. Defects in primary planning apraxia are characterized by disturbances in the ability to conceptually organize the required movement sequence and a general cognitive organizational disorder not restricted to motor behavior. The neural basis of this syndrome is in frontal pathology. In secondary planning apraxia, which is due to parietooccipital pathology, the difficulties in planning are the result of spatial disorientation. Execution apraxia is due to pathology of premotor areas and is characterized by an inability to perform an intended action due to disturbance in execution of the planned motor sequences. Unit apraxia is associated with pathology in the precentral and postcentral motor areas and results in problems in producing individual movements and limb positions, which are associated with loss of strength or loss of kinesthetic sense.

The distinction between planning and execution could also improve our understanding of the nature of MLD. In the study by Dewey and Kaplan (1994), three subgroups of children with MLD were identified: (1) one with deficits in motor sequencing; (2) another with deficits in balance, coordination, and gestural performance; and (3) a third group with deficits in all motor skill areas. The finding of a subgroup with a disturbance in motor sequencing was consistent with Roy's (1978) classification of primary planning apraxia and the finding of a subgroup with deficits in balance, coordination, and gestural performance was consistent with Roy's classification of executive apraxia. Thus, these findings suggest that for some children with MLD, the problem may be in formulating a plan of action. In other words, they have deficits in the strategic processes, which are associated with the neural activity that takes place before motor execution has begun. However, other children with MLD, may be able to formulate the plan but have difficulties in executing it effectively (Dewey, 2002).

The *perceptual–motor integration processes* can be seen as processes involved in *selecting* targets for movements. The posterior parietal cortex is the main structure involved in developing representations that serve as targets for movements. The premotor cortex, however, is also critical for visually guided movements. The posterior parietal cortex selects individual spatial targets, and the premotor cortex contributes to the execution of movements to these targets (Willingham, 1998).

The term *perceptual* is often used to describe the processes by which sensory information is registered, integrated, and interpreted. Most researchers in the MLD field assume that some disruption of perceptual and/or motor control mechanisms underlie the disorder. A meta-analysis of existing research findings (Wilson & McKenzie, 1998) showed that children with MLD performed worse than did control children on measures of information processing. Deficits were pronounced in complex visuospatial, visuoperceptual, and cross-modal perception measures. Because the processing of visual information provides the substrate for subsequent processing operations, impaired visual processing would be expected to result in problems in motor coordination.

Perceptual–motor subtypes have been reported in the studies that have investigated possible subtypes of MLD. As described earlier, Hoare (1994) described a subtype with specific difficulties on both visual and kinesthetic tasks. Another subtype displayed significant discrepancy between their kinesthetic and visual processing. We also found different subtypes with visuospatial and kinesthetic problems in our longitudinal study (Ahonen, 1990; Cantell et al., 1994, 2003). Interestingly, the term *somatodyspraxia* has been used to refer to a subgroup of children whose MLD is hypothesized to be due to poor somatosensory processing (Cermak, 1991). These children have difficulty in learning new tasks, but once learned, the task can be performed with adequate skill.

The *motor sequencing processes* are those processes involved in the activation of the supplementary motor area and basal ganglia. The left hemisphere seems to be dominant for movement sequencing and it is possible that it is dominant not only in learning to select movements in sequence but also in learning to select a limb movement that is appropriate for using a particular object (Leiguarda & Marsden, 2000). Furthermore, different neural systems are actively engaged in the preparation and generation of a sequential action depending on whether the sequence is a prelearned or a new one. In the execution of automatic and overlearned sequential movements, the supplementary motor area and basal ganglia are mainly involved. When sequences are very complex or new, prefrontal, premotor, and parietal mechanisms are used (Leiguarda & Marsden, 2000).

According to Williams (2002), the variability that is characteristic of the execution of movements carried out by children with MLD can be the result of their motor slowness and inconsistency. Furthermore, this can be seen as an indication of problems in the underlying central nervous system processes involved in organizing the upcoming movement sequences. In fact, one of the main features of MLD, especially dyspraxic problems, is the inability to learn or to perform serial voluntary movements to complete skilled acts (Deuel & Doar, 1992; Dewey & Kaplan, 1994).

The *dynamic processes* are those associated with the innervation of muscles (Willingham, 1998). The primary motor cortex codes movements in space—not specific muscle commands—that are projected via the interneurons in the spinal cord. These neurons project to motoneurons, which innervate muscles. Thus, spinal interneurons are likely candidates in the transformation between spatial and motor information.

Children with MLD seem to exhibit greater electromyographic activity than others when performing fine motor tasks, and there is a tendency to overuse muscles to fixate the joints for stability (Wilson & Trombly, 1984). Therefore, one reason for these children's variable movement patterns could be the inappropriate application of muscle force. It has been shown that there may be developmental differences in the input–output properties of the alpha motoneuron pool between children with and without MLD (Williams & Burke, 1995). Changes in sensory feedback and/or motoneuron excitability of the peripheral reflex loop, crossed-spinal pathways, and supraspinal pathways may be impaired in these children. The spinal and supraspinal influences are important because the successful performance of voluntary movements depends on the ability of the central nervous system (CNS) to regulate the excitability of the alpha motoneuron pool (i.e., the final common pathway).

In addition to the aforementioned four processes proposed by Willingham (see Figure 12.1), two additional processes could be added to his model, which could help in integrating the empirical findings concerning the motor problems of children with MLD. The first is *timing*; the second is *postural control*. Both of these processes are closely related to the functions of the cerebellum, which is involved in the regulation of balance, posture, gait, dynamic motor planning, fine motor control, and motor timing.

Rhythmic coordination or *timing* of movements is universally recognized as a common deficit in MLD. Furthermore, children with MLD do not show improvements in timing ability as they mature (Williams, 2002; Williams, Woollacott, & Ivry, 1992). They have difficulties establishing a given rate of tapping to an external stimulus and then maintaining the given rate when the external stimulus is no longer present. The link between different types of soft neurological signs and timing in children with MLD has been studied by Lundy-Ekman and colleagues (1991). They identified one group of children with soft signs indicative of cerebellar disorder and a second group with soft signs associated with basal ganglia dysfunction. Results on a motor-tapping task showed a consistent dissociation between groups. In contrast to the other children, the children with cerebellar signs were unable to maintain a steady tapping rate, similar to patients with lesions of the lateral cerebellum.

Postural control involves controlling the body's position in space for the dual purposes of stability and orientation. Postural stability, or balance, is the ability to maintain the body in equilibrium. The development of postural control is an essential aspect of the development of skilled actions, such as locomotion and manipulation (Shumway-Cook & Woollacott, 2001). One of the common features in children with MLD is poor balance and/or postural control, and it is possible that the poor balance is a major source of the problems underlying poor coordination in children with MLD (Williams et al., 1992). It appears that the difficulties seen in these children are not only in the executory or manipulative phase of the action but also in the positioning, postural, or preparatory phase.

Input from visual, somatosensory, and vestibular systems are important sources of information on the body's position and movement in space. Using a moving room paradigm, Wann, Mon-Williams, and Rushton (1998) found that children with MLD swayed significantly more than did the control children when asked to stand in a simple, upright position with eyes open. This suggests that children with MLD may be slow in developing the capacity to process proprioceptive input and to effectively integrate visual and proprioceptive information. Children with MLD have also been found to be significantly more variable than children without MLD in activating postural synergies to counteract anterior sway but not to backward sway (Williams & Woollacott, 1997). The postural control system of children with MLD tends to activate responses quickly on some occasions and extremely slowly on others. Such difficulties could be the result of a motor dysfunction in the flocculonodular system or in the vermal cerebellar structures, which typically result in disturbances in posture and balance.

Disparate Representation Principle

The second main principle in Willingham's (1998) theory is called the disparate representation principle. According to this principle, different cognitive components use different forms of representation. The brain uses multiple spatial frames of reference for planning movements. In so-called allocentric representations, objects' locations are coded relative to one another and these representations are dedicated to conscious perception. Anatomically this processing stream progresses ventrally to the temporal lobe.

Allocentric spatial representations are used for strategic processes in goal selection. Likewise, in *egocentric* representations, objects' locations are coded relative to some part of the body. These representations are dedicated to movement and are not open to awareness. Anatomically, this processing stream progresses dorsally into the parietal lobe. These egocentric spatial representations are used for perceptual–motor integration and sequencing.

As noted previously, visuoperceptual problems are common in children with MLD. Rösblad (2002) identified two research traditions on visual information processing and motor control in children with MLD. The first one could be described as studies of perception for apprehension and its relationship with movement control (i.e., figure–ground tests, shape and line discrimination, visual memory for shape, and reproduction of geometric patterns). These studies have shown that although children with MLD perform poorly on tests of visual perception, there is still a fundamental lack of understanding of how their performance on visuoperceptual tests affects motor control (Rösblad, 2002). The second tradition described by Rösblad is founded in studies of perception for action. In this research, the ability to use perceptual information for movement planning and control is tested, and movement outcome is often measured directly with various motion analysis systems. Studies of reaching fall within this tradition. Reaching can be divided into two functional components: the transport phase and the grasp phase. For the transport phase, visual information is needed for planning and programming the movement. In the grasp phase the control of the isometric fingertip forces applied to an object is important for proper execution of various hand tasks. Developmental studies have shown that small children use excessive grip force and a large safety margin (Forssberg et al., 1999). Pereira, Landgren, Gillberg, and Forssberg (2001) found that children with MLD exhibited disturbances of the basic coordination of forces in the initial transport phase of the movement, manifested by longer time latencies and higher force levels than those of the control group. Higher grip forces and safety margins and greater variation in the parametric control of the grip force were also documented for children with MLD. Van der Meulen, van der Gon, Gielen, Gooskens, and Willemse (1991) suggested that in reaching tasks with or without visual feedback, the problems of children with MLD could be explained by both less developed ability for anticipatory control and difficulties in using visual information. However, Rösblad and von Hofsten (1994) reported that the differences between MLD and control children were not in the use of visual feedback but in movement speed. They suggested that children with MLD moved consistently more slowly because anticipatory control strategies were less developed. Due to this inefficiency, children with MLD have to rely on feedback control (Rösblad, 2002). But what is the reason for the impaired capacity in anticipatory control?

New to the MLD field are a number of studies that are attempting to address this issue. They include studies of motor imagery in children with MLD (Katschmarsky, Cairney, Maruff, Wilson, & Currie, 2001; Maruff, Wilson, Trebilcock, & Currie, 1999; Wilson, Maruff, Ives, & Currie, 2001). These studies are based on the idea that imagined motor performance is subject to the same environmental and physiological constraints as real motor performance. Interestingly, results have indicated that the preparation and internal representation of volitional movements was impaired in children with MLD. Because this impairment occurred only for movements performed in imagination, it could not be attributed to motor output systems. This suggests that problems in programming force and timing, which result in an inability to generate accurate internal representations of volitional movements, may reflect an impaired ability to process efference copy or corollary discharge signals in the parietal lobes (Jordan, 1995).

Dual-Mode Principle

The third main principle in Willingham's (1998) theory is the dual-mode principle. According to this principle, all voluntary actions are initiated by a conscious environmental goal, but the subsequent transformations (i.e., perceptual–motor integration, sequencing, and dynamic process) generate representations for the movement outside awareness. The strategic process that is conscious is proposed to be dependent on attention, but the following processes are not. Usually, we use the conscious mode when performing an unfamiliar task, but when we get more experience, we move to the unconscious mode. This process is usually referred to as the development of automatization. The dual-mode principle proposes that even a well-practiced skill can be executed in a conscious, attention-demanding manner, similar to learning a novel skill.

In learning disability research, an "automatization deficit" has been proposed as one possible core deficit (Nicholson & Fawcett, 1990). The automatization hypothesis states that children with learning disabilities (especially dyslexia) have difficulties in becoming an expert in any skill that requires "automatic" performance and consequently suffer problems in fluency for any skill that should become automatic through extensive practice (Nicholson & Fawcett, 1990). Support for this hypothesis comes from findings showing that children with dyslexia often have problems in balance and motor skill learning (Nicholson & Fawcett, 2001). Fawcett and Nicolson (1999) found that up to 80% of a sample of 60 dyslexic children showed behavioral signs of cerebellar deficit. This is interesting because the neuropsychological basis for difficulties in the automatization of motor skills is proposed to be in cerebellum. In a PET study (Nicholson et al., 1999), brain activation was significantly lower for the dyslexic adults than for the controls in the right cerebellar cortex when learning a new sequence of finger movements. The question of the specific contribution of the cerebellum to motor learning and automatization, however, needs more research because it has also been proposed that the cerebellum does not necessarily contribute to learning of the motor skill itself but is engaged primarily in the modification of performance (Seidler et al., 2002).

MOTOR SKILL LEARNING
FROM A NEUROPSYCHOLOGICAL PERSPECTIVE

Willingham's (1998) theory proposes two key mechanisms that support motor skill learning. The first is *learning through strategic processes* so that more effective high-level goals or more effective spatial targets for movement are selected and sequenced. The improved selection of high-level goals results in improved strategy. Although being able to describe how to execute a task does not mean that one can actually do it, the theory predicts that the actor will be more successful with strategic knowledge than without it. The usefulness of strategic knowledge depends on its precision regarding spatial targets.

According to Gentile (1998), an action goal defines certain features of the environment as critical for successful task performance. Therefore, an action goal specifies a mapping function between the performer and the environment. Like Willingham, Gentile also assumes that this strategic or explicit learning process is open to conscious awareness. During this learning process an internal model of the motor skill is being developed and this internal model simulates the most important features of the performer's morphology and environmental constraints. Using this internal model it is possible to produce movements without customary environmental conditions being present—that is, pantomime performance.

In children with MLD, and more specifically those with disorders in gestural performance (Dewey, 1995), the difficulty in learning new gestures may be due to deficits in these strategic or explicit processes. Strategic learning is also related to the more general executive functions associated with the frontal systems. Therefore, children with MLD may have difficulties in executive functions (e.g., in planning, initiating, organizing, monitoring, or inhibiting motor behavior). These more general difficulties may also affect motor control and learning of new motor skills.

Willingham's second key mechanism is *learning through the tuning of perceptual–motor integration, sequencing, and dynamic processes* so that movements become more efficient for a particular task. It is proposed that learning via these tuning processes occurs only if a movement and the representation of the movement are produced at the same time. This type of learning occurs outside awareness. Gentile (1998) also states that in learning new functional skills the movement's shape structure is first perhaps "good enough" to meet task demands and achieve the goal but represents only a crude organization of force generation processes. With practice in implicit unconscious learning, the organization of active and passive force components is finely tuned. During early practice, there is high variability in force generation and feedback. According to Gentile, "this variability should be viewed as yielding fortuitous force production patterns that expand the range of options available to the system" (p. 10) and is in this sense a necessary and essential aspect of the implicit learning process.

According to Willingham's (1998) dual-mode principle, the unconscious mode of learning requires proprioceptive feedback but the conscious mode does not. This principle also assumes that conscious and unconscious modes are available at all times in learning new skills. However, in the early stages of practicing the unconscious mode cannot be used effectively. The task must be practiced consciously before fine-tuning of the sequencing, the perceptual–motor integration and the dynamic processes takes place. With practice or implicit learning, unconscious processes develop task-specific knowledge.

In children with MLD, neuromotor and perceptual–motor subsystems may be "inexperienced," and the tuning of these systems may be limited (Sporns & Edelman, 1993). We know also that children with MLD are quite often hypoactive in everyday life (Hands & Larkin, 2002). As a result, they may not be getting enough practice for implicit learning to occur. Our knowledge of early development in children with MLD is quite limited. But, because MLD is a developmental disability with neurodevelopmental backgrounds we assume that movement difficulties are present in the early phases of development. Thus, the possibilities for the tuning of perceptual–motor integration, sequencing, and dynamic processes and implicit learning could be reduced from very early age.

According to the neural separability principle, dissociations of motor skill should be observed so that if the child has problems in only one of the brain regions that support motor skill learning, only one motor skill learning process should be affected. This means that the child should be able to learn tasks that do not require a contribution from that process. For example, children with MLD and visuoperceptual difficulties may benefit from a different kind of motor task than those with kinesthetic problems. According to the theory, there is no general "motor learning center" which contributes to the learning of all the different types of motor skills.

Skills that are represented in the egocentric space require that proprioceptive information—especially information concerning the location of body parts—is available during learning. But it is also possible to learn new skills consciously in a strategic or explicit learning phase without performing them and thus without proprioception. This happens in observational learning and when mental imagery is used. Both modeling and imagery training, therefore, are promising approaches in helping children with MLD improve their ability to internally represent the visuospatial coordinates of intended movements and monitoring of efference copy signals (Wilson et al., 2001).

SUMMARY AND CONCLUSIONS

In the current chapter we presented an alternative perspective for conceptualizing motor problems in children. We suggest that the existing classifications do not successfully capture the inherent heterogeneity seen in these children and, more important, do not address the main challenge these children are confronted with (i.e., their inability to learn everyday motor skills). Therefore, in order to capture the motor behavior of these children, we adopted the term *motor learning disability* (see Hands & Larkin, 2002). In our view, a motor learning perspective offers an excellent theoretical basis for improved understanding of the underlying mechanisms of MLD. Moreover, it also provides the basis for theoretically sound interventions. By introducing Willingham's (1998) neuropsychological model of motor learning, we acknowledge the fact that there is a need for integrating the existing empirical knowledge on MLD with possible underlying brain mechanisms. The theory is unique in its capacity of explaining motor learning in terms of motor control processes and provides a rich source of testable hypotheses to be pursued in future research.

REFERENCES

Ahonen, T. (1990). *Developmental coordination disorders in children: A developmental neuropsychological follow-up study*. Doctoral dissertation, University of Jyvaskyla.

Aldenderfer, M. S., & Blashfield, R. K. (1984). *Cluster analysis*. Beverly Hills, CA: Sage.

American Psychiatric Association. (1987). *Diagnostic and statistical manual of mental disorders* (3rd ed., rev.). Washington, DC: Author.

American Psychiatric Association. (1994). *Diagnostic and statistical manual of mental disorders* (4th ed.). Washington, DC: Author.

Annell, A. L. (1949). School problems in children of average or superior intelligence: A preliminary report. *Journal of Mental Science, 95*, 901–909.

Ayres, J. A. (1972). *Sensory integration and learning disorders*. Los Angeles: Western Psychological Services.

Ayres, A. J. (1985). *Developmental apraxia and adult onset apraxia.* Torrance, CA: Sensory Integration International.

Bairstow, P. J., & Laszlo, J. I. (1989). Deficits in planning, control and recall of hand movements in children with perceptuo-motor dysfunction. *British Journal of Developmental Psychology, 7,* 251–273.

Blondis, T. A., Snow, J. H., Roizen, N. J., Opacich, K. J., & Accordo, P. J. (1993). Early maturation of motor-delayed children at school age. *Journal of Child Neurology, 8,* 323–329.

Brenner, M. W., & Gillman, S. (1966). Visuo-motor ability in school children—A survey. *Developmental Medicine and Child Neurology, 8,* 686–703.

Cantell, M., & Kooistra, L. (2002). Long-term outcomes of Developmental Coordination Disorder. In S. A. Cermak & D. Larkin (Eds.), *Developmental coordination disorder* (pp. 23–38). Albany, NY: Delmar Thomson Learning.

Cantell, M., Kooistra, L., & Larkin, D. (2001). Approaches to intervention for children with developmental coordination disorder. *New Zealand Journal of Disability Studies, 9,* 106–119.

Cantell, M. H., Smyth, M. M., & Ahonen, T. P. (1994). Clumsiness in adolescence: Educational, motor and social outcomes of motor delay detected at 5 years. *Adapted Physical Activity Quarterly, 11,* 115–129.

Cantell, M. H., Smyth, M. M. & Ahonen, T. P. (2003). Two distinct pathways for developmental coordination disorder: Persistence and resolution. *Human Movement Science, 22,* 413–431.

Cermak, S. A. (1985). Developmental dyspraxia. In E. A. Roy (Ed.), *Neuropsychological studies of apraxia and related disorders* (pp. 225–248). Amsterdam: North-Holland.

Cermak, S. A. (1991). Somatodyspraxia. In A. G. Fisher, E. A. Murray, & A. C. Bundy (Eds.), *Sensory integration: Theory and practice* (pp. 137–170). Philadelphia: Davis.

Cermak, S. A., Gubbay, S. S., & Larkin, D. (2002). What is developmental coordination disorder? In S. A. Cermak & D. Larkin (Eds.), *Developmental coordination disorder* (pp. 2–22). Albany, NY: Delmar Thomson Learning.

Cousins, M., & Smyth, M. M. (2003). Developmental coordination impairments in adulthood. *Human Movement Science, 22,* 433–459.

Dare, M. T., & Gordon, N. (1970). Clumsy children: A disorder of perception and motor organization. *Developmental Medicine and Child Neurology, 12,* 178–185.

David, R., Deuel, R., Ferry, P., Gascon, G., Golden, G., Rapin, I., et al. (1981). *Proposed nosology of disorders of higher cerebral function in children.* Minneapolis, MN: Child Neurology Society.

Dawdy, S. C. (1981). Pediatric neuropsychology: Caring for the developmentally dyspraxic child. *Child Neuropsychology, 3,* 30–37.

Denckla, M. B. (Ed.). (1984). *Developmental dyspraxia: The clumsy child.* Boston: University Park Press.

Denckla, M. B., & Roeltgen, D. P. (1992). Disorders of motor function and control. In I. Rapin & S. J. Segalowitz (Eds.), *Handbook of neuropsychology, Vol. 6: Child neuropsychology* (pp. 455–476). New York: Elsevier Science.

Deuel, R. (1992). Motor skill disorders. In S. Hooper, G. Hynd, & R. Mattison (Eds.), *Developmental disorders: Diagnostic criteria and clinical assessment* (pp. 239–281). Hillsdale, NJ: Erlbaum.

Deuel, R. K., & Doar, B. P. (1992). Developmental manual dyspraxia: A lesson in mind and brain. *Journal of Child Neurology, 7,* 99–103.

Dewey, D. (1995). What is developmental dyspraxia? *Brain and Cognition, 29,* 254–274.

Dewey, D. (2002). Subtypes of developmental coordination disorder. In S. A. Cermak & D. Larkin (Eds.), *Developmental coordination disorder* (pp. 40–68). Albany, NY: Delmar Thomson Learning.

Dewey, D., & Kaplan, B. J. (1992). Analysis of praxis task demands in the assessment of children with developmental motor deficits. *Developmental Neuropsychology, 8,* 367–379.

Dewey, D., & Kaplan, B. J. (1994). Subtyping of developmental motor deficits. *Developmental Neuropsychology, 1994*, 265–284.

Dewey, D., Kaplan, B. J., Wilson, B. N., & Crawford, S. G. (1999). *Developmental coordination disorder and developmental dyspraxia: Are we talking about the same thing?* Paper presented at 27th annual meeting of the International Neuropsychology Society, Boston.

Erhardt, P., McKinlay, I. A., & Bradley, G. (1987). Coordination screening for children with and without moderate learning difficulties: Further experience with Gubbay's tests. *Developmental Medicine and Child Neurology, 29*, 666–673.

Fawcett, A., & Nicholson, R. (1999). Performance of dyslexic children on cerebellar and cognitive tests. *Journal of Motor Behavior, 31*, 68–78.

Fitts, P. M., & Posner, M. I. (1967). *Human performance*. Belmont, CA: Brooks/Cole.

Fitzpatrick, D. (2003). The lived experience of physical awkwardness: Adults' retrospective views. *Adapted Physical Activity Quarterly, 20*, 279–298.

Ford, D. R. (1966). *Diseases of the nervous system in infancy, childhood and adolescents* (5th ed.). Springfield, IL: Thomas.

Forssberg, H., Kinoshita, H., Eliasson, A., Johansson, R., Westling, G., & Gordon, A. (1999). Development of human precision grip. II. Anticipatory control of isomentric forces for object's weight. *Experimental Brain Research, 90*, 393–398.

Fuster, J. (2000). Executive frontal functions. *Experimental Brain Research, 133*, 66–70.

Gentile, A. (1998). Implicit and explicit processes during acquisition of functional skills. *Scandinavian Journal of Occupational Therapy, 5*, 7–16.

Geuze, R., & Borger, H. (1993). Children who are clumsy: Five years later. *Adapted Physical Activity Quarterly, 10*, 10–21.

Gillberg, I. C., & Gillberg, C. (1989). Children with preschool minor neurodevelopmental disorders. IV: Behaviour and school achievement at age 13. *Developmental Medicine and Child Neurology, 31*, 3–13.

Goodgold-Edwards, S. A., & Cermak, S. A. (1990). Integrating motor control and motor learning concepts with neuropsychological perspectives on apraxia and developmental dyspraxia. *American Journal of Occupational Therapy, 44*, 431–439.

Greer, K. (1984). Physiology of motor control. In M. Smyth & A. Wing (Eds.), *The psychology of human movement* (pp. 17–46). London: Academic Press.

Gubbay, S. S. (1975a). *The clumsy child*. London: Saunders.

Gubbay, S. S. (1975b). Clumsy children in normal schools. *Medical Journal of Australia, 1*, 233–236.

Gubbay, S. S. (1985). Clumsiness. In J. A. M. Frederiks (Ed.), *Handbook of clinical neurology* (Vol. 2, pp. 159–167). Amsterdam: Elsevier.

Gubbay, S. S., Ellis, E., Walton, J. N., & Court, S. D. M. (1965). Clumsy children: A study of apraxic and agnosic defects in 21 children. *Brain, 88*, 295–312.

Hadders-Algra, M. (2002). Two distinct forms of minor neurological dysfunction: Perspectives emerging from a review of data of the Groningen Perinatal Project. *Developmental Medicine and Child Neurology, 44*, 561–571.

Hall, D. M. B. (1988). Clumsy children. *British Medical Journal, 296*, 375–376.

Hands, B., & Larkin, D. (2001). Developmental coordination disorder: A discrete learning disability. *New Zealand Journal of Disability Studies, 9*, 93–105.

Hands, B., & Larkin, D. (2002). Physical fitness and developmental coordination disorder. In S. Cermak & D. Larkin (Eds.), *Developmental coordination disorder* (pp. 172–184). Albany, NY: Delmar Thomson Learning.

Haubenstricker, J. (1982). Motor development in children with learning disabilities. *Journal of Physical Education, Recreation and Dance*, 41–43.

Henderson, S. E. (1987). The assessment of "clumsy children": Old and new approaches. *Journal of Child Psychology and Psychiatry, 28*, 511–527.

Henderson, S. E. (Ed.). (1993). *Motor development and minor handicap*. Cambridge, UK: Cambridge University Press.

Henderson, S. E., & Barnett, A. L. (1998a). The classification of specific motor coordination disorders in children: Some problems to be solved. *Human Movement Science, 17*, 449–470.

Henderson S. E., & Barnett, A. L. (1998b). Developmental movement disorders. In J. Rispens, T. A. van Yperen, & W. Yule (Eds.), *Perspectives on the classification of specific developmental disorders* (pp. 203–230). Dordrecht, Netherlands: Kluwer Academic.

Henderson, S. E., & Hall, D. (1982). Concomitants of clumsiness in young school children. *Developmental Medicine and Child Neurology, 24*, 448–460.

Hoare, D. (1994). Subtypes of developmental coordination disorder. *Adapted Physical Activity Quarterly, 11*, 158–169.

Hulme, C., Biggerstaff, A., Moran, G., & McKinlay, I. (1982). Visual, kinaesthetic and cross-modal judgments of length by normal and clumsy children. *Developmental Medicine and Child Neurology, 24*, 461–471.

Hulme, C., Smart, A., & Moran, G. (1982). Visual perceptual deficits in clumsy children. *Neuropsychologia, 20*, 475–481.

Iloeje, S. O. (1987). Developmental apraxia among Nigerian children in Enugor, Nigeria. *Developmental Medicine and Child Neurology, 29*, 502–507.

Ingram, T. (1963). Chronic brain syndromes in childhood other than cerebral palsy, epilepsy and mental defect. *Little Club Clinics in Developmental Medicine, 10*, 10–17.

Jongmans, M. J., Mercuri, E., Dubowitz, L. M. S., & Henderson, S. E. (1998). Perceptual–motor difficulties and their concomitants in six-year-old children born prematurely. *Human Movement Science, 17*, 629–654.

Jordan, M. (1995). Computational motor control. In M. Gazzaniga (Ed.), *The cognitive neurosciences* (pp. 597–609). Cambridge, MA: MIT Press.

Kadesjo, B., & Gillberg, C. (1999). Developmental coordination disorder in Swedish 7-year old children. *Journal of the Academy of Child and Adolescent Psychiatry, 38*, 820–828.

Kalverboer, A. (1988). Follow-up of biological high-risk groups. In M. Rutter (Ed.), *Psychosocial risk factors: Power of longitudinal data* (pp. 114–137). Cambridge, UK: Cambridge University Press.

Kalverboer, A. F., de Vries, H. J., & van Dellen, T. (1990). Social behavior in clumsy children as rated by parents and teachers. In A. F. Kalverboer (Ed.), *Developmental Biopsychology: Experimental and observational studies in children at risk* (pp. 257–269). Ann Arbor: University of Michigan Press.

Kaplan, B. J., Wilson, B. N., Dewey, D. M., & Crawford, S. G. (1998). DCD may not be a discrete disorder. *Human Movement Science, 17*, 471–490.

Katschmarsky, S., Cairney, S., Maruff, P., Wilson, P., & Currie, J. (2001). The ability to execute saccades on the basis of efference copy: Impairments in double-step saccade performance in children with developmental co-ordination disorder. *Experimental Brain Research, 136*, 73–78.

Keogh, J., Sugden, D., Reynard, C., & Calkins, J. (1979). Identification of clumsy children: Comparisons and comments. *Journal of Human Movement Studies, 5*, 32–41.

Knuckey, N., & Gubbay, S. (1983). Clumsy children: A prognostic study. *Australian Pediatric Journal, 19*, 9–13.

Larkin, D., & Parker, H. (2002). Task-specific intervention for Developmental Coordination Disorder: A systems view. In S. Cermak & D. Larkin (Eds.), *Developmental coordination disorder: Theory and practice* (pp. 234–247). Albany, NY: Delmar Thomson Learning.

Laszlo, J., & Bairstow, P. (1985). *Perceptual-motor behaviour: Developmental assessment and therapy*. London: Holt, Rinehart & Winston.

Laszlo, J. I., Bairstow, P. J., Bartrip, J., & Rolfe, U. T. (Eds.). (1988). *Clumsiness or perceptuo-motor dysfunction?* Amsterdam: Elsevier Science.

Laszlo, J., & Sainsbury, K. (1994). Adequate kinaesthetic development: prevention of perceptual-motor dysfunction or clumsiness. In J. van Rossum & J. Laszlo (Eds.), *Motor development: Aspects of normal and delayed development.* Amsterdam: VU University Press.

Lefebvre, C., & Reid, G. (1998). Prediction in ball catching by children with and without a developmental coordination disorder. *Adapted Physical Activity Quarterly, 15,* 299–315.

Leiguarda, R., & Marsden, C. (2000). Limb apraxia: Higher-order disorders of sensorimotor integration. *Brain, 123,* 860–879.

Lord, R., & Hulme, C. (1987a). Kinaesthetic sensitivity of normal and clumsy children. *Developmental Medicine and Child Neurology, 29,* 720–725.

Lord, R., & Hulme, C. (1987b). Perceptual judgments of normal and clumsy children. *Developmental Medicine and Child Neurology, 29,* 250–257.

Losse, A., Henderson, S. A., Elliman, D., Hall, D., Knight, E., & Jongmans, M. (1991). Clumsiness in children: Do they grow out of it? A 10-year follow-up study. *Developmental Medicine and Child Neurology, 33,* 55–68.

Lundy-Ekman, L., Ivry, R., Keele, S. W., & Woollacott, M. (1991). Timing and force control deficits in clumsy children. *Journal of Cognitive Neuroscience, 3,* 367–376.

Luria, A. R. (1973). *The working brain.* Baltimore: Penguin.

MacNab, J., Miller, L., & Polatajko, H. (2001). The search for subtypes of DCD: Is cluster analysis the answer? *Human Movement Science, 20,* 49–72.

Maruff, P., Wilson, P., Trebilcock, M., & Currie, J. (1999). Abnormalities of imagined motor sequences in children with developmental coordination disorder. *Neuropsychologia, 37,* 1317–1324.

May-Benson, T., Ingolia, P. & Koomar, J. (2002). Daily living skills and Developmental Coordination Disorder. In S. A. Cermak & D. Larkin (Eds.), *Developmental coordination disorder* (pp. 140–156). Albany, NY: Delmar Thomson Learning.

Miller, L. T., Polatajko, H. J., Missiuna, C. C., Mandich, A. D., & Macnab, J. J. (2001). A pilot trial of a cognitive treatment for children with developmental coordination disorder. *Human Movement Science, 20,* 183–210.

Missiuna, C. (1994). Motor skills acquisition in children with developmental coordination disorder. *Adapted Physical Activity Quarterly, 11,* 214–235.

Missiuna, C., & Mandich, A. (2002). Integrating motor learning theories into practice. In S. A. Cermak & D. Larkin (Eds.), *Developmental coordination disorder: Theory and practice* (pp. 221–233). Albany, NY: Delmar Thomson Learning.

Miyahara, M. (1994). Subtypes of students with learning disabilities based upon gross motor functions. *Adapted Physical Activity Quarterly, 11,* 368–382.

Mon-Williams, M., Pascal, E., & Wann, J. (1994). Opthalmic factors in developmental coordination disorder. *Adapted Physical Activity Quarterly, 11,* 170–178.

Morris, R., Blashfield, R., & Satz, P. (1981). Neuropsychology and cluster analysis: Problems and pitfalls. *Journal of Clinical Neuropsychology, 3,* 79–99.

Neumann, C., & Walker, E. (1996). Childhood neuromotor soft signs, behaviour problems and adult psychopathology. In T. Ollendic & R. Prinz (Eds.), *Advances in clinical child psychology* (Vol. 18, pp. 173–203). New York: Plenum Press.

Newell, K. (1986). Constraints on the development of coordination. In M. Wade & H. Whiting (Eds.), *Motor development in children: Aspects of coordination and control* (pp. 341–360). The Hague, The Netherlands: Nijhoff.

Nicholson, R., & Fawcett, J. (1990). Automaticity: A new framework for dyslexia research? *Cognition, 35,* 159–182.

Nicholson, R., & Fawcett, A. (2001). Dyslexia, learning and the cerebellum. In M. Wolf (Ed.), *Dyslexia, fluency and the brain* (pp. 159–187). Timonium, PA: York Press.

Nicholson, R., Fawcett, A., Berry, E., Jenkins, I., Dean, P., & Brooks, D. (1999). Association of abnormal cerebellar activation with motor learning difficulties in dyslexic adults. *Lancet, 353*, 1662–1667.

Orton, S. T. (1937). *Reading, writing and speech problems in children.* New York: Norton.

Pereira, H., Landgren, M., Gillberg, C., & Forssberg, H. (2001). Parametric control of fingertip forces during precision grip lifts in children with DCD (developmental coordination disorder) and DAMP (deficits in attention motor control and perception). *Neuropsychologia, 39*, 478–488.

Polatajko, H. J., Fox, A. M., & Missiuna, C. (1995). An international consensus on children with developmental coordination disorder. *Canadian Journal of Occupational Therapy, 62*, 3–6.

Rösblad, B. (2002). Visual perception in children with developmental coordination disorder. In S. A. Cermak & D. Larkin (Eds.), *Developmental coordination disorder* (pp. 104–116). Albany, NY: Delmar.

Rösblad, B., & von Hofsten, C. (1994). Repetitive goal-directed arm movements in children with developmental coordination disorders: Role of visual information. *Adapted Physical Activity Quarterly, 11*, 190–202.

Roy, E. (1978). Apraxia: A new look at an old syndrome. *Journal of Human Movement Studies, 4*, 191–210.

Schoemaker, M. M., Hijlkema, M. G. J., & Kalverboer, A. F. (1994). Physiotherapy for clumsy children: An evaluation study. *Developmental Medicine and Child Neurology*, 143–155.

Seidler, R., Purushotham, A., Kim, S., Ugurbil, K., Willingham, D., & Ashne, J. (2002). Cerebellum activation associated with performance change but not motor learning. *Science*, 2043–2046.

Seitz, R. J., Stephan, K. M., & Binkofski F. (2000). Control of action as mediated by the human frontal lobe. *Experimental Brain Research, 133*, 71–80.

Shumway-Cook, A., & Woolacott, M. (2001). *Motor control: Theory and practical applications* (2nd ed.). Baltimore: Lippincott, Williams & Wilkins.

Smyth, T. (1992). Impaired motor skill (clumsiness) in otherwise normal children: A review. *Child: Care, Health and Development, 18*, 283–300.

Smyth, T. R., & Glencross, D. J. (1986). Information processing deficits in clumsy children. *Australian Journal of Psychology, 38*, 13–22.

Soorani-Lunsing, R., Hadders-Algra, M., Huisjes, H., & Touwen, B. (1994). Neurobehavioural relationships after the onset of puberty. *Developmental Medicine and Child Neurology, 36*, 334–343.

Sporns, O., & Edelman, G. (1993). Solving Bernstein's problem: a proposal for the development of coordinated movement by selection. *Child Development, 64*, 960–981.

Sugden, D., & Keogh, J. (1990). *Problems in movement skill development.* Columbia: University of South Carolina Press.

Sugden, D. A., & Sugden, L. (1990). *The assessment and management of movement skills problems.* Leeds, UK: School of Education.

Touwen, B. (1993). Longitudinal studies on motor development: Developmental neurological considerations. In A. F. Kalverboer, B. Hopkins, & R. Geuze (Eds.), *Motor development in early and later childhood: Longitudinal approaches* (pp. 15–34). Cambridge, UK: Cambridge University Press.

van Dellen, T., & Geuze, K. H. (1988). Motor response programming in clumsy children. *Journal of Child Psychology and Psychiatry, 29*, 489–500.

van Dellen, T., Vaessen, W., & Schoemaker, M. (1990). Clumsiness: Definition and selection of subjects. In A. F. Kalverboer (Ed.), *Developmental biopsychology* (pp. 135–152). Ann Arbor: University of Michigan Press.

van der Meulen, J. H. P., van der Gon, J. J. D., Gielen, C. C. A. M., Gooskens, R. H. J. M., &

Willemse, J. (1991). Visuomotor performance of normal and clumsy children. I: Fast goal-directed arm-movements with and without visual feedback. *Developmental Medicine and Child Neurology, 33,* 40–54.

Wall, A. E., Reid, G., & Paton, J. (1990). *The syndrome of physical awkwardness.* Amsterdam: Elsevier Science.

Walton, J. N., Ellis, E., & Court, S. D. M. (1962). Clumsy children: Developmental apraxia and agnosia. *Brain, 85,* 603–612.

Wann, J. P., Mon-Williams, M., & Rushton, K. (1998). Postural control and coordination disorders: The swinging room revisited. *Human Movement Science, 17,* 491–513.

Williams, H. (2002). Motor control in children with developmental coordination disorder. In S. A. Cermak & D. Larkin (Eds.), *Developmental coordination disorder: Theory and practice* (pp. 117–137). Albany, NY: Delmar Thomson Learning.

Williams, H., & Burke, J. (1995). Conditioned patellar tendon reflex function in children with and without developmental coordination disorders. *Adapted Physical Activity Quarterly, 12,* 250–261.

Williams, H., & Woollacott, M. (1997). Characteristics of neuromuscular responses underlying posture control in clumsy children. *Motor Development: Research and Reviews, 1,* 8–23.

Williams, H. G., Woollacott, M. H., & Ivry, R. (1992). Timing and motor control in clumsy children. *Journal of Motor Behavior, 24,* 165–172.

Willingham, D. (1998). A neuropsychological theory of motor skill learning. *Psychological Review, 105,* 558–584.

Wilson, B., & Trombly, C. (1984). Proximal and distal function in children with and without sensory integrative dysfunction: An EMG study. *Canadian Journal of Occupational Therapy, 51,* 11–17.

Wilson, P., Maruff, P., Ives, S., & Currie, J. (2001). Abnormalities of motor and praxis imagery in children with DCD. *Human Movement Science, 17,* 491–513.

Wilson, P. H., & McKenzie, B. E. (1998). Information processing deficits associated with developmental coordination disorder: A meta-analysis of research findings. *Journal of Child Psychology and Psychiatry, 39,* 829–840.

Wilson, P. H., Thomas, P., & Maruff, P. (2002). Motor imagery training ameliorates motor clumsiness in children. *Journal of Child Neurology, 17,* 491–498.

World Health Organization. (1989). *The ICD-9 classification of mental and behavioural disorders: Clinical descriptions and diagnostic guidelines.* Geneva: Author.

World Health Organization. (1992). *The ICD-10 classification of mental and behavioural disorders: Clinical descriptions and diagnostic guidelines.* Geneva: Author.

Wright, H. C., & Sugden, D. A. (1996). A two-step procedure for the identification of children with developmental co-ordination disorder in Singapore. *Developmental Medicine and Child Neurology, 38,* 1099–1105.

Wright, H. C., & Sugden, D. A. (1998). A school based intervention programme for children with developmental coordination disorder. *European Journal of Physical Education, 3,* 35–50.

CHAPTER 13

Visuospatial, Kinesthetic, Visuomotor Integration, and Visuoconstructional Disorders

IMPLICATIONS FOR MOTOR DEVELOPMENT

PETER WILSON

At present, no single account exists that explains motor coordination difficulties in children. Furthermore, the manifestation of poor motor coordination is varied (Mon-Williams, Tresilian, & Wann, 1999; Wilson, Maruff, Ives, & Currie, 2001). For example, some children have specific problems with fine motor skills and others with gross motor, and others have problems across all performance domains. Heterogeneity at the motor outcome level suggests that a range of causal factors may need to be isolated in order to explain the various forms in which motor disorders occur. This view is consistent with systems approaches to motor behavior (e.g., Davis & Burton, 1991; Larkin & Hoare, 1992) and client-centered views of remediation (Miller, Polatajko, Missiuna, Mandich, & Macnab, 2001). Yet, many researchers remain aligned to the view that a discrete number of core deficits may best capture this variation, which is the approach adopted in this chapter.

Any useful theory that attempts to explain motor coordination difficulties must direct researchers to those factors most likely to explain why certain children fail to develop appropriate levels of motor skill. A guiding assumption for most *experimental* researchers is that motor impairments reflect disruption to normal neural processes (Losse et al., 1991). Theories of motor control and learning are used to model processing operations in the brain and to provide a conceptual framework for understanding atypical behavior. In this chapter, we draw on both information processing and neuroscience models to help understand the association between developmental disorders of motor learning on the one hand and disorders in visuospatial representation, kinesthesis, visuomotor integration, and visuoconstructional function on the other.

INFORMATION-PROCESSING DEFICITS
AND MOTOR DEVELOPMENT

The hierarchical structure of information-processing (IP) models allows investigation of different levels of motor control: action planning, response programming and on-line modulation, effector output, and feedback control. These models are attractive in the developmental area because of their conceptual simplicity and the promise that more effective remedial strategies might be developed for children with motor impairments as processing deficits are isolated (Schoemaker, Smits-Engelsman, & Kalverboer, 1998). In particular, the literature on developmental coordination disorder (DCD) is arguably the most informed for examining the relative contribution to motor development of perceptual, cognitive (decision and planning), and motor (programming and output) processes. The basic argument here is that if disorders in sensory and perceptual function are strongly associated with DCD, then such disorders might well be causal agents in cases in which motor development deviates from a normal developmental trajectory, as is clearly the case in children with DCD. As noted by Ahonen, Kooistra, Viholainen, and Cantell (Chapter 12, this volume), these children perform substantially below age norms and their level of motor difficulty is of such a magnitude that everyday activities (such as sports and schoolwork) are adversely affected. In this chapter we avoid walking over the same ground as Ahonen and colleagues (Chapter 12), who have already done such an excellent job of defining DCD and describing the neuropsychological functioning of children with this disorder. Rather, we draw on mainstream models of motor control and learning and selected research programs to explain how impairments of sensory and perceptual function have particular implications for motor development. As well, to better understand the time course of DCD, we refer to a developmental theory that describes how normal patterns of perceptuomotor function unfold.

The relative importance of motor versus nonmotor factors in the etiology of DCD has been an issue of ongoing debate. The term *nonmotor* is taken here to represent the processing of *perceptual* information in the service of action. The term *motor* is taken here to represent control processes that are responsible for selecting and programming an appropriate motor response in light of environmental input (Wilson & McKenzie, 1998). With respect to nonmotor factors, several different etiologies have been offered as accounting for DCD, each claiming a body of empirical support. These include visuoperceptual deficits, visuospatial representation deficits, deficits in kinesthetic function, and deficits in visuomotor integration. A meta-analysis of the DCD literature by Wilson and McKenzie (1998) attempted to identify IP factors that best characterize the disorder. The meta-analysis covered 50 studies published between 1974 and 1996, yielding 374 individual estimates of effect size. The IP categories investigated were visual processing, other perceptual processing (kinesthetic and cross-modal perception), and spatiotemporal parameters of movement planning and execution (e.g., reaction time, movement time, accuracy, and variability). The main deficit associated with DCD was found to be visuospatial processing. Regardless of whether a motor response was required or not, children with DCD had difficulties with visuospatial processing (Wilson & McKenzie, 1998). These included tasks such as length discrimination (e.g., Hulme, Biggerstaff, Moran, & McKinlay, 1982) and complex visuospatial tasks such as Block Design and Object Assembly from the Wechsler Intelligence Scale for

Children, third edition (WISC-III; Wechsler 1992). Examination of kinesthetic perception revealed a significant difference between children with and without DCD with a combined effect size in the moderate to high range. The effect size was found to be higher for those studies that involved active movement (e.g., Hulme, Biggerstaff, et al., 1982) than passive movement (e.g., Laszlo & Bairstow, 1983, 1985). The third and final factor that was found to have a moderate effect size in differentiating the two groups was cross-modal perception. Wilson and McKenzie (1998) suggested that this was consistent with the early work of Ayres (1972), who argued that children with motor coordination problems had difficulty integrating vestibular, proprioceptive, and tactile information.

Recently, researchers in the area of DCD have begun to merge IP theory with contemporary models in cognitive neuroscience in an effort to transcend the occasionally abstract conception of behavior that is associated with functional modeling. Our research program (e.g., Wilson & Maruff, 1999; Wilson et al., 2001), together with that of Sigmundsson, Ingvaldsen, and Whiting (1997) and Mon-Williams, Wann, and Pascal (e.g., 1999) are three notable examples. From the former, converging evidence is provided that deficits in the visuospatial representation of intended movements may provide a parsimonious explanation for motor clumsiness in children. This is described in the next section. We argue that this hypothesis can potentially unify many seemingly disparate findings in the motor development literature.

VISUOSPATIAL DEFICITS
IN DEVELOPMENTAL COORDINATION DISORDER:
THE INTERNAL REPRESENTATION OF MOTOR ACTS

One of the main difficulties in investigating the role of visuospatial processing in motor control involves specifying the particular informational constraints that are used to map prospective movements. In many cases an artificial separation is created between visual input and action systems. Only by understanding processes that help glue so-called percepts to effector (output) systems will our grasp of DCD be advanced. Moreover, in studies in which the presentation of the motor disturbance is described in basic chronometric terms (time on target, interresponse interval, etc.), researchers frequently put forward causal processes without directly testing them (Henderson, 1993). For example, using serial movement tasks, greater response variability in DCD across movement parameters has been suggested to reflect a problem in motor timing perhaps linked to cerebellar function (e.g., Geuze & Kalverboer, 1987, 1993). Although beyond the scope of the present chapter, it should be noted that more recent kinematic studies by Geuze and colleagues (e.g., Volman & Geuze, 1998a, 1998b) have transcended some of these difficulties by testing more specifically models of motor timing.

More recently, other researchers have also taken up a number of useful techniques for exploring the motor control system of children with DCD. Their major objective has been to isolate disruptions to those control processes that would, under normal circumstances, fine-tune the function of input–output systems. One example involves goal-directed movement in rich visual environments—the goal here is to better understand how space is represented in both egocentric and allocentric terms, and the nature of coordinate transformations that occur when objects in space are mapped onto potential trajectories for action. One method of enquiry involves simulated action; using a *visually guided pointing task*, for example, it has be shown that the impact of environmental constraints is preserved for children without motor difficulties but not for children with DCD (see below for a more detailed discussion). In another line of inquiry, the ability to sequence movements has been investigated using *serial reaction time* tasks. We have recently used the well-validated paradigm of Nissen and Bullemer (1987) to show that basic sequencing abilities appear intact in children with DCD (Wilson, Maruff, & Lum, 2003).

Importantly, we have seen the emergence of tasks, drawn from mainstream neuroscience, that are designed to tap selectively key processing networks in the central nervous system (CNS): for example, so-called dorsal stream operations responsible for location-centered analysis and ventral stream operations responsible for object-centered analysis (Jeannerod, 1997; Milner & Goodale, 1995). In the remainder of this section we explore several key examples of more contemporary approaches: (1) studies of (covert) orienting of visuospatial attention drawing on the neurocognitive model of Posner, Inoff, Friedrich, and Cohen (1987); (2) imagined or simulated action drawing on the representational model of Jeannerod (1996, 1997) and others (e.g., Crammond, 1997); and (3) the predictive control of eye movements drawing on the neurocomputational framework of Wolpert (1997). These lines of inquiry provide converging evidence that children with DCD appear to have difficulty representing the visuospatial coordinates of prospective actions. All these paradigms require that the performer generate internal representations of purposive motor acts, the only distinction being the scale of the movement: simple oculomotor plans for both covert and overt visual attention and the scaling of manual responses for simulated movement. Some disruption to the forward modeling of movement parameters would appear to provide a unifying explanation for the abnormal pattern of performance we describe. We argue that without adequate feedforward control, these children are forced to rely on (slower) afferent feedback when adjusting movements, a form of control that is inefficient particularly in complex or rapidly changing environments. Thus, this hypothesis would explain the slower and more variable performance of children with DCD across a range of tasks.

Visuospatial Attention

Visuospatial attention, as a preparatory process in motor control, has been investigated using the covert orienting of visual spatial attention task (COVAT). It provides a valid and reliable measure of the speed with which the focus of visual attention can be directed across the visual field without the use of eye movements (Posner, 1980). In this task, the child fixates on a central cross and then is cued as to the appearance of a target in one of two peripheral locations, one to each side of the fixation point. The target may appear either on the side indicated by the cue (valid trial) or on the opposite side (invalid trial). Peripheral cues are used to summon an *automatic* mode of orienting (subserved mainly by midbrain structures), while central symbolic cues summon a *controlled* mode (subserved mainly by cortical attentional zones, particularly the parietal lobe) (Rafal & Henik, 1994). Using this technique, we identified that attentional shifts in children with DCD did not differ from normal control children when initiated automatically by environmental signals. But, when shifts were initiated voluntarily, children with DCD displayed a deficit in the ability to disengage attention from incorrectly cued locations (Wilson, Maruff, & McKenzie, 1997). In a second COVAT study, we replicated this finding and showed that the deficit persisted irrespective of the amount of time allowed for voluntary attentional shifts (Wilson & Maruff, 1999). Interestingly, the pattern of COVAT deficits displayed by children with DCD mirrored closely those displayed by parietal patients. The parietal lobe is intimately involved in mapping visual-to-motor coordinates in space and in comparing feedforward information with afferent (visual and somatosensory) information (Anderson, Snyder, Bradley, & Xing, 1997; Jeannerod, 1997; Milner & Goodale, 1995).

Covert attentional shifts are thought to be tightly coupled to processes that subserve the programming of saccadic eye movements made to the location of visual cues (Maruff, Yucel, Stuart, Danckert, & Currie, 1999). Attentional processes of this type help set up coordinates in our three-dimensional representation of space that might serve as targets for prospective action or, indeed, for further visual sampling. In children with DCD, delayed disengagement of attention from invalid cues would severely impair their ability to code locations that might be valid targets for action. This in turn would interfere with the establishment of an accurate internal representation for an intended movement. This impairment is likely to be most pronounced in rich visual environments where task-irrelevant cues may interfere with the processes of coding the spatial layout in egocentric coordinates and the use of these coordinates to generate a feedforward action plan. Generation of the plan may be based on distorted egocentric coordinates or may be delayed as greater time may be required to sample all parts of the visual field. If the egocentric coordinates are distorted, any on-line adjustments that are made with reference to an efference copy (i.e., an "image" of how a movement is meant to unfold) would be poorly calibrated as the original template is inherently inaccurate. If the feedforward plan is delayed in production, however, later online adjustments may no longer be relevant to the current state of the environment (Wolpert, 1997). Thus, a deficit of internal modeling could explain why children with DCD find it difficult to negotiate novel and/or multiple task demands under time pressure (see Geuze & van Dellen, 1990; Henderson, Rose, & Henderson, 1992). In a more closed environment, when given sufficient time to allocate processing resources (and to negotiate any precue processing), performance deficits may be less pronounced.

Motor Imagery

The visuospatial representation of movements has been analyzed more closely using tasks that assess *motor imagery*. Motor imagery is a dynamic state that involves mental simulation of a motor action. The simulation of movement from a first-person perspective is thought to reflect the same processes by which overt movements are represented—that is, an egocentric coding of movement parameters (force and timing) that are scaled to the ambient environment (Jeannerod, 1999). Supporting this view are behavioral and neuroimaging studies that show that imagined motor performance is subject to the same environmental and physiological constraints as executed movements. In normal humans, for example, both the actual and imagined execution of motor sequences is constrained by the required timing and accuracy of those movements. This relationship (or *speed-for-accuracy trade-off*) is described by Fitts's law (Fitts, 1954). However, focal brain lesions, which give rise to abnormalities of executed motor performance, disrupt motor imagery.

Recently, we modified a visually guided pointing task (VGPT) and verified that actual and imagined movements conformed to Fitts's law in normal subjects (Maruff, Wilson, DeFazio, et al., 1999). The task requires that performers make a series of alternating movements between two (target) locations using a hand-held stylus. The distance between the two locations remains constant while the width of the target is varied between 1.9 and 30 millimeters. Target width is expressed as Index of Difficulty (ID) using Fitts's law. Using the same task in children with DCD, we found that executed motor sequences were slower than normal controls but still conformed to Fitts's law—a linear relationship between ID and MT (movement time). However, imagined motor sequences were not slower in children with DCD than in normal controls and did not conform to Fitts's law, unlike the imagined movements of the controls. Similar results have been shown for patients with parietal lobe lesions (Sirigu et al., 1996). This finding suggests that imagined movements were not constrained by the same environmental and physiological constraints as executed movements in children with DCD.

In a second study, we added an external load (1-kilogram weight) to the hand making the response (under both imagined and real conditions), in order to determine whether the performance of the children with DCD was attributable to inaccurate programming of relative force (Wilson et al., 2001). Like the earlier study, only real movements conformed to Fitts's law in the DCD group. Importantly, a group by condition interaction was found for the effect of load—for real movements, movement duration did not differ between load and no-load conditions for either group, while for imagined movements, movement duration increased under the load condition for the control group only. It was hypothesized that this weight-related slowing of imagined movements in the control group occurred because subjects were required to program a greater muscle force in order to overcome the additional weight when moving the stylus. When required to *actually* perform the pointing movements, this additional force allowed subjects to move at the same speed as when no weight was attached; this also occurred in the DCD group. Under most circumstances, however, increases in force are generally associated with increased movement duration (Decety, Jeannerod, & Prablanc, 1989). Thus, when control subjects were required only to imagine making a movement while carrying the load, the motor control system must have read the additional force calculation as representing that the duration of the movement should be increased. Therefore, imagined movements were slowed across all levels of item difficulty for these children. This calibration for force is independent of timing and has been shown to occur for normal adults under similar conditions where imagined movements are programmed under a weight constraint (see also Decety et al., 1989). This effect, however, was not observed in the DCD group, which suggests that the abnormality in motor imagery found in the children with DCD occurred because they had difficulty with representing *both* the timing and force component of imagined movements (Wilson et al., 2001). In the same study, visual (or nonmotor) imagery was shown to be normal on the Praxis Imagery Questionnaire. Because the VGPT required no overt motor movements, the abnormal performance of children with DCD reflects a deficit in cognitive function, most likely related to the internal representation of motor acts (or forward modeling of *efference copy*) (Maruff, Wilson, Trebilcock, & Currie, 1999).

Internal Modeling

Models of motor function define efference copy as a copy of the efferent motor command signal sent to CNS structures as a corollary of its transmission to the neuromuscular system (Crammond, 1997). This "copy" provides a template against which the expected sensory consequences of a movement can be compared, and the movement corrected, if necessary. In essence, the copy is a feedforward model of the visuospatial coordinates of a prospective action represented in kinematic terms—an "image" of how a movement is meant to unfold.

A study by Katschmarsky and colleagues (2001) tested whether children with DCD displayed an internal modeling deficit (IMD) by using an oculomotor paradigm known as the double-step saccade task (DSST). (Note that the more descriptive term IMD is used in preference to the term *efference copy deficit*, cited originally in Wilson et al. [2001]. IMD is used to denote specifically the type of motor control deficit we believe underlies DCD is most cases.) The DSST is a rapid successive tracking task whereby two target lights are flashed sequentially and then disappear. The first target appears for 140 msec and the second for 100 msec. Participants are required to make a saccade to the first target and then shift their eye gaze to the second target location. Because the second saccade starts from a different location (the end of the first saccade) from where the target was initially observed (from the fixation point), a spatial dissonance emerges between the retinal coordinates of the second target and the motor coordinates of the required saccade. It is argued that efference copy signals are used to determine the end position of the first saccade prior to the initiation of the second. Consistent with the hypothesis that children with DCD display an IMD, Katschmarsky and colleagues demonstrated that children with DCD had a specific impairment on the second saccade of the DSST, manifested as a decrease in accuracy. By comparison, exogenously controlled saccades (using a single-step prossacade task) were performed normally, as were first saccades on the DSST. Intriguingly, this pattern of results has been observed previously in parietal patients (Heide, Blankenburg, Zimmermann, & Kompf, 1995) whose performance on the COVAT (Petersen, Robinson, & Currie, 1989; Posner et al., 1987) and motor imagery tasks (Sirigu et al., 1996) is also similar to children with DCD.

Thus, there is converging evidence that children with DCD have difficulty processing the visuospatial properties of voluntary movements. In particular, there appears to be some disruption to the forward modeling of efference copy signals. Analyses of individual differences have revealed that the majority of DCD children in our samples (i.e., about 65–70%) exhibit deficits in visual representation of the types described previously.

The use of internal feedforward models to predict the consequences of action is an important theoretical concept in motor control (Wolpert, 1997). First, internal feedforward models contribute to volitional control by anticipating and canceling out the sensory consequences of a given movement enabling the mobile observer to distinguish between self-produced and externally induced motion. Second, these feedforward models also maintain the stability of motor systems in the face of sensorimotor feedback delays including slow parasympathetic nerve transmission times and psychological refractory periods. The predictive function of feedforward modeling enables actions to be modified and updated before sensory feedback is available. Feedforward models can be used to calculate potential error in the outcome of a movement, which can be used to alter the motor command, thus facilitating motor adaptation and learning. The parietal lobe is believed to be intimately involved in processing feedforward information from downstream motor areas by comparing this with visuospatial representations that specify action coordinates (Heide et al., 1995). Motor imagery would appear to map directly onto this predictive process by setting feedforward parameters for prospective movements, coded spatially, but also represented in terms of force and timing information. Thus, the IMD hypothesis provides a parsimonious explanation for the abnormal performance displayed by children with DCD on tasks where these children are required to use internal representations of motor acts (e.g., making covert shifts of attention, simulating movements, making eye movements to remembered locations, remembering movement sequences, and localizing an unseen finger) (Dwyer & McKenzie, 1994; Wilson & McKenzie, 1998).

More recently, the IMD hypothesis was tested by examining the efficacy of an imagery intervention designed to train the feedforward modeling of purposive actions. Children referred with motor coordination difficulties were assigned randomly to one three groups: imagery, perceptual–motor training (PMT), and wait-list control. The imagery training protocol, delivered in a multimedia format, was shown to be equally effective to PMT in facilitating the development of motor skill in the referred children. These results further strengthen the IMD hypothesis (see also Hill & Wing, 1999, for an examination of grip force modulation in DCD—deficits in feedforward planning are inferred). For those children who do not display deficits of this type, other types of cognitive dysfunction might be associated with poor motor coordination.

DEFICITS IN KINESTHETIC FUNCTION: PERCEPTUAL SENSITIVITY OR MULTIMODAL MAPPING?

Kinesthesis is the ability to apprehend the position in space of body parts and the force, timing, amplitude, and direction of movement using proprioceptive and vestibular input (McCloskey, 1978). Kinesthesis is regarded as an integral component of the sensory feedback loop in all motor actions. Such input is generated and monitored continuously, providing information about postural changes and the topography of the movement itself (Laszlo & Bairstow, 1985; Massaro, 1990). Both the acquisition and skilled performance of motor acts depend on kinesthesis, although the relative importance of feedback processing appears to vary according to the specific task and the expertise of the performer (Laszlo, 1990). It is often reported that the less skilled rely more heavily on feedback control, especially in the early stages of learning (Newell, 1991). It follows that disruptions to the development of kinesthetic perception may impede the normal development of motor skills. Here, we review some of the evidence bearing on this issue.

Studies of kinesthetic development are remarkably rare, especially those that inform our understanding of motor development. Those that do exist have focused mainly on children of school age. The traditional view has been that children younger than 6 years have a poorly developed sense of kinesthesis (e.g., Laszlo & Bairstow, 1985; von Hofsten & Rösblad, 1988) and that, in general, the greatest rate of development of kinesthesis occurs between 4 and 7 years of age (Coleman, Piek, & Livesey, 2001). However, while children of 7 years display adequate kinesthetic sensitivity, recent work suggests that it continues to develop over the adolescent years. Visser and Geuze (2000), for example, tested two groups of boys longitudinally, at 6-month intervals, the first group between the ages of 11½ and 14 years and the second between 14 and 16½ years. Results indicated improvement with age on a test of kinesthetic sensitivity, similar in magnitude to that observed in children between 5 and 12 years. Issues with the assessment of kinesthetic function, however, constrain our interpretation of these studies.

Studies of kinesthetic development have relied largely on tasks that may not be valid measures of kinesthesis and whose psychometric properties can be questioned. The most commonly used task has been the Kinesthetic Sensitivity Test (KST) (Laszlo & Bairstow, 1985). The KST was designed for use with school-age children. It involves two tasks, one designed to measure kinesthetic acuity (the ability to discriminate a passive arm movement) and the other kinesthetic perception and memory (the accuracy and memory of complex movement patterns, also involving arm movements). The latter, however, is more a test of cross-modal integration than kinesthetic perception (Elliott, Connelly, & Doyle, 1988). Subjects are required to trace around a stencil pattern using a hand-held stylus positioned under a masking box. At the completion of the movement, the pattern is rotated to a set angle. The masking box is then removed and the subject was required to reorient the pattern back to its original position. In other words, the child is asked to translate a kinesthetic representation of the pattern into a visual judgement of orientation. Thus, KST is not a pure measure of kinesthesis. Researchers have also noted that the reliability of the KST is poor, especially for children under 12 years of age (e.g., Lord & Hulme, 1987b; Visser & Geuze, 2000).

To address these concerns, Livesey and Parkes (1995) developed the Kinesthetic Acuity Test (KAT) for young children (ages 3–6 years). Unlike the KST, test–retest reliability of the KAT is very high ($r = .90$). Livesey and Coleman (1998) showed discriminant validity to be sound to the extent that performance on the KAT improved over early childhood from 3–5 years of age. The authors also reasoned that if kinesthetic acuity explains individual differences in motor ability, then variations in error scores on the KAT should correlate with measures of motor skill. Moderate correlations were shown between error scores and several measures of skill: static and dynamic balance, ball skills, and drawing. Whether this is a causal link remains unclear because the findings are based on correlational data only.

In a follow-up study using the KAT, Coleman et al. (2001) examined kinesthetic development longitudinally in children between 4 and 6 years of age. Using a large sample of children ($N = 291$), error scores and number correct on the KAT and subtests of the Wechsler Preschool and Primary Scale of Intelligence—Revised (WPPSI-R) (Block Design, Object Assembly, and Geometric Design) were used to predict motor ability (Movement Assessment Battery for Children; Movement ABC). The regression explained only 18.3% of the variance in Movement ABC scores. The amount of unique variance explained by KAT error and KAT number correct was very low (1.6 and 1.8 %, respectively). High overlap between predictors would account for this effect, although the exact magnitude was unclear because other estimates were not provided (e.g., simple correlations between variables). Importantly, children who were identified as being at risk for DCD (≤15th percentile on the Movement ABC) per-formed significantly worse than control children on the KAT at both initial testing and also 1 year later. This finding is consistent with earlier work by Laszlo and Bairstow (1983) for children in middle childhood and Piek and Coleman-Carman (1995) for older children (8–12 years), both of which used the KST. Similarly, the meta-analysis of Wilson and McKenzie (1998) showed that studies of kinesthetic perception and visuomotor integration in children with DCD reveal moderate effect sizes. Notwith-standing these results, even Coleman and colleagues (2001) have argued that the KAT (like the KST Memory Task) is more a test of visuomotor integration than pure kines-thesis. Thus, it may be more correct to argue that the mapping of kinesthetic with vi-sual space poses significant difficulty for children with DCD. This is discussed in some detail in the following section.

The results of training studies, which have investigated whether children with DCD display a kinesthetic deficit, have been mixed. Early work by Laszlo, Bairstow, and colleagues using the KST was encouraging (Bairstow & Laszlo, 1981; Laszlo & Bairstow, 1983; Laszlo, Bairstow, Bartrip, & Rolfe, 1988). They reported that only clumsy children who received kinesthetic training improved their level of motor per-formance compared to several groups of clumsy children given different treatments. More recent studies, however, have found only limited support for kinesthetic train-ing. Polatajko and colleagues (1995) found no effect of kinesthetic training on motor performance. Sims, Henderson, Hulme, and Morton (1996) showed that both treated and untreated groups of clumsy children improved their general motor performance at posttest. In a second study, Sims, Henderson, Morton, and Hulme (1996) found that kinesthetic training was no more effective than an alternative training regime that in-corporated several perceptual–motor tasks. In addition, other studies have failed to replicate Bairstow and Laszlo's (1981) findings (Elliott et al., 1988; Lord & Hulme, 1987b; Sugden & Wann, 1987). The poor reliability of the KST may account for some of the foregoing discrepancies (Lord & Hulme, 1987b); however, even more signifi-cant is the constrained mode of response used with the KST.

Recall that the KST requires that children perform a passive arm movement on the acuity task. The movement is thus *constrained* in that subjects do not control its initiation or termination. Only voluntary movements are potentially ballistic and pre-programmed and involve the generation of a true efference copy (Jones, 1981; Wolpert, 1997). This mode of action on location and ramp tasks would lead to more precise coding of limb-position information because children may better anticipate the consequences of their actions (Roy, 1978). Thus, we can predict that an *unconstrained* mode of response may facilitate kinesthetic coding by virtue of the contribution of feedforward information about limb position. In effect, the performer is learning to calibrate limb-position information with a self-generated (or internal) plan for action. Over repeated trials, it is likely that internal models for action can be trained to better approximate (kinesthetic) positional information arising from the movement itself. Be-cause motor imagery performed from a first-person perspective is thought to represent feedforward plans for action, this type of repeated learning may enhance the kines-thetic (or feeling) aspect of motor imagery, thereby further facilitating "perceptual" judgements in a cyclical manner. In sum, the training protocol used on the KST acuity task is clearly limited as a method for refining kinesthetic judgements.

ARE KINESTHETIC DEFICITS ASSOCIATED
WITH FORWARD MODELING?

Both visuospatial and kinesthetic modalities appear to contribute to an accurate (internal) model of how an intended movement will unfold (Blakemore, Goodbody, & Wolpert, 1998). While the parietal lobe is thought to subserve visuospatial modelling, the cerebellum is intimately involved in setting models for the timing of prospective actions (Wolpert, 1997). Wilson and colleagues (2001) have suggested that in DCD, the spatial, force, and timing characteristics of movement are all incorrectly coded when feedforward models of motor actions are generated. One hypothesis is that disruptions in the development of multimodal maps between motor and nonmotor representational systems may contribute to inaccurate feedforward models of efference copy. This would result in motor output that is not well integrated with the spatial and inertial constraints for action in one's immediate "workspace." Supporting this view is the observation that self-produced locomotion is normally responsible for fine-tuning the calibration of visual and proprioceptive space by enhancing access to flow cues (Berthenthal & Campos, 1989; Rieser, 1990). How this might be disrupted in other cases (and how feedforward modeling is affected) remains unclear but is a worthy topic for future research. Clearly, motor imagery training is one promising method for enhancing the multimodal integrity of efference copy—a combination of visualizing the action, imagining the look of the workspace, and "feeling" the limb may well enhance mapping between visual and proprioceptive space and predictive modeling.

DEFICITS IN VISUOMOTOR INTEGRATION: WHAT HAPPENS
WHEN VISUAL AND MOTOR SPACE DO NOT MATCH?

When we speak of visuomotor integration, we are really referring to the moving organism's tacit knowledge of the systematic covariation between visually and kinesthetically perceived space. Motor coordination depends intimately on the close calibration between the two such that changes in the structure of visually perceived space map onto changes in the flow of proprioceptive information via afferent pathways. Moreover, feedforward models need to provide some mechanism by which visuospatial and motor representations of intended actions are integrated as movements unfold. Most of the available information on the development of visuomotor integration comes from simple reproduction paradigms. (Note that studies of so-called crossmodal integration have focused largely on visual and motor modalities.) More recent work using a manual pointing task has elaborated on this early work.

Intersensory Integration Involving Simple Stimuli

Early reproduction studies using simple stimuli (such as line length) suggest that crossmodal integration (i.e., transforming information codes from one modality to another) tends to lag behind intramodal (i.e., translating information codes over time within the same modality) development during childhood, although the discrepancy between the two tends to abate with age. Hulme, Smart, Moran, and Raine (1983), for example, have shown that older children (9- and 10-year-olds) perform more accurately than do younger children (5- and 6-year-olds) when matching length information cross-modally. In addition, cross-modal performance was inferior to that within the visual and kinesthetic modalities for both age groups. In short, this and earlier studies (e.g., Connolly & Jones, 1970), suggest that processes of *simple* visuomotor translation develops rapidly over childhood but appears to lag behind intramodal ability up to about 11 years of age. Whether this lag places significant constraints on motor learning during this time is unclear.

Using the same paradigm, Hulme and colleagues (Hulme, Biggerstaff, et al., 1982; Hulme, Smart, & Moran, 1982; Hulme, Smart, & Raine, 1983) examined whether cross-modal development helps to explain individual differences in motor skill learning. The details of their work have been widely cited in the DCD literature. Briefly, their results showed no performance deficits on cross-modal tasks for children classified as "clumsy." Rather, there was a relative impairment in visual-to-visual matching, the magnitude of which was weak. Other studies that have used similar intersensory integration paradigms have found mild-to-moderate cross-modal deficits (Wilson & McKenzie, 1998).

Manual Pointing Tasks

We are now in the fortunate position to have a number of studies using the same, well-validated paradigm, the manual pointing task of von Hofsten and Rösblad (1988). What is intriguing about the set of studies are the diverse range of results and inferences, all drawn on the same or similar population.

The manual pointing task consists of a table with centrally located inlay, usually measuring about 20 square centimeters (Schoemaker et al., 2001). A large (A3) sheet of graph paper is attached to the undersurface of the table. Small dots are positioned on top of the inlay and serve as targets. The child sits directly in front of the table. He or she is required to place bulletin pins into the undersurface to locate the target dot as accurately as possible. This occurs under three conditions in which the type of perceptual information is varied: *vision-only condition* (V: P), *visual–proprioceptive condition* (VP: P) (the child places the index finger of his or her free hand on the dot and observes its location while placing the pin under the table), and *proprioceptive condition* (P: P) (like the former but with no visual cues to locate the target). Performance is measured as a distance error in both absolute and directional terms.

Children with DCD are more variable in their responses across a range of motor tasks (Wilson & McKenzie, 1998). Results from the manual pointing task are consistent with this observation. Regardless of the type of information/condition, manual pointing with the preferred hand was less consistent in children with DCD (e.g., Schoemaker et al., 2001; Smyth & Mason, 1997). However, the results for response accuracy are less clear.

There is inconsistent support for the hypothesis that children with DCD rely more heavily on visual information when regulating their movements (i.e., the view that response inaccuracy is compensated for by modifying trajectories on the basis of visual feedback) (van der Meulen, van der Gon, Gielin, Gooskens, & Willemse, 1991). Supporting this view, both Rösblad and von Hofsten (1992) and Smyth and Mason

(1997) showed that performance differences between children with DCD and controls were most pronounced in the proprioceptive condition. Contrary to these findings, Schoemaker and colleagues (2001) showed that although groups with and without DCD performed worse under this condition than did others, the increase in absolute error was similar for both groups (see also Mon-Williams, Wann, & Pascal, 1999). Minor differences in screening the children for motor disturbance may explain some of the discrepancy among these studies but certainly not all. When more homogenous DCD groups are tested, the main difficulties appear to be encountered in the visual condition. Mon-Williams, Wann, and Pascal (1999), for example, provide perhaps the most consistent set of data using a manual pointing task. They first chose to recruit a fairly homogeneous group of children in terms of the severity of DCD. They selected only those children in the bottom fifth percentile on motor ability for their age that experienced difficulties across the four domains of the Movement ABC. They showed that these children differed from controls on absolute error when the target location was coded in visual terms only. In the study by Shoemaker and colleagues, results approached significance in this same condition but also in the condition in which a combination of visual and proprioceptive information informed the pointing response. In children with specific hand–eye coordination problems (HECP), Sigmundsson and colleagues (1997) show that performance was compromised when targets were located using either a combination of visual and proprioceptive cues or proprioceptive only but only when using the nonpreferred hand. Sigmundsson, Whiting, and Ingvaldsen (1999) suggest that a deficit in processing spatial information within the right hemisphere might explain the pattern of performance observed in his studies.

Taken together, it can be inferred from these studies that children with DCD have the most difficulty mapping visual and visuoproprioceptive information about a target's location with the proprioceptive information supplied by the pointing hand. Whether this argument applies to both preferred and nonpreferred hands may depend on the type of group: DCD, HECP, or other. Patterns of results are least consistent when directional errors are considered. Again, differences in group composition and within-group variability on outcome measures cloud our interpretation.

VISUOCONSTRUCTIONAL DISORDERS: MOTOR SYMPTOM OR PROCESSING DEFICIT?

Visual construction refers to the ability to integrate isolated pieces of visual information into an ordered whole using a motoric response (Lezak, 1995). Graphic copying, WISC Object Assembly, and Block Design are some of the more commonly used tasks for assessing constructional ability and have been applied with equal vigor to the study of normal and atypical motor development. We consider first graphic copying as the prototypical task for assessing constructional ability.

As an output measure, copying confounds two aspects of functioning: visuospatial ability and motor skill (Dwyer & McKenzie, 1994; Heilbronner, 1992; Heilbronner, Buck, & Adams, 1989; Lezak, 1995). Thus, from the outset, we need to be clear about what level of analysis is being considered in relation to developmental motor disorders. For the child with motor impairments, poor graphic performance may reflect difficulties in visuospatial functioning, in the integrity of motor output systems, or in both. Consider first poor graphic skill at the symptom level. Of those children who are referred with motor coordination problems, poor graphic skills are a common feature. Indeed, copying and writing problems are perhaps the most frequently observed of all "symptoms" in children with DCD (Schoemaker et al., 2001; Smits-Engelsman, Niemeijer, & van Galen, 2001). These problems become especially apparent when children enter primary school and demands on the development of basic academic skills are made. Conservatively speaking, a group difference on measures of copying skill is consistent with the motor deficits that occur as part of the DCD syndrome.

As mentioned elsewhere, the meta-analysis of Wilson and McKenzie (1998) showed significant deficiencies in DCD on complex visuospatial tasks, regardless of motor involvement. Graphic tasks contributed a substantial number of effect sizes to the weighted estimates of difference between groups with and without DCD. Under most circumstances these involved the child copying geometric patterns of varying complexity under timed and untimed conditions. Measures of response latency, completion time, and accuracy were made. In general, the performance of children with DCD is worse than age-matched controls on most measures of accuracy. Effects for time are less consistent over studies (Dwyer & McKenzie, 1994; Wilson & McKenzie, 1998). Speed–accuracy trade-offs tend not to explain the pattern of deficits.

There is much descriptive evidence of inaccuracy on copying tasks where children with DCD are concerned. For example, these children have been shown to display more form and scale errors than controls when copying more complex stimuli (e.g., van Mier, Hulstijn, & Meulenbroek, 1994). They also experience particular difficulty reproducing figures with oblique lines, such as diamonds and cubes, and curved lines relative to figures with vertical and horizontal lines (Laszlo & Broderick, 1985, 1991; Lord & Hulme, 1988). A similar pattern of difficulty has been observed in young children ages 5–6 years compared with older children (Broderick & Laszlo, 1987, 1988), perhaps suggesting an immaturity in the development of visual constructional skills. Longitudinal studies are required to test this hypothesis more fully. The reproductions show particular evidence of poor global analysis of the spatial configuration of elements within the various stimulus designs (see Figure 13.1a). Moreover, poor (local) attention to detail is also frequently seen, most commonly in conjunction with poor global analysis (Figure 13.1c) but also sometimes in isolation (Figure 13.1b), perhaps reflecting poor visual attention and/or failure to persist with a task in which the frustration of poor fine-motor control is experienced.

Interestingly, judgments of visual discrimination appear to follow similar developmental trends to the ability to construct geometric patterns in copying tasks (Feeney & Stiles, 1996); similar strategies for analyzing spatial relations operate across both tasks and even young children have a basic ability to attend to both local and global properties of a spatial array. A reduced ability to analyze spatial relations may explain, in part, why children with poor motor coordination tend to perform poorly on *both* visuoperceptual and constructional tasks (Wilson & McKenzie, 1998).

Alternatively, their poor performance may reflect a reduced ability to map a visuospatial percept of an object in near space into an appropriate representation from which it can be reproduced kinesthetically. Copying is, after all, a task of visuomotor integration. The stimulus is perceived visually and then converted into a visuospatial

Stimulus   **Reproduction**

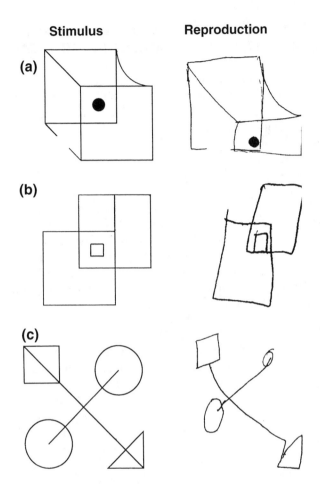

FIGURE 13.1. Graphic reproductions of children with developmental coordination disorder showing: (a) evidence of poor global analysis of the spatial configuration of elements within a stimulus design, (b) omission of local detail, and (c) a combination of (a) and (b).

representation that best preserves the spatial relationship between elements in the design. This representation must then be converted into a kinesthetic form, expressed ultimately as a set of precise motor outputs to the effector. Clearly, the precision with which this is achieved is highly dependent on the coupling between visual and kinesthetic space. In other words, copying performance involves the translation of visuospatial information about form and position into coordinates for graphic movements. The ability to make this translation between spatial codes accurately is thought not fully developed in younger children and either delayed or abnormal in those with DCD. This argument fits in nicely with our earlier analysis of imagery deficits in DCD. Fine-motor control—indexed by the ability to produce straight lines and lines of good continuation—is another aspect of performance in this case, one perhaps distinct from the spatial integrity of the graphic production itself (Feeney & Stiles, 1996).

TOWARD A UNIFYING ACCOUNT OF DISORDERS
OF MOTOR DEVELOPMENT IN CHILDREN

The development of theoretical models and treatment programs for children with problems of motor development has been limited by a lack of suitable brain–behavior models for motor dysfunction and by disagreement about the relative contributions of motor and cognitive impairment (Wilson & McKenzie, 1998). In the section on visuospatial disorders, we described a series of studies that suggest feedforward control processes might explain much of what we observe in the domain of motor incoordination. More specifically, problems in predictive coding of movement parameters (or forward modelling of efference copy) might provide a parsimonious explanation for DCD. This may translate into inaccurate feedforward models for prospective actions. Kinesthetic, visuomotor integration, and constructional disorders were then described, with reference to a (putative) common representational basis.

In terms of visuospatial coding, the IMD hypothesis outlined in this chapter does not seek to separate artificially the motor and cognitive contributions to the clinical presentation of developmental motor disorders (Katschmarksy et al., 2001; Wilson et al., 2001). Rather, we propose that the slow and variable motor performance that characterizes DCD reflects impairment in the processes associated with the forward modeling of efference copy (Wolpert, 1997). Normally, a feedforward model of efference copy allows the CNS to maintain the stability of motor systems despite delays in the availability of reafferent signals. This mechanism predicts and corrects the consequences of voluntary movements before reafferent feedback becomes available. An impairment in this operation would result in the evaluation of unfolding volitional motor acts being more reliant on slow reafferent motor signals rather than on the more efficient efference copy. This would add time and error to each step of any volitional motor sequences, a result consistent with clinical presentations and kinematic profiles of motor clumsiness in children (Katschmarsky et al., 2001; Schellekens, Scholten, & Kalverboer, 1983). One crucial behavior disrupted by an efference-copy deficit is motor imagery (e.g., Wilson et al., 2001). We saw that while children with DCD can generate sequences of motor movements in their imaginations, these are unconstrained by the biomechanical or environmental factors that operate for actual movements.

It was also noted that not all children in DCD samples exhibit visuospatial deficits of the type described previously, which raises the possibility that other types of cognitive dysfunction might also be associated with the disorder. From existing data, kinesthetic and cross-modal deficits are implicated, perhaps in a smaller proportion of DCD children (Wilson & McKenzie, 1998). However, the types of performance difficulties reported in these domains might equally be explained in terms of complex visuospatial and feedforward encoding. Conventional cross-modal tasks and those thought to tap kinesthetic function (such as the KST acuity task) were suggested to involve "knowledge" of the complex spatial calibration between visual and kinesthetic coordinate systems. It is thought that an accurate internal model for an intended action is predicated, to a large extent, on knowledge of or tacit experience with this calibration. Generation of an internal model based on aberrant visuospatial information would provide an inaccurate template against which the sensory consequences of an unfolding movement are assessed. This would, in turn, severely limit the on-line corrections that normally occur when movements go off trajectory or encounter unexpected perturbations (Wolpert, 1997). In short, an abnormality of efference copy may provide a parsimonious explanation for the abnormal performance found on a variety of tasks where children with poor motor coordination are required to use internal representations of motor acts: for example, remembering movements (see Dewey, 1993; Skorji & McKenzie, 1997), remembering drawings (e.g., Dwyer & McKenzie, 1994), or localizing an unseen finger (e.g., Mon-Williams, Wann, & Pascal, 1999). Deficiencies in exploratory behavior in infant development may explain, in part, the failure of some children to accurately calibrate visual and proprioceptive frames (Rourke, 1995) and to use this efficiently as a basis for feedforward encoding. These conjectures remain to be fully articulated but offer a unifying theme in the literature on developmental motor disorders.

The foregoing discussion does not rule out the possibility that alternate forms of dysfunction might also be found in subsamples of children with DCD. For example, dysfunction to the supplementary motor area and structures of the basal ganglia might explain the motor sequencing and selection problems that have also been ascribed to some children with developmental motor deficits (Lundy-Ekman, Ivry, Keele, & Woollacott, 1991). Lundy-Ekman showed a generalized timing control deficit in a subgroup of children with DCD who displayed cerebellar "soft signs." Force control deficits were evident in another subgroup with basal ganglia "soft signs." Cluster-analytic studies conducted at the process level are needed to clarify the existence or otherwise of these putative subgroups (Schoemaker et al., 1998; Wilson et al., 2001).

In sum, only by understanding the pathways to motor incoordination and the overlap between particular disruptions to neurocognitive processing and patterns of motor skill development will our causal models become rich and informative at the level of hypothesis testing and intervention. The arguments and tentative framework presented in this chapter can, we hope, make some contribution to this endeavor by providing a conceptual bridge between seemingly disparate findings.

REFERENCES

Anderson, R. A., Snyder, L. H., Bradley, D. C., & Xing, J. (1997). Multimodal representation of space in the posterior parietal cortex and its use in planning movements. *Annual Review of Neuroscience, 20*, 303–330.

Ayres, A. J. (1972). *Sensory integration and learning disorders*. Los Angeles: Western Psychological Services.

Bairstow, P. J., & Laszlo, J. I. (1981). Kinesthetic sensitivity to passive movements in children and adults, and its relationship to motor development and motor control. *Developmental Medicine and Child Neurology, 23*, 606–616.

Bertenthal, B. I., & Campos, J. J. (1990). A systems approach to the organizing effects of self-produced locomotion during infancy. *Advances in Infancy Research, 6*, 1–60.

Blakemore, S. J., Goodbody, S. J., & Wolpert, D. M. (1998). Predicting the consequences of our own actions: The role of sensorimotor context estimation. *Journal of Neuroscience, 18*, 7511–7518.

Broderick, P., & Laszlo, J. I. (1987). The drawing of squares and diamonds: A perceptual–motor task analysis. *Journal of Experimental Child Psychology, 43*, 44–61.

Broderick, P., & Laszlo, J. I. (1988). The effects of varying planning demands on drawing components of squares and diamonds. *Journal of Experimental Child Psychology, 45*, 18–27.

Coleman, R., Piek, J. P., & Livesey, D. J. (2001). A longitudinal study of motor ability and kinesthetic acuity in young children at risk of developmental coordination disorder. *Human Movement Science, 20*, 95–110.

Connolly, K., & Jones, B. (1970). A developmental study of afferent-reafferent integration. *British Journal of Psychology, 61*, 259–266.

Crammond, D. J. (1997). Motor imagery: Never in your wildest dream. *Trends in Neuroscience, 20*, 54–57.

Davis, W. E., & Burton, A. W. (1991). Ecological task analysis: Translating movement behavior theory into practice. *Adapted Physical Activity Quarterly, 8*, 154–177.

Decety, J., Jeannerod, M., & Prablanc, C. (1989). The timing of mentally represented actions. *Behavioral Brain Research, 34*, 35–42.

Dewey, D. (1993). Error analysis of limb and orofacial praxis in children with developmental motor deficits. *Brain and Cognition, 23*, 203–221.

Dwyer, C., & McKenzie, B. E. (1994). Visual memory impairment in clumsy children. *Adapted Physical Activity Quarterly, 11*,179–189.

Elliott, J. M., Connolly, K. J., & Doyle, A. J. R. (1988). Development of kinesthetic sensitivity and motor performance in children. *Developmental Medicine and Child Neurology, 30*, 80–92.

Feeney, S. M., & Stiles, J. (1996). Spatial analysis: An examination of preschoolers' perception and construction of geometric patterns. *Developmental Psychology, 32*, 933–941.

Fitts, P. M. (1954). The information capacity of the human motor system in controlling the amplitude of movement. *Journal of Experimental Psychology, 47*, 381–391.

Geuze, R. H., & Kalverboer, A. F. (1987). Inconsistency and adaptation in timing of clumsy children. *Journal of Motor Behavior, 20*(3), 341–367.

Geuze, R. H., & Kalverboer, A. F. (1993). Bimanual rhythmic coordination in clumsy and dyslexic children. In S. S. Valenti & J. B. Pittenger (Eds.), *Studies in perception and action*. Hillsdale, NJ: Erlbaum.

Geuze, R. H., & van Dellen, T. (1990). Auditory precue processing during a movement sequence in clumsy children. *Journal of Human Movement Studies, 19*, 11–24.

Heide, W., Blankenburg, M., Zimmermann, E., & Kompf, D. (1995). Cortical control of double-step saccades: Implications for spatial orientation. *Annals of Neurology, 38*, 739–748.

Heilbronner, R. L. (1992). The search for a "pure" visual memory test: Pursuit of perfection? *The Clinical Neuropsychologist, 6*, 105–112.

Heilbronner, R. L., Buck, P., & Adams, R. L. (1989). Factor analysis of verbal and nonverbal clinical memory tests. *Archives of Clinical Neuropsychology, 4*, 299–309.

Henderson, L., Rose, P., & Henderson, S. E. (1992). Reaction time and movement time in children with a developmental coordination disorder. *Journal of Child Psychology and Psychiatry, 33*, 895–905.

Henderson, S. E. (1993). Motor development and minor handicap. In A. F. Kalverboer, B. Hopkins, & R. H. Geuze, (Eds.) *Motor development in early and later childhood: Longitudinal approaches* (pp. 286–306). Cambridge, UK: Cambridge University Press.

Hill, E. L., & Wing, A. M. (1999). Coordination of grip force and load force in developmental coordination disorder: A case study. *Neurocase, 5*, 537–544.

Hulme, C., Biggerstaff, A., Moran, G., & McKinlay, I. (1982). Visual, kinesthetic and crossmodal judgements of length by normal and clumsy children. *Developmental Medicine and Child Neurology, 24*, 461–471.

Hulme, C., Smart, A., & Moran, G. (1982). Visual perceptual deficits in clumsy children. *Neuropsychologia, 20*, 475–481.

Hulme, C., Smart, A., Moran, G., & Raine, A. (1983). Visual, kinesthetic and cross-modal development: Relationships to motor skill development. *Perception, 12,* 477–483.

Jeannerod, M. (1996). Motor representations: One or many? *Behavioral and Brain Sciences, 19,* 759–765.

Jeannerod, M. (1997). *The cognitive neuroscience of action.* Oxford, UK: Blackwell.

Jeannerod, M. (1999). To act or not to act: Perspectives on the representation of actions. *Quarterly Journal of Experimental Psychology, 52,* 1–29.

Jones, B. (1981). The developmental significance of cross-modal matching. In R. D. Walk & H. L. Pick (Eds.), *Intersensory perception and sensory integration* (pp. 109–132). New York: Plenum Press.

Katschmarsky, S., Cairney, S., Maruff, P., Wilson, P. H., Tyler, P., & Currie, J. (2001). The ability to execute saccades on the basis of efference copy: Impairments in children with developmental coordination disorder. *Experimental Brain Research, 136,* 73–78.

Larkin, D., & Hoare, D. (1992). The movement approach: A window to understanding the clumsy child. In J. J. Summers (Ed.), *Approaches to the study of motor control and learning* (pp. 413–439). Amsterdam: Elsevier.

Laszlo, J. I. (1990). Child perceptuo-motor development: Normal and abnormal development of skilled behavior. In C. A. Hauert (Ed.), *Developmental psychology: Cognitive, perceptuomotor, and neuropsychological perspectives* (pp. 272–308). Amsterdam: Elsevier.

Laszlo, J. I., & Bairstow, P. J. (1983). Kinesthesis: Its measurement training and relationship to motor control. *Quarterly Journal of Experimental Psychology, 35,* 411–421.

Laszlo, J. I., & Bairstow, P. J. (1985). *Perceptual–motor behavior: Developmental assessment and therapy.* London: Holt, Rinehart & Winston.

Laszlo, J. I., Bairstow, P. J., Bartrip, J., & Rolfe, U. T. (1988). Clumsiness or perceptuomotor dysfunction? In A. M. Colley & J. R. Beech (Eds.), *Cognition and action in skilled behavior* (pp. 293–309). Amsterdam: Elsevier.

Laszlo, J. I., & Broderick, P. A. (1985). The perceptual-motor skill of drawing. In N. H. Freeman & M. V. Cox (Eds.), *Visual order: The nature and development of pictorial representation* (pp. 356–373). Cambridge, UK: Cambridge University Press.

Laszlo, J. I., & Broderick, P. (1991). Drawing and handwriting difficulties: Reasons for and remediation of dysfunction. In J. Wann, A. M. Wing, & N. Sovik (Eds.), *Development of graphic skills* (pp. 259–280). London: Academic Press.

Lezak, M. D. (1995). *Neuropsychological assessment* (3rd ed.). New York: Oxford University Press.

Livesey, D., & Coleman, R. (1998). The development of kinesthesis and its relationship to motor ability in preschool children. In J. P. Piek (Ed.), *Motor behavior and human skill: A multidisciplinary approach* (pp. 253–269). Champaign, IL: Human Kinetics.

Livesey, D. J., & Parkes, N. (1995). Testing kinesthetic acuity in preschool children. *Australian Journal of Psychology, 47,* 160–163.

Lord, R., & Hulme, C. (1987a). Kinesthetic sensitivity of normal and clumsy children. *Developmental Medicine and Child Neurology, 29,* 720–725.

Lord, R., & Hulme, C. (1987b). Perceptual judgements of normal and clumsy children. *Developmental Medicine and Child Neurology, 29,* 250–257.

Lord, R., & Hulme, C. (1988). Visual perception and drawing ability in clumsy and normal children. *British Journal of Developmental Psychology, 6,* 1–9.

Losse, A., Henderson, S. E., Elliman, D., Hall, D. Knight, E., & Jongmans, M. (1991). Clumsiness in children—Do they grow out of it? A 10-year follow-up study. *Developmental Medicine and Child Neurology, 33,* 55–68.

Lundy-Ekman L., Ivry, R., Keele, S., & Woollacott, M. (1991). Timing and force control deficits in clumsy children. *Journal of Cognitive Neuroscience, 3,* 367–376.

Maruff, P., Wilson, P. H., DeFazio, J., Cerritelli, B., Hedt, A., & Currie, J. (1999). Asymmetries between dominant and non-dominant hands in real and imagined motor task performance. *Neuropsychologia, 37,* 379–384.

Maruff, P., Wilson, P. H., Trebilcock, M., & Currie, J. (1999). Abnormalities of imagined motor sequences in children with developmental coordination disorder. *Neuropsychologia, 37,* 1317–1324.

Maruff, P., Yucel, M., Stuart, G., Danckert, J., & Currie, J. (1999). Facilitation and inhibition associated with the reflexive orienting of attention. *Neuropsychologia, 37,* 731–744.

Massaro, D. W. (1990). An information-processing analysis of perception and action. In O. Neumann & W. Prinz (Eds.), *Relationships between perception and action: Current approaches* (pp. 133–166). Berlin: Spinger-Verlag.

McCloskey, D. I. (1978). Kinesthetic sensibility. *Physiological Reviews, 58,* 763–813.

Miller, L. T., Polatajko, H. J., Missiuna, C., Mandich, A. D., & Macnab, J. J. (2001). A pilot trial of a cognitive treatment for children with developmental coordination disorder. *Human Movement Science, 20,* 183–210.

Milner, A. D., & Goodale, M. A. (1995). *The visual brain in action.* London: Oxford University Press.

Mon-Williams, M., Tresilian, J. R., & Wann, J. P. (1999). Perceiving limb position in normal and abnormal control: An equilibrium point perspective. *Human Movement Science, 18,* 397–419.

Mon-Williams, M. A., Wann, J. P., & Pascal, E. (1999). Visual-proprioceptive mapping in children with developmental coordination disorder. *Developmental Medicine and Child Neurology, 41,* 247–254.

Newell, K. (1991). Motor skill acquisition. *Annual Review of Psychology, 42,* 213–237.

Nissen, M. J., & Bullemer, P. (1987). Attentional requirements of learning: Evidence from performance measures. *Cognitive Psychology, 19,* 1–32.

Petersen, S. E., Robinson, D. L., & Currie, J. N. (1989). Influences of lesions parietal cortex on visual spatial attention in humans. *Experimental Brain Research, 76,* 267–280.

Piek, J. P., & Coleman-Carman, R. (1995). Kinesthetic sensitivity and motor performance of children with developmental coordination disorder. *Developmental Medicine and Child Neurology, 37,* 976–984.

Polatajko, H. J., Macnab, J. J., Anstett, B., Malloymiller, T., Murphy, K., & Noh, S. (1995). A clinical trial of the process-oriented treatment approach for children with developmental coordination disorder. *Developmental Medicine and Child Neurology, 37,* 310–319.

Posner, M. I. (1980). Orienting of attention. *Quarterly Journal of Experimental Psychology: Human Experimental Psychology, 32,* 3–25.

Posner, M. I., Inhoff, A. W., Friedrich, F. J., & Cohen, A. (1987). Isolating attentional systems: A cognitive-anatomical analysis. *Psychobiology, 15,* 107–121.

Rafal, R., & Henik, A. (1994). The neurology of inhibition: Integrating controlled and automatic processes. In D. Dagenbach & T. H. Carr (Eds.), *Inhibitory processes in attention, memory, and language* (pp. 1–51). San Diego, CA: Academic Press.

Rieser, J. J. (1990). Development of perceptual-motor control while walking without vision: The calibration of perception and action. In H. Bloch & B.I. Bertenthal (Eds.), *Sensory-motor organisations and development in infancy and early childhood* (pp. 379–408). Dordrecht: Kluwer Academic.

Rösblad, B., & von Hofsten, C. (1992). Perceptual control of manual pointing in children with motor impairments. *Physiotherapy Theory and Research, 8,* 223–233.

Rourke, B. P. (1995). *Syndrome of nonverbal learning disabilities: Neurodevelopmental manifestations.* New York: Guilford Press.

Roy, E. (1978). Apraxia: A new look at an old syndrome. *Journal of Human Movement Studies, 4,* 191–210.

Schellekens, J. M. H., Scholten, C. A., & Kalverboer, A. F. (1983). Visually guided hand movements in children with minor neurological dysfunction: Response time and movement organization. *Journal of Child Psychology and Psychiatry, 24,* 89–102.

Schoemaker, M. M., Smits-Engelsman, B. C. M., & Kalverboer, A. F. (1998). The classification of specific motor disorders: Implications for intervention. In J. Rispens, T. A. van Yperen, & W. Yule (Eds.), *Perspectives on the classification of specific developmental disorders* (pp. 231–244). Dordrecht: Kluwer Academic.

Schoemaker, M. M., van der Wees, M., Flapper, B., Verheij-Jansen, N., Scholten-Jaegers, S., & Geuze, R. H. (2001). Perceptual skills of children with developmental coordination disorder. *Human Movement Science, 20,* 111–133.

Sigmundsson, H., Ingvaldsen, R. P., & Whiting, H. T. A. (1997). Inter- and intra-sensory modality matching in children with eye-hand co-ordination problems. *Experimental Brain Research, 114,* 492–499.

Sigmundsson, H., Whiting, H. T. A., & Ingvaldsen, R. P. (1999). Putting your foot in it! A window into clumsy behavior. *Behavioral Brain Research, 102,* 131–138.

Sims, K., Henderson, S. E., Hulme, C., & Morton, J. (1996). The remediation of clumsiness. I An evaluation of Laszlo's kinesthetic approach. *Developmental Medicine and Child Neurology, 38,* 976–987.

Sims, K., Henderson, S. E., Morton, J., & Hulme, C. (1996). The remediation of clumsiness. II. Is kinesthesis the answer? *Developmental Medicine and Child Neurology, 38,* 988–997.

Sirigu A., Duhamel, J. R., Cohen, L., Pillon, B., Dubois B., & Agid, Y. (1996). The mental representation of hand movements after parietal cortex damage. *Science, 273,* 1564–1567.

Skorji, V., & McKenzie, B. E. (1997). How do children who are clumsy remember modelled movements? *Developmental Medicine and Child Neurology, 39,* 404–408.

Smits-Engelsman, B. C. M., Niemeijer, A. S., & van Galen, G. P. (2001). Fine motor deficiencies in children diagnosed as DCD based on poor grapho-motor ability. *Human Movement Science, 20,* 161–182.

Smyth, M. M., & Mason, U. C. (1997). Planning and execution of action in children with and without developmental coordination disorder. *Journal of Child Psychology and Psychiatry and Allied Disciplines, 38,* 1023–1037.

Sugden, D., & Wann, C. (1987). The assessment of motor impairment in children with moderate learning difficulties. *British Journal of Educational Psychology, 57,* 225–236.

van der Meulen, J. H. P., van der Gon, J. J. D., Gielen, C. C. A. M., Gooskens, R. H. J. M., & Willemse, J. (1991). Visuomotor performance of normal and clumsy children. I: Fast goal-directed arm-movements with and without visual feedback. *Developmental Medicine and Child Neurology, 33,* 40–54.

van Mier, H., Hulstijn, W., & Meulenbroek, R. G. J. (1994). Movement planning in children with motor disorders: Diagnostic implications of pattern complexity and previewing in copying. *Developmental Neuropsychology, 10,* 231–254.

Visser, J., & Geuze, R. H. (2000). Kinesthetic acuity in adolescent boys: A longitudinal study. *Developmental Medicine and Child Neurology, 42,* 93–96.

Volman, M. J. M., & Geuze, R. H. (1998a). Relative phase stability of bimanual and visuomotor rhythmic coordination patterns in children with developmental coordination disorder. *Human Movement Science, 17,* 541–572.

Volman, M. J. M., & Geuze, R. H. (1998b). Stability of rhythmic finger movements in children with developmental coordination disorder. *Motor Control, 2,* 34–60.

von Hofsten, C., & Rösblad, B. (1988). The integration of sensory information in the development of precise manual pointing. *Neuropsychologia, 26,* 805–821.

Wechsler, D. (1992). *Manual for the Wechsler Intelligence Scale for Children* (3rd ed.). New York: Psychological Corporation.

Wilson, P. H., & Maruff, P. (1999). Deficits in the endogenous control of covert visuospatial attention in children with developmental coordination disorder. *Human Movement Science, 18*, 421–442.

Wilson, P. H., Maruff, P., Ives, S., & Currie, J. (2001). Abnormalities of motor and praxis imagery in children with developmental coordination disorder. *Human Movement Science, 20*, 135–159.

Wilson, P. H., Maruff, P., & Lum, J. (2003). Procedural learning in children with developmental coordination disorder (DCD). *Human Movement Science, 22*, 515–526..

Wilson, P. H., Maruff, P., & McKenzie, B. E. (1997). Covert orienting of attention in children with developmental coordination disorder. *Developmental Medicine and Child Neurology, 39*, 736–745.

Wilson, P. H., & McKenzie, B. E. (1998). Information processing deficits associated with Developmental Coordination Disorder: A meta-analysis of research findings. *Journal of Child Psychology and Psychiatry and Allied Disciplines, 39*, 829–840.

Wolpert, D. (1997). Computational approaches to motor control. *Trends in Cognitive Science, 1*, 209–216.

CHAPTER 14

Processing Deficits in Children with Movement and Attention Problems

JAN P. PIEK

THELMA M. PITCHER

Understanding the underlying deficits in children with motor coordination problems, termed *developmental coordination disorder* (DCD) in the fourth edition of the *Diagnostic and Statistical Manual of Mental Disorders* (DSM-IV; American Psychiatric Association, 1994), is complex as DCD is a heterogeneous condition in terms of its movement disabilities (Henderson & Barnett, 1998). Children with DCD can have problems with fine motor abilities such as writing or tying a shoelace, with gross motor abilities such as running and climbing, or with both fine and gross motor abilities. For children to be diagnosed with DCD, their motor impairment needs to be "sufficient to produce functional performance deficits not explicable by the child's [chronological] age or intellect, or by other diagnosable neurological or psychiatric disorders" (Polatajko, Fox, & Missiuna 1995, p. 5).

In addition to its heterogeneity, DCD has been found to be comorbid with a variety of disorders including attention-deficit/hyperactivity disorder (Kaplan, Wilson, Dewey, & Crawford, 1998; Piek, Pitcher, & Hay, 1999) and reading disability (Kaplan et al., 1998; Ramus, Pidgeon, & Frith, 2003). Recently, research has focused on the link between DCD and attention-deficit/hyperactivity disorder (ADHD). Children with ADHD are characterized by persistent symptoms of inattention and/or hyperactivity–impulsivity that are not consistent with their developmental level and are maladaptive (DSM-IV; American Psychiatric Association, 1994). Three subtypes of ADHD have been identified by DSM-IV: predominantly inattentive type (ADHD-PI), predominantly hyperactive–impulsive type (ADHD-HI), and combined type (ADHD-C) (i.e., combined inattentive and hyperactive/impulsive symptoms). Recently, Pitcher, Piek, and Hay (2003) found a high percentage of movement problems in all three subtypes, with 58% of ADHD-PI, 49% of ADHD-HI, and 47% of ADHD-C children with motor performance in the lower 15th percentile of a standard movement assessment battery. These proportions are quite similar despite evidence to suggest that the three subtypes of ADHD are genetically distinct disorders (Levy, McStephen, & Hay, 2001). The percentage of children with DCD (i.e., in the lower 5th percentile) was also high for each group, namely, 42% for the ADHD-PI group, 31% for the ADHD-HI group, and 29% for the ADHD-C group. These findings are not surprising given that a relationship between ADHD and motor dysfunction has been demonstrated throughout the ADHD literature (e.g., Barkley, 1990; Doyle, Wallen, & Whitmont, 1995; Lerer, Lerer, & Artner, 1977; McMahon & Greenburg, 1977; Parry, 1996; Piek et al., 1999; Shaywitz & Shaywitz, 1984; Stewart, Pitts, Craig, & Dieruf, 1966; Szatmari, Offord, & Boyle, 1989; Whitmont & Clark, 1996).

Comorbidity between DCD and ADHD has not been well recognized by DSM-IV (American Psychiatric Association, 1994). Within the differential diagnoses section for DCD, the motor skill problems of children with ADHD are regarded as being "usually due to distractibility and impulsiveness, rather than to motor impairment" (p. 54), although a dual diagnosis for both disorders may be given. Our recent findings (Pitcher et al., 2003), however, demonstrate that poor fine motor ability associated with ADHD cannot be attributed to inattentive or hyperactive/impulsive symptomatology. Of concern is that although DSM-IV links ADHD and motor incoordination within the differential diagnosis section for DCD, there is no reciprocal recognition of the motor skills disorders (i.e., DCD) within the differential diagnosis section for ADHD: The possibility of dual diagnoses is not indicated. DSM-IV's position in relation to dual diagnosis may be clinically disadvantageous as the long-term outcome for children with a comorbid condition (i.e., ADHD with DCD) may be less positive than for those children with only ADHD or DCD (Gillberg, 1992).

An alternative diagnostic system that identifies the possibility of a dual diagnosis is the "deficits in attention, motor control, and perception" model (DAMP) (Airaksinen et al., 1991, cited in Gillberg, 1998). DAMP is viewed as an overarching concept that encompasses "combinations of motor control and perceptual problems in conjunction with attentional problems encountered in children who do not show mental retardation or cerebral palsy" (Gillberg, 1995, p. 139). It includes areas of attention, gross and fine motor skills, perceptual ability, and speech/language dysfunction (Gillberg, 1992). Gillberg (1998) argued that few studies have examined the relationship between these core features despite them being "linked in a meaningful way" for over 100 years (p. 108). From a DAMP perspective, it is important to provide separate diagnoses for children with DCD and ADHD, in order to have a greater insight into the underlying problems of each disorder. It is the aim of this chapter to investigate these underlying problems by examining the relationship between perceptual, motor, and attentional deficits in children with either a single diagnosis of DCD or ADHD or the combined diagnosis of DCD and ADHD.

A popular theoretical approach used by cognitive psychologists to investigate human functioning (Schmidt & Lee, 1999), and in particular deficits in functioning in disorders such as DCD and ADHD, is the information-processing approach. This approach considers perception as the "input" stage of information processing, which involves the registration, integration, and interpretation of sensory information (Wilson & McKenzie, 1998). In the response–selection stage, a decision is made on what response is needed, and the final motor or output processes involve the organization and initiation of the appropriate response or motor program.

INFORMATION-PROCESSING DEFICITS IN CHILDREN
WITH DEVELOPMENTAL COORDINATION DISORDER

An extensive review of information-processing deficits in children with DCD can be found in Chapter 13 (Wilson, this volume). A meta-analysis by Wilson and McKenzie (1998) demonstrated that significant visuospatial, kinesthetic, and cross-modal deficits exist for children with DCD, with visuospatial deficits having the largest effect size. Our own research has supported this finding. We found that school-age children with DCD are poorer on subtests of Performance IQ from the Wechsler Intelligence Scale for Children, third edition (WISC-III: Wechsler, 1992), especially those requiring complex visuospatial tasks such as block design and object assembly (Piek & Coleman-Carman, 1995). Furthermore, our recent research (Coleman, Piek, & Livesey, 2001) indicates that this is also the case for younger children ages 4–6 years when tested on the Wechsler Preschool and Primary Scale of Intelligence—Revised (WPPSI-R: Wechsler, 1989). In this study, children with DCD performed more poorly than did control children on the subtests of object assembly, geometric design, and block design. In both of these studies we also examined kinesthetic acuity in children with and without DCD. Again, in support of Wilson and McKenzie's findings, children with DCD were poorer at the kinesthetic acuity tasks.

None of these studies, however, controlled for possible comorbidity with ADHD. Could the deficits identified be a result of inattention or hyperactivity/impulsivity caused by comorbid ADHD? The following section examines literature that has investigated information processing deficits in children with ADHD.

INFORMATION-PROCESSING DEFICITS IN CHILDREN
WITH ATTENTION-DEFICIT/HYPERACTIVITY DISORDER

An examination of the literature on information processing deficits in children with ADHD has produced mixed results. Few studies have investigated kinesthetic ability in children with ADHD. Whitmont and Clark (1996) investigated kinesthetic acuity and fine motor skills in a group of children with ADHD using the Kinaesthetic Acuity Test (Livesey & Parkes, 1995). The children with ADHD had both significantly poorer kinesthetic acuity and poorer fine motor ability than did the control group. A significant but weak association was shown between the two variables. The authors also found a strong association between fine motor skill deficits and severity of ADHD pathology as measured by the Hyperactivity Index of the Conners Rating Scales ($r = -.57$, $p = .005$, one-tailed) (Goyette, Conners, & Ulrich, 1978).

Subsequent to Whitmont and Clark (1996), we investigated kinesthetic sensitivity in children with either ADHD-PI or ADHD-C and control children and found no significant difference in group performance on the kinesthetic tasks (Piek et al., 1999). However, a number of factors leave a comparison of the two studies in doubt. First, different assessment devices were used, as our study measured kinesthetic sensitivity using the Kinaesthetic Sensitivity Test (Laszlo & Bairstow, 1985). In addition, we included an ADHD-PI group. Although not formally assessed, Whitmont and Clark (1996) reported that none of the ADHD group would have fulfilled the criteria for ADHD-PI (i.e., all were either ADHD-HI or ADHD-C). They did not address the issue of subtype variability in performance. Neither study separated the ADHD groups into those with or without DCD. Hence, it is unclear whether the different findings can be explained in terms of the presence or absence of an underlying motor disorder in the two different samples of children with ADHD.

Visuomotor processing difficulties have been found to differentiate children with ADHD from control children in some studies (e.g., Moffitt & Silva, 1988; Oie & Rund, 1999; Raggio, 1999). Raggio (1999) found that a group of 26 preadolescent children with ADHD-C scored significantly lower than the normative sample scores on the Bender–Gestalt test (Bender, 1983). Oie and Rund (1999) found poorer performance for their group of boys with ADHD (DSM-III-R; American Psychiatric Association, 1987) than for the control group (note: mixed-gender control group) on Part B of the Trail Making Test (Reitan & Wolfson, 1993) and WISC-R Digit Symbol subtest (Wechsler, 1974), although these results are more reflective of difficulties with attention and speed of information processing (Groth-Marnat, 1997) rather than perceptual organization. In contrast, Carlson, Lahey, and Neeper (1986) did not find any significant visuomotor skill differences on the Beery Visual–Motor Integration test which involved copying 24 geometric designs of increasing complexity (Berry, 1967). In this study, children were identified using the DSM-III-R category. This earlier categorization identified two major subtypes: (1) children with hyperactivity (ADD-H) and (2) children without hyperactivity (ADD-WO) who had core deficits in attention and impulsivity (Cantwell & Baker, 1992; Carlson, 1986; Schaughency & Hynd, 1989). Again, most of these studies did not consider a dual diagnosis of ADHD and DCD, and therefore did not examine the impact of each disorder on visuomotor processing.

Recently, Pitcher (2001) investigated information processing deficits in children with all three subtypes of ADHD (American Psychiatric Association, 1994) and a comparison group using the Performance IQ (PIQ) subtests from the WISC-III (Wechsler, 1992) to examine visuospatial processing and processing speed. The PIQ subtests can be used to separately assess Perceptual Organization (subtests of picture completion, picture arrangement, block design, and object assembly), and Processing Speed (subtests of coding and symbol search). Pitcher found that all three ADHD subtypes had significantly poorer PIQ scores than the comparison group, and the findings could not be directly attributable to general lower intelligence as all groups were statistically equivalent in terms of their prorated Verbal IQ scores.

When the PIQ scores were examined separately for Perceptual Organization and Processing Speed, the three ADHD groups were significantly poorer than the comparison group for Processing Speed but not for Perceptual Organization. The finding for Processing Speed supports other studies which have identified children with ADHD as having slower Processing Speed than comparison children (Mayes, Calhoun, & Crowell, 1998; Pennington & Ozonoff, 1996; Schwean & Saklofske, 1998). Processing speed (a measure of mental and motor speed) is "sensitive to change over time . . . [and the] . . . one factor score that is most likely to be lower in ADHD children as a group" (Schwean & Saklofske, 1998, p. 95). However, an unexpected finding was that no significant subtype differences were evident. According to Sattler (1992), the Processing Speed factor "appears to reflect the ability to employ a high degree of concentration and attention in processing information rapidly by scanning an array" (pp. 1045–1046). As such, it was expected that children with subtypes including inattentive symptomatology (i.e., ADHD-PI and ADHD-C) would be more likely to score more poorly on the Processing Speed factor. However, this was not found to be the case. It should be pointed out, however, that, according to the categorical definitions, children in the hyperactive subtype can also have up to five inattentive symptoms which could produce ambiguous results.

Consequently, Pitcher (2001) also employed a dimensional approach by using standard multiple regression to examine the relationship between ADHD symptomatology (i.e., total inattention score and total hyperactive–impulsive score) and PIQ scores. It was found that inattentive symptomatology and not hyperactive–impulsive symptomatology predicted PIQ, in particular Processing Speed. Furthermore, Pitcher reported that inattentive symptomatology did not predict either Verbal IQ (VIQ) or Perceptual Organization. Attention appears to be a key variable in understanding information-processing deficits in children with ADHD. Also, given its relationship with motor control (e.g., Dewey, Kaplan, Crawford, & Wilson, 2002; Piek et al., 1999), it is also an important variable to consider in children with DCD.

ATTENTION

William James (1890, cited in Summers & Ford, 1995) defined attention as, "the taking possession by the mind, in clear and vivid form, of one out of what seem several simultaneously possible objects or trains of thought" (p. 64). This definition raises the concept of selectivity (Summers & Ford, 1995) and as Schmidt (1988) has described, the ability to attend to different stimuli is a finite characteristic of our conscious capacity to process information. Selectivity helps to avoid cognitive overload and is determined by an individual's ability to direct attention toward the most important stimuli while modulating the intensity of attention required for each stimulus (i.e., external or internal) (Summers & Ford, 1995).

Attention has been alternatively described as the rate of information processing within the working memory system (Schiffrin & Schneider, 1977, cited in Sergeant & van der Meere, 1990). A theoretical point of conjecture arises when efforts are directed toward using attention theory to pinpoint the location of an information-processing limitation in the input-to-output sequence (Keele, 1973). Keele (1973) suggested that instead of attention being viewed as "point specific," its role is better conceived of as one of a "control process for the flow of information" (p. 57). From an information-processing approach, attention assists the process of stimuli recognition, response selection, and response organization as compatible memory traces are accessed, selected, and assimilated and incompatible activities are attenuated (Keele, 1973). Where the parameters for a response have already been identified and are awaiting execution (e.g., in a simple reaction time task), attention may also be responsible for the maintenance of the intended response between the period of response formulation to response initiation (Goodrich, Henderson, Allchin, & Jeevaratnam, 1990). Imposition of a secondary task and increased task complexity can interfere with the attentional requirements (or load) and delay response (Summers & Ford, 1995). Moreover, a reduced ability to disengage attention can result in less proficient performance (Summers & Ford, 1995; Wilson, Maruff, & McKenzie, 1997).

An individual's capacity to attend may be influenced by his or her state of arousal or alertness, with research demonstrating that increased arousal leads to an inverted

U-shape capacity (Kahneman, 1973, cited in Summers & Ford, 1995). Increased arousal may also lead to the "activation of additional resources," thereby increasing capacity (Summers & Ford, 1995, p. 75). Sergeant and others (Sanders, 1983; Sergeant, 2000; van der Meere, 1996) view attentional resources as being fundamentally entrenched within a broader information-processing-based, cognitive–energetical system. This model details a multistate regulatory function system, describing three key processing levels (i.e., evaluation mechanisms, energetical mechanisms, and processing stages) that are heavily influenced by the role of attention processes (see Pribram & McGuiness, 1975; Sanders, 1983; Sergeant, 2000; van der Meere, 1996). The energetical systems of arousal, effort, and activation modulate the processing stage operations (Tannock, 1998; van der Meere, 1996). The processing stage level involves "encoding, search, decision and motor organisation" (Sternberg, 1969, cited in Sergeant, 2000, p. 8).

Attention, and an ability to attend selectively have been described as basic and essential prerequisites for skilled performance and are influential in motor learning (Summers & Ford, 1995; Wilson et al., 1997). Attention is especially important during the learning of new movement sequences when the activity of the areas of the brain not engaged by the task is, by a process of selective attention, thought to be "depressed" to reveal a reduction in activity (Jenkins, Brooks, Nixon, Frackowiak, & Passingham, 1994). Specific areas of the frontal and parietal lobes have been implicated in separate functions of selective attention (Posner & Dehaene, 1994). Furthermore, a movement with well-defined, consistent parameters in terms of output expectations will, over time and with practice, gradually require less attentional resources in order to achieve a similar standard of performance. Attention as a limited capacity central processor has long been linked with discussion about automation of movement (Fitts & Posner, 1967). A regular consensus is that the "capacity limitations evident under controlled processing may not apply when the task becomes automated" (Summers & Ford, 1995, p. 73). That is, automated processing decreases the demand for selective attentional resources. Interestingly, studies have shown that the learning of motor sequences with some unique elements can take place in the presence of distraction, while the repetition of previously learned elements in different orders within a sequence requires attention (Cohen, Ivry, & Keele, 1990; Keele & Jennings, 1992). Cohen and colleagues (1990) suggested that this was due to the attentional demands associated with hierarchical processing of the parts of the learned elements into different representations for action.

DEFICITS IN CHILDREN WITH ATTENTION-DEFICIT/ HYPERACTIVITY DISORDER WITH AND WITHOUT DEVELOPMENTAL COORDINATION DISORDER

The relationship between motor difficulties and problems of attention is evident within reviews of the history and correlates of ADHD (see Barkley, 1998; Gillberg, 1995; Rosenthal & Allen, 1978; Sandberg & Barton, 1996; Taylor, 1998). It is not surprising then that several studies have demonstrated that inattentive symptomatology, and not hyperactive–impulsive symptomatology, of children with ADHD is a potent predictor of poor motor performance (McGee, Williams, & Silva, 1985; Piek et al.,

1999). The link between ADHD and motor functioning is of key interest as there is evidence indicating greater impairment and less optimistic longer-term outcomes for individuals with the comorbid condition (i.e., DAMP; Gillberg, 1992).

Information-Processing Deficits

In line with the DAMP model, Pitcher (2001) investigated Perceptual Organization and Processing Speed in boys with ADHD who either did or did not have comorbid DCD. Three groups of boys ages between 8 and 12 years were examined. The first group (ADHD/DCD) included 55 boys who met the criteria for any of the three ADHD subtypes (DSM-IV) and a "DCD" categorization (i.e., performance on the Movement Assessment Battery for Children ≤15th percentile; Henderson & Sugden, 1992). A second group consisted of 49 boys with an ADHD diagnosis but no "DCD" diagnosis. This group of boys had "pure" ADHD (acording to DSM-IV) but with unspecified subtypes (n = 49). The comparison group comprised boys without either ADHD or DCD (n = 31).

Children with the dual diagnosis of ADHD and DCD had significantly lower scores on Perceptual Organization than the comparison group. However, children with the single diagnosis of ADHD did not differ from either the comparison group or the group with dual diagnoses on Perceptual Organization. Unlike children with DCD (e.g., Coleman et al., 1997, 2001; Wilson & McKenzie, 1998), Perceptual Organization did not appear to be the source of the lowered PIQ in children with a single diagnosis of ADHD. This supports the findings of a meta-analysis carried out by Pennington and Ozonoff (1996) who examined information-processing deficits and, specifically, executive functioning, in 18 different studies. Executive functioning (EF) describes aspects of information processing that manage complex, controlled behaviors as opposed to automatic actions and include planning action sequences, working memory, and the ability to delay or inhibit particular responses (Hughes & Graham, 2002). Pennington and Ozonoff examined 60 EF measures used across the 18 studies. Forty of these demonstrated significantly worse performance in the ADHD groups compared with the control groups. In contrast, of the 19 measures that examined visuospatial organization, only four demonstrated significant differences between the control and ADHD groups. As with the findings of Pitcher (2001), studies that utilized the block design and object assembly from the WISC-III did not find group differences.

It is also worth noting that in a recent study (Piek et al., in press), we compared children with DCD and a control group on three tasks measuring EF. Children with DCD were no worse than the control children on tasks that measure response inhibition (e.g., go/no-go task and goal-neglect task), although the DCD children were poorer on a task that assessed working memory in addition to behavioral inhibition (trailmaking/memory updating task), even when attention was controlled. Overall, these findings suggest that response inhibition may be a process that is disrupted in ADHD but not DCD, whereas visuospatial organization is a process that is disrupted in DCD but not ADHD.

As described earlier, poor Processing Speed in children with ADHD has been found in previous research. Pennington and Ozonoff (1996) examined this variable in their meta-analysis and found that ADHD groups were consistently poorer on the subtests of coding and symbol search compared with control groups. This was supported by Pitcher (2001), who found that children with the single diagnosis of ADHD were significantly poorer on Processing Speed than the comparison group. Children with the dual diagnosis of ADHD and DCD had significantly lower scores on Processing Speed than the comparison group but were also significantly poorer than the single-diagnosis group with ADHD. This is consistent with Gillberg's (1992) assertion that the outcome for children with a dual diagnosis is considerably poorer than for children with a single diagnosis.

Deficits in Timing and Force Control

There is no doubt as to the importance of timing and force control in the production of coordinated movement, and there has been increasing interest in these issues with respect to children with ADHD. The findings for children with DCD indicate problematic timing functions in sequential tapping tasks (e.g., Lundy-Ekman, Ivry, Keele, & Woollacott, 1991; Missiuna, 1994; Williams, Woollacott, & Ivry, 1992), which generally manifest in greater variability and inconsistency in both time-interval measures and movement duration (Geuze, 1990; Geuze & Kalverboer, 1987, 1994). The neural localization of a central timing deficit has been hypothesized to be within the cerebellum (Williams et al., 1992), with some evidence that the basal ganglia may influence variability in force production (Lundy-Ekman et al., 1991). The temporal relationship between the agonist and antagonist bursts of the muscles required for sequential movement may be impeded, or may result in greater variability, as a result of an imprecise timekeeper mechanism (Marsden, 1977, cited in Lundy-Ekman et al., 1991). While some of these studies have noted flaws (see Kalverboer, 1998; Kooistra, Snijders, Schellekens, Kalverboer, & Geuze, 1997; Schoemaker, Smits-Engelsman, & Kalverboer, 1998), they do emphasize the issue of central timing. In contrast to those studies implicating a central timing mechanism (e.g., Geuze & Kalverboer, 1987, 1994; Lundy-Ekman et al., 1991; Williams et al., 1992), output deficits associated with motor execution have also been linked with motor dysfunction (e.g., Kooistra, Schellekens, Schoemaker, Vulsma, & van der Meere, 1998; Kooistra et al., 1997; Piek & Skinner, 1999).

According to Barkley (1997), timing difficulties in children with ADHD are linked to EF and are a hypothesized outcome of working-memory problems stemming from inhibitory deficits. These deficits are associated with the prefrontal cortex. Hyperactive children have been found to be less able than controls to estimate time intervals (Cappella, Gentile, & Juliano, 1977), although recent research has indicated that their time estimation abilities are intact but they are "impaired in timing their motor output" (Rubia, Taylor, Taylor, & Sergeant, 1999, p. 1237). We (Pitcher, Piek, & Barrett, 2002) investigated these factors in children with ADHD utilizing a sequential tapping task employed by Piek and Skinner (1999) for children with DCD. This approach is similar to that originally described by Semjen and colleagues (Semjen & Garcia-Colera, 1986; Semjen, Garcia-Colera, & Requin, 1984), and modified by Piek, Glencross, Barrett, and Love (1993). We demonstrated that the ADHD-PI and ADHD-C but not ADHD-HI subtypes had significantly longer movement time and higher peak force than did the comparison children, and greater variability that was not associated directly with the complexity of the movement sequence. That is, only the subtypes with inattentive symptomatology were affected. Slower tapping speed and inattentive symptomatology have been linked in past research (McGee et al., 1985), although this link in the current study may have been influenced by the type of task used. That is, it required distributive planning (Garcia-Colera & Semjen, 1988; Semjen & Garcia-Colera, 1986; Semjen et al., 1984), which emphasizes the role of on-line processing in that not all movement parameters within the sequence are preprogrammed or automatic. The influence of inattention on the current study's task requirement for on-line motor processing has not previously been documented. Some interactive effect is likely to be evident given that previous research with children with ADHD has shown that "controlled processing tasks differentiated groups better than did automated tasks" (Carte, Nigg, & Hinshaw, 1996, p. 481).

Pitcher and colleagues (2002) also investigated differences in timing and force control between groups with either a single diagnosis of ADHD or a dual diagnosis of ADHD and DCD, and compared the results with a control group. Both the group with ADHD and the group with ADHD/DCD had significantly longer movement times (as measured by the intertap intervals) than the control group but did not differ significantly from each other. However, children with the dual diagnosis of ADHD and DCD had significantly longer reaction times and higher peak force than did comparison children. This was not the case for the children with ADHD only who did not differ from the control group on these variables. Again, this demonstrates that a child with a dual diagnosis has unique difficulties to those with a single diagnosis of ADHD.

There are several possible processes that may result in the difference in peak force for a child with both ADHD and DCD. Based on the earlier findings, it is possible that poor perceptual organization may have contributed to the higher peak force output. An alternate explanation may be drawn from the recent hypothesis that timing and force difficulties for children with DCD may occur due to impaired processing of the "efference copy" (Wilson, Maruff, Ives, & Currie, 2001), which is a copy of the efferent motor commands. It is linked to the parietal lobe. An "efference-copy deficit" would lead to an inhibition of both error detection/correction and subsequent motor commands (Wilson et al., 2001). These suggestions certainly warrant the further investigation of force control in children with subtypes of ADHD, DCD, and their comorbid condition.

CONCLUSIONS

Given the links between motor difficulties, ADHD, and inattention, the results from studies reporting on DSM-IV subtypes of ADHD will remain difficult to interpret if comorbid motor deficits are not identified. The findings for children with both ADHD and DCD demonstrate that this comorbid relationship results in poorer performance on measures of PIQ, reaction time, and peak force compared with children with a single diagnosis of ADHD. Children with a dual diagnosis appear to have significant difficulties with both Perceptual Organization and Processing Speed tasks compared with both the comparison group and children with a single diagnosis of ADHD with no significant motor problems. Processing Speed and movement time difficulties were also evident for children with a single diagnosis of ADHD. Perceptual Organization has previously been identified as a factor that "provides the best estimate of cognitive potential" (Schwean & Saklofske, 1998, p. 100). Pitcher's (2001) finding that VIQ was lower for children with a dual diagnosis further emphasizes the poorer cognitive potential in this group.

The profile for the children with both ADHD and DCD is, in many ways, reflective of the performance of children with DCD. Children with DCD have been found to have longer and more variable reaction times in a range of experimental tasks (e.g., Geuze, 1990; Henderson, Rose, & Henderson, 1992; Piek & Skinner, 1999; Piek et al., in press). They have also been found to have greater difficulty processing information in preparation for the response (van Dellen & Geuze, 1988), which has alternatively been described as related to response organization (or motor programming) (Smyth & Glencross, 1986). Henderson and colleagues (1992) proposed that children with DCD have low stimulus–response compatibility and that this deficit contributes to their coordination difficulties by overtaxing the child's attentional resources, especially during high-demand activities (Henderson et al., 1992). Other studies have also reported longer movement duration times for children with DCD and identified that inefficient processing of visual feedback compounded aiming inaccuracies (van der Meulen, van der Gon, Gielen, Gooskens, & Willemse, 1991a, 1991b). These outcomes may also be linked to perceptual organization and cross-modal integration of information (e.g., Coleman et al., 2001; Wilson & McKenzie, 1998).

The aforementioned findings for Processing Speed, Perceptual Organization, and timing and force variables may provide an explanation for inconsistencies of previous research with children on ADHD, in particular those with inattentive symptomatology, where the underlying motor difficulties have remained unassessed. Perceptual Organization and peak force were only affected in the ADHD/DCD group and not the ADHD group. If children with comorbid DCD are not identified in research on ADHD, it will confound studies that involve tasks that require visuospatial or motor skills.

The highest correlation between IQ and ADHD symptomatology variables occurred between processing speed and inattention. Thus, an interesting and important relationship between inattentive symptomatology and the scores for PIQ and Processing Speed has been established. Of equal importance is the finding that hyperactive–impulsive symptomatology does not appear to predict any of the intelligence factors. Also, inattentive symptomatology did not significantly predict VIQ or Perceptual Organization. As Buitelaar and van Engeland (1996) have pointed out, the "pathogenetic mechanisms of the link between inattention and either general or specific cognitive impairments are as yet incompletely explored" (p. 60).

In conclusion, in investigating information processing, and timing and force mechanisms that are disrupted in children with ADHD and DCD, we have identified common mechanisms that are disrupted in both disorders (namely Processing Speed and movement time). However, there also appears to be processes unique to children with ADHD (namely response inhibition) and DCD (Perceptual Organization and movement force). Hence, to design appropriate intervention strategies for these children, it is imperative that we identify what specific problems these children are having. Identification of comorbid conditions such as DCD in children with ADHD and, likewise, comorbid conditions such as ADHD in children with DCD is an essential prerequisite to any treatment program.

REFERENCES

American Psychiatric Association. (1987). *Diagnostic and statistical manual of mental disorders* (3rd ed., rev.). Washington, DC: Author.

American Psychiatric Association. (1994). *Diagnostic and statistical manual of mental disorders* (4th ed.). Washington, DC: Author.

Barkley, R. A. (1990). *Attention-deficit/hyperactivity disorder: A handbook for diagnosis and treatment.* New York: Guilford Press.

Barkley, R. A. (1997). Behavioral inhibition, sustained attention, and executive functions: Constructing a unifying theory of ADHD. *Psychological Bulletin, 121,* 65–94.

Barkley, R. A. (1998). *Attention-deficit/hyperactivity disorder: A handbook for diagnosis and treatment* (2nd ed.). New York: Guilford Press.

Bender, L. A. (1983). *A visual motor gestalt test and its clinical use.* Bethesda, MD: American Orthopsychiatry Association.

Berry, K. E. (1967). *Developmental Test of Visual–Motor Integration.* Chicago: Follett Educational.

Buitelaar, J. K., & van Engeland, H. (1996). Epidemiological approaches. In S. Sandberg (Ed.), *Monographs in child and adolescent psychiatry: Hyperactivity disorders of childhood* (pp. 26–68). Cambridge, UK: Cambridge University Press.

Cantwell, D. P., & Baker, L. (1992). Attention deficit disorder with and without hyperactivity: A review and comparison of matched groups. *Journal of the American Academy of Child and Adolescent Psychiatry, 31*(3), 432–438.

Cappella, B., Gentile, J. R., & Juliano, D. B. (1977). Time estimation by hyperactive and normal children. *Perceptual and Motor Skills, 44,* 787–790.

Carlson, C. L. (1986). Attention deficit disorder without hyperactivity: A review of preliminary experimental evidence. In B. B. Lahey & A. E. Kazdin (Eds.), *Advances in clinical child psychology* (Vol. 9, pp. 153–175). New York: Plenum Press.

Carlson, C. L., Lahey, B. B., & Neeper, R. (1986). Direct assessment of the cognitive correlates of attention deficit disorders with and without hyperactivity. *Journal of Psychopathology and Behavioral Assessment, 8*(1), 69–86.

Carte, E. T., Nigg, J. T., & Hinshaw, S. P. (1996). Neuropsychological functioning, motor speed, and language processing in boys with and without ADHD. *Journal of Abnormal Child Psychology, 24,* 481–499.

Cohen, A., Ivry, R., & Keele, S. W. (1990). Attention and structure in sequence learning. *Journal of Experimental Psychology: Learning, Memory and Cognition, 16,* 17–30.

Coleman, R., Piek, J. P., & Livesey, D. J. (1997). Kinaesthetic acuity in preprimary children at risk of developmental coordination disorder. *Australian Educational and Developmental Psychologist, 14,* 80–86.

Coleman, R., Piek, J. P., & Livesey, D. J. (2001). A longitudinal study of motor ability and kinaesthetic acuity in young children at risk of development coordination disorder. *Human Movement Science, 20,* 95–110.

Dewey, D., Kaplan, B. J., Crawford, S. G., & Wilson, B. N. (2002). Developmental coordination disorder: Associated problems in attention, learning and psychosocial adjustment. *Human Movement Science, 21,* 905–918.

Doyle, S., Wallen, M., & Whitmont, S. (1995). Motor skills in Australian children with attention deficit hyperactivity disorder. *Occupational Therapy International, 2,* 229–240.

Fitts, P. M., & Posner, M. I. (1967). *Human performance.* Belmont,CA: Wadsworth.

Garcia-Colera, A., & Semjen, A. (1988). Distributed planning of movement sequences. *Journal of Motor Behavior, 20,* 341–367.

Geuze, R. H. (1990). Variability of performance and adaptations to changing task demands in clumsy children. In A. F. Kalverboer (Ed.), *Developmental biopsychology: Experimental and observational studies in children at risk* (pp. 207–222). Ann Arbor: University of Michigan Press.

Geuze, R. H., & Kalverboer, A. F. (1987). Inconsistency and adaptation in timing of clumsy children. *Journal of Motor Behavior, 20*(3), 341–367.

Geuze, R. H., & Kalverboer, A. F. (1994). Tapping a rhythm: A problem of timing for children who are clumsy and dyslexic? *Adapted Physical Activity Quarterly, 11*, 203–213.

Gillberg, C. (1992). Deficits in attention, motor control and perception, and other syndromes attributed to minimal brain dysfunction. In J. Aicardi (Ed.), *Diseases of the nervous system in childhood. Clinics in developmental medicine: No. 115-118* (pp. 1321–1337). London: MacKeith Press.

Gillberg, C. (1995). Deficits in attention, motor control and perception, and other syndromes attributed to minimal brain dysfunction. In C. Gillberg (Ed.), *Clinical child neuropsychiatry* (pp. 138–172). Cambridge, UK: Cambridge University Press.

Gillberg, C. (1998). Hyperactivity, inattention and motor control problems: prevalence, comorbidity and background factors. *Folia Phoniatrica et Logopaedica, 50*(3), 107–117.

Goodrich, S., Henderson, S. E., Allchin, N., & Jeevaratnam, A. (1990). On the peculiarity of simple reaction time. *Quarterly Journal of Experimental Psychology, 42A*, 763–775.

Goyette, C. H., Conners, C. K., & Ulrich, R. F. (1978). Normative data on revised Conners parent and teacher rating scales. *Journal of Abnormal Child Psychology, 6*, 221–236.

Groth-Marnat, G. (1997). *Handbook of psychological assessment* (3rd ed.). New York: Wiley.

Henderson, L., Rose, P., & Henderson, S. E. (1992). Reaction time and movement time in children with a developmental coordination disorder. *Journal of Child Psychology and Psychiatry, 33*(5), 895–905.

Henderson, S. E., & Barnett, A. L. (1998). The classification of specific motor coordination disorders in children: Some problems to be resolved. *Human Movement Science, 17*, 449–469.

Henderson, S. E., & Sugden, D. A. (1992). *Movement Assessment Battery for Children.* New York: Psychological Corporation/Harcourt.

Hughes, C., & Graham, A. (2002). Measuring executive functions in childhood: Problems and solutions. *Child and Adolescent Mental Health, 7, 131–142.*

Jenkins, I. H., Brooks, D. J., Nixon, P. D., Frackowiak, R. S. J., & Passingham, R. E. (1994). Motor sequence learning: A study with positron emission tomography. *Journal of Neuroscience, 14*, 3775–3790.

Kalverboer, A. F. (1998). On the relevance of specific classifications of disorders with a particular focus on DCD, developmental coordination disorder. In J. Rispens, T. A. V. Yperen, & W. Yule (Eds.), *Perspectives on the classification of specific developmental disorders* (pp. 265–278). Dordrecht, Netherlands: Kluwer Academic.

Kaplan, B. J., Wilson, B. N., Dewey, D., & Crawford, S. G. (1998). DCD may not be a discrete disorder. *Human Movement Science, 17*, 471–490.

Keele, S. W. (1973). Mechanisms of attention. In E. C. Carterette & M. P. Friedman (Eds.), *Handbook of perception* (Vol. 9, pp. 1–68). New York: Academic Press.

Keele, S. W., & Jennings, P. J. (1992). Attention in the representation of sequence: Experiment and theory. *Human Movement Science, 11*, 125–138.

Kooistra, L., Schellekens, J. M. H., Schoemaker, M. M., Vulsma, T., & van der Meere, J. J. (1998). Motor problems in children with early-treated congenital hypothyroidism: A matter of failing cerebellar motor control? *Human Movement Science, 17*, 609–628.

Kooistra, L., Snijders, T. A. B., Schellekens, J. M. H., Kalverboer, A. F., & Geuze, R. H. (1997). Timing variability in children with early-treated congenital hypothyroidism. *Acta Psychologica, 96*(1–2), 61–73.

Laszlo, J. I., & Bairstow, P. J. (1985). *Kinaesthetic Sensitivity Test.* London: Holt, Rinehart & Winston.

Lerer, R. J., Lerer, M. P., & Artner, J. (1977). The effects of methylphenidate on the handwriting of children with minimal brain dysfunction. *Journal of Pediatrics, 91*(1), 127–132.

Levy, F., McStephen, M., & Hay, D.A. (2001). Diagnostic genetics of ADHD symptoms and subtypes. In F. Levy & D. A. Hay (Eds)., *Attention, genes and ADHD* (pp. 35–57). Sydney, Australia: MacMillan.

Livesey, D. J., & Parkes, N.-A. (1995). Testing kinaesthetic acuity in preschool children. *Australian Journal of Psychology, 47*(3), 160–163.

Lundy-Ekman, L., Ivry, R., Keele, S., & Woollacott, M. (1991). Timing and force control deficits in clumsy children. *Journal of Cognitive Neuroscience, 3*(4), 367–376.

Mayes, S. D., Calhoun, S. L., & Crowell, E. W. (1998). WISC-III Freedom from Distractibility as a measure of attention in children with and without attention deficit hyperactivity disorder. *Journal of Attention Disorders*, (4), 217–227.

McGee, R., Williams, S. M., & Silva, P. A. (1985). Factor structure and correlates of ratings of inattention, hyperactivity, and antisocial behavior in a large sample of 9-yr-old children from the general population. *Journal of Consulting and Clinical Psychology, 53*, 480–490.

McMahon, S. A., & Greenburg, L. M. (1977). Serial neurologic examination of hyperactive children. *Pediatrics, 59*(4), 584–587.

Missiuna, C. (1994). Motor skill acquisition in children with developmental coordination disorder. *Adapted Physical Activity Quarterly, 11*, 214–235.

Moffitt, T., & Silva, P. (1988). Self-reported delinquency, neuropsychological deficit and history of attention deficit disorder. *Journal of Abnormal Child Psychology, 16*(5), 553–569.

Oie, M., & Rund, B. R. (1999). Neuropsychological deficits in adolescent-onset schizophrenia compared with attention deficit hyperactivity disorder. *American Journal of Psychiatry, 156*(8), 1216–1222.

Parry, T. (1996). Multiple stimuli disorganisation syndrome: Treatment and management of children with attentional disorders. *Australian Educational and Developmental Psychologist, 13*(1), 56–58.

Pennington, B. F., & Ozonoff, S. (1996). Executive functions and development psychopathology. *Journal of Child Psychology and Psychiatry and Allied Disciplines, 37*, 51–87.

Piek, J. P., & Coleman-Carman, R. (1995). Kinaesthetic sensitivity and motor performance of children with developmental co-ordination disorder. *Developmental Medicine and Child Neurology, 37*, 976–984.

Piek, J. P., Dyck, M. J., Nieman, A., Anderson, M., Hay, D., Smith, L. M., et al. (in press). The relationship between motor coordination, executive functioning and attention in school aged children. *Archives of Clinical Neuropsychology*.

Piek, J. P., Glencross, D. J., Barrett, N. C., & Love, G. L. (1993). The effect of temporal and force changes on the patterning of sequential movements. *Psychological Research, 55*, 116–123.

Piek, J. P., Pitcher, T. M., & Hay, D. A. (1999). Motor coordination and kinaesthesis in boys with attention deficit hyperactivity disorder. *Developmental Medicine and Child Neurology, 41*(3), 159–165.

Piek, J. P., & Skinner, R. A. (1999). Timing and force control during a sequential tapping task in children with and without motor coordination problems. *Journal of the International Neuropsychological Society, 5*, 320–329.

Pitcher, T. M. (2001). *Motor performance and motor control in children with subtypes of attention deficit hyperactivity disorder.* Unpublished doctoral dissertation, Curtin University of Technology, Perth, Australia.

Pitcher, T. M., Piek, J. P., & Barrett, N. C. (2002). Timing and force control in boys with attention deficit hyperactivity disorder: Subtype differences and the effect of comorbid developmental coordination disorder. *Human Movement Science, 21*, 919–945.

Pitcher, T. M., Piek, J. P., & Hay, D. A. (2003). Fine and gross motor ability in boys with attention deficit hyperactivity disorder. *Developmental Medicine and Child Neurology, 45,* 525–535.

Polatajko, H. J., Fox, A. M., & Missiuna, C. (1995). An international consensus on children with developmental coordination disorder. *Canadian Journal of Occupational Therapy, 62,* 3–6.

Posner, M. I., & Dehaene, S. (1994). Attentional networks. *TINS, 17,* 75–79.

Pribram, K. H., & McGuiness, D. (1975). Arousal, activation and effort in the control of attention. *Psychological Review, 82,* 116–149.

Raggio, D. J. (1999). Visuomotor perception in children with attention deficit hyperactivity disorder-combined type. *Perceptual and Motor Skills, 88,* 448–450.

Ramus, F., Pidgeon, E., & Frith, U. (2003). The relationship between motor control and phonology in dyslexic children. *Journal of Child Psychology and Psychiatry, 44,* 712–722.

Reitan, R. M., & Wolfson, D. (1993). *The Halstead–Reitan Neuropsychological Test Battery: Theory and clinical interpretation.* Tucson, AZ: Neuropsychology Press.

Rosenthal, R. H., & Allen, T. W. (1978). An examination of attention, arousal, and learning dysfunction of hyperkinetic children. *Psychological Bulletin, 85,* 689–715.

Rubia, K., Taylor, A., Taylor, E., & Sergeant, J. A. (1999). Synchronization, anticipation, and consistency in motor timing of children with dimensionally defined attention deficit hyperactivity behaviour. *Perceptual and Motor Skills, 89,* 1237–1258.

Sandberg, S., & Barton, J. (1996). Historical development. In S. Sandberg (Ed.), *Monographs in child and adolescent psychiatry: Hyperactivity disorders of childhood* (pp. 1–25). Cambridge, UK: Cambridge University Press.

Sanders, J. A. (1983). Toward a model of stress and human performance. *Acta Psychologica, 53,* 61–97.

Sattler, J. M. (1992). *Assessment of children: WISC-III and WPPSI-R supplement.* San Diego, CA: Author.

Schaughency, E. A., & Hynd, G. W. (1989). Attentional control systems and the attention deficit disorders (ADD). *Learning and Individual Differences, 1*(4), 423–449.

Schmidt, R. A. (1988). *Motor control and learning: A behavioral emphasis* (2nd ed.). Champaign, IL: Human Kinetics.

Schmidt, R. A., & Lee, T. D. (1999). *Motor control and learning* (3rd ed.). Champaign, IL: Human Kinetics.

Schoemaker, M. M., Smits-Engelsman, B. C. M., & Kalverboer, A. F. (1998). The classification of specific motor disorders: Implications for intervention. In J. Rispens, T. A. V. Yperen, & W. Yule (Eds.), *Perspectives on the classification of specific developmental disorders* (pp. 231–244). Dordrecht, The Netherlands: Kluwer Academic.

Schwean, V. L., & Saklofske, D. H. (1998). WISC-III assessment of children with attention deficit/hyperactivity disorder. In A. Prifitera & D. Saklofske (Eds.), *WISC-III clinical use and interpretation: Scientist–practitioner perspectives* (pp. 91–118). San Diego, CA: Academic Press.

Semjen, A., & Garcia-Colera, A. (1986). Planning and timing of finger-tapping sequences with a stressed element. *Journal of Motor Behavior, 18,* 287–322.

Semjen, A., Garcia-Colera, A., & Requin, J. (1984). On controlling force and time in rhythmic movement sequences: The effect of stress location. In J. G. L. Allen. (Ed.), *Timing and time perception* (Vol. 423, pp. 168–182). New York: Annals of the New York Academy of Sciences.

Sergeant, J. (2000). The cognitive–energetic model: An empirical approach to attention-deficit hyperactivity disorder. *Neuroscience and Biobehavioral Reviews, 24,* 7–12.

Sergeant, J. A., & van der Meere, J. (1990). Attention deficit disorder: A paradigmatic approach. In A. F. Kalverboer (Ed.), *Developmental biopsychology: Experimental and observational studies in children at risk* (pp. 39–67). Ann Arbor: University of Michigan Press.

Shaywitz, S. E., & Shaywitz, B. A. (1984). Diagnosis and management of attention deficit disorder: A pediatric perspective. *Pediatrics Clinics of North America, 31*(2), 429–457.

Smyth, T. R., & Glencross, D. J. (1986). Information processing deficits in clumsy children. *Australian Journal of Psychology, 38*(1), 13–22.

Stewart, M. A., Pitts, F. N., Craig, A. G., & Dieruf, W. (1966). The hyperactive child syndrome. *American Journal of Orthopsychiatry, 36*, 861–867.

Summers, J., & Ford, S. (1995). Attention in sport. In T. Morris & J. Summers (Eds.), *Sport psychology: Theory, application and issues.* Milton, Brisband, Australia: Wiley.

Szatmari, P., Offord, D. R., & Boyle, M. H. (1989). Correlates, associated impairments, and patterns of service utilization of children with attention deficit disorders: Findings from the Ontario child health study. *Journal of Child Psychology and Psychiatry, 30*(2), 205–217.

Tannock, R. (1998). Attention deficit hyperactivity disorder: Advances in cognitive, neurobiologic, and genetic research. *Journal of Child Psychology and Psychiatry, 39*, 65–99.

Taylor, E. (1998). Clinical foundation of hyperactivity research. *Behavioural Brain Research, 94*, 11–24.

van der Meere, J. (1996). The role of attention. In S. Sandberg (Ed.), *Monographs in child and adolescent psychiatry: Hyperactivity disorders of childhood* (pp. 111–148). Cambridge, UK: Cambridge University Press.

van der Meulen, J. H. P., van der Gon, D. J. J., Gielen, C. C. A. M., Gooskens, R. H. J. M., & Willemse, J. (1991a). Visuomotor performance of normal and clumsy children. I: Fast goal-directed arm-movements with and without visual feedback. *Developmental Medicine and Child Neurology, 33*, 40–54.

van der Meulen, J. H. P., van der Gon, D. J. J., Gielen, C. C. A. M., Gooskens, R. H. J. M., & Willemse, J. (1991b). Visuomotor performance of normal and clumsy children II: Arm tracking with and without visual feedback. *Developmental Medicine and Child Neurology, 333*, 118–129.

Wechsler, D. (1974). *Manual for the Wechsler Intelligence Scale for Children—Revised.* New York: Psychological Corp.

Wechsler, D. (1989). *Manual for the Wechsler Preschool and Primary Scale of Intelligence—(Revised).* New York: Psychological Corp.

Wechsler, D. (1992). *Manual for the Wechsler Intelligence Scale for Children* (3rd ed.). New York: Psychological Corp.

Whitmont, S., & Clark, C. (1996). Kinaesthetic acuity and fine motor skills in children with attention deficit hyperactivity disorder: A preliminary report. *Developmental Medicine and Child Neurology, 38*, 1091–1098.

Williams, H. G., Woollacott, M. H., & Ivry, R. (1992). Timing and motor control in clumsy children. *Journal of Motor Behavior, 24*, 165–172.

Wilson, P. H., Maruff, P., & McKenzie, B. (1997). Covert orientating of visuospatial attention in children with developmental coordination disorder. *Developmental Medicine and Child Neurology, 39*, 736–745.

Wilson, P. H., Maruff, P., Ives, S., & Currie, J. (2001). Abnormalities of motor and praxis imagery in children with DCD. *Human Movement Science, 20*, 135–159.

Wilson, P. H., & McKenzie, B. E. (1998). Information processing deficits associated with developmental coordination disorder: A meta-analysis of research findings. *Journal of Child Psychology and Psychiatry, 39*, 829–840.

CHAPTER 15

Understanding the "Graphia" in Developmental Dysgraphia

A DEVELOPMENTAL NEUROPSYCHOLOGICAL PERSPECTIVE FOR DISORDERS IN PRODUCING WRITTEN LANGUAGE

VIRGINIA W. BERNINGER

Children with motor problems are likely to have difficulty in learning to write, but so are some children without motor problems. In this chapter, I discuss research and clinical issues related to writing development in children with severe motor disorders and in children with disabled writing development in which subtle motor processes, as well as nonmotor processes, play a role.

WRITING IN INDIVIDUALS WITH MOTOR IMPAIRMENT

Severe Motor Impairment

Static Neuromotor Encephalopathy

Cerebral palsy is nonprogressive damage to the motor pathways in the central nervous system of congenital or early postnatal origin. In the most severe forms of cerebral palsy, children never acquire normal ability to use their limbs for ambulation, their hands for play with objects, or their mouths or fingers for linguistic communication. Although considerable research has focused on use of alternative communication systems with children having severe cerebral palsy, many of these communication systems use nonlinguistic symbols. Such alternative communication systems cannot be used to communicate via written language that has syntactic and discourse structures as well as vocabulary items. Ability to use language-based communication systems depends greatly on the user's level of cognitive development, which for individuals with severe cerebral palsy may be in the normal range (Berninger, Gans, St. James, & Connors, 1988; Berninger & Hart, 1992) but is very likely to be below the normal range (McCarty, St. James, Berninger, & Gans, 1986). Ability to use language-based communication systems also depends greatly on the user's aural language development. Phonemic and lexical skills needed to read and spell, and thus operate word processing programs, tend not to be as developed as discourse comprehension skills in those with normal intelligence despite severely impaired motor skills (Berninger & Gans, 1986). Computer technology may bypass severe motoric limitations, but the user's cognitive and language skills also need to be considered in designing alternative language-based communication systems (for guidelines to consider, see Berninger & Amtmann, 2003). Little systematic research has been conducted on the cognitive, aural language, and literacy development of well-defined samples of individuals with severe motor impairment. Longitudinal research is particularly needed to understand the normal course of their written language development when appropriate technology for alternative communication is and is not used in their literacy instruction.

Progressive Neuromotor Encephalopathy

Children with muscular dystrophy lose previously acquired motoric skills, including handwriting. During the decline, which occurs over time, the goal should be accommodation—that is, devising strategies for optimal use of pencil or keyboard given the child's current neuromotor status. These accommodations need to be monitored and changed as the neuromotor status changes. The same holds for other forms of progressive neurological disease affecting motor function.

Mild to Moderate Nonprogressive Motor Impairments

More prevalent than the severe motor impairments are the milder impairments that include motor coordination disorders, dyspraxia (impaired gesturing), and neurological soft signs (Denckla & Roeltgen, 1992).

Motor Coordination Disorder

Sometimes referred to as the clumsy child syndrome (Dewey & Kaplan, 1990; Gubbay, 1975), and more recently as developmental coordination disorder (American Psychiatric Association, 1994), this disorder involves difficulty in coordinating motor movements despite normal intelligence. Clear guidelines do not exist for differentiating this disorder from the milder forms of cerebral palsy, and consensus on definitional issues is lacking (Denckla & Roeltgen, 1992). Seldom do motor coordination difficulties occur in isolation; they tend to be found in children with attention deficit, hyperactivity, and/or learning disability (Denckla & Roeltgen, 1992). Consequently, written language development has not been studied in children selected just for motor clumsiness.

Dyspraxia

According to Denckla and Roeltgen (1992), the literature on developmental dyspraxia does not have clear findings because sometimes children with perceptual–motor dysfunction are included and sometimes they are excluded in research studies. Research progress is also hampered by lack of consensus on definitional issues.

Neurological Soft Signs

In contrast to neurological hard signs that are associated with lesions in specific brain sites, soft signs are not associated with known physiological or anatomical impairment (Taylor, 1987). Although nearly 100 soft signs have been described in the literature, these seem to have nonspecific behavioral significance in that they occur in a variety of clinical populations, including but not restricted to learning disabilities and psychiatric disorders (Tupper, 1987). However, Berninger and Rutberg (1992) found specific relationships between writing and three of four selected for affecting finger function (for finger repetition and finger succession, see Denckla, 1973, 1974, and Wolff, Gunnoe, & Cohen, 1983; for finger lifting and finger spreading, see Wolff et al., 1983) in an unreferred sample of 50 girls and 50 boys in first, second, and third grade. Finger repetition, finger succession, and finger lifting predicted handwriting but not spelling. Finger succession was related to composition. Of the four measures, only finger succession, which also had the best interrater and test–retest reliability, assesses planning and executing sequential finger movements. Such sequential movements are needed in producing letters in isolation and in written communication. A soft sign that should be studied in future research on the relationships between subtle motor function and writing is the choreiform twitch (Wolff & Hurwitz, 1966).

Dysgraphia

Most of the research on this disorder has been done with acquired dysgraphia in adults. Acquired linguistic dysgraphia (impaired ability to make word and letter choices) is differentiated from acquired motor dysgraphia (impaired ability to form letters) (Roeltgen & Heilman, 1985). Denckla and Roeltgen (1992) proposed, based on acquired dysgraphia, a model of developmental dysgraphia that has six components: a graphemic buffer, a graphemic system, an allographic store, motor planning, praxia, and visuomotor integration. Motor planning is necessary for controlling the relative size of strokes and alignment of letters on lines, praxia is necessary for the hand movements involved in executing letter production, and visuospatial integration plays a role in placing letters on paper or monitor. The graphemic buffer is where letters are held in working memory while motor plans are planned and executed (e.g., Ellis, 1982). This buffer is susceptible to disruption by disordered attention (Hillis & Caramazza, 1989), explaining why some children with attention deficit have extreme difficulty with handwriting. The graphemic system guides motor planning in letter production (Rothi & Heilman, 1981). The allographic store houses case forms (upper and lower) and style forms (manuscript and cursive). "Slips of the pen" (Ellis, 1979) reflect errors in accessing or retrieving these allographs. The next section discusses research on developmental dysgraphia from the perspective of cognitive studies of writing.

WRITING IN INDIVIDUALS
WITHOUT SEVERE MOTOR IMPAIRMENT

The current federal mandate in the United States for every child to be a reader at the end of third grade has missed an equally important opportunity for helping every child reach developmentally appropriate writing milestones by the third grade as well. The view that children first learn to read in the primary grades and then learn to write in the upper elementary and middle school years is no longer supported by research (Berninger, 2000). Reading and writing are best learned in an integrated manner from the beginning of formal literacy instruction (e.g., Clay, 1982), even if the developmental trajectory for reading and writing differs and writing takes longer to reach full maturity (Kellogg, 1994). A systematic line of research spanning over a decade at the University of Washington has traced the neurodevelopmental origins of later written expression problems to the primary grades (for a review of this research, see Berninger, 1994, 2000; Berninger & Amtmann, 2003; Berninger & Graham, 1998). Because such early identification and intervention are not happening, the incidence of writing problems in students in the early grades escalates by middle childhood and adolescence, and the size of the increase is alarming (Hooper, Swartz, Wakely, de Kruif, & Montgomery, 2002). A line of research begun at Children's Hospital in Boston (e.g., Levine, Oberklaid, & Meltzer, 1981) and continued at the University of North Carolina at Chapel Hill (e.g., Hooper et al., 1993, 1994, 2002; Sandler et al., 1992) is identifying the neurodevelopmental factors contributing to writing in middle childhood and adolescence. Because schools rely heavily on group-administered achievement tests with multiple-choice format, many students with specific writing disabilities are not identified and served (Sandler et al., 1992), especially prior to the transition to the upper elementary grades when writing requirements increase exponentially.

Children who exhibit deficits in orthographic coding, fine motor planning, and automaticity of letter retrieval and production are at risk for problems in fluency and quality of written expression of ideas not only during the primary grades but also throughout the elementary school years (e.g., Abbott & Berninger, 1993; Graham, Berninger, Abbott, Abbott, & Whitaker, 1997). Both handwriting (Berninger, Vaughn, Abbott, Abbott, et al., 1997b; Graham, Harris, & Fink, 2000) and spelling (Berninger, Vaughan, Abbott, Brooks, et al., 1998; Graham, Harris, & Fink, 2002) problems identified during the early primary grades are responsive to early intervention. There may be a critical developmental period early in schooling in which writing problems should be identified and treated because they are most easily treated during this developmental window (Berninger, 1994). Children whose handwriting and spelling problems are not identified and treated during the critical developmental period in the primary grades are likely to suffer from developmental dysgraphia during the rest of their schooling. Developmental dysgraphia is a disorder in which a student struggles in learning to write, in contrast to acquired dysgraphia in which previously normal writing function is lost in specific ways. Developmental dysgraphia is a specific dissociation in the functional writing system of individuals whose overall motor, sensory, language, cognitive, and social/emotional development is in the normal range for age, but their transcription skills (handwriting and spelling) are significantly underdeveloped compared to verbal reasoning and ability to generate ideas; the deficient transcription skills compromise the higher-level processes in written composition. Although overall motor development may fall in the normal range, subtle motor inefficiencies may compromise writing development (see section on soft signs).

"Dysgraphia" is a Greek word that means impaired writing. The stem *graph* refers both to the hand function in writing and to the letters used in the writing system to represent the phonemes of the language. The fine motor system used to produce the letters is thus often referred to as the graphomotor system. From the perspective of the working brain (Luria, 1973), the functional writing system draws on many more brain systems than the motor system. In keeping with the focus of this volume on the motor system, the contribution of the graphomotor system to the functional writing system is discussed first before providing a brief overview of the other brain systems that support the text generation and self-regulation components of the functional writing system. These include sensory, levels of language, cognitive, memory, attention, executive function, and reading systems. Finally, issues of differential and branching diagnosis, treatment, and prognosis are considered for developmental dysgraphia in the broader context of developmental disabilities and medical disorders as well as a specific, higher-order writing disability.

Contribution of the Graphomotor System to Transcription

Language has no end organs and, therefore, teams with the sensory and motor systems to make contact with the external world (Liberman, 1999). Language by "hand" is a functional brain system in which the internal language code teams with the fine motor system that controls hand movement. This functional system emerges in development with the fundamental graphic act when the infant or toddler first uses a writing implement to leave a trace on paper, a wall, or other writing surface (Gibson & Levin, 1975). Language by "ear" is a functional system in which language teams with the auditory sense; it begins with the first auditory sensation from spoken language. Language by "mouth" is a functional system in which language teams with the oral–motor system; it begins with the first vocal utterance. Language by "eye" is a functional system in which language teams with the visual sense; it begins with the first time a child looks at a book and also listens as an adult or older child reads the book orally. Language by "ear," "mouth," "eye," and "hand" are on their own developmental trajectories but interact with each other and draw on common and unique brain systems (Berninger, 2000). Language by ear and language by eye are not inverses of each other (Mattingly, 1972); also, language by eye and by hand are not inverses of each other (Read, 1981). Each of these functional systems for aural language, oral language, reading, and writing are unique functional systems with their own internal organization and developmental history (Berninger, 2000).

One component of transcription—automaticity of letter retrieval and production—is the major constraint on beginning writing development (for review of evidence, see Berninger, 1994, 2000) and the best predictor of both compositional fluency (amount written under timed conditions) and compositional quality (based on ratings of content and organization) (Graham et al., 1997). Graphomotor processes (planning and control during execution) affect the quality of the letter production and thus its legibility (Rutberg, 1998; Weintraub & Graham, 2000), which is necessary but not sufficient; transcription must also become automatic (e.g., Berninger et al., 1992; Jones & Cristensen, 1999). Orthographic coding and memory retrieval processes affect the automaticity of letter production (i.e., the ability to produce legible letters rapidly and with minimal conscious attention). Abbott and Berninger (1993) included both graphomotor tasks and orthographic coding tasks as predictors in a structural equation model in which the outcome was automaticity of letter production: Only the path from the orthographic coding factor to the outcome was statistically significant, but the model fit well when the graphomotor processes were included and contributed to the outcome indirectly via the orthographic coding factor. Indicators for the orthographic coding factor were tasks that required children to hold briefly exposed written words in short-term memory and then make judgments about whether a specific letter or letter group was in the word or whether a second letter string matched the first word exactly. Orthographic coding may take place in a graphemic buffer in working memory.

The important point is that handwriting is *"language* by hand," which uses the graphomotor system to produce visible language, but neither handwriting nor composing is merely a motor act. Language by hand relies greatly on internal representations of letter forms and written words that must be retrieved from memory during the writing process. Whether this internal representation is stored in a grapheme buffer just at output (Ellis, 1982) or at input, too, requires further research. Following a learning phase in which the graphomotor skills for letter production are acquired, the graphomotor skills typically become automatized—if they do not, a child is at risk for writing disability. First, the behavioral research on motor processes in handwriting is reviewed, and then recent *in vivo* brain imaging research is discussed that is shedding light on how different neural circuitry is involved in the initial motor learning and in the subsequent automatization of motor skills.

Motor Processes in Handwriting

Graham and Weintraub (1996) credit the increased research activity worldwide on handwriting to five factors: (1) growing interest in basic research on motor control processes, (2) advances in computer technology that permit reliable and precise study of handwriting movements, (3) more sophisticated theoretical models of the handwriting process, (4) increased concern with teaching handwriting to special education students many of whom have writing problems, and (5) formation of the International Graphonomics Society for the study of handwriting. Most of the research on the motor processes in handwriting is based on adult, skilled writers. On the one hand, the shape of letters produced depends somewhat on the specific muscles used in a particular writing task. On the other hand, the shape of letters produced often does not depend on the specific muscles used in a particular writing task. Thus, motor programs probably include both muscle-specific representations for ordered sequences for certain kinds of muscle movements and abstract representations for plans that are not muscle-specific. From the perspective of brain, both primary projection areas of motor cortex, which exert muscle-specific effects, and association areas of motor cortex, which do not exert muscle-specific effects, are likely to be involved. Although considerable evidence points to the letter as the basic unit of production, rather than component strokes of the letter or units larger than the single letter, motor planning seems to exert effects on production units beyond the single letter: Timing for producing a target letter is more influenced by the preceding letter than the letter that follows the target letter. Motor control processes in handwriting are organized sequentially and hierarchically but also operate in parallel. For behavioral evidence for each of these generalizations and further information, see review by Graham and Weintraub (1996).

Research on developing children indicates that initially children mix letter-like forms and pictorial representations and spontaneously produce drawings that accompany their early written productions. Initially they draw their letters, often from the bottom up. With sufficient practice, normally developing writers switch from controlled, strategic production of letters to automatic retrieval and production of letters (see Goodnow, 1977). Normal variation in how children hold their pencils has been well validated and does not seem to predict the legibility or speed of their handwriting (Berninger, Vaughan, Abbott, Abbott, et al., 1997; Graham & Weintraub, 1996). Girls tend to have more legible (Graham & Weintraub, 1996) and automatic (Berninger & Fuller, 1992) letter production. This gender superiority may not be entirely due to the well-documented finding that girls have better fine motor skills; it may also be due to gender differences in how letters are coded in the brain—that is, left-hemispheric verbal coding or right-hemispheric geometric coding (see Berninger & Fuller, 1992)—but further research is needed on this issue. Visuomotor integration either has correlations of low magnitude with handwriting or is not correlated with handwriting in normally developing beginning writers (for review, see Graham & Weintraub, 1996) but may be a strong predictor of handwriting later in schooling for those children who have severe handwriting impairment and probably some degree of possibly undiagnosed motor impairment (Weintraub & Graham, 2000). Although visual perception is not a good predictor of handwriting skill (Yost & Lesiak, 1980), orthographic coding in short-term memory, as operationalized in our programmatic research (Berninger, 2001a), is an excellent predictor of handwriting and other writing skills for both normally developing samples (Abbott & Berninger, 1993) and samples with dyslexia and dysgraphia (Berninger, Abbott, Thomson, & Raskind, 2001).

In Vivo Brain Imaging of Graphomotor Processes

Finger Function

A finger succession maneuver (touching thumb against each finger in sequence, Denckla, 1974), which is a reliable and valid predictor of beginning writing (Berninger & Rutberg, 1992), increased blood flow more in supplementary motor areas than did repetitive touches to the same finger without the sequential component (Shibasaki et al., 1993). This result is consistent with the finding that the supplementary motor area is involved in organizing forthcoming movements in complex motor sequences that require a precise timing plan (Gerloff, Corwell, Chen, Hallett, & Cohen, 1997). Activation of lactate (a brain chemical detected on magnetic spectroscopic imaging) increased in putamen and globus pallidus on the contralateral side while adults performed finger opposition movements (Kuwabara, Watanabe, Tsuji, & Yuasa, 1995).

Motor Learning

Mishkin (e.g., Mishkin, 1982; Mishkin & Appenzeller, 1987) proposed, based on primate research, that different neural pathways may be involved in cognitive learning than are involved in skills that have become habits (i.e., are automatized). Raichle and colleagues (1994) confirmed that such is the case for human verbal skills (generating verbs for visually presented nouns) before and after they are practiced. Van Mier, Tempel, Perlmutter, Raichle, and Petersen (1998) provided additional support for a shift in neural pathways after practice—in this case for graphomotor learning. Adults were scanned while they moved a pen through novel mazes or square patterns and then again after they practiced these continuous tracing tasks. Half used their right hand and half used their left hand. For the most part the same areas of brain were activated whether the right or left hand was used, consistent with abstract motor plans not being tied to specific muscle movements; however, hand used was related to activation in primary motor cortex and anterior cerebellum, consistent with some involvement of circuits that are tied to specific muscle movements (see prior section on behavioral research on motor learning). Rescanning, after participants practiced tracing for 10 minutes outside the magnet, detected changes in supplementary motor areas and left cerebellum. Van Mier and colleagues concluded that the anterior cerebellum was probably involved in motor execution, but the decreased activation in left cerebellum after practice was the result of learning. Van Mier and colleagues' findings mesh with accumulating evidence that the cerebellum is involved in not only motor control processes but also learning. Although cerebellum activates during motor learning, basal ganglia appear to activate only after overlearning (automatization) (Mazziotta, Grafton, & Woods, 1991).

For visual motor sequence learning, frontal areas activate more in early learning, whereas parietal areas activate more after practice (Sakai et al., 1998). Nicholson and colleagues (1999) used the same task as Jenkins, Brooks, Nixon, Frackowiak, and Passingham (1994) to replicate the Jenkins et al. finding that cerebellum is involved in motor sequence learning. Before scanning, participants learned (via auditory feedback for correct presses) and practiced a sequence of eight finger presses with their eyes closed; during scanning they learned a new sequence. Cerebellar function increased for both the prelearned and novel motor sequence, but more so during learning, confirming the role of the cerebellum in both new learning and automatization of practiced skills. Cerebellar circuits may be involved in a precise timing mechanism for the computations involved in motor learning and other cognitive processes (Ivry & Keele, 1989).

Exactly how brain structures and/or functions involved in finger movements, motor learning, and timing mechanisms may explain the problems of developmental dysgraphia requires further research. The current work based on normal skilled adults discussed in this section can serve as a starting point for such research on writing problems for those with developmental dysgraphia and/or other conditions.

Contribution of Other Brain Systems to Writing

Sensory Systems

Under normal circumstances, writers receive visual feedback from what they have written. This feedback may be helpful but not necessary (Graham & Weintraub, 1996). Visual feedback may be less necessary if letter production is automatized, but further research is needed on this issue. Writers also receive feedback from the kinesthetic, proprioceptive, and vestibular sensory systems. The kinesthetic receptors in skin transmit touch information from the writing instrument or keyboard to spinal cord, brain stem, ventral posterior lateral nucleus in thalamus, and primary somatosensory cortex in parietal lobe. In separate pathways the proprioception sense, which has receptors in muscles and joints as well as skin, conveys information about position and movement of the hand to primary somatosensory cortex. In the vestibular system, the semicircular canals detect head turns and orient body movement to the three planes in space; and the otolith organs detect linear movements. Together, the vestibular organs help maintain smoothness of movements of hand and eye. Exactly which of these sensory mechanisms may contribute causally to specific kinds of writing problems in students with well-defined developmental profiles and medical problems has received little research attention. However, these sensory mechanisms are likely to have an impact on the graphomotor processes more directly than other processes of the functional writing system, especially the language, cognition, and executive functions. Sensorimotor integration, as assessed by finger localization and finger recognition, also is related to written language learning to some degree (see Berninger & Rutberg, 1992).

Levels of Language Subsystems

The text generation component of the functional writing system translates generated ideas into language representations in memory, which then must be transcribed into written language via hand. The text generation process draws on many different levels of language (word selection, sentence construction, and discourse structure that is genre-specific) in this idea-to-language translation process. However, the translation process is not complete until language representations in memory are transformed into written language on paper or computer monitor. The transcription component of the functional writing system draws on letter production (a sublexical process) and spelling (a lexical process that in turn may draw on sublexical phonological, orthographic, and morphological processes) to complete this translation process. Beginning and developing writers exhibit intraindividual differences in their facility at the various levels of language involved in text generation and transcription (Berninger, 1994). Some of these individual differences within the same writer are normal variation, whereas some involve such marked dissociations (uneven development) that they fall outside the normal range and compromise writing development. Electrosurgical techniques have shown that different levels of language are represented in different parts of the distributed language systems in the brain (e.g., Ojemann, 1991). *In vivo* structural imaging has also contributed to current understanding of the neural architecture of language systems (Leonard, 1998). *In vivo* functional brain imaging research has demonstrated that the language system includes considerably more circuitry than the classic Wernicke-Broca's network based on autopsy studies suggested (e.g., see, Binder, Frost, Hammeke, Rao, & Cox, 1996; Mesulam, 1990). Research is needed to clarify exactly how circuitry for language is shared across language by ear, language by mouth, language by eye, and language by hand and how each of these functional systems draws uniquely on nonlanguage processes and is organized differently to achieve its hallmark goals.

Children with dysgraphia may have problems in handwriting only, spelling only, or both handwriting and spelling (Berninger, Abbott, et al., 2001). Spelling problems are easier to remediate in children who have only spelling problems than in those who have spelling and handwriting problems (Berninger, Abbott, Rogan, et al., 1998). Although children whose word reading problems are remediated may have persisting spelling problems, other children have spelling problems without word reading problems (e.g., Berninger, Abbott, Whitaker, Sylvester, & Nolen, 1995). Children with both word reading and spelling problems do not respond to spelling treatment until they have reached a certain level of word reading skill (Brooks, Vaughan, &

Berninger, 1999). Despite a myth that spelling is a purely visual skill, genetics research has shown that phonological short-term memory and phoneme–grapheme correspondence are important components of the phenotype for spelling disability (e.g., Hsu, Wijsman, Berninger, Thomson, & Raskind, 2002; Wijsman et al., 2000) as behavioral research has shown for reading disability (e.g., Wagner & Torgesen, 1987). Just as word reading is a language function that draws on orthographic and phonological processes, spelling is a language function that draws on phonological and orthographic processes (Berninger, Vaughan, Abbott, Brooks, et al., 1998; Chomsky, 1979; Foorman, Francis, Novy, & Liberman, 1991; Jenner et al., 2001; Matsuo et al., 2000; Treiman & Bourassa, 2000; Wood, Flowers, Buchsbaum, & Tallal, 1991; Venezky, 1970, 1999), and disabilities may occur in the phonological-to-orthographic translation process at the lexical or sublexical level (Roeltgen & Heilman, 1984). Further research is needed as to whether spelling problems are related to temporal asynchronies (Breznitz, 2002) or imprecise timing mechanisms in integrating phonological and orthographic codes (Wolf, Bowers, & Biddle, 2000). In normal spelling development, strategies (Varnhagen, 1994) give way to automatic retrieval (Steffer, Varnhagen, Friesen, & Treiman, 1998), but the process may not become automatized in individuals with spelling disability, resulting in long-term memory retrieval problems (Dreyer, Luke, & Melican, 1994). Morphological processes are less studied but equally important in spelling (Bryant, Nunes, & Bindman, 1997; Carlisle, 1988; Leong, 2000; Nagy, Diakidoy, & Anderson, 1993; Tyler & Nagy, 1989).

Cognitive System

Idea generation sets the writing process in motion (Kellogg, 1994) but little is known about how ideas are generated in the brain. Sometimes writers write about what they have read, but other times they self-generate their text entirely based on their own imagination. The brain processes involved in imagination (envisioning what does not exist, a future-oriented process) have not been as well investigated as memory (recreating the past) but are just as important in understanding writing.

Memory Systems

Researchers have devised numerous ways to categorize subprocesses of memory function (Lyon & Krasnegor, 1996), but mostly the distinction among short-term, long-term, and working memory has been applied to writing research. Not only long-term (Hayes & Flower, 1980) but also working memory (McCutchen, 1996) is involved in writing. The working-memory span predicts composing skill of developing writers and more so with increasing age (McCutchen, 1996), but timing limitations (Berninger, 1999) may be as important as capacity limitations operationalized by the load (Jonides et al., 1997) in working memory during the composing process. Because of the temporal constraints in working memory, instruction for treating written language disorders should be aimed at all components of the functional writing system close in time within the same lessons (e.g., Berninger, 1998b; Berninger et al., 1995). Short-term memory appears to play a greater role in spelling, whereas working memory appears to play a greater role in composing (Swanson & Berninger, 1996). As writers mature, they improve in ability to transform the contents retrieved from long-term memory to the audience and writing goals (Scardamalia & Bereiter, 1986).

Attentional System

The anterior component of the attention system that is involved in planning and producing responses and the conflict management component (anterior cingulate) of the attentional system (Mesulam, 1990) probably play major roles in the functional writing system. Handwriting is more likely to be compromised by the anterior component of the attentional system that influences motor processes involved in written output, whereas composing is more likely to be influenced by the conflict management component that monitors and resolves conflict, which is inevitable given the many different processes that must be juggled during the complex composing process. Some children with attention-deficit/hyperactivity disorder who also have handwriting problems show dramatic improvement in handwriting when given stimulant medication (e.g., Lerer, Lerer, & Artner, 1977). Further research is needed on the relationship between attention and effective treatment (both instructional and psychopharmacological) for handwriting and composing problems in children with attentional difficulties. Writing development should be closely monitored in any child with attentional deficit.

Executive Functions

The most influential model of the cognitive processes in writing identified three component processes that operate recursively rather than sequentially: planning, translating, and reviewing/revising. Of these, the first and last are also executive functions, which depend greatly on frontal (especially prefrontal) brain regions (e.g., Casey et al., 1997; Hooper et al., 2002; Smith & Jonides, 1999), which are among the last to myelinate (e.g. Huttenlocher, 1979; Klingberg, Vaidya, Gabrieli, Mosely, & Hedehus, 1999) and reach functional maturity (e.g., Chugani, Phelps, & Mazziotta, 1987). See Hooper and colleagues (2002) for the first report in literature to demonstrate that performance on standard neuropsychological measures of executive functions, based on Denckla's (1996) model, explains some of the variance in writing ability. Good and poor writers differ in the initiation and set-shift domains, and executive functions become increasingly important over the course of writing development (Hooper et al., 2002). Thus, writing instruction during the elementary school years should provide both explicit other-regulation by adults of the cognitive processes in writing (e.g., teacher modeling and scaffolding or guided assistance, e.g., Berninger et al., 1995) and explicit instruction in strategies for self-regulation of these processes (e.g., Graham, 1997; Graham & Harris, 1996; Graham, MacArthur, & Schwartz, 1995; Harris & Graham, 1996; Wong, 1997) for the purpose of helping students eventually transition to self-regulation of these processes (cf. Zimmerman & Reisenberg, 1997).

Reading System

In children and adults with dyslexia and dysgraphia, the level to which word reading is developed constrains the level to which spelling develops, and the level to which reading comprehension is developed constrains the level to which composing develops (Berninger, Abbott, et al., 2001). How the developing writing system draws on the developing reading system is a subject of ongoing research in several research groups including ours. Full understanding of these issues will require not only assessment data but also instructional studies that better support inferences about causal mechanisms.

Nature–Nurture Interactions

A survey of K–6 teachers in the United States (see Graham & Weingtraub, 1996) found that only 36% of the teachers had received training in how to teach handwriting during their teacher education program. Only 80% of schools required instruction in handwriting, and in those schools instructional time varied from a low of 30 minutes to a high of 60 minutes, on average, per week. In addition, the process writing movement (e.g., Graves, 1975) and whole-language movement in literacy instruction (e.g., Britton, 1978) have deemphasized explicit instruction in handwriting (see Graham & Weintraub, 1996) and emphasized instead functional communication for authentic purposes. Taken together, some writing problems, especially those related to basic ability to produce alphabet letters accurately and automatically, may be related to instructional issues. However, both twin and family genetics studies have provided evidence of a genetic basis for spelling disability (for a review, see Raskind, 2001). In our family genetics study of dyslexia and dysgraphia, spelling showed an aggregation pattern highly consistent with a genetic basis (Raskind, Hsu, Berninger, Thomson, & Wijsman, 2001), but to date handwriting has not. We have modified our phenotyping battery in order to explore more fully what the genetic factors in handwriting might be, especially in regard to graphomotor planning, quality of letter form representation, and executive functions regulating memory search. Currently we are also pursuing research on the different genetic mechanisms that may be contributing to the combined reading and spelling disability phenotype versus the spelling-disability-only phenotype. Identifying the genetic mechanisms in written language disorders is a challenge because of the nature–nurture interactions throughout the preschool and school years for disorders that change their phenotypical expression across development. Neuropsychologists should maintain a nature–nurture interaction perspective in assessing and planning treatment for students with specific written language disorders (Berninger, 1994; Berninger & Richards, 2002).

Diagnosis and Treatment

Differential and Branching Diagnosis

Diagnosis of writing problems has lagged behind diagnosis of reading problems (e.g., Hooper et al., 2002). Writing disorders are heterogeneous in terms of both the components of the functional writing system that are affected (e.g, handwriting, spelling, and composing) and the underlying neurodevelopmental processes that are affected (Berninger et al., 1995; Sandler et al., 1992). Sandler and colleagues (1992) identified four subtypes of writing disabilities based on cluster analyses in a referred sample: fine motor and linguistic deficits, visual spatial deficits, attention and memory deficits, and sequencing deficits.

Developmental dysgraphia is an appropriate diagnosis only if other diagnoses such as mental retardation, autism, pervasive developmental disorder, and developmental language disorder, according to the fourth edition of the *Diagnostic and Statis-*

tical Manual of Mental Disorders (DSM-IV; American Psychiatric Association, 1994), can be ruled out, and medical conditions that involve static or progressive damage to the central or peripheral nervous systems (e.g., cerebral palsy or muscular dystrophy) are not present. Individuals with any of these developmental or medical conditions may have writing problems, but their problems are not specific to writing: The etiology, effective treatment, and prognosis for their writing problems are not the same as for individuals with developmental dysgraphia or other specific writing disability. The etiology, treatment, and prognosis may also differ for students with developmental dysgraphia and slower learners who fall just within the lower limits of the normal range in all developmental domains including writing. Future research on diagnosis and treatment of writing problems will most likely be interpretable and applicable to practice if samples are well defined on the basis of developmental profiles across motor, language, cognition, memory, attention, executive, social/emotional, and academic functions as well as possible medical conditions. (See Berninger, 2001b, for an analogous case for grounding the differential diagnosis of developmental dyslexia in profiles across multiple developmental domains.) One form of specific writing disability, which is related to deficits in working memory and executive function, affects only high-level composing processes rather than low-level transcription and usually becomes evident during the middle school or high school grades when the writing requirements of the curriculum increase.

Table 15.1 offers an update of how to do branching diagnosis for writing disabilities (Berninger & Whitaker, 1993) using the Process Assessment of the Learner Test Battery for Reading and Writing (PAL-RW) (Berninger, 2001a), which can also be used as part of a broader three-tier model for preventing and treating writing disabilities through screening for early intervention, progress monitoring, and differential diagnosis and individual treatment planning for persisting reading and writing problems (Berninger, 1998b, 2002; Berninger, Stage, Smith, & Hildebrand, 2001). Both the *PAL Guides for Reading and Writing Intervention* (Berninger, 1998a) and the *Manual for the PAL-RW Test* point the examiner in the direction of research-supported interventions linked to specific assessment measures and test results. These assessment tools are based on research and norming procedures that excluded individuals with severe motor disabilities. Research is needed on whether these measures can be used, with or without modifications, in populations with well-defined motor disabilities. Table 15.2 offers a conceptual framework for diagnosis of specific writing disability in individuals for whom mental retardation, autism, pervasive developmental disorder, and primary language disorder can be ruled out. The PAL assessment-intervention system is aimed at prevention and treatment of writing problems in the elementary grades. The STRANDS (survey of teenage readiness and neurodevelopmental status) system (Hooper & Levine, 2001; Levine & Hooper, 2001) is aimed at adolescents with writing problems.

Treatment

Considerable research has been conducted on pedagogy for teaching writing, especially at the sixth-grade levels and above (e.g., Hillocks, 1986), on the cognitive processes in skilled writing (e.g., Alamargot & Chanquoy, 2001; Hayes & Flower, 1980; Kellogg, 1994), and on normal writing development (e.g., Berninger, 1994; Berninger,

TABLE 15.1. Branching Diagnosis of Specific Writing Disability[a]

Assess component writing skill with this achievement measure	If writing skill falls in deficient or at-risk range, also give this process measure
Handwriting legibility with PAL-RW Copying Tasks A and B	Fine motor processes (PAL-RW finger repetition, finger succession, finger localization, finger recognition, and fingertip writing)
Handwriting automaticity with PAL-RW Alphabet Writing Task	Orthographic coding (for whole words, letter in a word, and letter cluster in a word)
	Fine motor processes (PAL-RW finger repetition, finger succession, finger localization, finger recognition, and fingertip writing)
	Rapid automatic naming (RAN) for letters
Dictated spelling with WIAT II spelling	Orthographic coding for whole words, letter in a word, and letter cluster in a word
	Phonological coding for syllables, phonemes, rimes
	Orthographic word choice
	RAN for words prorated WISC-III Verbal IQ (Verbal Comprehension Factor)
Functional spelling with PAL-RW criterion-referenced measure for spelling in composition in Appendix D	Same as for dictated spelling plus finger succession
Compositional fluency with WIAT II Written expression (number of words) or PAL-RW criterion-referenced measure for compositional fluency in Appendix D	Same as for alphabet writing, dictated and functional spelling plus rapid automatic switching between words and numbers (set shift task)
Compositional quality with WIAT II Written expression (holistic or analytical coding scheme)	Same as for compositional fluency

[a] Using the *Wechsler Individual Achievement Test, Second edition* (WIAT II; Psychological Corporation, 2001) and *Process Assessment of the Learner Test Battery for Reading and Writing* (PAL-RW; Berninger, 2001a) measures, which are based on the University of Washington writing research program on writing and writing–reading connections and the *Wechsler Intelligence Scale for Children—Third edition* (WISC-III; Psychological Corporation, 1991). See *PAL-RW Test Manual* (Berninger, 2001a), *PAL Guides for Intervention* (Berninger, 1998b), and *PAL Research-Supported Reading and Writing Lessons* (Berninger & Abbott, 2003) for interventions linked to these assessment measures. See Berninger (1998b, 2002; Berninger et al., 2001a) for other test instruments that can also be used in diagnosis of specific reading and writing disabilities.

TABLE 15.2. Differential Diagnosis of Specific Writing Disability

Level I. Cross-domain developmental profile (motor, cognition, language, socioemotional/ behavioral, and attention/executive functions)

If criteria for mental retardation, autism, pervasive developmental disorder, or specific language impairment (see DSM-IV criteria) are met, make the relevant diagnosis and note any medical conditions affecting the motor system (e.g., cerebral palsy or muscular dystrophy). Developmental dysgraphia should only be diagnosed in the absence of these other diagnoses or medical conditions because its etiology, treatment, and prognosis may differ from other writing disorders. However, writing interventions described in the *PAL Intervention Guides* (Berninger, 1998b) and the *PAL Research-Supported Reading and Writing Lesson Plans* (Berninger & Abbott, 2003) may be modified to meet the needs of any writing disorder, as long as student progress is monitored and evaluated using multimodal assessment (see Chapter 10 of the *PAL Guides*). Expectations for reasonable progress and learning outcomes need to be modified depending on developmental disability and/or medical condition. More research is needed on treatment and prognosis for writing problems in children with specific developmental and/or medical conditions.

Level II. Component(s) of functional writing system affected[a,b]
Diagnose *developmental dysgraphia if* no Level I diagnosis is made and

   (a) *handwriting legibility and/or automaticity* falls in the deficient or at-risk category
   (b) *dictated spelling* falls in the deficient or at-risk category and below the level expected based on verbal reasoning ability; or
   (c) criteria for both handwriting (a) and spelling (b) disability are met

Diagnose *higher-order specific writing problem if* no Level I diagnosis is made, whether or not criteria for developmental dysgraphia are met, *and if*

   (a) *compositional fluency* falls in the deficient or at-risk category and below the level expected based on verbal reasoning ability; or
   (b) *compositional quality* falls in the deficient or at-risk category and below the level expected based on verbal reasoning ability

Note: Some children may have mixed developmental dysgraphia and higher-order specific writing problem, affecting transcription and composition skills.

Level III. Affected neurodevelopmental processes related to writing

The following neurodevelopmental processes should also be assessed and deficiencies noted because they may have implications for etiology, treatment, and prognosis

   (a) graphomotor skills (execution, control, and planning) or sensorimotor skills (initial sensory coding, related sensory perception, and sensory-motor integration)
   (b) orthographic, phonological, and morphological coding/awareness
   (c) attention (if possible, differentiate posterior, anterior, and cingulate components, Mesulam, 1990)
   (d) executive functions (planning and goal setting, maintaining on-task behaviors, self-monitoring, and revising)
   (e) memory (short-term, long-term, and working)

[a] See *PAL-RW Test Manual* for criteria for deficient ($\leq$20th percentile) and at-risk (> 20th to $\leq$40th percentile) categories.
[b] Students with developmental dysgraphia are also likely to have impaired higher-order writing skills but with treatment may show greater growth in the higher-order composing than lower-order transcription skills (see Brooks et al., 1999).

Fuller, & Whitaker, 1997; Langer, 1986; Scardamalia & Bereiter, 1986; special issue of *Educational Psychologist*, see Graham & Harris, 2000). Less has focused on instructional techniques for students with well-defined developmental and neuro-developmental profiles, but see Wong (1998) for an overview of effective instructional for writing in general for students with learning disabilities. For research-supported instructional interventions that are grounded in models of neuroscience and designed for transcription problems and transfer to translation processes, see Berninger (1998a, 1998b, 1998c). Prompting children to study numbered arrow cues for sequential pencil strokes *and* to write letters from memory was the most effective treatment in increasing accuracy and automaticity of letter production in first graders with poor handwriting (Berninger, Vaughan, Abbott, Abbott, et al., 1997). Coupling explicit instruction in alphabetic principles (from phonemes to spelling units) with modeling the lexical and onset-rime units in words was the most effective treatment in improving spelling in second graders with poor spelling (Berninger, Vaughan, et al., 1998). As children progress in spelling development, both assessment and intervention need to take into account multiple linguistic cues including phonological, morphological, and orthographic ones (Henry, 2003; Masterson, Apel, & Wasowicz, 2003).

Instructional design principles that have emerged from our research include the following: (1) design instruction to automatize lower-level transcription skills, (2) teach for transfer of low-level transcription skills to high-level composing skills, and (3) teach to all components of the functional writing system close in time within the same lesson because of temporal constraints in working memory that may interfere with connections forming among the components of the functional writing system (for further information, see Berninger, 1998b). Some children may need instruction aimed at motor control before instruction aimed at automatization. *Big Strokes for Little Folks* (Rubell, 1995), which is grounded in neurodevelopmental principles, integrates training in motor control with explicit instruction in forming alphabet letters. The Center for Learning and Behavior at the University of Maryland has developed and validated lesson plans for handwriting instruction (Graham et al., 2000). The *PAL Research-Supported Reading and Writing Lessons* (Berninger & Abbott, 2003), which are based on peer-reviewed research that can be implemented, with or without individual tailoring, by psychologists and other professionals (Lesson Sets 3–5, 7–8, 10, and 13–14 focus on writing), incorporated the foregoing design principles.

For a critical review of use of computer technology in designing instructional interventions for students with writing disabilities, see MacArthur (1999, 2000) and MacArthur, Ferretti, Okolo, and Cavalier (2001). Although computer technology holds great promise for helping students with specific written language disorders acquire writing skills, our clinical experience has shown that underlying neuro-developmental processes also affect how students use technology (Berninger & Amtmann, 2003). For example, students who do poorly on the finger succession task (Berninger, 2001a; Berninger & Rutberg, 1992; Denckla, 1973) often have considerable difficulty in using computer keyboards as well. Students with spelling disability often cannot use spell checks because (1) spell checks do not recognize the kinds of errors they make (e.g., additions, omissions, or substitutions of phonemes or other phonological units especially in medial portions of polysyllabic words), and (2) they cannot choose among the alternatives offered when a spelling error is detected. Computer technology may pose added challenges rather than quick solutions for students who have not only writing problems but also *selective* motor planning, language, attention, executive function, and/or working-memory problems despite otherwise normal motoric, linguistic, and cognitive development (see Berninger & Amtmann, 2003).

CONCLUSIONS

More research is needed on writing development in individuals with and without motor disabilities. In this research both motor and nonmotor processes (e.g,, language, attention, working memory, and executive functions) that affect writing development should be studied. In some cases the effects of severe motor disabilities on writing are obvious, whereas in other cases developing writers may have subtle motor inefficiencies that are only apparent on formal assessment but nonetheless influence the writing acquisition process.

ACKNOWLEDGMENTS

Grant Nos. HD 25858-11 and P50 HD 33812-06 from the National Institute of Child Health and Human Development (NICHD) supported preparation of this chapter and some of the reported research.

REFERENCES

Abbott, R., & Berninger, V. (1993). Structural equation modeling of relationships among developmental skills and writing skills in primary and intermediate grade writers. *Journal of Educational Psychology, 85*, 478–508.

Almargot, D., & Chanquoy, L. (2001). *Through the models of writing*. Dordrecht, The Netherlands: Kluwer Academic.

American Psychiatric Association. (1994). *Diagnostic and statistical manual of mental disorders* (4th ed.). Washington, DC: Author.

Berninger, V. W. (1994). *Reading and writing acquisition: A developmental neuropsychological perspective*. Madison, WI: Brown.

Berninger, V. W. (1998a). *Handwriting lessons program in process assessment of the learner (PAL) intervention kit*. San Antonio, TX: Psychological Corp.

Berninger, V. W. (1998b). *Process assessment of the learner: Guides for reading and writing intervention*. San Antonio, TX: Psychological Corp.

Berninger, V. W. (1998c). *Talking letters program in process assessment of the learner (PAL) intervention kit*. San Antonio, TX: Psychological Corp.

Berninger, V. W. (1999). Coordinating transcription and text generation in working memory during composing: Automatized and constructive processes. *Learning Disability Quarterly, 22*, 99–112.

Berninger, V. W. (2000). Development of language by hand and its connections to language by ear, mouth, and eye. *Topics of Language Disorders, 20*, 65–84.

Berninger, V. W. (2001a). *Process assessment of the learner (PAL) test battery for reading and writing (PAL-RW)*. San Antonio, TX: Psychological Corp.

Berninger, V. W. (2001b). Understanding the lexia in dyslexia. *Annals of Dyslexia, 51*, 23–48.

Berninger, V. W. (2002). Best practices in reading, writing, and math assessment-intervention links: A systems approach for schools, classrooms, and individuals. In A. Thomas & J.

Grimes (Eds.), *Best practices in school psychology* (Vol. 4, pp. 851–865). Bethesda, MD: National Association of School Psychologists.

Berninger, V. W., & Abbott, S. (2003). *PAL research-supported reading and writing lessons.* San Antonio, TX: Psychological Corp.

Berninger, V. W., Abbott, R., Rogan, L., Reed, L., Abbott, S., Brooks, A., et al. (1998). Teaching spelling to children with specific learning disabilities: The mind's ear and eye beat the computer or pencil. *Learning Disability Quarterly, 21,* 106–122.

Berninger, V. W., Abbott, R., Thomson, J., & Raskind, W. (2001). Language phenotype for reading and writing disability: A family approach. *Scientific Studies in Reading, 5,* 59–105.

Berninger, V. W., Abbott, R., Whitaker, D., Sylvester, L., & Nolen, S. (1995). Integrating low-level skills and high-level skills in treatment protocols for writing disabilities. *Learning Disability Quarterly, 18,* 293–309.

Berninger, V. W., & Amtmann, D. (2003). Preventing written expression disabilities through early and continuing assessment and intervention for handwriting and/or spelling problems: Research into practice. In H. L. Swanson, K. R. Harris, & S. Graham (Eds.), *Handbook of learning disabilities* (pp. 345–363). New York: Guilford Press.

Berninger, V. W., & Fuller, F. (1992). Gender differences in orthographic, verbal, and compositional fluency: Implications for diagnosis of writing disabilities in primary grade children. *Journal of School Psychology, 30,* 363–382.

Berninger, V. W., Fuller, F., & Whitaker, D. (1997). A process model of writing development across the life span. *Educational Psychology Review, 8,* 193–238.

Berninger, V. W., & Gans, B. (1986). Language profiles in nonspeaking individuals of normal intelligence with severe cerebral palsy. *Augmentative and Alternative Communication, 2,* 45–50.

Berninger, V. W., Gans, B., St. James, P., & Connors, T. (1988). Modified WAIS-R for patients with speech and/or hand dysfunction. *Archives of Physical Medicine and Rehabilitation, 69,* 250–255.

Berninger, V. W., & Graham, S. (1998). Language by hand: A synthesis of a decade of research on handwriting. *Handwriting Review, 12,* 11–25.

Berninger, V. W., & Hart, T. (1992). A developmental neuropsychological perspective for reading and writing acquisition. *Educational Psychologist, 27,* 415–434.

Berninger, V. W., & Richards, T. (2002). *Brain literacy for educators and psychologists.* New York: Academic Press.

Berninger, V. W., & Rutberg, J. (1992). Relationship of finger function to beginning writing: Application to diagnosis of writing disabilities. *Developmental Medicine and Child Neurology, 34,* 155–172.

Berninger, V. W., Stage, S., Smith, D., & Hildebrand, D. (2001). Assessment for reading and writing intervention: A three-tier model for prevention and remediation. In J. Andrews, D. Saklofske, & H. Janzen (Eds.), *Handbook of psychoeducational assessment: Ability, achievement, and behavior in children* (pp. 195–223). New York: Academic Press.

Berninger, V. W., Vaughan, K., Abbott, R., Abbott, S., Brooks, A., Rogan, L., et al. (1997). Treatment of handwriting fluency problems in beginning writing: Transfer from handwriting to composition. *Journal of Educational Psychology, 89,* 652–666.

Berninger, V. W., Vaughan, K., Abbott, R., Brooks, A., Abbott, S., Reed, E., et al. (1998). Early intervention for spelling problems: Teaching spelling units of varying size within a multiple connections framework. *Journal of Educational Psychology, 90,* 587–605.

Berninger, V. W., & Whitaker, D. (1993). Theory-based, branching diagnosis of writing disabilities. *School Psychology Review, 22,* 623–642.

Berninger, V. W., Yates, C., Cartwright, A., Rutberg, J., Remy, E., & Abbott, R. (1992). Lower-level developmental skills in beginning writing. *Reading and Writing: An Interdisciplinary Journal, 4,* 257–280.

Binder, J., Frost, J., Hammeke, S., Rao, S., & Cox, R. (1996). Function of the left planum temporale in auditory and linguistic processing. *Brain, 119*, 1239–1247.

Breznitz, Z. (2002). Asynchrony of visual–orthographic and auditory-phonological word recognition processes: An underlying factor in dyslexia. *Journal of Reading and Writing, 15*, 15–42.

Britton, J. (1978). The composing processes and the functions of writing. In C. Cooper & D. Odell (Eds.), *Research on composing. Points of departure* (pp. 13–28). Urbana, IL: NCTE.

Brooks, A., Vaughan, K., & Berninger, V. (1999). Tutorial interventions for writing disabilities: Comparison of transcription and text generation processes. *Learning Disability Quarterly, 22*, 183–191.

Bryant, P., Nunes, T., & Bindman, M. (1997). Children's understanding of the connection between grammar and spelling. In B. A. Blachman (Ed.), *Foundations of reading acquisition and dyslexia: Implications for early intervention* (pp. 219–240). Mahwah, NJ: Erlbaum.

Carlisle, J. (1988). Knowledge of derivational morphology and spelling ability in fourth, sixth, and eighth graders. *Applied Psycholinguistics, 9*, 247–266.

Casey, B., Trainor, R., Giedd, J., Vauss, Y., Vaituzis, C., Hamburger, S., et al. (1997). The role of anterior cingulate in automatic and controlled processes: A developmental neuroanatomical study. *Developmental Psychobiology, 30*, 61–69.

Chomsky, C. (1979). Reading, writing, and phonology. *Harvard Educational Review, 40*, 287–309.

Chugani, H., Phelps, M., & Mazziotta, J. (1987). Positron emission tomography study of human brain functional development. *Annals of Neurology, 22*, 487–497.

Clay, M. (1982). Research update. Learning and teaching writing: A developmental perspective. *Language Arts, 59*, 65–70.

Denckla, M. (1973). Development of speed in repetitive and successive finger movements in normal children. *Developmental Medicine and Child Neurology, 15*, 635–645.

Denckla, M. (1974). Development of motor co-ordination in normal children. *Developmental Medicine and Child Neurology, 16*, 729–741.

Denckla, M. (1996). A theory and model of executive function: A neuropsychological perspective. In G. R. Lyon & N. Krasnegor (1996). *Attention, memory, and executive function* (pp. 263–278). Baltimore: Brookes.

Denckla, M., & Roeltgen, D. (1992). Disorders of motor function and control. In I. Rapin & S. Segalowitz (Eds.), *Handbook of neuropsychology* (Vol. 8, pp. 455–476). Dordrecht, The Netherlands: Elsevier Science.

Dewey, D., & Kaplan, B. (1990). Motor coordination in clumsy children. *Journal of Experimental Clinical Neuropsychology, 12*, 96.

Dreyer, L., Luke, S., & Melican, E. (1994). Children's acquisition and retention of word spellings. In V. W. Berninger (Ed.), *The varieties of orthographic knowledge II: Relationships to phonology, reading, and writing* (pp. 291–320). Dordrecht, The Netherlands: Kluwer Academic.

Ellis, A. (1979). Slips of the pen. *Visible Language, 13*, 265–282.

Ellis, A. (1982). Spelling and writing (and reading and speaking). In A. Ellis (Ed.), *Normality and pathology in cognitive functioning* (pp. 301–330). London: Erlbaum.

Foorman, B., Francis, D., Novy, D., & Liberman, D. (1991). How letter–sound instruction mediates progress in first-grade reading and spelling. *Journal of Educational Psychology, 83*, 456–469.

Gerloff, C., Corwell, B., Chen, R., Hallett, M., & Cohen, L. (1997). Stimulation over the human supplementary motor area interferes with the organization of future elements in complex motor sequences. *Brain, 120*, 1587–1602.

Gibson, E., & Levin, H. (1975). *The psychology of reading*. Cambridge, MA: MIT Press.

Goodnow, J. (1977). *Children drawing*. Cambridge, MA: Harvard University Press.

Graham, S. (1997). Executive control in the revising of students with learning and writing difficulties. *Journal of Educational Psychology, 89*, 223–234.

Graham, S., Berninger, V., Abbott, R., Abbott, S., & Whitaker, D. (1997). The role of mechanics in composing of elementary school students: A new methodological approach. *Journal of Educational Psychology, 89*, 170–182.

Graham, S., & Harris, K. (1996). Addressing problems in attention, memory, and executive functioning: An example from self-regulated strategy development. In G. R. Lyon & N. Krasnegor (Eds.), *Attention, memory, and executive function* (pp. 349–365). Baltimore: Brookes.

Graham, S., & Harris, K. (2000). Writing development: Introduction to special issue. *Educational Psychologist, 35*, 1–2.

Graham, S., Harris, K., & Fink, B. (2000). Is handwriting causally related to learning to write? Treatment of handwriting problems in beginning writers. *Journal of Educational Psychology, 92*, 620–633.

Graham, S., Harris, K., & Fink, B. (2002). Contributions of spelling instruction to the spelling, writing, and reading of poor spellers. *Journal of Educational Psychology, 94*, 687–698.

Graham, S., MacArthur, C., & Schwartz, S. (1995). Effects of goal setting and procedural facilitation on the revising behavior and writing performance of students with writing and learning problems. *Journal of Educational Psychology, 87*, 230–240.

Graham, S., & Weintraub, N. (1996). A review of handwriting research: Progress and prospects from 1980 to 1994. *Educational Psychology Review, 8*, 7–87.

Graves, D. (1975). An examination of the writing processes of seven year-old children. *Research in the Teaching of English, 9*, 227–241.

Harris, K., & Graham, S. (1996). *Making the writing process work: Strategies for composition and self-regulation* (2nd ed.). Cambridge, MA: Brookline Books.

Hayes, J., & Flower, L. (1980). Identifying the organization of the writing process. In L. W. Gregg & E. R. Sternberg (Eds.), *Cognitive processes in writing* (pp. 3–30). Hillsdale, NJ: Erlbaum.

Henry, M. (2003). *Unlocking literacy. Effective decoding and spelling instruction.* Baltimore: Brookes.

Hillis, A., & Caramazza, A. (1989). The grapheme buffer and attentional mechanisms. *Brain and Language, 36*, 208–235.

Hillocks, G. (1986). *Research on written composition: New directions for teaching.* Urbana, IL: National Conference on Research in English.

Hooper, S. L., & Levine, M. (2001). *STRANDS: Survey of teenage readiness and neurodevelopmental status manual. Administration, scoring, and interpretation.* Boston: Educators Publishing Service.

Hooper, S., Montgomery, J., Swartz, C., Reed, M., Sandler, A., Levine, M., et al. (1994). Measurement of written expression. In G. R. Lyon (Ed.), *Frames of reference for the assessment of learning disabilities. New views on measurement issues* (pp. 375–417). Baltimore: Brookes.

Hooper, S., Swartz, C., Montgomery, J., Reed, M., Brown, T., Wasileski, T., et al. (1993). Prevalence of writing problems across three middle school samples. *School Psychology Review, 22*, 608–620.

Hooper, S., Swartz, C., Wakely, M., deKruif, R., & Montgomery, J. (2002). Executive functions in elementary school children with and without problems in written expression. *Journal of Learning Disabilities, 35*, 57–68.

Hsu, L., Wijsman, E., Berninger, V., Thomson, J., & Raskind, W. (2002). Familial aggregation of dyslexia phenotype II: Paired correlated measures. *American Journal of Medical Genetics/Neuropsychiatric Section, 114*, 471–478.

Huttenlocher, P. (1979). Synaptic density in human frontal cortex: Developmental changes and the effects of aging. *Brain Research, 163*, 195–205.

Ivry, R., & Keele, S. (1989). Timing functions of the cerebellum. *Journal of Cognitive Neuroscience, 1*, 136–152.

Jenkins, I., Brooks, D., Nixon, P., Frackowiak, R., & Passingham, R. (1994). Motor sequence learning: A study with positron emission tomography. *Journal of Neuroscience, 14,* 3775–3790.

Jenner, A., Pugh, K., Mencl, W., Fowler, A., Shankweiler, D., Shaywitz, B., et al. (2001, June). *Neuronal pathways associated with phonologic-to-orthographic mapping (spelling).* Boulder, CO: Society for the Scientific Study of Reading.

Jones, D., & Christensen, C. (1999). The relationship between automaticity in handwritng and students' ability to generate written text. *Journal of Educational Psychology, 91,* 44–49.

Jonides, J., Schumacher, E., Smith, E., Lauber, E., Awh, E., Minoshima, S., et al. (1997). Verbal working memory load affects regional brain activation as measured by PET. *Journal of Cognitive Neuroscience, 9,* 462–475.

Kellogg, R. T. (1994). *The psychology of writing.* New York: Oxford University Press.

Klingberg, T., Vaidya, C., Gabrieli, J., Mosely, M., & Hedehus, M. (1999). Myelination and organization of the frontal white matter in children: A diffusion tensor MRI study. *Neuroreport, 10,* 2817–2821.

Kuwabara, T., Watanabe, H., Tsuji, S., & Yuasa, T. (1995). Lactate rise in the basal ganglia accompanying finger movements: A localized ^{1}H-MRS study. *Brain Research, 670,* 326–328.

Langer, J. (1986). *Children reading and writing: Structures and strategies.* Norwood, NJ: Ablex.

Lerer, R., Lerer, M., & Artner, J. (1977). The effects of methylphenidate on the handwriting of children with minimal brain dysfunction. *Journal of Pediatrics, 91,* 127–132.

Leonard, C. (1998). Neural mechanisms of language. In H. Cohen (Ed.), *Neuroscience for rehabilitation* (2nd ed., pp. 349–368). New York: Raven Lippincott.

Leong, C. K. (2000). Rapid processing of base and derived forms of words and grades 4, 5, and 6 children's spelling. *Reading and Writing: An Interdisciplinary Journal, 12,* 277–302.

Levine, M., & Hooper, S. (2001). *Survey of teenage readiness and neurodevelopmental status. (STRANDS).* Boston: Educators Publishing Service.

Levine, M., Oberklaid, F., & Meltzer, L. (1981). Developmental output failure: A study of low productivity in school-age children. *Pediatrics, 67,* 18–25.

Liberman, A. (1999). The reading researcher and the reading teacher need the right theory of speech. *Scientific Studies of Reading, 3,* 95–111.

Luria, A. R. (1973). *The working brain.* NewYork: Basic Books.

Lyon, G. R., & Krasnegor, N. (Eds.). (1996). *Attention, memory, and executive function.* Baltimore: Brookes.

MacArthur, C. (1999). Overcoming barriers to writing: Computer support for basic writing skills. *Reading and Writing Quarterly, 15,* 169–192.

MacArthur, C. (2000). New tools for writing: Assistive technology for students with writing difficulties. *Topics in Language Disorders, 20,* 85–100.

MacArthur, C., Ferretti, R., Okolo, C., & Cavalier, A. (2001). Technology applications for students with literacy problems: A critical review. *Elementary School Journal, 101,* 273–301.

Masterson, J., Apel, K., & Wasowicz, J. (2003). *SPELL. Spelling Performance Evaluation for Language and Literacy* [Spelling assessment software for grade 2 through adult] [Online]. Available from www.learningbydesign.com.

Matsuo, K., Nakai, T., Kato, C., Moriya, T., Isoda, H., Takehara, Y., et al. (2000). Dissociation of writing processes: Functional magnetic resonance imaging during writing of Japanese ideographic characters. *Cognitive Brain Research, 9,* 281–286.

Mattingly, I. (1972). Reading, the linguistic process, and linguistic awareness. In J. Kavanagh & I. Mattingly (Eds.), *Language by ear and by eye: The relationship between speech and reading* (pp. 133–147). Cambridge, MA: MIT Press.

Mazziotta, J., Grafton, S., & Woods, R. (1991). The human motor system studied with PET measurements of cerebral blood flow: topography and motor learning. In N. Lassen, D. Ingvar, M. Raichle, & L. Friberg (Eds.), *Brain work and mental activity. Alfred Benzon Symposium, 31,* 280–290.

McCarty, S., St. James, P., Berninger, V., & Gans, B. (1986). Assessment of intellectual functioning across the life span in severe cerebral palsy. *Developmental Medicine and Child Neurology, 28*, 369–372.

McCutchen, D. (1996). A capacity theory of writing: Working memory in composition. *Educational Psychology Review, 8*, 299–325.

Mesulam, M. (1990). Large-scale neurocognitive networks and distributed processing for attention, language, and memory. *Annals Neurology, 28*, 597–613.

Mishkin, M. (1982). A memory system in the monkey. *Philosophical Transactions of the Royal Society of London, B298*, 85–95.

Mishkin, M., & Appenzeller, T. (1987, June). The anatomy of memory. *Scientific American*, 80–89.

Nagy, W., Diakidoy, I., & Anderson, R. (1993). The acquisition of morphology: Learning the contribution of suffixes to the meaning of derivatives. *Journal of Reading Behavior, 25*, 15–170.

Nicholson, R., Fawcett, A., Berry, E., Jenkins, I., Dean, P., & Brooks, D. (1999). Association of abnormal cerebellar activation with motor learning difficulties in dyslexic adults. *Lancet, 353*, 1662–1667.

Ojemann, G. (1991). The cortical organization of language. *Journal of Neuroscience, 11*, 2281–2287.

Psychological Corporation. (1991). *Wechsler Intelligence Test for Children, third edition (WISC-III)*. San Antonio, TX: Author.

Psychological Corporation. (2001). *Wechsler Individual Achievement Test, second edition (WIAT2)*. San Antonio, TX: Author.

Raichle, M., Fiez, J., Videen, T., MacLeod, A., Pardo, J., Fox, P., et al. (1994). Practice-related changes in human brain functional anatomy during nonmotor learning. *Cerebral Cortex, 4*, 8–26.

Raskind, W. (2001). Current understanding of the genetic basis of reading and spelling disability. *Learning Disability Quarterly, 24*, 141–157.

Raskind, W., Hsu, L., Berninger, V., Thomson, J., & Wijsman, E. (2001). Familial aggregation of dyslexia phenotypes. *Behavior Genetics, 30*, 385–395.

Read, C. (1981). Writing is not the inverse of reading for young children. In C. Frederickson & J. Domminick (Eds.), *Writing: The nature, development, and teaching of written communication* (Vol. 2, pp. 105–117). Hillsdale, NJ: Erlbaum.

Roeltgen, D., & Heilman, K. (1984). Lexical agraphia. Further support for the two-system hypothesis of linguistic agraphia. *Brain, 107*, 811–827.

Roeltgen, D., & Heilman, K. (1985). Review of agraphia and proposal for an anatomically based neuropsychological model of writing. *Applied Psycholinguistics, 6*, 205–230.

Rothi, L., & Heilman, K. (1981). Alexia and agraphia with spared spelling and letter recognition abilities. *Brain and Language, 12*, 1–13.

Rubell, B. (1995). *Big strokes for little folks*. San Antonio, TX: Therapy Skill Builders.

Rutberg, J. (1998). *A comparison of two treatments for remediating handwriting disabilities*. Unpublished doctoral dissertation, University of Washington.

Sakai, K., Hikosaka, O., Miyauchi, S., Takino, R., Sasaki, Y., & Putz, B. (1998). Transition of brain activations from frontal to parietal areas in visuomotor sequence learning. *Journal of Neuroscience, 18*, 1827–1840.

Sandler, A., Watson, T., Footo, M., Levine, M., Coleman, W., & Hooper, S. (1992). Neurodevelopmental study of writing disorders in middle childhood. *Developmental and Behavioral Pediatrics, 13*, 17–23.

Scardamalia, M., & Bereiter, C. (1986). Research on written composition. In M.C. Wittrock (Ed.), *Handbook of research on teaching* (3rd ed., pp. 778–803). New York: Macmillan.

Shibasaki, H., Sadatom N., Lyskow, H., Yonekura, U., Honda, M., Nagamine, T., et al. (1993). Both primary motor cortex and supplementary motor area play an important role in complex finger movement. *Brain, 116*, 1387–1398.

Smith, E., & Jonides, J. (1999). Storage and executive processes in the frontal lobes. *Science, 283*, 1657–1661.

Steffler, D, Varnhagen, C., Friesen, C., & Treiman, R. (1998). There's more to children's spelling than the errors they make: Strategic and automatic processes for one-syllable words. *Journal of Educational Psychology, 90*, 492–505.

Swanson, H. L., & Berninger, V. (1996). Individual differences in children's working memory and writing skills. *Journal of Experimental Child Psychology, 63*, 358–385.

Taylor, H. G. (1987). The meaning and value of soft signs in the behavioral sciences. In D. E. Tupper (Ed.), *Soft neurological signs* (pp. 297–335). New York: Grune & Stratton.

Treiman, R., & Bourassa, D. (2000). The development of spelling skill. *Topics in Language Disorders, 20*, 1–18.

Tupper, D. (1987). The issues with soft signs. In D. Tupper (Ed.), *Soft neurological signs* (pp. 1–16). Orlando, FL: Grune & Stratton.

Tyler, A., & Nagy, W. (1989). The acquisition of English derivational morphology. *Journal of Memory and Language, 28*, 649–667.

van Mier, H., Temple, L., Perlmutter, J., Raichle, M., & Petersen, S. (1998). Changes in brain activity during motor learning measured with PET: Effects of hand performance and practice. *Journal of Neurophysiology, 80*, 2177–2199.

Varnhagen, C. (1994). Children's spelling strategies. In V. W. Berninger (Ed.), *The varieties of orthographic knowledge II: Relationships to phonology, reading, and writing* (pp. 251–290). Dordrecht, The Netherlands: Kluwer Academic.

Venezky, R. (1970). *The structure of English orthography*. The Hague: Mouton.

Venezky, R. (1999). *The American way of spelling*. New York: Guilford Press.

Wagner, R., & Torgesen, J. (1987). The nature of phonological processing and its causal role in the acquisition of reading skills. *Psychological Bulletin, 101*, 192–212.

Weintraub, N., & Graham, S. (2000). The contribution of gender, orthographic, finger function, and visual-motor processes to the prediction of handwritten status. *Occupational Therapy Journal of Research, 20*, 121–140.

Wijsman, E., Peterson, D., Leutennegger, A., Thomson, J., Goddard, K., Hsu, L., et al. (2000). Segregation analysis of phenotypic components of learning disabilities I. Nonword memory and digit span. *American Journal of Human Genetics, 67*, 631–546.

Wolf, M., Bowers, P., & Biddle, K. (2000). Naming-speed processes, timing, and reading A conceptual review. *Journal of Learning Disabilities, 33*, 387–407.

Wolff, P., Gunnoe, C., & Cohen, C. (1983). Associated movements as a measure of developmental age. *Developmental Medicine and Child Neurology, 25*, 417–429.

Wolff, P., & Hurwitz, I. (1966). The choreiform syndrome. *Developmental Medicine and Child Neurology, 8*, 160–165.

Wong, B. (1997). Research on genre-specific strategies for enhancing writing in adolescents with learning disabilities. *Learning Disability Quarterly, 20*, 140–159.

Wood, F., Flowers, L., Buchsbaum, M., & Tallal, P. (1991). Investigation of abnormal left temporal functioning in dyslexia through rCBF, auditory evoked potentials, and positron emission tomography. *Reading and Writing: An Interdisciplinary Journal, 3*, 379–393.

Yost, L., & Lesiak, M. (1980). The relationship between performance on the Developmental Test of Visual Perception and handwriting ability. *Education, 101*, 75–77.

Zimmerman, B., & Reisenberg, R. (1997). Becoming a self-regulated writer: A social cognitive perspective. *Contemporary Educational Psychology, 22*, 73–101.

PART IV

ISSUES AND APPLICATIONS

CHAPTER 16

Hand Preference, Manual Asymmetry, and Manual Skill

MERRILL HISCOCK
LYNN CHAPIESKI

An extreme degree of manual asymmetry in a child is a source of concern for two reasons. First, functional impairment of one hand would limit the child's success in activities that require adroitness with both hands. More important, it might indicate an underlying brain abnormality. Lesser degrees of asymmetry, however—those that are presumed to fall within normal limits—have few practical implications and no known clinical significance. A modicum of asymmetry might even be regarded as advantageous. The "dominance" of one hand, as indicated by preferential use and superior skill, is often considered to be desirable, especially if the right hand is the dominant one (see Harris, 1980, for a historical review).

Clearly the extensive literature on manual asymmetry and hand preference is attributable to something other than the practical implications of being slightly more skilled and more practiced with one hand than with the other. Much of the interest in manual asymmetry has been motivated by theoretical concerns, and particularly by questions about handedness as a correlate of the manner in which language and other cognitive functions are represented in the brain (Corballis, 1991; Hardyck & Petrinovich, 1977; Harris, 1992).

Our focus here is somewhat different. Although we revisit some of the topics that have interested other neuropsychologists, especially the concept of pathological left-handedness, our ultimate concern is motor characteristics of children rather than cognitive characteristics. In particular, we use the neuropsychological literature on handedness as a starting point in exploring various aspects of the relationship between manual asymmetry and manual skill.

The plan of the chapter is straightforward. First, we review the concepts and methodological issues that bear directly on the evidence pertaining to human handedness. Then we discuss the literature that specifically concerns handedness and motor skill in children. Finally, we summarize what we do and do not know about the implications of children's handedness.

BASIC CONCEPTS

Hand Preference

The problems encountered in defining hand preference are manifold. When people declare themselves to be right- or left-handed, they usually are reporting the hand used for writing (Crovitz & Zener, 1962). But the hand used for writing is subject to social pressure and therefore may not indicate a true biological hand preference (Teng, Lee, Yang, & Chang, 1976). Furthermore, handwriting is a skill that came into existence long after right-handedness had become the hominid norm (see McManus, 1999). Indeed, a substantial number of people exhibit a dissociation between writing hand and throwing hand (Gilbert & Wysocki, 1992).

If classification of hand preference is based on an assortment of manual activities (e.g., writing, throwing, brushing the teeth, cutting with a knife, and lifting the lid of a box), a number of psychometric questions arise. How many items should be included in an inventory of activities, and how should those items be selected? Are some items more reliable and valid than others? If so, should those items be weighted more heavily than others? Should bimanual activities (e.g., sweeping with a broom) be included along with unimanual activities? Do items concerning footedness, eyedness, and earedness enhance the usefulness of a handedness inventory? To what degree is each activity affected by environmental influences? Should respondents be required to rate the strength of their hand preference for each activity or only to indicate a right- or left-hand preference?

The various handedness inventories that have been published reflect many different positions with respect to these questions (cf. Annett, 1970a; Beukelaar & Kroonenberg, 1983; Chapman & Chapman, 1987; Coren & Porac, 1978; Healey, Liederman, & Geschwind, 1986; Oldfield, 1971; Peters, 1998; Plato, Fox, & Garruto, 1984; Porac, Coren, Steiger, & Duncan, 1980; Raczkowski, Kalat, & Nebes, 1974; Steenhuis & Bryden, 1989; White & Ashton, 1976). Some questionnaires have as few as 4 items but others contain more than 50. Some ask respondents to rate the strength of their preference for each activity, but others require only a left versus right response. Some inventories employed factor analysis to categorize items and one is based on a hierarchical classification process known as association analysis. Scores from some questionnaires are converted to a laterality quotient (LQ), whereas other questionnaires are designed to yield discrete handedness categories instead of a continuous distribution. In short, there is no universally accepted procedure for measuring hand preference.

Among the most important issues in measuring hand preference by self-report is how to categorize people (i.e., what decision rules to use for dividing people into handedness groups). Peters (1992) has shown that, depending on the criterion chosen for right-handedness, the percentage of right-handers in a sample of university students may range from 13 to 91%. Admittedly, this large range of percentages stems from extremely divergent definitions of right-handedness. The 13% prevalence was obtained by classifying individuals as right-handers only if they indicated that they always use the right hand for each of 12 activities, whereas the 91% estimate was obtained by relaxing the criterion to include everyone with an overall score on the right-handed side of the scale's midpoint. The contrasting percentages, however, do accentuate the point that samples of left- and right-handers may not be comparable across different studies when different criteria are used to define the handedness groups. The findings also illustrate quite vividly that there are degrees of handedness. Hand preference is not a simple dichotomous attribute that could be reported unequivocally in response to a question on a survey. Annett (1970a) has remarked that "to talk about asymmetry in terms of left and right might be like talking about height in terms of 'tall' and 'short' " (p. 316). Hand preference depends, to a large degree, on the investigator's operational definition.

If it is not satisfactory to categorize hand preference as left or right, it may be useful instead to differentiate right-handers from individuals who report either a left-hand preference or no consistent hand preference for performing a specified number of activities. The distinction between right-handers and non-right-handers is a convenient one that has become quite prevalent in neuropsychology (e.g., Rasmussen & Milner, 1975; Witelson, 1980). It presumes, of course, that different forms of deviation from unambiguous right-handedness are comparable—that is, that strong left-handers are indistinguishable neurologically from individuals who have no hand preference.

Alternatively, the dichotomy of right-handed versus non-right-handed may be replaced by a trichotomous classification scheme in which strong right-handers and strong left-handers are distinguished not only from each other but also from mixed-handers (who also have been referred to as ambidextrous, ambilateral, ambilevous, inconsistent, or indeterminate, although these terms have diverse connotations). The trichotomy of right-, left-, and mixed-handedness has the disadvantage of confounding the polarity of hand preference with the strength of preference (Bryden & Steenhuis, 1991). Nevertheless, the trichotomous classification system is commonly used, especially in studies of children (e.g., Annett, 1967, 1983; Gabbard, Hart, & Gentry, 1995; Peters & Durding, 1978). Following the tradition of Samuel Orton (1937), studies of children often begin with the expectation that mixed-handers will perform below the level of both right-handers and left-handers. In other words, a firmly established hand preference is hypothesized to indicate an advantageous neural organization irrespective of the hand that is preferred.

Asymmetry of Manual Skill

A somewhat different set of problems confronts the investigator who chooses to measure or classify manual asymmetry on the basis of skill differences between the hands. One of the problems is how to define and sample adequately the multiple dimensions of motor and perceptual–motor ability. In some studies, researchers focus their attention on a single task such as finger tapping (Peters & Durding, 1978) or peg moving (Annett, Hudson, & Turner, 1974). However, even within a task, the direction of manual asymmetries may reverse as critical elements of the task are altered (Todor & Doane, 1978). Clinical neuropsychologists often assess finger-tapping speed, grip strength, and dexterity in moving pegs (Lezak, 1995), but those three tasks certainly do not cover the full spectrum of motor performance. Research with adults indicates that there may be as many as 10 independent dimensions of motor skill (Barnsley & Rabinovitch, 1970; Fleishman, 1972). We do not know the dimensionality of motor skill in children, nor do we know whether the factor structure changes throughout development.

The reliability of measures of motor skill asymmetry is a major problem. In testing seven different measures of motor skill in normal adults, Provins and Cunliffe (1972) found that even though the retest reliability of dominant-hand performance was statistically significant in all instances, the difference between hands was statistically significant for only two measures (cursive writing and finger tapping). Other studies have yielded a wide range of reliability coefficients for performance differences between hands (Annett et al., 1974; Hiscock & Kinsbourne, 1980; Shankweiler & Studdert-Kennedy, 1975; Todor & Doane, 1977). The reliability of dominant hand performance typically is higher than that of the nondominant hand, and the reliability of the right-minus-left difference is lower than that of either hand's performance (see Annett et al., 1974)

Given the uncertain reliability of right-minus-left difference scores, it is not surprising that the correlation between asymmetry scores obtained from different tasks tends to be low and sometimes not significantly different from zero (Carlier et al., 1996; Eling, 1983; Rigal, 1992). Even when statistically significant, the magnitude of the correlations tends to be modest. For example, in a study of 126 adults with diverse hand preferences, Eling found a correlation of .42 between peg-moving asymmetry and grip-strength asymmetry. Correlations between peg-moving asymmetry and different measures of finger-tapping speed asymmetry ranged from .19 to .42. Curt, Maccario, and Dellatolas (1992) reported a correlation of .45 between asymmetry scores from two manual tasks that were administered to young children. Annett (1992) found correlations ranging from .38 to .60 between peg-moving asymmetry and asymmetry scores from three group tests ("dotting" circles, connecting circles with a line, and punching holes in circles) that were administered to samples of primary and secondary school children. The corresponding correlations for young adults ranged from .44 to .65. Annett's correlation coefficients were all statistically significant but, as pointed out by Carlier and colleagues (1996), her group tests were designed to resemble the peg-moving task.

Despite the modest size of the typical association among asymmetry scores for different tasks, stronger correlations may be observed under special circumstances. For instance, in a sample of children with left hemiplegia, the correlations among asymmetry scores for finger tapping, Purdue Pegboard, and grip strength ranged between .78 and .83 (Hiscock, Hiscock, Benjamins, & Hillman, 1989a). The correlations for children with right hemiplegia ranged from .25 to .39, which is more commensurate with correlations found in the general population.

Practice effects may influence performance asymmetries. Any biologically based advantage of the dominant hand for a particular activity is likely to be amplified by preferential use of that hand for that activity. Conversely, intensive practice on a bimanual task such as typing may obliterate or even reverse a natural difference between the hands in proficiency (Hiscock, Caroselli, & Wood, in press; Provins & Glencross, 1968). Even novel laboratory tasks may be contaminated by practice effects to the extent that proficiency in highly practiced everyday activities transfers to the laboratory task being evaluated. The question of practice effects is complicated further by contradictory evidence about the transfer of training from one hand to the other, from bimanual to unimanual tasks, and from unimanual to bimanual tasks (Shulze, Lüders, & Jäncke, 2002).

The measurement of manual skill asymmetry is complicated by a conundrum that is inherent in all laterality research, namely, how to determine the magnitude of a left-versus-right difference when the overall level of performance varies across participants and between groups. The problem is this: The magnitude of differences between the hands (right minus left, or R-L) may vary with overall performance (right plus left, or R+L), and the covariance between R-L and R+L may or may not be theoretically meaningful. A positive association between R-L and R+L in a sample of children might indicate that the right hand shows more improvement than the left as children grow older (e.g., Miller, 1982). A negative association might indicate that the left hand tends to "catch up" with the right hand during development (e.g., Blank, Miller, & von Voß, 2000). Alternatively, a relationship between R-L and R+L could be a range artifact (i.e., a floor effect in the case of a positive association and a ceiling effect in the case of a negative association). For this reason, correlations between R-L and R+L must be interpreted cautiously (cf. Annett, 2002; Zung, 1985).

Distortion of scores by floor effects is a potential problem in studies of young children's motor performance because poor performance with the dominant hand restricts the range of the asymmetry score. The dominant hand performs so poorly as to leave little room for a difference between the dominant and nondominant hands. Conversely, a ceiling effect may be present when older children perform at a level that approaches the psychometric or biomechanical upper limit of performance. If a child performs close to that upper limit with the nondominant hand, the asymmetry score will be small because the dominant hand cannot perform much better. Both floor and ceiling effects might occur, in different age groups, within the same experiment.

The Relationship between Hand Preference and Manual Asymmetry

It is not surprising that studies usually find a significant association between hand preference and manual asymmetry (e.g., Annett, 1970a; Barnsley & Rabinovitch, 1970; Bishop, 1989; McManus, Kemp, & Grant, 1986; Nalcaci, Kalaycioglu, Cicek, & Genc, 2001; Peters, 1998; Todor & Doane, 1977; Todor & Kyprie, 1980). The relationship is evident in children as well as in adults (e.g., Annett, 1970b; Annett & Turner, 1974; Curt et al., 1992; Finlayson & Reitan, 1976; Hiscock, Kinsbourne, Samuels, & Krause, 1985; Kee, Gottfried, Bathurst, & Brown, 1987; Miller, 1982; Peters & Durding, 1978; Rigal, 1992). In a study of children between the ages of 6 and 11 years, a brief handedness assessment predicted the direction of manual asymmetry with 100% accuracy (Hiscock et al., 1985). Of 73 children who showed a right-hand preference for writing and four of eight other activities, every child finger tapped faster with the right hand than with the left. In another study of finger tapping in children, Peters and Durding (1978) reported a correlation of .965 between hand-preference group (from a total of nine ordered groups) and mean left-minus-right difference in the intertap interval. Todor and Doane (1977), however, reported that the relationship between hand preference and relative hand proficiency in adults varied with the difficulty of the task being performed. The correlation was weakest at moderate to high levels of task difficulty.

Hand preference and manual skill are not always related in predictable ways. Tan (1992) reported that strength of hand preference in left-handed adults is correlated with right-hand performance but not left-hand performance on peg-moving and dot-filling tasks. McManus and colleagues (1986) found hand differences between left- and right-handers in finger-tapping speed but not regularity of finger tapping. (This dissociation is contradicted by other evidence, e.g., Peters & Durding, 1978; Todor & Kyprie, 1980.) Kimura and Vanderwolf (1970) found that right-handed adults are more adept at flexing single fingers or pairs of fingers on the left hand than on the right hand. Ingram (1975) subsequently reported similar findings for a sample of 98 right-handed children of ages 3, 4, and 5 years. Roy and MacKenzie (1978) reported a left-hand superiority of right-handed adults on a task requiring accurate positioning of the thumb.

In young children, hand preference may be difficult to distinguish from a skill difference between the hands. If an infant holds a rattle longer with the right hand than with the left, or squeezes harder with the right hand (Caplan & Kinsbourne, 1976; Hawn & Harris, 1983; Petrie & Peters, 1980), does that asymmetry indicate a preference for the right hand or does it indicate a right-hand skill advantage? Maybe the differentiation of a motor preference from a skill asymmetry in the young infant is not a meaningful question.

The score distributions for hand preference and manual skill asymmetry typically have contrasting shapes. Handedness inventories yield scores that have strong negative skew (i.e., a piling up of scores on the right-hand pole) (Annett, 1970b, 1972; Curt et al., 1992; Miller, 1982; Oldfield, 1971). Sometimes the distributions are described as J-shaped, a term that acknowledges a minor concentration of scores at the left-hand end of the spectrum as well as the much larger concentration at the right-hand end. In contrast, R-L scores from skill tests such as finger tapping and peg moving tend to be distributed in an approximately normal fashion (Annett, 1972, 1992; Bryden, 1982; Curt, De Agostini, Maccario, & Dellatolas, 1995; Curt et al., 1992; Peters & Durding, 1978; Rigal, 1992; Woo & Pearson, 1927).

On closer examination of manual asymmetry scores, it seems that the scores are actually distributed as unimodal, bell-shaped curves for each hand-preference group (Annett, 1992, 2002). When scores for left- and right-handers are pooled and the respective means are relatively close together, the small bell-shaped distribution for left-handers is obscured by the much larger bell-shaped distribution for right-handers. This gives the appearance of a single normal distribution, which has long been considered to be the true distribution of manual asymmetry scores. However, as the means become more disparate (or the within-group variability is reduced), two separate bell-shaped distributions may be observed, one for each hand-preference group (Annett, 1992; Curt et al., 1992; Tapley & Bryden, 1985). Whether skill asymmetry scores are better represented as a single distribution or as two (or more) distributions depends on the manual task on which performance is measured as well as subject characteristics. Curt and colleagues (1992) found that even though a single normal curve fit the distribution of asymmetries on a circle-marking task for children between 2½ and 3½ years of age, two normal curves provided a better fit for the scores of older children. Irrespective of age group, a single normal curve provided a satisfactory fit for the distribution of asymmetries on a peg-moving task.

Even though a simple measure of hand preference is sometimes sufficient to predict the direction of performance asymmetry, much remains to be learned about the relationship between preference and skill. As noted previously, a substantial number of right-handed writers throw with the left hand, and an even greater proportion of left-handers throw with the right hand (Gilbert & Wysocki, 1992). Peters (1990) found that inconsistent left-handers tend to be stronger with the right hand than with the left. Peters (1998) has shown, more generally, that the correlation between hand preference and skill asymmetry is weaker for individuals with inconsistent hand preferences than for those with consistent preferences. This principle applies to both right- and left-handers, but it becomes apparent only when the assessment of hand preference is sensitive to differences in the consistency of preferences. Another complication is differential practice for the left and right hands. The relationship between hand preference and skill sometimes can be modified by practice, as evidenced by differences between unpracticed and practiced right-handers in hand differences on a typewriting task (Provins & Glencross, 1968), but the effects of practice are not always that straightforward. Schulze and colleagues (2002) found that 2 hours of unimanual practice on a peg-moving task, distributed over 4 weeks, benefited the untrained hand almost as much as the trained hand.

The established associations between hand preference and performance are mostly categorical rather than parametric. The literature tells us more about the direction of skill asymmetries in left- and right-handers than about the quantitative relationship between strength of hand preference and magnitude of performance asymmetry (e.g., Miller, 1982). The paucity of data about the strength of the associations presumably stems from the nonnormal shape of the hand-preference distribution, a consequent lack of agreement about how to quantify or categorize hand preference, and the limited reliability and concurrent validity of performance tasks. When hand preference is defined in terms of dichotomous or trichotomous categories, it is not possible to obtain anything more than a first approximation to the actual relationship between preference and asymmetrical skill.

Other unanswered questions are developmental in nature. Does preference arise from a difference between the hands in fine motor skill or, as suggested by Kimura and Vanderwolf (1970), does the association between preference and skill stem from some other mechanism? How general is the early relationship between hand preference and manual skill? Can the dimensions of preference and skill be differentiated early in life? These questions can be addressed by examining the developmental course of hand preferences and manual skills.

NORMAL DEVELOPMENT OF HAND PREFERENCE AND MANUAL ASYMMETRY

Manual asymmetries have been reported in very young infants. Yet, a child may show considerable variability in manifest handedness over the first 4 years of life, and some fluctuation may persist after that. In the words of Gesell and Ames (1947), "From four years on, the dominant hand is used mostly, but in some cases even at seven years there is a transient period of use of the non-dominant hand or of both hands together" (p. 157). As one might expect of a characteristic that has early-emerging components but requires as much as 7 years to stabilize, the development of handedness is neither simple nor well understood. Even though hand preference runs in families and is widely assumed to be genetically influenced (e.g., Annett, 2002; Corballis, 1980,

1983; McManus, 1999; McManus & Bryden, 1992), multiple factors undoubtedly contribute to an individual's handedness. Those factors are thought to include intrauterine and postnatal postural asymmetries as well as maternal handedness, which influences the way in which the mother holds and interacts with the infant (Michel, 1981, 1992, 2001; Previc, 1991; Provins, 1992).

Infants grasp objects for a longer time with the right hand than with the left (Caplan & Kinsbourne, 1976; Hawn & Harris, 1983; Petrie & Peters, 1980). This asymmetry has been observed in children as young as 17 days. The right arm tends to be more active than the left during the first 3 months of life (Coryell & Michel, 1978; Liederman, 1983; von Hofsten, 1982). Despite conflicting reports about early asymmetries in precision grasping, object manipulation and reaching, the right hand is generally preferred throughout the first 4 months of life for "directed, target-related" acts (Young, Segalowitz, Corter, & Trehub, 1983). Observations to the contrary may reflect a tendency of infants to engage in more nondirected activity (e.g., passive holding, reflexive movements, hand and finger movements in the absence of arm movements) with the left hand than with the right during this period. Furthermore, Liederman (1983) has suggested that when more left- than right-hand activity is seen in response to stimulation, it may very well reflect a decrease in ongoing right-hand activity rather than an increase in left-hand activity. Thus, according to Liederman, the left-sided bias reported in some studies of infant arm movements (e.g., McDonnell, Anderson, & Abraham, 1983) represents a generalized disinhibition of left-arm movement, which reflects the immaturity of the left arm relative to the right.

The development of handedness and manual asymmetry is neither "a unitary phenomenon nor an invariant one" (Young, Corter, Segalowitz, & Trehub, 1983, p. 8). In some instances, the developmental course of handedness for a particular activity can be characterized as (1) early asymmetry, (2) its subsequent disappearance, and (3) its ultimate reemergence and stabilization (Young, Corter, et al., 1983). Even though the changes over time presumably reflect structural and functional changes in the neural substrate of that activity, the functional significance of the behavior nonetheless may remain constant (Peters, 1983a, 1983c). Conversely, according to Peters, a superficial constancy in the topography of a movement may mask a shift in underlying processes. Peters's first proposition is supported by evidence of a temporal linkage between hand preference and language milestones. Discontinuities in the developmental course of manual asymmetry coincide with transitions between stages of language development (Ramsay, 1983, 1984, 1985). Cyclic changes in manifest handedness have been attributed to fluctuations in the degree to which speech interferes with use of the dominant hand (Bates, O'Connell, Vaid, Sledge, & Oakes, 1986). Such interference is thought to be due to the proximity of these two control processes in "functional cerebral space" (Kinsbourne & Hicks, 1978) within the same hemisphere. On the basis of a correlation between language competence and right-hand bias in children between the ages of 13 and 28 months, Bates et al. concluded that speech interferes maximally with right-hand activity while children are mastering a new problem in language development. When the problem is mastered, interference abates and the right-hand bias reverts to its usual level, at which it remains until the next problem in language development is encountered. If Bates et al. are correct, the apparent developmental changes in hand use reflect changes in language functioning that interact with a relative invariant manual asymmetry.

Two principles of special relevance to this chapter can be derived from the literature on the early development of manual asymmetry. One of these is the concept that the normal development of handedness depends on a multiplicity of factors. Its genetic basis notwithstanding, handedness does not simply unfold according to a genetic blueprint (Michel, 2001). Instead, the development of manual asymmetry depends on a dynamic interaction among various biological, genetic, and experiential variables. In the words of Liederman (1983), "Most behavior will be dominated by the left hemisphere–right hand—but this is due to the conjoint influence of many factors that themselves can operate relatively independently, rather than a single mechanism that reveals itself over time" (p. 89). In the next section, we consider the intrusion of pathological factors into the developmental process.

The other principle of interest is that hand preferences tend to be erratic during a protracted period of development. As Liederman (1983) has said about infancy, "Lateral preferences often fluctuate, the proportion of right-sidedness is lower than in adulthood, and there may even be periods when left-sidedness is predominant" (p. 71). Inconsistent hand use reportedly continues to the age of 28 months (Bates et al., 1986) and even to 4 years and beyond (Gesell & Ames, 1947; Gudmundsson, 1993; Öztürk et al., 1999). Perhaps variability in hand preference that persists beyond the age of 4 years or so is a marker for maturational delay of the central nervous system. Coren, Searleman, and Porac (1986) have reported that even as adolescents, left-handers lag behind right-handers in physical development. Unfortunately, Coren et al. did not indicate whether physical immaturity is associated specifically with inconsistent left-handedness.

PATHOLOGICAL LEFT-HANDEDNESS

Non-right-handers are overrepresented in diverse anomalous populations ranging from mentally retarded and epileptic individuals to children with learning disabilities and alcoholic adults (Annett, 2002; Coren, 1990, 1993; Harris, 1980; Harris & Carlson, 1988; Herron, 1980). A simple explanation for this is that left-handedness is the consequence of brain pathology (Gordon, 1920). A contemporary form of this hypothesis rests on a reported association among birth stress, brain damage, and non-right-handedness (Bakan, 1971, 1977, 1990; Bakan, Dibb, & Reed, 1973). Bakan has proposed that non-right-handedness is a manifestation of a "continuum of reproductive casualty" (Pasamanick & Knobloch, 1966), which is to say that deviation from right-handedness is one of many potential consequences of adverse prenatal and perinatal factors. Associated outcomes range from the relatively mild, such as learning disabilities, to the more severe, such as cerebral palsy and mental retardation. The behavioral anomalies observed in most left-handers sampled from the general population would, of course, fall on the mild end of the spectrum. Even though Bakan's hypothesis is difficult to disprove, the supporting evidence is unconvincing (Harris & Carlson, 1988; Schwartz, 1990).

Another hypothesis, more complex and detailed than Bakan's, has been offered by Geschwind and his colleagues (Geschwind & Behan, 1982; Geschwind & Galaburda, 1985a, 1985b, 1985c, 1987) to explain, among other phenomena, the reported associations between non-right-handedness and adverse behavioral characteristics. The crux of the Geschwind–Behan–Galaburda hypothesis is the idea that exposure of the fetal brain to elevated testosterone levels alters the development of the left hemisphere. This in turn has many implications for the development of the right hemisphere and other brain structures and for the immune system. Among the predicted behavioral consequences are anomalies of language development and atypical handedness. Although the empirical evidence has been largely unsupportive, the Geschwind–Behan–Galaburda hypothesis has had enormous impact on neuropsychology and has inspired a large number of empirical studies (see Bryden, McManus, & Bulman-Fleming, 1994, and associated commentaries).

If all left-handedness were the consequence of early brain pathology or a cascade of adverse developmental events stemming from a single neuroendocrinological anomaly, one might predict that large samples of left-handers would be lower in IQ than right-handers and that variability would be greater among left-handers. In fact, the results of several large-scale studies indicate that left- and right-handers in the general population are equal in IQ (Briggs, Nebes, & Kinsbourne, 1976; Hardyck, Petrinovich, & Goldman, 1976; Newcombe & Ratcliff, 1973; Roberts & Engle, 1974), and one such study even indicates that left-handers are less variable (Newcombe & Ratcliff, 1973). An interesting footnote to the debates over the Bakan hypothesis and the Geschwind–Behan–Galaburda model is the report by Hicks and Dusek (1980) that 578 gifted elementary school children were significantly *less* likely to have a preference for the right hand than were 391 nongifted children.

If left- and right-handers in the general population differ only with respect to hand preference, then why do left-handers appear to be overrepresented in clinical populations? The paradox suggests the existence of two subtypes of left-handers: "natural" left-handers and "pathological" left-handers. This dichotomy could account for the elevated prevalence of left-handers in clinical populations, while accommodating evidence that the great majority of left-handers are as intelligent, healthy, and behaviorally competent as right-handers.

According to the concept of pathological left-handedness (Gordon, 1920; Hécaen & Ajuriaguerra, 1964; Orsini & Satz, 1986; Satz, 1972, 1973; Silva & Satz, 1979), the number of natural left-handers in various clinical populations is enhanced by disproportionately high numbers of genotypic right-handers who have become left-handed as a consequence of early brain damage. The damage that effects a shift from right- to left-handedness also increases the risk of intellectual deficit or other adaptive limitations (see Bullard-Bates & Satz, 1983, for an example). The increased risk is not a consequence of left-handedness; rather, the increased risk and the left-handedness are consequences of the early brain damage (e.g., Satz, Strauss, Wada, & Orsini, 1988). The same logic would imply that early brain damage sometimes produces a shift from left- to right-handedness. Indeed this may occur, but the number of right-handers produced by this mechanism would be limited even if right-sided damage were as common as left-sided damage. Only natural left-handers would be candidates for switching to right-handedness and, besides, the relatively small number of pathological right-handers would be difficult to find in the huge pool of natural right-handers (Satz, 1973; Schonblom, 1977). Moreover, right-sided damage to the fetal or neonatal brain is less common than left-sided damage (see Harris & Carlson, 1988).

One difficulty with the concept of pathological left-handedness is the absence of definitive criteria for differentiating pathological from natural non-right-handers, especially in the general population (McManus, 1983). Different investigators have suggested a variety of markers for pathological left-handedness, which include a strong preference for the left hand (Hiscock & Hiscock, 1990); clumsiness of the non-preferred (right) hand (Bishop, 1984; Gillberg, Walderström, & Rasmussen, 1984); relatively small size of the right hand and foot (Satz, Orsini, Saslow, & Henry, 1985); and a noninverted writing posture (Hiscock & Hiscock, 1990). These criteria imply that pathological left-handedness is nothing more than a subtle form of right-sided hemiplegia, which makes the concept circular with respect to handedness and motor skill.

The concept of pathological left-handedness can be invoked to account for the elevated prevalence of non-right-handedness that has been found in studies of the mentally retarded (e.g., Batheja & McManus, 1985; Bradshaw-McAnulty, Hicks, & Kinsbourne, 1984; Hicks & Barton, 1975; see Pipe, 1990, for a review). Bradshaw-McAnulty and colleagues (1984) reported that non-right-handedness is more common in the severely retarded than in the moderately retarded. Moreover, these investigators failed to find a substantial correlation between the hand preference of children with mental retardation and the hand preference of their parents. Even though these findings support the concept of pathological left-handedness in a broad sense, the neuropathology leading to mental retardation—whether associated with Down syndrome or another etiology—is unlikely to be unilateral (Harris & Carlson, 1988). Consequently, Batheja and McManus (1985) proposed a "neurobiological noise" model of non-right-handedness in which adverse biological influences may disrupt the individual's development of right-handedness. As pointed out by Harris and Carlson (1988), this model differs from Satz's (1972, 1973) version of pathological left-handedness in that the Batheja and McManus model does not require unilateral neuropathology. Various forms of pathology may lead to an elevated level of "biological noise," which, in turn, increases the likelihood of a deviation from right-handedness.

Much of the discrepancy between the positions of McManus and Satz has been resolved by a revision of Satz's model of pathological left-handedness to include a category of ambiguous handedness (AH). Satz and his colleagues (Satz, Soper, & Orsini, 1988; Satz, Soper, Orsini, Henry, & Zvi, 1985; Soper & Satz, 1984; Soper et al., 1986; Soper, Satz, Orsini, Van Gorp, & Green, 1987) identified a subgroup of individuals with AH among individuals with autism, as well as nonautistic individuals with mental retardation. People in the AH category tended to show inconsistent hand preference even for the same task. The AH subgroup is distinct from groups of ambidextrous individuals (people with mixed- or inconsistent-handedness), whose hand preference is inconsistent across tasks but consistent with respect to the same task at different times (Satz et al., 1988). Satz and his colleagues attribute AH to severe, bilateral early brain damage that precludes the normal development of manual dominance. Consequently, ambiguous handedness, with its bilateral and presumably diffuse etiology, bears at least a superficial resemblance to Batheja and McManus's concept of pathological left-handedness.

The distinction between natural and pathological (or ambiguous) non-right-handedness is useful for two reasons. First, it accounts for the apparent contradiction between the elevated prevalence of non-right-handedness in clinical populations and the absence of any association between non-right-handedness and abnormality in the general population. Second, it implies that deviation from right-handedness in clinical populations is a consequence of the neuropathology that underlies the abnormality. However, as noted by Kinsbourne (1988), any adverse outcome that can be attributed to pathological left-handedness in genotypic right-handers might also be attributed to a higher risk of that pathology in genotypic left-handers. In other words, it is difficult to disprove the alternative proposal that left-handers are more vulnerable than right-handers to a variety of disorders. The source of the pathology could be endogenous or exogenous.

Even if the hypothesis of greater risk among left-handers were shown to be correct, left-handedness per se would not be viewed as the source of adverse outcomes. One could still maintain the distinction between affected left-handers, who are at risk for a disorder and acquire the disorder, and normal left-handers, who are at risk for the disorder but do not acquire it. As long as the source of the disorder is dissociable from left-handedness per se, one would expect to find two subtypes of left-hander—one with and one without the disorder in question. This leads us back to the practical question of how to distinguish natural left-handers from pathological left-handers (including genotypic left-handers who have been affected by pathology). Several ways of subtyping non-right-handers have been suggested.

IDENTIFYING SUBGROUPS OF LEFT-HANDERS

Handwriting Posture

Levy and Reid (1976, 1978) proposed that the position of the hand when engaged in cursive writing indicates the neural organization of language and motor control. The noninverted writing posture that characterizes most right-handers was claimed to reflect left-hemispheric language representation and contralateral control of writing. Similarly, a noninverted writing posture in left-handers was thought to indicate right-hemispheric language and contralateral motor control. However, the majority of left-handers write with the hand in an inverted (or hooked) position, which, according to Levy and Reid, is associated with left-sided language representation and ipsilateral control of the left hand. Much of the subsequent evidence, however, has cast doubt on the relationship between handwriting posture and language representation (cf. Guiard & Millerat, 1984; Levy, 1982, 1984; Peters, 1983b; Peters & McGrory, 1987; Smith & Moscovitch, 1979; Weber & Bradshaw, 1981). Especially damaging to the hypothesis of Levy and Reid is a series of failures to find differences between inverted and noninverted writers in speech lateralization as determined via the intracarotid sodium Amytal test (Ajersch & Milner, 1983; Strauss, Wada, & Kosaka, 1984; Volpe, Sidtis, & Gazzaniga, 1981).

Even if it reveals nothing about language representation, handwriting posture might imply something about motor control. Various investigators have reported differences in motor skill between adults who write with inverted posture and those who use a noninverted posture (Gregory & Paul, 1980; Parlow, 1978; Parlow & Kinsbourne, 1981; Peters & McGrory, 1987; Todor, 1980). The exact nature of the between-group difference, however, varies across studies and the results in aggregate do not lead to any straightforward interpretation (see Peters, 1983b). In addition, the positive findings are counterbalanced by negative findings (Peters, 1983b; Peters & McGrory, 1987).

One of the more interesting findings from the literature on inverted and non-inverted handwriting in adult left-handers is that noninverted writers are more adept than inverted writers in writing with the nonpreferred posture (Peters & McGrory, 1987). This finding supports previous suggestions by Herron (1980) and Peters (1983b) that the inverted posture is an adaptation to the mechanical demands of left-to-right cursive writing. In other words, some left-handers learn to use the inverted writing position as an advantageous alternative to the "default option" of the noninverted posture that is more appropriate for right-handers than for left-handers.

If inverted writing posture is the "technically superior" posture for left-handers (Peters, 1983b), then normal left-handed children might be inclined to shift from a noninverted to an inverted writing posture at some point in their development. Yet there is only mixed evidence that a developmental shift of this kind actually occurs. Peters and Pedersen (1978) and Bryson and Macdonald (1984) did find a dramatic increase in the prevalence of inverted writers between grades 1–4 and grades 5 and 6 in their cross-sectional studies of left-handed Canadian children. In contrast, Peters (1986) observed no age-related change in German elementary school children. Across the range of grades 1–5, 62.6% of the left-handed German children wrote with an inverted hand position. When a difference in writing posture between girls and boys is found, it is the boys who more frequently use the inverted writing posture, and this is true of right-handed children as well as left-handed children (Allen & Wellman, 1980).

The rather sparse evidence from studies of children seems to fit Peters' (1983b, 1986, 1995) conclusion that writing posture is determined by sociocultural influences (e.g., orientation of the paper, the direction in which letters are slanted, and the age at which cursive writing is learned) rather than by neurological factors. If boys in some cultures are more likely than girls to adopt the advantageous inverted posture, perhaps it is only because boys are more likely to deviate from the externally imposed norm of noninverted writing. Nonetheless, a finding by Hiscock, Hiscock, Benjamins, and Hillman (1989b) suggests that limitations of fine motor control may preclude, or at least delay, adoption of the inverted writing posture. In this study, every child in a sample of 29 children with right hemiplegia wrote with a noninverted posture. The children, who ranged in age from 4 to 14 years, tended to score below average on tests of motor skill even with the left hand. Thus, assuming that damage was not restricted to the left hemisphere in these children with cerebral palsy, one might speculate that the inverted writing posture is unlikely to be an option for left-handed children if the right hemisphere has been compromised by early pathology.

Familial Sinistrality

Left-handers may be distinguished from each other on the basis of whether or not left-handedness runs in their families. It is often assumed that individuals with familial sinistrality (FS+) are more likely to have a genetic basis for their left-handedness than are individuals with no family history of left-handedness (FS-). The assumed importance of familial sinistrality is not without empirical support. LeMay (1977), for instance, found that FS- left-handers had structural asymmetries of the brain that resembled those of right-handers. Only the brains of FS+ left-handers were likely to diverge from the pattern of asymmetry observed in brains of right-handers. Hécaen and Sauguet (1971), in a clinical study, found corresponding differences in language representation between FS+ and FS- left-handers. Again the FS+ left-handers were more likely to deviate from the norm for right-handers.

Familial sinistrality has been considered in numerous studies of visual and auditory laterality, but the results have been notable only for their inconsistency (e.g., Bryden, 1973; Hines & Satz, 1971; Hiscock & Mackay, 1985; Lake & Bryden, 1976; McKeever, Seitz, Hoff, Marino, & Diehl, 1983; Springer & Searleman, 1980; Zurif & Bryden, 1969). In his review of dichotic listening results, Bryden (1988) concluded that FS has no major effect on dichotic listening asymmetry. McManus and Bryden (1992) expressed a more general conclusion: "There certainly is no justification for the belief that FS divides the left-handed population into those who are 'naturally' left-handed and those who are 'pathologically' left-handed" (pp. 134–135).

Some of the variability across FS studies may be attributable to difficulties in the measurement of FS. Many respondents may not have correct information about the hand preferences of all their first-degree relatives (Hiscock & Cole, 2004). In addition, as Bishop (1980b) has pointed out, the probability of FS+ varies with number of first-degree relatives. A child who has 10 siblings is much more likely to have a left-hander in the family than is a child with only one sibling.

Difficulties with the concept of FS go beyond measurement problems. Dozens of clinical and experimental studies of FS have been reviewed and critiqued by McKeever (1990), who acknowledged that "there is considerable noise in the data" and suggested that familial sinistrality "is probably confounded, in some critical but unknown ways, with other effective variables" (p. 401). McKeever argued that neither FS+ nor FS- is a homogeneous category, and that both categories need to be decomposed into subgroups representing different combinations of genetic, pathological, and environmental influences on handedness.

Consistency of Handedness

An obvious means of subclassifying left-handers is to divide them according to the degree, or strength, of their preference for the left hand (Grimshaw & Bryden, 1994). Bryden and his colleagues have argued that the strength and inflexibility (i.e., resistance to modification) of a person's hand preference may be a more fundamental biological attribute than the direction of preference (cf. Bryden, 1987; Bryden & Steenhuis, 1991; McManus & Bryden, 1992). Some investigators have found differences between weak and strong left-handers on tests of perceptual laterality (Dee, 1971; Knox & Boone, 1970; Satz, Achenbach, & Fennell, 1967). Unfortunately, the direction of the differences has not been uniform across studies, and even the definition of consistency is a matter of dispute. Consistency may be quantified by adding strength-of-preference ratings across various activities, thereby intermixing consistency across activities and consistency within each activity (Peters, 1998). Alternatively, consistency may be defined in terms of congruence across activities irrespective of the strength of preference for each activity (Annett, 2002; Peters & Pang, 1992).

In 1987, Ponton reported that inconsistent left-handers outperformed consistent left-handers and right-handers on a number of performance tasks, including counting aloud and making specified sequential movements with the hand and arm. Groups were defined according to the number of left-hand responses made to a specified set of eight items from a hand-preference questionnaire. Although Peters and Servos (1989) failed to replicate Ponton's findings, they did find a dissociation between asymmetry of strength and asymmetry of fine motor skill in the inconsistent left-handed group. Inconsistent left-handers performed better with the left hand than with the right hand on tasks requiring manual speed and control, but they exhibited more strength in the right hand than in the left. Subsequent studies by Peters (1990) and Peters and Pang (1992) confirmed that inconsistent left-handers are stronger on the right side despite their greater skill with the left hand. In addition, most inconsistent left-handers throw with the right hand, and their throwing accuracy is greater with the right hand than with the left.

When defined by self-reported hand preference according to Ponton's (1987) criteria, inconsistent left-handers constitute approximately 50% of the left-handed population and thus about 5% of the general population (Peters & Pang, 1992). Peters and Pang note that these percentages are compatible with Geschwind and Galaburda's (1985a, 1985b, 1985c) speculation, based on work by Gesell and Ames (1947), that about 5% of the population might show an anomalous dissociation between the lateralization of systems for controlling proximal and distal musculature. A similar distinction has been invoked to characterize sex differences in motor skill. Women tend to perform better than men on fine motor tasks, which involve control over the distal musculature, whereas men tend to perform better than women on throwing tasks and other "targeting" tasks, which depend primarily on control over the proximal muscles (Kimura, 1999). Despite the potential explanatory power of the proximal versus distal distinction, Peters and Pang's (1992) data failed to support the prediction that many inconsistent left-handers would show a left-sided superiority for finger tapping (distal musculature) and a right-sided superiority for arm tapping (proximal musculature). Inconsistent left-handers displayed a left-sided superiority for both tasks.

Throwing is a particularly interesting manifestation of handedness because of its putative significance in human evolution (Calvin, 1991) and also because of the large sex differences in throwing that materialize early in development (Kimura, 1999; Thomas & French, 1985). Although less than 2% of right-handed writers throw with the left hand, approximately one-third of left-handed writers throw with the right hand (Gilbert & Wysocki, 1992; McManus, Porac, Bryden, & Boucher, 1999). Thus, right-throwing left-handedness represents a common phenomenon, and one that awaits explanation at the neurological level. Annett (2002), using a sample of 1,849 children and adults, examined the asymmetry of peg-moving speed in subgroups based on all possible combinations of writing hand and throwing hand. She found that both preferred writing hand and preferred throwing hand independently predicted asymmetry of peg moving, but writing hand was the better predictor. Annett's findings support Peters's (1998) claim that asymmetries of motor skill are greater for consistent than for inconsistent left-handers. The same findings also imply that it may be useful for some purposes to define consistency simply as a concordance between hand preference for throwing and for writing.

Footedness

Some other manifestations of motor or postural asymmetry have been suggested as bases for defining subgroups of right- and left-handers (McManus & Bryden, 1992). Among them are the manner of interlacing the fingers when the hands are clasped, the manner in which the arms are folded, and the way in which a person crosses his or her legs. A more promising alternative index of motor asymmetry is footedness, or the congruity between handedness and footedness (see Peters, 1988, for a review). Even though footedness is correlated with handedness, the correlation is not perfect, especially among left-handers (e.g., Annett, 2002; Annett & Turner, 1974; Peters & Durding, 1979; Porac & Coren, 1981), and the developmental course of foot preference appears to differ from that of hand preference (Gabbard, 1993). The measurement of foot preference and skill is not without its methodological and interpretive difficulties; however, the study of footedness holds promise for several reasons. First, foot preference has been claimed to be more closely related than hand preference to measures of language lateralization (Elias & Bryden, 1998; Searleman, 1980). Second, foot and leg performance are highly sensitive to neurologically based problems of motor control (Peters, 1988), and third, foot asymmetries are less susceptible to social pressures than are hand asymmetries (Chapman, Chapman, & Allen, 1987).

RELATIONSHIP BETWEEN CHILDREN'S HAND PREFERENCE AND MANUAL SKILL

The literature we have summarized thus far provides a context for evaluating and interpreting the relatively modest number of studies that have investigated the association between handedness and manual performance in children sampled from the general population and from various clinical populations. For example, the neuropsychological literature on pathological left-handedness helps us to understand the motivation for studies in which right- and non-right-handed children are compared. Whether justified or not, there is a prevalent expectation that non-right-handed children will be motorically slower or clumsier than their right-handed peers. Yet, the same literature provides ample reason not to assume that non-right-handed children constitute a homogeneous population.

Children in the General Population

Table 16.1 summarizes studies of motor skill in unselected samples of children. One salient feature of this set of studies is the diversity of criteria for forming groups of children. Of the 19 studies summarized in the table, 15 categorized children on the basis of hand preference. However, the criteria for hand preference ranged from the hand used for writing (Bishop, 1980a) to the child's score on a 22-item handedness questionnaire (Bhushan, Dwivedi, Mishra, & Mandal, 2000). Children in three studies were grouped according to the consistency of lateral preference across hand and eye or hand, eye, and foot (Flick, 1966; Horine, 1968; Keogh, 1972) and, in the remaining study, stability of hand preference over time served as the criterion for classifying children (Gottfried & Bathurst, 1983). The number of groups derived from the various criteria ranged from two to four.

If any general pattern were apparent in this aggregation of studies, it would be a tendency for good overall manual performance in young children to be associated with relatively strong hand preference or consistent hand use across tasks. Two reports indicate a positive association between motor skill and well-established hand dominance

TABLE 16.1. Consistency of Hand Preference Related to Motor Skill

Study	Subjects	Asymmetry characteristic	Performance characteristic	Findings
Flick (1966)	453 normal children, 3–4 yr	Hand used for copying and pegboard tasks; sighting dominance assessed with hole test	3 copying tests from the Stanford–Binet and Merrill–Palmer tests; 2 mazes from the Porteus Mazes	LH with left-eye dominance scored below RH and below LH with right-eye dominance on copying tests and mazes
Horine (1968)	Normal 10-yr-old boys (77 purely right sided, 99 predominantly right sided, 30 mixed, 14 purely or predominantly left sided)	Laterality of eye, hand, and foot use on variety of motor tasks	Gross motor skills	No group differences
Keogh (1972)	Normal preschool children between 48 and 71 mo of age (43 consistent lateral usage, 36 inconsistent lateral usage)	Consistency of hand, foot, and eye use	Pattern Drawing Test and Draw-A-Person Test	No group differences
Kaufman, Zalma, & Kaufman (1978)	Normal children, 2–9 yr (967 RH, 42 LH)	Consistency of hand use across 4 activities	5 tests of gross and fine motor coordination (McCarthy [1972] Motor Scale)	For younger children only (2½–4½ yr), the dominance-established children scored higher on the motor tasks
Peters & Durding (1978)	Normal children, 5–13 yr (434 RH, 31 LH, 48 ambidextrous)	Hand used for 7 activities	Tapping a microswitch device with the index finger (10 10-sec trials with each hand)	Ambidextrous children were significantly slower than either RH or LH; no difference between RH and LH
Bishop (1980a)	Unselected children, 8–9 yr (147 RH, 23 LH)	Hand used for writing	Tracing a square with pen, using preferred and nonpreferred hand	A higher proportion of LH than RH performed in the bottom 20% of children with respect to performance of the nonpreferred hand

(continued)

TABLE 16.1. *(continued)*

Study	Subjects	Asymmetry characteristic	Performance characteristic	Findings
Gottfried & Bathurst (1983)	Normal children at 30, 36, and 42 mo of age (24 stable males, 24 unstable males, 23 stable females, 18 unstable females)	Stability of hand preference on drawing task assessed every 6 mo between the ages of 18 and 42 mo	Motor Scale from the McCarthy Scales	Stable females performed better than unstable females at 36 mo; no difference at any age between stable and unstable males
Kilshaw & Annett (1983)	Normal children, 3½–15 yr (230 consistent RH, 63 mixed RH, 53 LH)	Hand used for 5–7 activities	Annett et al. (1974) peg-moving task	Groups differed in speed of performance with the nonpreferred hand; LH faster than mixed RH; mixed RH faster than consistent RH; no differences with the preferred hand
Bishop (1984)	9,731 11-yr-olds (8,891 RH, 840 LH) from a national longitudinal survey	Hand used for drawing and throwing	Marking squares with a pencil and transferring matches from one box to another	A higher proportion of LH than RH performed in the bottom 5% of children with respect to performance of the nonpreferred hand on match transferring but not square marking
Gillberg, Walenström, & Rasmussen (1984)	Normal children at ages 9.4–10.4 yr (46 RH, 45 LH matched for sex)	Hand used for writing and drawing	Tracing a square with pen, using preferred and nonpreferred hand (same as Bishop, 1980)	A higher proportion of LH than RH performed in the bottom 33% of children with respect to performance of the nonpreferred hand
Tan (1985)	Normal children, 4–5 yr (41 matched RH-LH pairs and 24 matched RH-no hand preference [NH] pairs)	Number of activities, out of 13, performed with the right hand, left hand, and both hands	McCarthy (1972) Motor Scale, augmented by 9 measures of fine motor skill	No difference in aggregate motor score between the 41 LH and 41 matched RH; the 24 NH scored lower than the 24 matched RH; the difference was attributed to the low scores of NH boys

Study	Sample	Preference measure	Performance task	Findings
Rigal (1992)	Normal children, 6–9 yr (55–109 RH, 0–13 LH, 6–73 ambidextrous, depending on hand preference criteria)	Hand used to perform each of 10 activities	Performance with each hand on tests of aiming, finger tapping, finger dexterity, arm–hand steadiness, strength, and handwriting	No difference among groups in total performance (preferred hand plus nonpreferred hand) on any test
Gabbard, Hart, & Kanipe (1993)	Normal children, 4–6 yr (114 consistent RH, 8 consistent LH and 38 inconsistent in their hand use)	Hand preference on 2 trials of 3 motor tasks	Finger tapping	No relationship between consistency of hand preference and tapping speed
Gabbard & Hart (1995)	Normal children at ages 4–6 yr (24 RH, 24 LH matched for sex and age)	Hand used for 3 activities; foot used for 3 activities	Rate of finger tapping and foot tapping	No difference in rate of hand and foot tapping (combined data)
Gabbard, Hart, & Gentry (1995)	Normal 4- to 6-yr-olds (24 RH, 24 mixed, 24 LH)	Hand preference on 2 trials of 3 motor tasks	Finger tapping task	No group differences
Iteya, Gabbard, & Hart (1995)	Normal 4- to 6-yr-olds (45 left-footed, 45 mixed-footed; 46 right-footed; 46 LH, 46 mixed-handed, 46 RH)	Foot preference on 2 trials of 2 motor tasks; hand preference on 2 trials of 2 motor tasks	3 upper-limb, 3 lower-limb, and 3 whole body motor tasks	No relationship between foot preference and motor performance; no relationship between hand preference and motor performance
Karapetsas & Vlachos (1997)	Normal 5- to 12-yr-olds (420 LH, 420 RH)	Laterality quotient calculated from hand preference questionnaire	Copying Rey-Osterrieth Complex Figure	RH outperformed LH
Bhushan, Dwivedi, Mishra, & Mandal (2000)	Normal male secondary school students (10 RH, 10 mixed-handers, 10 LH)	Grouped by laterality index calculated from 22-item preference questionnaire	Mirror-drawing task	Mixed-handers completed the task in less time than RH or LH
Giagazoglou, Fotiadou, Angelopoulou, Tsikoulas, & Tsimaras (2001)	Normal 4- to 6-yr-olds (31 LH, 31 RH)	Hand preference on 13 motor tasks	2 motor subscales from the Griffiths Test No. II	No relationship of handedness to gross motor abilities; RH outperformed LH on fine motor tasks

Note. RH, right-handed children; LH, left-handed children.

in young children (Kaufman, Zalma, & Kaufman, 1978; Tan, 1985), and a third study shows better performance in females whose hand preference was stable over time (Gottfried & Bathurst, 1983). All these findings pertain to children between the ages of 2½ and 5½ years. However, the positive findings are offset by the repeated failures of Gabbard and his colleagues to find any performance deficiency in mixed-handed children between the ages of 4 and 6 years (Gabbard et al., 1995; Gabbard, Hart, & Kanipe, 1993; Iteya, Gabbard, & Hart, 1995). For instance, Gabbard and colleagues (1993) found no difference in finger-tapping speed between 122 4- to 6-year-olds who showed consistent hand preferences for writing, throwing a ball, and stacking cubes and 38 other children who were less consistent. Although consistency was defined in such a way as to confound consistency across activities with stability over trials, that is not problematic in light of the negative outcome. It seems likely that the confounding of those two aspects of consistency would have increased the prospects of finding a difference among groups.

In addition to the three positive outcomes based on children below the age of 6 years, Peters and Durding (1978) reported a similar result for children between the ages of 5 and 13. Peters and Durding's 48 ambidextrous children finger tapped more slowly than did either 31 left-handers or 434 right-handers. No significant difference between left- and right-handers was found. This study is notable because of the relatively large sample size and because of the care with which finger-tapping rate was measured. Not only were tap-to-tap intervals measured with millisecond precision, but each child performed five tapping trials with each hand. Nevertheless, it is difficult to assess the meaningfulness of a 7.5% between-group difference in speed on a single task, especially when the finding has not been replicated. Also, it should be noted that Kilshaw and Annett (1983) reported dissimilar results in their study of peg-moving speed in children between the ages of 3½ and 15 years. Mixed right-handers in that study performed faster than consistent right-handers but slower than left-handers.

Bhushan and colleagues (2000) reported that male adolescents with relatively weak hand preferences performed a mirror-tracing task faster than did strong right- or left-handers. This finding is difficult to interpret because of the atypical task, which requires a reversal of the usual motor responses to visual cues. The results may indicate only that there are special circumstances in which weak manual dominance is advantageous.

If the evidence is inconclusive with respect to strength or consistency of handedness, it is largely negative with respect to differences between right- and left-handers. Right-handers outperformed left-handers in two of the studies summarized in Table 16.1 (Giagazoglou, Fotiadou, Angelopoulou, Tsikoulas, & Tsimaras, 2001; Karapetsas & Blachos, 1997), and left-handers outperformed right-handers in one study (Kilshaw & Annett, 1983). Nonetheless, comparisons between the two groups more commonly have yielded no significant difference. Nonsignificant differences in lower-limb performance tend to favor left-handers over right-handers (Gabbard & Hart, 1995; Iteya et al., 1995). No obvious aspect of subject classification (e.g., age or the operational definition of manual asymmetry) or dependent variable (e.g., fine motor vs. gross motor performance; speed vs. accuracy) can account satisfactorily for the diversity of outcomes.

Of particular interest are the three related studies by Bishop (1980a, 1984) and Gillberg and colleagues (1984). Bishop (1980a) asked an unselected sample of English

8- and 9-year olds to trace a square path while staying within the parallel lines that defined the boundaries of the path. Performance was quantified according to the number of times the child crossed the boundaries. Left-handers were overrepresented among the children who scored in the lowest 20% with the nonpreferred hand but not among children who scored in the lowest 20% with the preferred hand (even though the performance of the preferred hand was correlated at $r = .54$ with performance of the nonpreferred hand). The overrepresentation of left-handers among poor-performing children might be attributable to pathological left-handedness, as the poor performers were more likely than other children to have a positive neurological history. The poor-performing children also had lower mean scores on measures of IQ and reading ability.

In a subsequent study based on an enormous sample of 11-year-olds, Bishop (1984) replicated the central finding of her 1980 study. Specifically, she found an excess number of left-handers among children whose skill in using the nondominant hand fell in the bottom 5% for the sample. The children who performed poorly on a match-moving task with the nondominant hand were more likely than other children to have a history of neurological disorders and seizures. However, the findings pertain only to performance on a task that required the child to transfer matches from one container to another. Poor performance on the other motor task—making pencil marks in each of a series of squares—was not associated with left-handedness.

A study of Swedish 10-year-olds by Gillberg and colleagues (1984) further confirmed Bishop's finding of a surplus of left-handers among children who perform poorly with the nondominant hand. Beginning with a sample of 985 children from the third grade of 21 public schools in the city of Göteborg, the investigators randomly selected 45 left-handers and 46 right-handers for inclusion in the study. Left-handed children were identified from teachers' observations of left-hand writing and drawing. (Nonidentified children apparently were assumed to be right-handed.) Bishop's square-tracing task yielded poor performance, as defined by a high number of errors or slow performance with the nonpreferred hand, in 44% of left-handers but only 22% of right-handers. As in Bishop's studies, poor performance with the dominant hand was not significantly more frequent in left-handers than in right-handers even though there was a substantial correlation ($r = .65$) between left-and right-hand performance. Gillberg and colleagues also found that poor performance with the nondominant hand was associated with concurrent neurological dysfunction as well as a history of prenatal and neonatal risk factors, poor academic achievement, and elevated teacher ratings of behavioral problems.

Both Bishop (1980a) and Gillberg and colleagues (1984) found that left-handers with poor motor skill in the nondominant right hand resembled right-handers significantly more than other left-handers in the frequency of FS. This finding, along with the various indications of neurological risk factors and behavioral abnormality, suggests that the left-handed children who were found to be especially clumsy or slow with the right hand might constitute a subgroup of pathological left-handers within the general population of left-handers. It should be pointed out, however, that large initial samples of children were required in order for the few putative pathological left-handers to be identified. Also, it should be noted that each of the three studies—two by Bishop and one by Gillberg and colleagues—used different criteria for low performance on the motor task and not all motor tasks yield a surplus of left-handers among poor performers. Consequently, even though the three studies succeed in demonstrating the existence of probable pathological left-handed children in the general population, the studies provide primarily a conceptual basis, rather than specific criteria, for identifying such children in a nonclinical sample of children. We do not know which motor tasks may prove to be the most useful for that purpose, nor do we know where to draw the line between normal and subnormal performance with the nonpreferred hand.

A paper published in 2001 by Gabbard, Helbig, and Gentry is not included in Table 16.1 because it provides no information about manual skill. Nonetheless, it suggests an important way in which left- and right-handers seem to differ. Gabbard and colleagues asked normal left- and right-handed 5- to 7-year-olds to reach out and grasp a foam cube that was positioned at various locations within the child's left and right hemispace. Children in both handedness groups used their dominant limb to reach the cube when it was on the side ipsilateral to the dominant hand but often switched to the nondominant limb when the cube was on the opposite side. Right-handed children, however, were more likely to reach across the midline to the contralateral side with their dominant hand. In other words, the right-handers showed a stronger preference for the dominant limb. This finding is commensurate with evidence that right-handed children perform better than left-handed children with the dominant hand but not as well with the nondominant hand (e.g., Peters & Durding, 1978).

Children in Clinical Samples

The elusiveness of a relationship between non-right-handedness and performance deficits in the general population does not mitigate against the concept of pathological left-handedness. On the contrary, if only some non-right-handedness is pathological, one would expect to find a markedly increased prevalence of left- and mixed-handedness only among individuals with known or suspected abnormalities in brain development. There is, as noted previously, abundant evidence that non-right-handedness is more common in a number of clinical populations, as well as evidence of various disorders of motor function in such populations (Denckla & Roeltgen, 1992).

Left-handedness has been reported to be twice as common in individuals with epilepsy as in the general population (Milner, Branch, & Rasmussen, 1964; Satz, Yanowitz, & Wilmore, 1984). Left-handedness also appears to be about twice as common in the mentally retarded as in cognitively normal individuals (Bradshaw-McAnulty et al., 1984; Pipe, 1988, 1990; Silva & Satz, 1979). Data reported by Soper and colleagues (1986), however, suggest that many of the individuals with mental retardation who are classified as either left- or right-handed may actually be mixed or ambiguous in their handedness.

Pervasive developmental disorder also has been associated with an increased incidence of non-right-handedness (Fein, Humes, Kaplan, Lucci, & Waterhouse, 1984; Fein, Waterhouse, Lucci, Pennington, & Humes, 1985; Satz, Soper, & Orsini, 1988; Tsai, 1982). Tsai (1982), for instance, found that, although only 10.3% of autistic individuals between the ages of 5 and 23 years were left-handed, 47.1% showed mixed handedness for five common unimanual activities. Hauck and Dewey (2001) likewise found an elevated prevalence of ambiguous handedness, and no consistent left-handedness, in 20 children with autism between the ages of 2 and 7 years. With respect to hand preferences, the children with autism in Hauck and Dewey's study resembled younger normal children more closely than children of their own age with nonspecific developmental delays. Only the children with autism, however, showed an association between lack of clear hand preference and low scores on measures of motor and cognitive ability. The findings were interpreted by the investigators as support for the hypothesis of bilateral brain dysfunction in autism.

O'Callaghan, Burn, Mohay, Rogers, and Tudehope (1993a, 1993b) examined the hand preference and motor development of children with extremely low birth weights as well as children with higher birth weights who had been ventilated mechanically following birth. Hand preference was assessed by parental report and observed preference for drawing and hammering. Motor development was assessed by a physiotherapist. In this sample of children, left-handedness occurred in 34% of the extremely low-birth-weight infants.

Reports of non-right-handedness in clinical groups with less obvious brain dysfunction have not been as consistent. Although most studies of children with developmental language disorders have failed to find an elevated frequency of non-right-handedness (Bishop, 1990; Preis, Schittler, & Lenard, 1997), there is some evidence of an increased frequency of non-right-handedness in children with more severe language disorders (Neils & Aram, 1986). The findings for children with reading and other learning disabilities have also been variable (Bishop, 1983; Dean, Schwartz, & Smith, 1981; Fennell, Satz, & Morris, 1983; Hardyk et al., 1976; Harris, 1979; O'Donnell, 1983; Satz & Fletcher, 1987). Beaumont (1976) and Yamamoto and Hatta (1982) found an unusually high prevalence of non-right-handedness among children diagnosed as having minimal brain damage.

If non-right-handedness is a marker for brain dysfunction, then those individuals in clinical populations who are left- or mixed-handed should also be the most impaired. Non-right-handedness in clinical populations does seem to be associated with greater cognitive impairments. Satz, Soper, and Orsini (1988) reviewed a number of studies which indicate that the elevated frequency of left-handedness among the mentally retarded is more pronounced among those with lower levels of intellectual functioning. Similarly, Satz and colleagues concluded that individuals with autism who have mixed or ambiguous handedness are more impaired cognitively than individuals with stronger handedness. Hauck and Dewey's (2001) findings for children with autism are consistent with this conclusion. Within the extremely low birth weight infants studied by O'Callaghan and colleagues. (1993a, 1993b), those who had mixed-handedness had lower levels of intellectual functioning at 6 years of age than did either those who were strong right- or left-handers. Handedness, however, did not have any relationship with motor ability in this instance.

CONCLUSIONS

Seemingly ubiquitous claims of associations between non-right-handedness and behavioral abnormality notwithstanding, one is hard-pressed to find a consistently adverse consequence of non-right-handedness in the general population. This negative conclusion, which has been stated repeatedly with respect to intellectual consequences, applies as well to motor consequences. It is possible that during the lengthy and fluctuating course of motor development, children who lag behind their peers or are tested while transitioning from one linguistic stage to another may exhibit temporarily an indeterminate or inconsistent hand preference along with subaverage motor skill. There is, however, little reason to suspect a persistent deficiency in the manual skills of non-right-handers in the general population. Only one study indicates that ambidextrous children above the age of 5 years might be disadvantaged in motor performance.

Even the few positive findings for young children in the general population are suspect, partly because the number of published studies is small, and partly because no one knows the true frequency of studies with negative outcomes. It seems plausible that significant differences between children with consistent and inconsistent hand preferences are more likely to be reported than are negative findings. This is Rosenthal's (1979) "file drawer problem." Any positive finding obtained by chance (Type I error) most likely would be published, whereas a much larger number of negative outcomes would not be published. It also is conceivable that, given the numerous possible ways of classifying children, some investigators may capitalize on chance by reporting findings based on criteria that yield significant differences while disregarding other classification criteria that yield no between-group differences.

In the absence of a general theory of handedness (Peters, 1995; Todor & Smiley, 1985), there is no compelling reason to suspect that the lack of a clear hand preference or skill asymmetry would be disadvantageous. Admittedly, the instances of association between inconsistent handedness and poor motor skill in Table 16.1 might be used to promote the characterization of mixed-handers as individuals with two nondominant hands. That concept is problematic, even though Todor and Doane (1978) did identify a group of bilaterally unskilled adults whom they called "ambisinistrals." Offsetting the 12 ambisinistrals, however, was a group of 21 ambidextrals, whose performance with both hands was comparable to that of the right hand of right-handers. Thus, even though there are normal adults who perform as if they had two nondominant hands, other ambilateral adults perform as if they had two dominant hands. Only if the former individuals outnumber the latter would one expect to find a depressed level of skill in unselected mixed-handers. We are unaware of any studies of normal children in which mixed-handers have been divided into ambisinistral and ambidextral subtypes.

The work of Bishop (1980a, 1984), as corroborated by Gillberg and colleagues (1984), constitutes a critical nexus between studies of handedness in normal children and studies of handedness in clinical populations. Apparently there is an association between left-handedness and poor motor performance in the general population of children, but its revelation is not a straightforward matter. The investigator must begin with a large sample (or entire population) of children in order to find an adequate number of left-handers. The next step is to administer to the children a manual task that is sufficiently sensitive to detect relatively minor degrees of motor impairment in the nondominant hand. Among the impaired children will be found an elevated prevalence of left-handers, and it is these left-handers who will have a history of neurological abnormalities or risk factors, academic problems, behavioral problems, and so on. These children are the elusive pathological left-handers in the general population. In effect, Bishop's approach identifies pathological left-handers by searching for X + LH, where X is poor performance with the nondominant hand and LH is manifest left-hand preference.

Despite the large initial sample (or population) sizes in the Bishop and Gillberg and colleagues studies, the ultimate yield of putative pathological left-handers was small and, perhaps for that reason, there were almost no statistically significant differences between left- and right-handers within the poorly performing group. Consequently, it remains to be seen whether "X + LH" provides more information than "X" alone. In other words, the factor associated with adverse neurological and behavioral circumstances seems to be poor performance in the non-dominant hand, irrespective of whether the child is left-handed or right-handed.

Diversity in handedness, and in sidedness more generally, is a more complex and multifaceted phenomenon than it first appeared to be. Knowing that a child is left-handed, whether the child is drawn from the general population or from a clinical population, adds little or nothing to our ability to predict the child's overall motor proficiency. Yet, the data are rather sparse, and we may be justified in reserving judgment about the implications of left-handedness. We sympathize with Bax (1980), who gave the following advice to pediatric neurologists.

> Where does all this leave the clinician? He or she must emphasize that usually sinistrality is of no significance, and that most left-handers do as well as right-handers. There is certainly no need to alarm parents of left-handed children, but perhaps one should keep the caution in one's own mind to examine the left-handed child a little more carefully than his right-handed brother or sister. (p. 568)

Neuropsychological researchers and theorists have examined the problem of non-right-handedness extensively, and even though their main emphasis has been placed on language representation, the neuropsychological approach has been helpful in defining some issues of potential relevance to the study of motor skill in non-right-handers (Harris, 1992). The concept of pathological left-handedness may be the most important of those issues, but the neuropsychological perspective has also influenced (1) the measurement of handedness and motor asymmetry, (2) the characterization of the early development of motor asymmetry, and (3) the identification of subtypes of non-right-handers. If knowledge about motor skill in right- and non-right-handed children remains fragmentary, it is not because neuropsychological studies have proven to be unfruitful but, rather, because neuropsychological concepts and methods have yet to be applied broadly to the study of children's hand preference and manual skill.

It is ironic that a phenomenon as commonplace and self-evident as human handedness should have attracted so much scholarly attention, and that the major questions about handedness should have proven, thus far, so intractable. But progress has been made, and more advances will be evident as additional information accumulates.

REFERENCES

Ajersch, M. K., & Milner, B. (1983). Handwriting posture as related to cerebral speech lateralization, sex, and writing hand. *Human Neurobiology, 2,* 143–145.

Allen, M., & Wellman, M. M. (1980). Hand position during writing, cerebral laterality and reading: Age and sex differences. *Neuropsychologia, 18,* 33–40.

Annett, M. (1967). The binomial distribution of right, mixed and left handedness. *Quarterly Journal of Experimental Psychology, 19,* 327–333.

Annett, M. (1970a). The classification of hand preference by association analysis. *British Journal of Psychology, 61,* 303–320.

Annett, M. (1970b). The growth of manual preference and speed. *British Journal of Psychology, 61,* 545–558.

Annett, M. (1972). The distribution of manual asymmetry. *British Journal of Psychology, 63,* 343–358.

Annett, M. (1983). Hand preference and skill in 115 children of two left-handed parents. *British Journal of Psychology, 74,* 17–32.

Annett, M. (1992). Five tests of hand skill. *Cortex, 28,* 583–600.

Annett, M. (2002). *Handedness and brain asymmetry: The right shift theory.* East Sussex, UK: Psychology Press.

Annett, M., Hudson, P. T. W., & Turner, A. (1974). The reliability of differences between the hands in motor skill. *Neuropsychologia, 12,* 527–531.

Annett, M., & Turner, A. (1974). Laterality and the growth of intellectual abilities. *British Journal of Educational Psychology, 44,* 37–46.

Bakan, P. (1971). Birth order and handedness. *Nature, 229,* 195.

Bakan, P. (1977). Left-handedness and birth order revisited. *Neuropsychologia, 15,* 837–839.

Bakan, P. (1990). Nonright-handedness and the continuum of reproductive casualty. In S. Coren (Ed.), *Left-handedness: Behavioral implications and anomalies* (pp. 33–74). Amsterdam: North-Holland.

Bakan, P., Dibb, G., & Reed, P. (1973). Handedness and birth stress. *Neuropsychologia, 11,* 363–366.

Barnsley, R. H., & Rabinovitch, M. S. (1970). Handedness: Proficiency versus stated preference. *Perceptual and Motor Skills, 30,* 344–362.

Bates, E., O'Connell, B., Vaid, J., Sledge, P., & Oakes, L. (1986). Language and hand preference in early development. *Developmental Neuropsychology, 2,* 1–15.

Batheja, M., & McManus, I. C. (1985). Handedness in the mentally handicapped. *Developmental Medicine and Child Neurology, 27,* 63–68.

Bax, M. (1980). Left hand, right hand. *Developmental Medicine and Child Neurology, 22,* 567–568.

Beaumont, J. G. (1976). The cerebral laterality of "minimal brain damaged" children. *Cortex, 12,* 373–382.

Beukelaar, L. J., & Kroonenberg, P. M. (1983). Towards a conceptualization of hand preference. *British Journal of Psychology, 74,* 33–45.

Bhushan, B., Dwivedi, B. B., Mishra, R., & Mandal, M. K. (2000). Performance on a mirror-drawing task by non-right-handers. *Journal of General Psychology, 127,* 271–277.

Bishop, D. V. M. (1980a). Handedness, clumsiness and cognitive ability. *Developmental Medicine and Child Neurology, 22,* 569–579.

Bishop, D. V. M. (1980b). Measuring familial sinistrality. *Cortex, 16,* 311–313.

Bishop, D. V. M. (1983). How sinister is sinistrality? *Journal of the Royal College of Physicians of London, 17,* 161–172.

Bishop, D. V. M. (1984). Using non-preferred hand skill to investigate pathological left-handedness in an unselected population. *Developmental Medicine and Child Neurology, 26,* 214–226.

Bishop, D. V. M. (1989). Does hand proficiency determine hand preference? *British Journal of Psychology, 80,* 191–199.

Bishop, D. V. M. (1990). Handedness, clumsiness and developmental language disorders. *Neuropsychologia, 28,* 681–690.

Blank, R., Miller, V., & von Voß, H. (2000). Human motor development and hand laterality: A kinematic analysis of drawing movements. *Neuroscience Letters, 295,* 89–92.

Bradshaw-McAnulty, G., Hicks, R. E., & Kinsbourne, M. (1984). Pathological left-handedness and familial sinistrality in relation to degree of mental retardation. *Brain and Cognition, 3,* 349–356.

Briggs, G. G., Nebes, R. D., & Kinsbourne, M. (1976). Intellectual differences in relation to personal and family handedness. *Quarterly Journal of Experimental Psychology, 28,* 591–601.

Bryden, M. P. (1973). Perceptual asymmetry in vision: Relation to handedness, eyedness, and speech lateralization, *Cortex, 9,* 418–435.

Bryden, M. P. (1982). *Laterality: Functional asymmetry in the intact brain.* New York: Academic Press.

Bryden, M. P. (1987). Handedness and cerebral organization: Data from clinical and normal populations. In D. Ottoson (Ed.), *Duality and unity of the brain* (pp. 55–70). Harmondsworth, UK: Macmillan.

Bryden, M. P. (1988). An overview of the dichotic listening procedure and its relation to cerebral organization. In K. Hugdahl (Ed.), *Handbook of dichotic listening: Theory, methods and research* (pp. 1–43). Chichester, UK: Wiley.

Bryden, M. P., McManus, I. C., & Bulman-Fleming, M. B. (1994). Evaluating the empirical support for the Geschwind-Behan-Galaburda model of cerebral lateralization. *Brain and Cognition, 26,* 103–167.

Bryden, M. P., & Steenhuis, R. E. (1991). Issues in the assessment of handedness. In F. L. Kitterle (Ed.), *Cerebral laterality: Theory and research* (pp. 35–51). Hillsdale, NJ: Erlbaum.

Bryson, S., & MacDonald, V. (1984). The development of writing posture in left-handed children and its relation to sex and reading skills. *Neuropsychologia, 22,* 91–94.

Bullard-Bates, P. C., & Satz, P. (1983). A case of pathological left-handedness. *International Journal of Clinical Neuropsychology, 5,* 128–129.

Calvin, W. H. (1991). *The throwing madonna: Essays on the brain.* New York: Bantam.

Caplan, P. J., & Kinsbourne, M. (1976). Baby drops the rattle: Asymmetry of duration of grasp by infants. *Child Development, 47,* 532–536.

Carlier, M., Spitz, E., Vacher-Lavenu, M. C., Villeger, P., Martin, B., & Michel, F. (1996). Manual performance and laterality in twins of know chorion type. *Behavior Genetics, 26,* 409–417.

Chapman, J. P., Chapman, L. J., & Allen, J. J. (1987). The measurement of foot preference. *Neuropsychologia, 25,* 579–584.

Chapman, L. J., & Chapman, J. P. (1987). The measurement of handedness. *Brain and Cognition, 6,* 175–183.

Corballis, M. C. (1980). Is left-handedness genetically determined? In J. Herron (Ed.), *Neuropsychology of left-handedness* (pp. 159–176). New York: Academic Press.

Corballis, M. C. (1983). *Human laterality.* New York: Academic Press.

Corballis, M. C. (1991). *The lopsided ape: Evolution of the generative mind.* New York: Oxford University Press.

Coren, S. (Ed.). (1990). *Left-handedness: Behavioral implications and anomalies.* Amsterdam: Elsevier.

Coren, S. (1993). *The left-hander syndrome: The causes and consequences of left-handedness.* New York: Vintage Books.

Coren, S., & Porac, C. (1978). The validity and reliability of self-report items for the measurement of lateral preference. *British Journal of Psychology, 69,* 207–211.

Coren, S., Searleman, A., & Porac, C. (1986). Rate of physical maturation and handedness. *Developmental Neuropsychology, 2,* 17–23.

Coryell, J. F., & Michel, G. F. (1978). How supine postural preferences of infants can contribute toward the development of handedness. *Infant Behavior and Development, 1,* 245–257.

Crovitz H. F., & Zener, K. (1962). A group test for assessing hand and eye dominance. *American Journal of Psychology, 75*, 271–276.

Curt, F., De Agostini, M., Maccario, J., & Dellatolas, G. (1995). Parental hand preference and manual functional asymmetry in preschool children. *Behavior Genetics, 25*, 525–536.

Curt, F., Maccario, J., & Dellatolas, G. (1992). Distributions of hand preference and hand skill asymmetry in preschool children: Theoretical implications. *Neuropsychologia, 30*, 27–34.

Dean, R. S., Schwartz, N. H., & Smith, L. S. (1981). Lateral preference patterns as a discriminator of learning difficulties. *Journal of Consulting and Clinical Psychology, 49*, 227–235.

Dee, H. L. (1971). Auditory asymmetry and strength of manual preference. *Cortex, 7*, 236–245.

Denckla, M. B., & Roeltgen, D. P. (1992). Disorders of motor function and control. In I. Rapin & S. J. Segalowitz (Eds.), *Handbook of neuropsychology, Vol. 6, Section 10: Child neuropsychology (Part 1)* (pp. 455–476). Amsterdam: Elsevier.

Elias, L., & Bryden, M. P. (1998). Footedness is a better predictor of language laterality than handedness. *Laterality, 3*, 41–45.

Eling, P. (1983). Comparing different measures of laterality: Do they relate to a single mechanism? *Journal of Clinical Neuropsychology, 5*, 135–147.

Fein, D., Humes, M., Kaplan, E., Lucci, D., & Waterhouse, L. (1984). The question of left hemisphere dysfunction in infantile autism. *Psychological Bulletin, 95*, 258–281.

Fein, D., Waterhouse, L., Lucci, D., Pennington, B., & Humes, M. (1985). Handedness and cognitive functions in pervasive developmental disorders. *Journal of Autism and Developmental Disorders, 15*, 323–333.

Fennell, E. B., Satz, P., & Morris, R. (1983). The development of handedness and dichotic ear listening asymmetries in relation to school achievement: A longitudinal study. *Journal of Experimental Child Psychology, 35*, 248–262.

Finlayson, M. A. J., & Reitan, R. M. (1976). Handedness in relation to measures of motor and tactile–perceptual functions in normal children. *Perceptual and Motor Skills, 43*, 475–481.

Fleishman, E. A. (1972). On the relation between abilities, learning, and human performance. *American Psychologist, 27*, 1017–1032.

Flick, G. L. (1966). Sinistrality revisited: A perceptual-motor approach. *Child Development, 37*, 613–622.

Gabbard, C. (1993). Foot laterality during childhood: A review. *International Journal of Neuroscience, 72*, 175–182.

Gabbard, C., & Hart, S. (1995). Foot performance of right- and left-handers: A question of environmental influence. *Perceptual and Motor Skills, 80*, 671–674.

Gabbard, C., Hart, S., & Gentry, V. (1995). A note on trichotomous classification of handedness and fine-motor performance in children. *Journal of Genetic Psychology, 156*, 97–104.

Gabbard, C., Hart, S., & Kanipe, D. (1993). Hand preference consistency and fine motor performance in young children. *Cortex, 29*, 749–753.

Gabbard, C., Helbig, C. R., & Gentry, V. (2001). Lateralized effects on reaching by children. *Developmental Neuropsychology, 19*, 41–51.

Geschwind, N., & Behan, P. (1982). Left-handedness: Association with immune disease, migraine, and developmental learning disorder. *Proceedings of the National Academy of Science, 79*, 5097–5100.

Geschwind, N., & Galaburda, A. M. (1985a). Cerebral lateralization: Biological mechanisms, associations and pathology: A hypothesis and a program for research, I. *Archives of Neurology, 42*, 428–459.

Geschwind, N., & Galaburda, A. M. (1985b). Cerebral lateralization: Biological mechanisms, associations and pathology: A hypothesis and a program for research, II. *Archives of Neurology, 42*, 521–552.

Geschwind, N., & Galaburda, A. M. (1985c). Cerebral lateralization: Biological mechanisms, associations and pathology: A hypothesis and a program for research, III. *Archives of Neurology, 42*, 634–654.

Geschwind, N., & Galaburda, A. M. (1987). *Cerebral lateralization.* Cambridge, MA: MIT Press.

Gesell, A., & Ames, L. B. (1947). The development of handedness. *Journal of Genetic Psychology, 70*, 155–175.

Giagazoglou, P., Fotiadou, E., Angelopoulou, N., Tsikoulas, J., & Tsimaras, V. (2001). Gross and fine motor skills of left-handed preschool children. *Perceptual and Motor Skills, 92*, 1122–1128.

Gilbert, A. N., & Wysocki, C. J. (1992). Hand preference and age in the United States. *Neuropsychologia, 30*, 601–608.

Gillberg, C., Walenström, E., & Rasmussen, P. (1984). Handedness in Swedish 10-year-olds. Some background and associated factors. *Journal of Child Psychology and Psychiatry, 25*, 421–432.

Gordon, H. (1920). Left-handedness and mirror writing, especially among defective children. *Brain, 43*, 313–368.

Gottfried, A. W., & Bathurst, K. (1983). Hand preference across time is related to intelligence in young girls, not boys. *Science, 221*, 1074–1076.

Gregory, R., & Paul, J. (1980). The effects of handedness and writing posture on neurological test results. *Neuropsychologia, 18*, 231–235.

Grimshaw, G. M., & Bryden, M. P. (1994). Are there meaningful handedness subtypes? *International Neuropsychology Society Program and Abstracts*, 68.

Gudmundsson, E. (1993). Lateral preference of preschool and primary school children. *Perceptual and Motor Skills, 77*, 819–828.

Guiard, Y., & Millerat, F (1984). Writing postures in left-handers: Inverters are hand crossers. *Neuropsychologia, 22*, 535–538.

Hardyck, C., & Petrinovich, L. F. (1977). Left-handedness. *Psychological Bulletin, 84*, 385–404.

Hardyck, C., Petrinovich, L., & Goldman, R. (1976). Left-handedness and cognitive deficit. *Cortex, 12*, 266–279.

Harris, A. J. (1979). Lateral dominance and reading disability. *Journal of Learning Disabilities, 12*, 57–63.

Harris, L. J. (1980). Left-handedness: Early theories, facts, and fancies. In J. Herron (Ed.), *The neuropsychology of left-handedness* (pp. 3–78). New York: Academic Press.

Harris, L. J. (1992). Left-handedness. In I. Rapin & S. J. Segalowitz (Eds.), *Handbook of neuropsychology, Vol. 6, Section 10: Child Neuropsychology (Part 1)* (pp. 145–208). Amsterdam: Elsevier.

Harris, L. J., & Carlson, D. F. (1988). Pathological left-handedness: An analysis of theories and evidence. In D. L. Molfese & S. J. Segalowitz (Eds.), *Brain lateralization in children: Developmental implications* (pp. 289–372). New York: Guilford Press.

Hauck, J. A., & Dewey, D. (2001). Hand preference and motor functioning in children with autism. *Journal of Autism and Developmental Disorders, 31*, 265–277.

Hawn, P. R., & Harris, L. J. (1983). Hand differences in grasp duration and reaching in two and five month old infants. In G. Young, S. J. Segalowitz, C. M. Corter, & S. E. Trehub (Eds.), *Manual specialization and the developing brain* (pp. 331–348). New York: Academic Press.

Healey, J. M., Liederman, J., & Geschwind, N. (1986). Handedness is not a unidimensional trait. *Cortex, 22*, 33–53.

Hécaen, H., & Ajuriaguerra, J. (1964). *Left-handedness.* New York: Grune & Stratton.

Hécaen, H., & Sauguet, J. (1971). Cerebral dominance in left-handed subjects. *Cortex, 7*, 19–48.

Herron, J. (1980). Two hands, two brains, two sexes. In J. Herron (Ed.), *The neuropsychology of left-handedness* (pp. 233–260). New York: Academic Press.

Hicks, R. A., & Dusek, C. M. (1980). The handedness distributions of gifted and non-gifted children. *Cortex, 16,* 479–481.

Hicks, R. E., & Barton, A. (1975). A note on left-handedness and severity of mental retardation. *Journal of General Psychology, 127,* 323–324.

Hines, D., & Satz, P. (1971). Superiority of right visual half-fields in right-handers for recall of digits at varying rates. *Neuropsychologia, 9,* 21–25.

Hiscock, C. K., Hiscock, M., Benjamins, D., & Hillman, S. (1989a). Motor asymmetries in hemiplegic children: Implications for the normal and pathological development of handedness. *Developmental Neuropsychology, 5,* 169–186.

Hiscock, C. K., Hiscock, M., Benjamins, D., & Hillman, S. (1989b). Writing posture in right hemiplegic children. *Cortex, 25,* 683–686.

Hiscock, M., Caroselli, J. S., & Wood, S. (in press). Concurrent counting and typing: Lateralized interference depends on a difference between the hands in motor skill. *Cortex.*

Hiscock, M., & Cole, L. C. (2004). *Auditory and manual asymmetry: Correlated dimensions of laterality?* Manuscript in preparation.

Hiscock, M., & Hiscock, C. K. (1990). Laterality in hemiplegic children: Implications for the concept of pathological left-handedness. In S. Coren (Ed.), *Left-handedness: Behavioral implications and anomalies* (pp. 131–152). Amsterdam: Elsevier.

Hiscock, M., & Kinsbourne, M. (1980). Asymmetry of verbal–manual time sharing in children: A follow-up study. *Neuropsychologia, 18,* 151–162.

Hiscock, M., Kinsbourne, M., Samuels, M., & Krause, A. E. (1985). Effects of speaking upon the rate and variability of concurrent finger tapping in children. *Journal of Experimental Child Psychology, 40,* 486–500.

Hiscock, M., & Mackay, M. (1985). The sex difference in dichotic listening: Multiple negative findings. *Neuropsychologia, 23,* 441–444.

Horine, L. E. (1968). An investigation of the relationship of laterality groups to performance on selected motor tests. *Research Quarterly, 39,* 90–95.

Ingram, D. (1975). Motor asymmetries in young children. *Neuropsychologia, 13,* 95–102.

Iteya, M., Gabbard, C., & Hart, S. (1995). Patterns of limb laterality and gross-motor agility in children. *Perceptual and Motor Skills, 81,* 623–626.

Karapetsas, A. B., & Vlachos, F. M. (1997). Sex and handedness in development of visuomotor skills. *Perceptual and Motor Skills, 85,* 131–140.

Kaufman, A. S., Zalma, R., & Kaufman, N. L. (1978). The relationship of hand dominance to the motor coordination, mental ability, and right-left awareness of young normal children. *Child Development, 49,* 885–888.

Kee, D. W., Gottfried, A. W., Bathurst, K., & Brown, K. (1987). Left-hemisphere language specialization: Consistency in hand preference and sex differences. *Child Development, 58,* 718–724.

Keogh, B. K. (1972). Preschool children's performance on measures of spatial organization, lateral preference, and lateral usage. *Perceptual and Motor Skills, 34,* 299–302.

Kilshaw, D., & Annett, M. (1983). Right and left-hand skill I: Effects of age, sex and hand preference showing superior skill in left-handers. *British Journal of Psychology, 74,* 253–268.

Kimura, D. (1999). *Sex and cognition.* Cambridge, MA: MIT Press.

Kimura, D., & Vanderwolf, C. H. (1970). The relation between hand preference and the performance of individual finger movements by left and right hands. *Brain, 93,* 769–774.

Kinsbourne, M. (1988). Sinistrality, brain organization, and cognitive deficits. In D. L. Molfese & S. J. Segalowitz (Eds.), *Brain lateralization in children: Developmental implications* (pp. 259–279). New York: Guilford Press.

Kinsbourne, M., & Hicks, R. E. (1978). Functional cerebral space: A model for overflow, transfer and interference effects in human performance. In J. Requin (Ed.), *Attention and performance* (Vol. 7, pp. 345–362). Hillsdale, NJ: Erlbaum.

Knox, A. W., & Boone, D. R. (1970). Auditory laterality and tested handedness. *Cortex, 6,* 164–173.

Lake, D. A., & Bryden, M. P. (1976). Handedness and sex differences in hemispheric asymmetry. *Brain and Language, 3,* 266–282.

LeMay, M. (1977). Asymmetries of the skull and handedness. *Journal of the Neurological Sciences, 32,* 243–253.

Levy, J. (1982). Handwriting posture and cerebral organization: How are they related? *Psychological Bulletin, 91,* 589–608.

Levy, J. (1984). A review, analysis, and some new data on hand–posture distributions in left-handers. *Brain and Cognition, 3,* 105–127.

Levy, J., & Reid, M. (1976). Variations in writing posture and cerebral organization. *Science, 194,* 337–339.

Levy, J., & Reid, M. (1978). Variations in cerebral organization as a function of handedness, hand posture in writing and sex. *Journal of Experimental Psychology: General, 107,* 119–144.

Lezak, M. D. (1995). *Neuropsychological assessment* (3rd ed.). New York: Oxford University Press.

Liederman, J. (1983). Mechanisms underlying instability in the development of hand preference. In G. Young, S. J. Segalowitz, C. M. Corter, & S. E. Trehub (Eds.), *Manual specialization and the developing brain* (pp. 71–92). New York: Academic Press.

McDonnell, P. M., Anderson, V. E. S., & Abraham, A. (1983). Asymmetry and orientation of arm movements in 3 to 8 week old infants. *Infant Behavior and Development, 6,* 287–298.

McKeever, W. F. (1990). Familial sinistrality and cerebral organization. In S. Coren (Ed.), *Left-handedness: Behavioral implications and anomalies* (pp. 373–412). Amsterdam: Elsevier.

McKeever, W. F., Seitz, K. S., Hoff, A. L., Marino, M. F., & Diehl, J. A. (1983). Interacting sex and familial sinistrality characteristics influence both language lateralization and spatial ability in right handers. *Neuropsychologia, 21,* 661–668.

McManus, I. C. (1983). Pathologic left-handedness: Does it exist? *Journal of Communication Disorders, 16,* 315–344.

McManus, I. C. (1999). Handedness, cerebral lateralization, and the evolution of language. In M. C. Corballis & S. E. G. Lee (Eds.), *The descent of mind: Psychological perspectives on hominid evolution* (pp. 194–217). Oxford, UK: Oxford University Press.

McManus, I. C., & Bryden, M. P. (1992). The genetics of handedness, cerebral dominance and lateralization. In I. Rapin & S. J. Segalowitz (Eds.), *Handbook of neuropsychology, Vol. 6, Section 10: Child neuropsychology (Part 1)* (pp. 115–144). Amsterdam: Elsevier.

McManus, I. C., Kemp, R. I., & Grant, J. (1986). Differences between fingers and hands in tapping ability: Dissociation between speed and regularity. *Cortex, 22,* 461–473.

McManus, I. C., Porac, C., Bryden, M. P., & Boucher, R. (1999). Eye-dominance, writing hand and throwing hand. *Laterality, 4,* 173–192.

Michel, G. F. (1981). Right-handedness: A consequence of infant supine head-orientation preference? *Science, 212,* 685–687.

Michel, G. F. (1992). Maternal influences on infant hand-use during play with toys. *Behavior Genetics, 22,* 163–175.

Michel, G. F. (2001). A developmental–psychobiological approach to developmental neuropsychology. *Developmental Neuropsychology, 19,* 11–32.

Miller, C. A. (1982). Degree of lateralization as a hierarchy of manual and cognitive skill levels. *Neuropsychologia, 20,* 155–162.

Milner, B., Branch, C., & Rasmussen, T. (1964). Observations on cerebral dominance. In A. V. S. de Reuck & M. O'Connor (Eds.), *Ciba Foundation Symposium: Disorders of Language* (pp. 200–204). Boston: Little, Brown.

Nalcaci, E., Kalaycioglu, C., Cicek, M., & Genc, Y. (2001). The relationship between handedness and fine motor performance. *Cortex, 37,* 493–500.

Neils, J. R., & Aram, D. M. (1986). Handedness and sex of children with developmental language disorders. *Brain and Language, 28,* 53–65.

Newcombe, F., & Ratcliff, G. (1973). Handedness, speech lateralization and ability. *Neuropsychologia, 11,* 399–407.

O'Callaghan, M. J., Burn, V. R., Mohay, H. A., Rogers, Y., & Tudehope, D. I. (1993a). Handedness in extremely low birth weight infants: Aetiology and relationship to intellectual abilities, motor performance, and behaviour at four and six years. *Cortex, 29,* 629–637.

O'Callaghan, M. J., Burn, V. R., Mohay, H. A., Rogers, Y., & Tudehope, D. I. (1993b). The prevalence and origins of left hand preference in high risk infants, and its implications for intellectual, motor and behavioural performance at four and six years. *Cortex, 29,* 617–627.

O'Donnell, J. (1983). Lateralized sensorimotor asymmetries in normal, learning-disabled and brain-damaged young adults. *Perceptual and Motor Skills, 57,* 227–232.

Oldfield, R. C. (1971). The assessment and analysis of handedness: The Edinburgh Inventory. *Neuropsychologia, 9,* 97–113.

Orsini, D. L., & Satz, P. (1986). A syndrome of pathological left-handedness: Correlates of early left hemisphere injury. *Archives of Neurology, 43,* 333–337.

Orton, S. T. (1937). *Reading, writing, and speech problems in children.* New York: Norton.

Öztürk, C., Durmazlar, N., Ural, B., Karaagaoglu, E., Yalaz, K., & Anlar, B. (1999). Hand and eye preference in normal preschool children. *Clinical Pediatrics, 38,* 677–680.

Parlow, S. (1978). Differential finger movements and hand preference. *Cortex, 14,* 608–611.

Parlow, S. E., & Kinsbourne, M. (1981). Handwriting posture and manual motor asymmetry in sinistrals. *Neuropsychologia, 19,* 687–696.

Pasamanick, B., & Knobloch, H. (1966). Retrospective studies on the epidemiology of reproductive causality: Old and new. *Merrill-Palmer Quarterly of Behavior, 12,* 7–26.

Peters, M. (1983a). Differentiation and lateral specialization in motor development. In G. Young, S. J. Segalowitz, C. M. Corter, & S. E. Trehub (Eds.), *Manual specialization and the developing brain* (pp. 141–159). New York: Academic Press.

Peters, M. (1983b). Inverted and noninverted left-handers compared on the basis of motor performances and measures related to the act of writing. *Australian Journal of Psychology, 35,* 405–416.

Peters, M. (1983c). Lateral bias in reaching and holding at six and twelve months. In G. Young, S. J. Segalowitz, C. M. Corter, & S. E. Trehub (Eds.), *Manual specialization and the developing brain* (pp. 367–374). New York: Academic Press.

Peters, M. (1986). Incidence of left-handed writers and the inverted writing position in a sample of 2194 German elementary school children. *Neuropsychologia, 24,* 429–433.

Peters, M. (1988). Footedness: Asymmetries in foot preference and skill and neuropsychological assessment of foot movement. *Psychological Bulletin, 103,* 179–192.

Peters, M. (1990). Subclassification of non-pathological left-handers poses problems for theories of handedness. *Neuropsychologia, 28,* 279–289.

Peters, M. (1992). How sensitive are handedness prevalence figures to differences in handedness classification procedures? *Brain and Cognition, 18,* 208–215.

Peters, M. (1995). Handedness and its relation to other indices of cerebral lateralization. In R. J. Davidson & K. Hugdahl (Eds.), *Brain asymmetry* (pp. 183–214). Cambridge, MA: MIT Press.

Peters, M. (1998). Description and validation of a flexible and broadly usable handedness questionnaire. *Laterality, 3,* 77–96.

Peters, M., & Durding, B. M. (1978). Handedness measured by finger tapping: A continuous variable. *Canadian Journal of Psychology, 32,* 257–261.

Peters, M., & Durding, B. M. (1979). Footedness of left- and right-handers. *American Journal of Psychology, 92,* 133–142.

Peters, M., & McGrory, J. (1987). The writing performance of inverted and noninverted right- and left-handers. *Canadian Journal of Psychology, 41,* 20–32.

Peters, M., & Pang, J. (1992). Do "right-armed" left-handers have different lateralization of motor control for the proximal and distal musculature? *Cortex, 28,* 391–399.

Peters, M., & Pedersen, K. (1978). Incidence of left-handers with inverted writing position in a population of 5920 elementary school children. *Neuropsychologia, 16,* 743–746.

Peters, M., & Servos, P. (1989). Performance of subgroups of left-handers and right-handers. *Canadian Journal of Psychology, 43,* 341–358.

Petrie, B. F., & Peters, M. (1980). Handedness: Left/right differences in intensity of grasp response and duration of rattle holding in infants. *Infant Behavior and Development, 3,* 215–221.

Pipe, M.-E. (1988). Atypical laterality and retardation. *Psychological Bulletin, 104,* 343–347.

Pipe, M.-E. (1990). Mental retardation and left-handedness: Evidence and theories. In S. Coren (Ed.), *Left-handedness: Behavioral implications and anomalies* (pp. 293–318). Amsterdam: Elsevier.

Plato, C. C., Fox, K. M., & Garrruto, R. M. (1984). Measures of lateral functional dominance: Hand dominance. *Human Biology, 56,* 259–275.

Ponton, C. W. (1987). Enhanced articulatory speed in ambidexters. *Neuropsychologia, 25,* 305–311.

Porac, C., & Coren, S. (1981). *Lateral preferences and human behavior.* New York: Springer-Verlag.

Porac, C., Coren, S., Steiger, J. H., & Duncan, P. (1980). Human laterality: A multidimensional approach. *Canadian Journal of Psychology, 34,* 91–96.

Preis, S., Schittler, P., & Lenard, H.-G. (1997). Motor performance and handedness in children with developmental language disorder. *Neuropediatrics, 28,* 324–327.

Previc, F. H. (1991). A general theory concerning the prenatal origins of cerebral lateralization in humans. *Psychological Review, 98,* 299–334.

Provins, K. A. (1992). Early infant motor asymmetries and handedness: A critical evaluation of the evidence. *Developmental Neuropsychology, 8,* 325–365.

Provins, K. A., & Cunliffe, P. (1972). The reliability of some motor performance tests of handedness. *Neuropsychologia, 10,* 199–206.

Provins, K. A., & Glencross, D. J. (1968). Handwriting, typewriting and handedness. *Quarterly Journal of Experimental Psychology, 20,* 282–289.

Raczkowski, D., Kalat, J. W., & Nebes, R. (1974). Reliability and validity of some handedness questionnaire items. *Neuropsychologia, 12,* 43–47.

Ramsay, D. S. (1983). Unimanual hand preference and duplicated syllable babbling in infants. In G. Young, S. J. Segalowitz, C. M. Corter, & S. E. Trehub (Eds.), *Manual specialization and the developing brain* (pp. 161–176). New York: Academic Press.

Ramsay, D. S. (1984). Onset of duplicated syllable babbling and unimanual handedness in infancy: Evidence for developmental change in hemispheric specialization? *Developmental Psychology, 20,* 64–71.

Ramsay, D. S. (1985). Fluctuations in unimanual hand preference in infants following the onset of duplicated syllable babbling. *Developmental Psychology, 21,* 318–324.

Rasmussen, T., & Milner, B. (1975). Clinical and surgical studies of the cerebral speech areas in man. In K. J. Zülch, O. Creutzfeldt, & G. C. Galbraith (Eds.), *Cerebral localization* (pp. 238–257). Berlin: Springer-Verlag.

Rigal, R. A. (1992). Which handedness: Preference or performance. *Perceptual and Motor Skills, 75,* 851–866.

Roberts, J., & Engle, A. (1974). Family background, early development, and intelligence of children 6–11 years. In *National Center for Health Statistics, Data from National Health Survey, Series II, No. 142* (DHEW Publication No. HRA 75–1624). Washington, DC: U.S. Government Printing Office.

Rosenthal, R. (1979). The "file drawer problem" and tolerance for null results. *Psychological Bulletin, 86,* 638–641.

Roy, E. A., & MacKenzie, C. (1978). Handedness effects in kinesthetic spatial location judgements. *Cortex, 14,* 250–258.

Satz, P. (1972). Pathological left-handedness: An explanatory model. *Cortex, 8,* 121–137.

Satz, P. (1973). Left-handedness and early brain insult: An explanation. *Neuropsychologia, 11,* 115–117.

Satz, P., Achenbach, K, & Fennell, E. (1967). Correlations between assessed manual laterality and predicted speech laterality in a normal population. *Neuropsychologia, 5,* 295–310.

Satz, P., & Fletcher, J. M. (1987). Left-handedness and dyslexia: An old myth revisited. *American Journal of Pediatrics, 12,* 291–298.

Satz, P., Orsini, D. L., Saslow, E., & Henry, R. R. (1985). Early brain injury and pathological left-handedness: Clues to a syndrome. In D. F. Benson & E. Zaidel (Eds.), *The dual brain: Hemispheric specialization in the human* (pp. 117–125). New York: Guilford Press.

Satz, P., Soper, H. V., & Orsini, D. L. (1988). Human hand preference: Three nondextral subtypes. In D. L. Molfese & S. J. Segalowitz (Eds.), *Brain lateralization in children: Developmental implications* (pp. 281–287). New York: Guilford Press.

Satz, P., Soper, H. V., Orsini, D. L., Henry, R. R., & Zvi, J. C. (1985). Handedness subtypes in autism. *Psychiatric Annals, 15,* 447–451.

Satz, P., Strauss, E., Wada, J., & Orsini, D. L. (1988). Some correlates of intra- and interhemispheric speech organization after left focal brain injury. *Neuropsychologia, 26,* 345–350.

Satz, P., Yanowitz, J., & Wilmore, J. (1984). Early brain damage and lateral development. In R. Bell, J. Elias, R. Green, & J. Harvey (Eds.), *Interfaces in psychology* (pp. 87–107). Lubbock: Texas Tech Press.

Schonblom, J. E. (1977). On the probability of pathological right-handedness. *Cortex, 13,* 213–214.

Schulze, K., Lüders, E., & Jäncke, L. (2002). Intermanual transfer in a simple motor task. *Cortex, 38,* 805–815.

Schwartz, M. (1990). Left-handedness and prenatal complications. In S. Coren (Ed.), *Left-handedness: Behavioral implications and anomalies* (pp. 75–97). Amsterdam: Elsevier.

Searleman, A. (1980). Subject variables and cerebral organization. *Cortex, 16,* 239–254.

Shankweiler, D., & Studdert-Kennedy, M. (1975). A continuum of lateralization for speech perception? *Brain and Language, 2,* 212–225.

Silva, D., & Satz, P. (1979). Pathological left-handedness: Evaluation of a model. *Brain and Language, 7,* 8–16.

Smith, L. C., & Moscovitch, M. (1979). Writing posture, hemispheric control of movement and cerebral dominance in individuals with inverted and noninverted hand postures during writing. *Neuropsychologia, 17,* 637–644.

Soper, H. V., & Satz, P. (1984). Pathological left-handedness and ambiguous handedness: A new explanatory model. *Neuropsychologia, 22,* 511–515.

Soper, H. V., Satz, P., Orsini, D. L., Henry, R. R., Zvi, J. C., & Schulman, M. (1986). Handedness patterns in autism suggest subtypes. *Journal of Autism and Developmental Disorders,* *16,* 155–167.

Soper, H. V., Satz, P., Orsini, D. L., Van Gorp, W. G., & Green, M. F. (1987). Handedness distribution in a residential population with severe or profound mental retardation. *American Journal of Mental Deficiency, 92,* 94–102.

Springer, S. P., & Searleman, A. (1980). Left-handedness in twins: Implications for the mechanisms underlying cerebral asymmetry of function. In J. Herron (Ed.), *Neuropsychology of left-handedness* (pp. 139–158). New York: Academic Press.

Steenhuis, R. E., & Bryden, M. P. (1989). Different dimensions of hand preference that relate to skilled and unskilled activities. *Cortex, 25,* 289–304.

Strauss, E., Wada, J., & Kosaka, B. (1984). Writing hand posture and cerebral dominance for speech. *Cortex, 20,* 143–147.

Tan, L. E. (1985). Laterality and motor skills in four-year-olds. *Child Development, 56,* 119–124.

Tan, U. (1992). The relation of hand preference to hand performance in left-handers: Importance of the left brain. *International Journal of Neuroscience, 65,* 1–10.

Tapley, S. M., & Bryden, M. P. (1985). A group test for the assessment of performance between the hands. *Neuropsychologia, 23,* 215–221.

Teng, E. L., Lee, P., Yang, K., & Chang, P. C. (1976). Handedness in a Chinese population: Biological, social, and pathological factors. *Science, 193,* 1148–1150.

Thomas, J. R., & French, K. E. (1985). Gender differences across age in motor performance: A meta-analysis. *Psychological Bulletin, 98,* 260–282.

Todor, J. (1980). Sequential ability of left-handed inverted and noninverted writers. *Acta Psychologica, 44,* 165–173.

Todor, J. I., & Doane, T. (1977). Handedness classification: Preference versus proficiency. *Perceptual and Motor Skills, 45,* 1041–1042.

Todor, J. I., & Doane, T. (1978). Handedness and hemispheric asymmetry in the control of movements. *Journal of Motor Behavior, 10,* 295–300.

Todor, J. I., & Kyprie, P. M. (1980). Hand differences in the rate and variability of rapid tapping. *Journal of Motor Behavior, 12,* 57–62.

Todor, J. I., & Smiley, A. L. (1985). Performance differences between the hands: Implications for studying disruption to limb praxis. In E. A. Roy (Ed.), *Neuropsychological studies of apraxia and related disorders* (pp. 309–344). Amsterdam: North-Holland.

Tsai, L. Y. (1982). Handedness in autistic children and their families. *Journal of Autism and Developmental Disorders, 12,* 421–423.

Volpe, B. T., Sidtis, J. T., & Gazzaniga, M. S. (1981). Can left-handed writing posture predict cerebral language laterality? *Archives of Neurology, 38,* 637–638.

von Hofsten, C. (1982). Eye-hand coordination in the newborn. *Developmental Psychology, 18,* 450–461.

Weber, A. M., & Bradshaw, J. L. (1981). Levy and Reid's neurological model in relation to writing hand/posture: An evaluation. *Psychological Bulletin, 90,* 74–88.

White, K., & Ashton, R. (1976). Handedness assessment inventory. *Neuropsychologia, 14,* 261–264.

Witelson, S. F. (1980). Neuroanatomical asymmetry in left-handers: A review and implications for functional asymmetry. In J. Herron (Ed.), *Neuropsychology of left-handedness* (pp. 79–113). New York: Academic Press.

Woo, T. L., & Pearson, K. (1927). Dextrality and sinistrality. *Biometrika, 19,* 192–198.

Yamamoto, M., & Hatta, T. (1982). Handedness and imbalance lateralization on the tapping test in MBD children. *International Journal of Neuroscience, 17,* 215–218.

Young, G., Corter, C. M., Segalowitz, S. J., & Trehub, S. E. (1983). Manual specialization and the developing brain: An overview. In G. Young, S. J. Segalowitz, C. M. Corter, & S. E. Trehub (Eds.), *Manual specialization and the developing brain* (pp. 3–12). New York: Academic Press.

Young, G., Segalowitz, S. J., Corter, C. M., & Trehub, S. E. (Eds). (1983). *Manual specialization and the developing brain*. New York: Academic Press.

Zung, B. J. (1985). Left-right comparison and children's performance on sensorimotor tests. *Journal of Clinical Psychology, 41*, 788–795.

Zurif, E., & Bryden, M. P. (1969) Familial handedness and left-right differences in auditory and visual perception. *Neuropsychologia, 7*, 179–187.

CHAPTER 17

Constraints in Neuromotor Development

REINT H. GEUZE

For over 100 years theories have been advanced to explain motor development. These range from the early nativist and behavioristic theories to information-processing theories and more recently theories that acknowledge the importance of the interaction between the organism and its environment as a main driving force in motor development. Of these latter theories, those that consider development to be a process of self-organization resulting in nonlinear change are generally termed *dynamic systems theories* (see Thelen & Smith, 1994). In this chapter, I adopt the dynamic systems approach as the unifying theory underlying the developmental mechanisms in the neuromotor system. The goal of this chapter is to provide a brief overview of the important principles in development from a dynamic systems perspective and introduce the concept of constraints. This is followed by a review of the development of associated movements. The framework will be used to address the issue of associated movements and their significance as neuromotor constraints in the development of coordination.

THEORETICAL ISSUES

Early Self-Organization

According to the dynamic systems approach, the process of self-organization and selection is assumed to be the most powerful drive in the development of the motor system. Higher levels of organization are characterized by an increasing level of flexibility and integration, enabling the systems units to adapt to changing task demands by forming temporary synergies. This self-organizational process of development evolves spontaneously but is of course subject to *internal constraints*, such as biological growth, genetically induced changes, and *environmental constraints*. Interaction between the distinctive subsystems and with the environment is essential for the development of the sensory–motor system. Moreover, some criterion of functionality is assumed to govern the processes of self-organization and selection. Prechtl (1993) discusses the functionality of the emerging movement patterns *in utero*. For example, the functionality of early movements is that they help to shape the joints and bones of the skeleton and are necessary for the normal development of the muscles.

Edelman's (1987) theory of neural group selection conceives of plasticity as a continuing property of the neural system. According to this theory, changing the weights of neural connections, or loss or outgrowth of dendrite connections, can result in short- and long-term changes. Thus, this theory can account for the almost immediate adaptation to changing task demands seen in individuals, as well as the functional reorganization seen in patients after cerebral ischemia or limb amputation.

Within the dynamic systems framework, *development* can be defined as the result of a self-organizing process of interaction between biological growth (maturation if you like) and spontaneous learning (exploration), generally in the direction of increasing functionality. It is characterized by a relatively slow rate of change. *Learning* can be distinguished from development as the process of change that is independent of biological growth. It is based on relatively fast changes of neural connections. In the case of structural or functional deficits, functional reorganization is assumed to be subject to the same principles of self-organization and functional directiveness.

Constraints

The concept of constraints is very important for the understanding of development and related deficits because it links the functional organization at the neural level with the functional capacities and limitations at the behavioral level. Constraints emerge from specific synergies or functional neural coupling between muscles or muscle groups. Newell (1986) proposed three categories of constraints that interact and determine the resulting coordination and control at the behavioral level: (1) *organismic constraints*, which refer to limitations within the system (e.g., limited muscle force or information-processing capacities)—they may be divided in two types: (a) *structural constraints* that are relatively time independent; they refer to "hard-wired" constraints in the perceptual-motor system (i.e., limited muscle force, perceptional constraints, and limited speed of neural signal transduction due to incomplete myelination); (b) *functional constraints* that are relatively time dependent; they depend on current weights of connections in the neural networks and are relatively easily adapted through experience and learning (i.e., when children learn new complex skills by imitation, training, or instruction in a relatively short time); (2) *environmental constraints*, which are due to external influences on the system, such as the gravity and resistance of the water while swimming, rearing patterns, or the cultural conditions in which the child matures; environmental constraints reflect the more permanent ambient conditions that influence the task and motor development; and (3) *task constraints*, which are due to the specific demands of the task and require a specific sort of coordination (e.g., handling a pair of scissors and picking up a glass of water); task constraints may relate to the goal of the task, the way the task is to be executed (e.g., fast or slow), and the characteristics of the objects and implements used in the task.

During development the organismic constraints change as a result of biological change and because of their continuous interaction with the environment. The functional constraints may change due to learning and experience. Because of their plasticity, they enable the system to acquire functional skills and to adapt to changing task demands. Both structural and functional constraints may be involved in motor performance and movement disorder. In the following sections the focus is on specific types of organismic constraints that are present during the development of coordination. These constraints manifest as associated movements that is, unwanted action during the performance of different motor tasks.

Coordination

At the level of motor behavior, coordination manifests itself as cooperation between parts of the body in an efficient and purposeful way. But how do we accomplish such a complex task? The problem of coordination is not self-evident as the human body has more than 700 muscles and some 70 joints that somehow need to be controlled. It is generally assumed that the precise control of each individual muscle is too large a load for our brain (Bernstein, 1984). Bernstein (1984) formulated the movement problem as follows: "The coordination of movement is the process of mastering redundant degrees of freedom of the moving organ into a controllable system" (p. 355). This is assumed to occur through the emergence of *coordinative ensembles* (Tuller, Turvey, & Fitch, 1982), a term introduced to denote the stable temporary functional relationships that exist between muscles during a certain task. The control of an ensemble is relatively simple because it acts as a unit. Newell (1986) extended the basic notion of emerging control by specifying coordination and control, and the development of skill as follows: (1) *coordination* is the process of constraining the degrees of freedom such that goal-directed behavior emerges; (2) *control* is the setting of parameters that specify the movement (e.g., choice of velocity or forcefulness of the movements); and (3) *skill* is the optimal parameterization of the control; it implies that the perceptual–motor system is optimally tuned to the goal of the movement.

These concepts and theories, when applied to motor development, may now be summarized as follows. Perceptual–motor development is the result of the continuous interaction between biological growth and environmental influences, which leads through self-organization to an increasingly functional movement repertoire. During early development the main driving factor is biological growth, with increasing environmental influences after birth. As the rate of change of the biological factors diminishes, the environmental influences become stronger. Environmental influences also become stronger because of the organism's increased capacity to handle external information as it matures. During childhood, the external influences become dominant. The distinct functional units of the neuromotor system (e.g., motor units or, at a higher level, coordinative structures) may be inhibited or coupled in an increasingly functional way. This adaptive capacity of the system is constrained by biological growth (structural constraints) and by the plasticity of the neural networks (functional constraints). How organismic constraints may change with age and develop differentially or at a slower rate in case of deficits is illustrated in the following section using the phenomena of associated movements.

ASSOCIATED MOVEMENTS

Coordination requires that functional parts of the neuromotor system act cooperatively, while other parts of the system should remain inactivated. For a specific task, the functional units become coupled dynamically. It is important that the activation patterns do not spread through the neural system because involuntary movement of other parts of the system can disturb the intended movement. Moreover, associated movements waste energy. Inhibition of the nonfunctional parts of the system, therefore, may be as important as the activation of the task-relevant part. However, many associated movements do not interfere with task execution.

The term *associated movement* refers to the phenomenon of irrelevant involuntary movement, which accompanies, but is not necessary for, executing a specific movement or adopting a posture. They are referred to as soft neurological signs and various terms have been used for this phenomenon (i.e., *synkinetic movement, comovement, overflow movement*, and *mirror movement*). They reflect internal or organismic constraints of the neuromotor system and have been linked with possible neurological dysfunction and behavioral disorders (e.g., Abercrombie, Lindon, & Tyson, 1964; Peters, 1987; Reitz & Müller, 1998; Shaffer, 1978; Taylor, 1987; Touwen, 1979; Tupper, 1987; Walshe, 1923).

Associated movements are often observed in infants and young children. Their appearance decreases with age and most disappear later in childhood (Connolly & Stratton, 1968; Lazarus & Todor, 1987; Wolff, Gunnoe, & Cohen, 1983). Wolff and colleagues (1983) argued that their incidence may be used as a measure of developmental age in clinical populations. The observation of associated movements is part of most neurodevelopmental tests, either as specific test items (Abercrombie et al., 1964; Connolly & Stratton, 1968) or as an assessment of co-movement during other tests of development of neuromotor function (Peters, 1987; Touwen, 1979) (see Barnett & Peters, Chapter 4, this volume, and Tupper, 1987, for a more detailed discussion of neurodevelopmental tests).

In the following sections, I first present a description of the main types and characteristics of associated movements. This presentation is followed by a review of the developmental data on the frequency of their occurrence, their significance as markers for developmental delay and neurological damage, and their relationship to localize neurological damage.

Types of Associated Movement

Co-movement of limbs not involved in task execution has been classified in several ways. Examples are co-movement of the contralateral arm or homologous finger, also termed *mirror movement* (Reitz & Müller, 1998) or *identical associated movement* (Zülch & Müller, 1969), and co-movement of the neighboring fingers, termed *affiliative movements*. In general, if a co-movement occurs in nonhomologous parts of the body at the ipsilateral or the contralateral side, these are called ipsilateral or contralateral associated movements, respectively. In specific tasks, associated movements can occur on both the ipsilateral and contralateral sides. Another type of associated movement manifests as overflow to other body parts, without specific lateralization. Linkages have been found between mouth and fingers and between feet and arms/hands (Noterdaeme, Amorosa, Ploog, & Scheimann, 1988). Some examples of finger–mouth linkage are the following: the mouth-opening finger-spreading phenomenon (Touwen, 1979), when opening the mouth wide a response of spreading the fingers of both hands of the passively stretched arms is elicited; protruding the tip of the tongue during writing with effort; and finger opposition with typical responses in the mouth area (Noterdaeme et al., 1988). Examples of foot–arm/hand linkage are the synkineses in the arms during stress gaits (Connelly & Stratton, 1968; Wolff et al., 1983) and heel–toe alternation or toe tapping which may produce associated movements in the contralateral hand (Noterdaeme et al., 1988). Table 17.1 presents a list of tasks used to induce associated movements, a short description of the typical associated response, factors that influence the response, and the references.

Factors That Affect Associated Movement

An important finding in studies with children is the effect of exerted force on the occurrence of associated movements (Lazarus & Todor, 1987, 1991; Todor & Lazarus, 1986). The amount of force in the passive hand increases with the level of force in the active hand (Todor & Lazarus, 1986), an effect which has also been found in adults, albeit to a lesser degree (Zijdewind & Kernell, 2001). Todor and Lazarus (1986) studied isometric squeezing of thumb and index finger in 7- to 8-year-old children. As the force of unilateral squeezing increased, the force between these digits in the passive hand increased with a power of about 2.6, and at maximum force the level of the associated response reached levels between 13% and 63% of the active hand. In adults, this range was 0.4–16.1%. It was concluded that this finding was due to an increase of irradiation to neurons of the homologous muscles of the passive hand that are closely connected to the active neurons. Apparently this irradiation effect is not compensated for by stronger inhibition of the homologous muscles. There is clear evidence now that during sustained, effortful contractions, the outflow to the contralateral hemisphere is increased due to reduced transcallosal inhibition. Effort-induced mirror contractions are thus the result of disinhibition of the contralateral crossed projections rather than disinhibition of ipsilateral uncrossed pathways (Arányi & Rösler, 2002).

Different neural pathways that are not necessarily controlled by a single developmental mechanism probably mediate the various kinds of associated movements. The coactivation of mirror movements, for example, involves crossed motor pathways, whereas synkineses from stress gaits (i.e., motor irradiations to heterologous muscles of the upper limbs) probably involve ipsilateral motor pathways (Wolff et al., 1983). Other relevant factors that influence associated movements are hand (i.e., in right-handed children associated movements are more intense in the right hand than the left hand) and hand order (i.e., associated movements are more intense if the passive hand has been active just before) (Todor & Lazarus, 1986), feedback (i.e., associated movements are suppressed by auditory feedback regarding the activity of the passive hand) (Lazarus & Todor, 1991), sex (i.e., females show slightly fewer associated movements than males) (Largo et al., 2001), and task complexity (i.e., more complex tasks elicit more associated movements) (Largo et al., 2001). In an endurance test, it was found that the strength of associated movement also depends on fatigue (Arányi & Rösler, 2002; Zijdewind & Kernell, 2001). Adults exerting long-lasting abduction force with their index finger at 30% of maximum voluntary contraction showed a progressive in-

TABLE 17.1. Studies of Factors Influencing the Occurrence of Associated Movements

Task	Measure	Associated response	Influencing factors	Subjects (age/n)	Authors (year)
Isometric squeezing, thumb–index finger	Force at 25–100% MVF Observed assoc. mov.	Homologous contr. Heterologous mov.	MVF, hand, hand order	7–8 yr; N = 42	Todor & Lazarus (1986)
Isometric squeezing, thumb–index finger	Force at 50–100% MVF Observed assoc. mov.	Homologous contr. Heterologous mov.	Age 6 yr, 5 mo vs. other	6 yr, 5 mo; 8 yr, 5 mo; 10 yr, 4 mo; 12 yr, 4 mo; 16 yr, 5 mo; total N = 140	Lazarus & Todor (1987)
Isometric squeezing, thumb–index finger	Force at 75% MVF	Homologous contr. Heterologous contr.	Age, feedback	6 yr, 7 mo; 8 yr, 9 mo; 10 yr, 6 mo; 12 yr, 5 mo; 16 yr, 8 mo; 5 × 10 boys	Lazarus & Todor (1991)
Elbow flex. against fixed load	EMG biceps, triceps	< 6 yr contralateral antagonist > 7 yr contralateral agonist	Age	3–4 yr, 5–7 yr, 8–14 yr, adult; N = 5, 7, 8, 1?	Missiuro (1963)
Clip-pinching test Finger-spreading test Finger-lifting test Walk on outside of feet	Observed assoc. mov.	Contralateral thumb mov. Fail or contralateral mov. Associated mov. Arms pron./sup. or stretch	Age, type of task	4 yr, 9 mo–15 yr, 8 mo; N = 68	Connolly & Stratton (1968)
Finger-lifting test Finger-spreading test Timed motor tests (N = 6) Stress gaits[a]	Observed assoc. mov. mirror + contralat. overflow Observed assoc. mov.	Mirror + affiliative mov. Mirror + affiliative mov. Mirror mov. Arms/hands pron./sup., flex./ext.	Age, type of task	5 yr, 5 mo; 6 yr, 5 mo; 2×, N = 50; longitudinal 3× at interval of 6 mo	Wolff et al. (1983)
Timed motor tests Diadochokinesis Pegboard Jumping Stress gaits[a]	Observed duration and degree of assoc. mov.	Contralateral mov. Contralateral mov. Contralateral mov. Upper extremity? Arms pron./sup. and hand flex.	Age, sex, task complexity	5 yr, 8 mo; 7 yr, 2 mo; 9 yr, 3 mo; 12 yr, 5 mo; 15 yr, 0 mo; 18 yr, 1 mo; total N = 662; 50% male, 50% female	Largo et al. (2001)
Clip-pinching test Finger-lifting test	Observed assoc. mov.	Contralateral mov. Homolateral mov. Contralateral mov.	Age, type of task, CP	Control 6 yr, 9 yr N = 45; CP, handicapped, 7 yr, 5 mo–17 yr, 8 mo, N = 50	Abercrombie et al. (1964)

Note. flex., flexion; ext., extension; pron., pronation; sup., supination; assoc., associated; mov., movement; MVF, maximum voluntary force; CP, cerebral palsy; EMG, electromyogram; contr., contraction.

[a] Walking on heels, toes, outer side of the feet, and inner side of the feet.

394

crease of the unintended associated force measured at the contralateral index finger
(Zijdewind & Kernell, 2001).

Development of Associated Movements

Because the infant cannot be instructed to perform tasks unilaterally, associated movements are difficult to assess, although they can be observed in spontaneous behavior
(e.g., when the infant grasps an object unimanually). Moreover, the incidence of associated movements is highly variable at a young age, and consequently the clinical predictive value is limited. Most developmental neurological examinations of associated
movements, therefore, are not suitable for children under 3 years of age.

The common finding among developmental studies of children 3–18 years of age
has been a decrease of associated movements with chronological age. This decrease is,
however, nonlinear, task dependent, and variable between individual children (Connolly & Stratton, 1968; Largo et al., 2001; Lazarus & Todor, 1987, 1991). In other
words, each of the functions tested followed a characteristic course of development in
normal children. With respect to age 3 important results have been reported: (1) the
age effect is nonlinear; (2) the onset of the decrease of associated movements is variable between children and tasks; and (3) the rate of decrease is variable between children and tasks. This large variability suggests that children may follow individual
pathways of development with respect to the disappearance of associated movements.
Based on the rather unique developmental trajectory that each task shows (different
onsets and rates), it may be concluded that it is unlikely that a common neurodevelopmental factor is responsible for the decrease in occurrence of associated movement (Largo et al., 2001; Wolff et al., 1983).

The following paragraphs present a short summary of developmental trends for
the main tasks used to elicit these associated movements. For a detailed overview of
the main developmental trends for different tasks that can elicit mirror movements and
synkineses, the reader is referred to Lazarus and Todor (1987), Connolly and
Stratton (1968) and the recent extensive normative data set of Largo and colleagues
(2001).

Mirror Movements

Mirror movements can be observed in limbs contralateral to the one used in the task.
Among the tasks used in the upper extremities are isometric finger pinching, finger lifting, finger spreading, and diadochokinesis. A variety of measures have been used to
quantify the mirror movements. From the observed behavior, measures such as frequency of occurrence and estimation of the degree are noted. Quantitative measures
used include duration to perform 20 movements and measured force level. Two studies have used unilateral squeezing of the thumb and finger or fingers (Connolly &
Stratton, 1968; Lazarus & Todor, 1987) to assess mirror movements. Connolly and
Stratton had children pinch a bulldog clip, which was too strong to open up completely between the thumb and other fingers. It may be assumed that children had to
use maximum force for this task. Both the dominant and the nondominant hand were
tested on one trial each. The passive hand was in a symmetrical position with the
thumb opened. The movement of the thumb of the passive hand was observed. At the

age of 5 years, more than 95% of the children showed mirror movements. At the age of 15 years, only 4% of the children pinched the clip with observable contralateral movement. The developmental trend showed a linear decrease ($R^2 = .87$), with an onset of the decrease of mirror movements commencing at 4.3 years and disappearing by 17.3 years (author's statistics on the data from Connolly & Stratton, 1968). Lazarus and Todor (1987) redesigned the test so that they could measure the force between thumb and index finger when squeezing two levers isometrically. Children pinched the levers with their right hand with visual feedback of the required force level and just held the second pair of levers with their other hand. At 100% of maximum voluntary force (MVF), comparable to the aforementioned study, the developmental trend showed that mirror force was substantial. A decrease from 36% of MVF at 6½ years to 19% at 16½ years of age, with the main decrease between 6½ and 8½ years (author's statistics: quadratic trend $R^2 = .82$) was noted. At lower levels of force, (e.g., at 50% MVF), the level of mirror force dropped to 16% of MVF at 6½ years and less than 5% MVF at 8½ years and above. The findings of these two studies indicated that the mirror movements decrease with age. However, the rate of decrease in mirror movements with age differs across the two studies.

Finger lifting is another task commonly used to elicit mirror movements. Typically, the subject rests the hands and fingers flat on the table and lifts the finger that is pointed to. Any movement of the homologous finger is scored (Connolly & Stratton, 1968; Wolff et al., 1983). The middle and the ring fingers are most sensitive to associated movement. Connolly and Stratton reported a quadratic trend for the middle finger with an estimated onset at 3 years and substantial improvement between 4 and 8 years. For the ring finger a linear decrease of mirror movement between 5 and 15 years from 95 to 56% was found. The study by Wolff and colleagues showed that the percentage of children with mirror movements between 5½ and 7½ years was below 10% and decreased when one looked at the middle finger. When the ring finger was investigated associated movements decreased from 45 to 3% between 5½ and 7½ years. The difference in frequency of occurrence of mirror movement between the two studies may be explained by the use of different criteria for scoring mirror movement, with Wolff et al. using stricter ones. Both studies found that fourth-finger mirror movements disappeared later in development than those displayed by the third finger. A point of critique with respect to the finger-lifting task is that subjects may use different strategies to prevent the associated movement. The occurrence of associated movement may be different if subjects press the other fingers firmly down on the table while lifting the indicated finger, compared to a relatively relaxed state of the other fingers when lifting the target finger. The studies reported earlier did not attempt to control for such strategy differences.

Finger spreading requires the subject to spread two fingers of one hand while keeping the other fingers together. The hands rest on the table, palm down, and the assessor indicates the fingers to be spread. Connolly and Stratton (1968) found that the incidence of mirror movements was above 90% in children between 5 and 9 years of age, decreased in children between the ages of 9 and 12 years, and leveled off at about 55% in children between 12 and 15 years of age. Wolff and colleagues (1983) reported a decrease in mirror movements in children between 5½ and 7½ years from 50 to 15% for the second and third fingers and from 70 to 60% for the third and fourth fingers. Again differences in task and criteria likely account for different findings of these two studies. Connolly and Stratton had children stretch out their hands while performing the task, and they used a pass (correct spreading of fingers without associated movement), fail (associated movement in either hand) scoring system. Wolff and colleagues studied finger spreading with hands placed on a table, and scored contralateral and ipsilateral or affiliative associated movements separately.

Diadochokinesis was studied by Largo and colleagues (2001). In this well-known test, the child is standing with the upper arms hanging down, the elbows touching the body, and the lower arms stretched forward at an angle of 90 degrees. The child is asked to quickly pronate and supinate the hand and lower arm of a single limb (Touwen, 1979). At the age of 5 years, few children (8%) showed no signs of mirror movement, 35% showed barely visible mirror movements, 48% showed moderate mirror movements, and 8% showed marked mirror movements. At the age of 18 years, these percentages were 50%, 44%, 6%, and 0%, respectively.

In many tasks that elicit associated movements, affiliative movements or nonspecific overflow can be observed in contralateral or ipsilateral limb segments. These have been less accurately reported in most studies. The study by Wolff and colleagues (1983) indicated that their frequency of occurrence is task dependent: They may be as common as the mirror movements (i.e., in finger lifting and walking on toes or heels) or may occur less frequently (i.e., in finger spreading and walking on inner or outer soles). Like the specific associated movements, their incidence decreases with age.

Synkineses from stress gaits may be elicited when children walk on their toes, their heels, the outer soles, or the inner soles of their feet. Table 17.2 lists the synkinetic responses to these stress gaits. Three developmental studies have reported on these synkinetic responses (Connolly & Stratton, 1968, walking on outer soles only; Largo et al., 2001; Wolff et al., 1983). Wolff and colleagues (1983) distinguish between definite synkinetic responses in arms and hands, which mimic the posture assumed by the legs and feet and nonspecific overflow, when the movements of arms and hands do not mimic the gait posture. Largo and colleagues measured the percentage of time during a 6-second walk that the subjects mimicked the posture in arms and hands and calculated developmental trends for "present nearly all of the time" and "only present for a short period." Figures 17.1 and 17.2 summarize the developmental data for the percentage of children with synkinesis from the tests of walking on toes and

TABLE 17.2. Synkinetic Responses in Arms and Hands to Stress Gaits

Type of stress gait	Response in arms	Response in hands
Walking on toes	Extension of the arms	Ventroflexion of the hands and the wrist in backward direction
Walking in heels	Extension of the arms	Dorsiflexion of the hands in forward direction
Walking on outer soles	Elevation of the shoulders, flexion of the elbow	Ventroflexion of the hands, extension of the fingers
Walking on inner soles	Adduction of the arms to the body, extension of the elbows	Dorsiflexion of the wrists, extension of the fingers

Note. Data from Wolff, Gunnoe, and Cohen (1983).

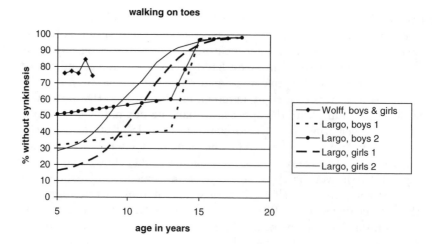

FIGURE 17.1. Percentage of children without synkinetic responses elicited by walking on toes. From Wolff et al. (1983) and Largo et al. (2001). Copyright 1983, 2001 by MacKeith Press. Adapted by permission. In the data set of Largo et al. children below the bottom line are free of associated movement, children above the top line have the typical synkinetic response all the time during 6 seconds of stress walking. In between the lines children show the synkinetic response during a proportion of the task.

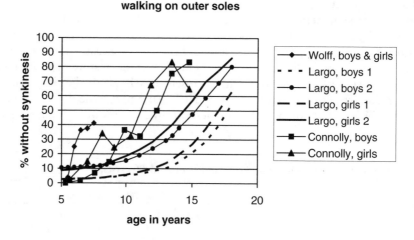

FIGURE 17.2. Percentage of children without synkinetic responses elicited by walking on outer soles of the feet. From Connolly and Stratton (1968), Wolff et al. (1983), and Largo et al. (2001). Copyright 1968, 1983, and 2001 by MacKeith Press. Adapted by permission. In the data set of Largo et al. children below the bottom line are free of associated movement, children above the top line have the typical synkinetic response all the time during 6 seconds of stress walking. In between the lines children show the synkinetic response during a proportion of the task.

walking on outer soles. Unfortunately, the three studies present developmental trends that are incompatible. For the age range of 5½ to 7½ years for walking on toes, Largo and colleagues and Wolff and colleagues find hardly any change in the incidence of definite synkinesis, but the percentage of children without signs of synkinesis is much higher in the Wolff and colleagues study. Only when the incidence of nonspecific overflow is added does the Wolff and colleagues normative data for 5½ to 7½ years (55% without associated movements) come closer to the Largo and colleagues normative data for this age range (33% without associated movements). Walking on outer soles also shows clear differences in developmental rate among the studies. There was also no agreement about sex differences in the developmental trajectories of these stressed walking patterns. Wolff and colleagues report that sex differences were not significant. In the other two studies, girls were found to have an earlier onset of the decrease of associated movements compared to boys. It appears then that differences in the criteria that define associated movements on these tasks and the methods of observation are likely responsible for the lack of agreement. The study by Largo and colleagues used video recording and made the observations from video. This enabled them to classify the synkinesis semiquantitatively and test for interobserver reliability. The other studies used direct observation and did not test for interrater reliability.

Recently, transcranial magnetic stimulation (TMS), a new method for the assessment of associated movements, has been examined. This method has been used to investigate the ipsilateral and contralateral connections of the motor cortices more directly. Studies with patients with abnormalities of the corpus callosum revealed transcallosal inhibition to be absent or delayed in these patients (Meyer, Rorichr, Grafin von Einsiedel, Kruggel, & Weindl, 1995). Other investigations have found that by focusing TMS on the hand area of the motor cortex at a position that evokes the largest motor potentials in the hand muscles, ipsilateral and contralateral electromyogram (EMG) responses can be evoked (Ziemann et al., 1999). In a study of 50 healthy 3- to 10-year-old children, which used TMS, ipsilateral motor evoked potentials were found in proximal and distal muscles of the arm with a 10–12 ms longer latency than the contralateral responses in two-thirds of the children (Reitz, Kass-Iliyya, & Müller, 1997). Ipsilateral projecting corticospinal or corticorubrospinal connections can explain these ipsilateral responses. These connections are likely the cause of increasing transcallosal inhibition during development (Reitz & Müller, 1998) and were not found in children over 9 years of age (Reitz et al., 1997). Future research is needed, however, to determine if this method is applicable to other synkineses.

Associated Movements as Markers for Developmental Delay or Neurological Impairment

Clinical interest in associated movements has arisen from the idea that they either reflect a delay in neurological maturation when they do not decrease and then disappear with age (Touwen, 1979) or are the expression of a neurological deficit, as they may emerge after acquired damage (Hashimoto, Shindo, & Yanagisawa, 2001). However, the actual clinical significance of associated movements during development is less clear-cut. First, the large developmental variability in onset and in the rate of decrease of associated movements makes it hard to use them for clinical purposes. Second, their functional significance is not well established. Third, in most cases, there is no sound relationship with localized structural damage. There is, however, a clear association between a number of developmental disorders and the presence of associated movements. In the following paragraphs, I present a number of examples.

Congenital mirror movements without any other neurological abnormality are rare. This condition, which can be observed from the first months after birth, is characterized by an extreme symmetry in hand or arm movements and an inability to perform unimanual movements. Ruggieri, Amartino, and Fejerman (1999) present the case of a 4-year-old boy with congenital mirror movements, who dropped things from one hand when trying to pick up an object with the other. The father reported that he himself had similar difficulties since childhood but had managed with time to partially control and even inhibit these mirror movements. Clearly, in these cases, the mirror movements affected functional behavior and its development. Reitz and Müller (1998) compared congenital mirror movements of a 4-year-old child with normative data. The child presented with distinct mirror movements in the hand and fingers, which occurred symmetrically on both sides, and without a similar phenomenon in the lower limbs. The mirror movements were elicited by focal TMS above the hand area of the motor cortex at a position that evoked the largest motor potentials in the hand muscles. Unilateral stimulation evoked bilateral EMG responses, which had strikingly identical latencies, and mirror movements with simultaneous onset. In contrast, normal children showed 10–12 ms transcallosal delay between ipsilateral and contralateral activation. The most likely explanation put forward by the authors is that the congenital mirror movements were due to ipsilateral corticospinal connections. These present a structural constraint that may seriously affect functional coordination. The authors concluded that these findings argue against a common neural mechanism for congenital mirror movements and associated mirror movements. Maegaki and colleagues (2002) report functional magnetic resonance imaging (fMRI) and TMS studies of a child and an adult with congenital mirror movement in hands and fingers. fMRI showed bilateral activation of the primary sensorimotor cortices during unilateral hand squeezing. Longitudinal TMS data of the child collected at ages 5-11, 7-8, and 8-8 provided evidence of differential developmental changes in ipsilateral and contralateral responses in hand and forearm muscles.

Another syndrome with associated movements is hemiplegic cerebral palsy. Using TMS, Carr, Harrison, and Stephens (1993) found evidence of reorganization in novel ipsilateral pathways from the undamaged motor cortex to the hemiplegic hand in 65% of the patients. Half of these patients showed intense mirror movements, whereas, the remaining patients did not have intense mirror movements. Based on the effects of digital nerve stimulation and the cross-correlation analysis of the EMGs of these patients, Carr and colleagues concluded that corticospinal axons had branched abnormally and projected bilaterally to homologous motor neuron pools in those patients who displayed mirror movements, while in those that did not display mirror movements no evidence of branching was found. In patients with congenital hemiparesis, Staudt and colleagues (2002) provided evidence that the type of corticospinal reorganization depends on the extent of the brain lesion. They propose that involvement of the ipsilateral hemisphere can be of the premotor type (i.e., without ipsilateral motor projections but with significant activation of ipsilateral premotor areas), or of the primary motor type (i.e., with abnormal ipsilateral corticospinal projections to the paretic hand).

Partial or complete hemispherectomy is sometimes performed as a treatment for children with severe drug-resistant epilepsy due to congenital or acquired disease. Holloway and colleagues (2000) studied the reorganization of sensorimotor function in children after hemispherectomy (age range 6–19 years, at least 1 year after surgery). The consequence of this surgery was of course a full or partial hemiplegia. Eight patients had congenital brain damage (first seizure on average at 1 year, 7 months), and nine with acquired disease had sustained their initial insult at the age of 1 year or older (mean age of insult 4 years, 4 months). Sensorimotor functions of the hand were studied using fMRI during passive movement (only in four patients in each group), somatosensory evoked potentials using median nerve stimulation, and behavioral tests such as moving pegs, force production, and finger tapping at maximum rate. Both hands were tested. Of the nine patients with acquired disease none showed any residual motor function in the affected limb. All the patients with congenital disease and hemispherectomy showed some residual sensory function in the affected hand. Four of them had some residual force production. Of these four patients, three demonstrated residual motor function on peg moving and finger tapping and mirror movements. Three explanations are suggested for the ipsilateral residual function after hemispherectomy: (1) there may be strengthening of remaining ipsilateral pathways promoted by functional demand; (2) there may be novel axonal sprouting resulting in new functional pathways; or (3) the inhibitory influence from the opposite hemisphere does not develop and ipsilateral pathways remain functioning as the cortex matures. These three mechanisms may be interpreted as functional reorganization (i.e., an attempt of the central nervous system to restore some of the functionality that was lost by the disease and the hemispherectomy). With respect to residual motor function, this was present only in half of the children with congenital disease, which indicates that the functional reorganization is most likely if it is required very early in development. The finding that associated movements were present in three of four cases with residual function in the affected arm suggests that ipsilateral pathways may be involved in residual sensorimotor function.

Associated movements also may occur as a comorbid phenomenon to behavioral disorders, such as learning disorders, which do not have a clear neurological defect. They are noted as one of the neurological soft signs and are found more frequently in these populations than in the typical population (Touwen, 1979). Studies have reported an association with speech and language problems (Klipcera, Wolff, & Drake, 1981; Noterdaeme et al., 1988) and with risk factors for development, such as low birth weight (Leitner et al., 2000) and congenital hypothyroidism (Bargagna et al., 2000). At present, little can be said about the underlying neurological deficit and the predictive value of the associated movements in these cases. Touwen (1987) and Taylor (1987), in their discussions of the meaning of soft neurological signs, draw the conclusion that associated movements do not have an undisputed neurological significance or clinical value. Only in individual cases and in conjunction with other information can a particular set of soft neurological signs be a significant indicator of specific neural dysfunction.

Some Consequences for Intervention

It is clear that congenital mirror movements may interfere with skilled manual performance. For adolescent boys with severe learning disabilities, persistence of mirror
movements also poses a problem for the development of skilled motor performance. In
contrast, synkineses do not seem to have a direct effect on motor performance (Wolff
et al, 1983). Thus, in the case of persistent mirror movements that interfere with daily
activities, intervention is desirable. But are mirror movements modifiable? The most
direct evidence is reported by Ruggieri and colleagues (1999): The father of the 4-year-
old boy with severe congenital mirror movements remembered having suffered similar
problems at an early age; he had learned with time, to partially control and even inhibit these mirror movements. Other evidence comes from Lazarus and Todor (1991),
who found that feedback reduced the mirror force level in the contralateral hand. Holloway and colleagues (2000) interpret the partial functionality of the affected hand
more than 1 year after hemispherectomy as a sign of functional reorganization of the
ipsilateral neural pathways. This evidence converges to support the conclusion that
mirror movements are susceptible to intervention.

CONCLUSION

This chapter began with a discussion of the view that the developing sensorimotor system is a dynamic system with self-organizing properties influenced by internal and external constraints. The changing nature of organismic constraints was explored
through the phenomena of associated movements. The development and significance
of associated movements were reviewed. It was concluded that the general notion that
associated movements or mirror movements disappear by the age of 10 years is wrong.
Most of them are task dependent. Each type of associated movement follows its own
developmental pathway, and some do not disappear until adulthood and may still be
elicited under certain conditions. Their interference with the normal development of
motor competence seems to be limited, except for the case of congenital mirror movements. In this latter case, ipsilateral connections form a structural constraint. There is
evidence that even these constraints may be changed with training and effort, which
offers possibilities for intervention. Overall, research findings indicate that that the
neuromotor system is subject to organismic constraints that change with age and experience.

REFERENCES

Abercrombie, M. L. J., Lindon, R. L., & Tyson, M. C. (1964). Associated movements in normal
    and physically handicapped children. *Developmental Medicine and Child Neurology, 6,*
    573–580.
Arányi, Z., & Rösler, K. M. (2002). Effort-induced mirror movements. A study of transcallosal
    inhibition in humans. *Experimental Brain Research, 145,* 76–82.
Bernstein, N. (1984). Some emergent problems of the regulation of motor acts. In H. T. A.
    Whiting (Ed.), *Human motor actions: Bernstein reassessed* (pp. 343–371). Amsterdam:
    North-Holland.

Bargagna, S., Canepa, G., Costagli, C., Dinetti, D., Mareschi, M., Millepiedi, S., et al. (2000). Neurophysiological follow-up in early treated congenital hypothyroidism: A problem oriented approach. *Thyroid, 10*, 243–249.

Carr, L. J., Harrison, A. L., & Stephens, J. A. (1993). Patterns of central motor reorganisation in hemiplegic cerebral palsy. *Brain, 116*, 1223–1247.

Connolly, K., & Stratton, P. (1968). Developmental changes in associated movements. *Developmental Medicine and Child Neurology, 10*, 49–56.

Edelman, G. M. (1987). *Neural Darwinism: The theory of neural group selection.* New York: Basic Books.

Hashimoto, T., Shindo, M., & Yanagisawa, N. (2001). Enhanced associated movements in the contralateral limbs elicited by brisk voluntary contraction in choreic disorders. *Clinical Neurophysiology, 122*, 1612–1617.

Holloway, V., Gadian, D. G., Vargha-Kadem, F., Porter, D. A., Boyd, S. G., & Connelly, A. (2000). The reorganisation of sensorimotor function in children after hemispherectomy. A functional MRI and somatosensory evoked potential study. *Brain, 123*, 2423–2444.

Klipcera, C., Wolff, P. H., & Drake, C. (1981). Bimanual co-ordination in adolescent boys with reading retardation. *Developmental Medicine and Child Neurology, 23*, 617–624.

Largo, R. H., Caflisch, J. A., Hug, F., Muggli, K., Molnar, A. A., & Molinari, L. (2001). Neuromotor development from 5 to 18 years. Part 2: Associated movements. *Developmental Medicine and Child Neurology, 43*, 444–453.

Lazarus, J. C., & Todor, J. I. (1987). Age differences in the magnitude of associated movement. *Developmental Medicine and Child Neurology, 29*, 726–733.

Lazarus, J. C., & Todor, J. I. (1991). The role of attention in the regulation of associated movement in children. *Developmental Medicine and Child Neurology, 33*, 32–39.

Leitner, Y., Fattal-Valevski, A., Geva, R., Bassan, P. H., Posner, E., Kutai, M., et al. (2000). Six-year follow-up of children with intrauterine growth retardation: Long-term, prospective study. *Journal of Child Neurology, 15*,781–786.

Maegaki, Y., Seki, A., Suzaki, I., Sugihara, S., Ogawa, T., Amisaki, T., et al. (2002). Congenital mirror movement: A study of functional MRI and transcranial magnetic stimulation. *Developmental Medicine and Child Neurology, 44*, 838–843.

Meyer, B. U., Rorichr, S., Grafin von Einsiedel, H., Kruggel F., & Weindl, A. (1995). Inhibitory and excitatory interhemispheric transfers between motor cortical areas in normal humans and patients with abnormalities of the corpus callosum. *Brain, 118*, 429–440.

Missiuro, W. (1963). Studies on developmental stages of children's reflex reactivity. *Child Development, 34*, 33–41.

Newell, K. M. (1986). Constraints on the development of coordination. In M. G. Wade & H. T. A. Whiting (Eds.), *Motor development in children: Aspects of coordination and control* (pp. 341–360). Dordrecht, The Netherlands: Nijhoff.

Noterdaeme, M., Amorosa, H., Ploog, M., & Scheimann, G. (1988). Quantitative and qualitative aspects of associated movements in children with specific developmental speech and language disorders and in normal pre-school children. *Journal of Human Movement Studies, 15*, 151–169.

Peters, J. E. (1987). A special or soft neurological examination for school age children. In D. E. Tupper (Ed.), *Soft neurological signs* (pp. 369–379). Orlando, FL: Grune & Straton.

Prechtl, H. F. R. (1993). Principles of early motor development in the human. In A. F. Kalverboer, B. Hopkins, & R. H. Geuze (Eds.), *Motor development in early and later childhood: Longitudinal approaches* (pp. 35–50). Cambridge, UK: Cambridge University Press.

Reitz, M., Kass-Iliyya, F., & Müller, K. (1997). Are ipsilateral corticospinal connections a correlate to associated movements? *Electroencephalogaphy and Clinical Neurophysiology, 102*, 51P.

Reitz, M., & Müller, K. (1998). Differences between "congenital mirror movements" and "associated movements" in normal children: A neurophysiological case study. *Neuroscience Letters, 256,* 69–72.

Ruggieri, V., Amartino, H., & Fejerman, N. (1999). Movimientos en espejo congenitos. Tres nuevoscasos de una rara entidad [Congenital mirror movements. Three new cases of a rare condition]. *Revista de Neurologia, 29,* 731–735.

Shaffer, D. (1978). "Soft" neurological signs and later psychiatric disorder—A review. *Journal of Child Psychology and Psychiatry, 19,* 63–65.

Staudt, M., Grodd, W., Gerloff, C., Erb, M., Stitz, J., & Krägeloh-Mann, I. (2002). Two types of ipsilateral reorganization in congenital hemiparesis. A TMS and fMRI study. *Brain, 125,* 2222–2237.

Taylor, H. G. (1987). The meaning and value of soft signs in the behavioral sciences. In D. E. (Ed.), *Soft neurological signs* (pp. 297–335). Orlando, FL: Grune & Straton.

Thelen, E., & Smith, L. B. (1994). *A dynamic systems approach to the development of cognition and action.* Cambridge, MA: MIT Press.

Todor, J. I., & Lazarus, J. I. (1986). Exertion level and the intensity of associated movements. *Developmental Medicine and Child Neurology, 28,* 205–212.

Touwen, B. C. L. (1979). *Examination of the child with minor neurological dysfunction.* Philadelphia: Lippincott.

Touwen, B. C. L. (1987). The meaning and value of soft signs in neurology. In D. E. Tupper (Ed.), *Soft neurological signs* (pp. 281–295). Orlando, FL: Grune & Straton.

Tuller, B., Turvey, M. T., & Fitch, H. L. (1982). The Bernstein perspective: II. The concept of linkage or co-ordinative structure. In J. A. S. Kelso (Ed.), *Human motor behavior: An introduction* (pp. 15–34). Hillsdale, NJ: Erlbaum.

Tupper, D. E. (1987). The issues with soft signs. In D. E. Tupper (Ed.), *Soft neurological signs* (pp. 1–16). Orlando, FL: Grune & Straton.

Walshe, F. M. R. (1923). On certain tonic or postural reflexes in hemiplegia, with special reference to the so-called "associated movements." *Brain, 46,* 1–37.

Wolff, P. H., Gunnoe, C. E., & Cohen, C. (1983). Associated movements as a measure of developmental age. *Developmental Medicine and Child Neurology, 25,* 546–549.

Ziemann, U., Ishii, K., Borgheresi, A., Yaseen, Z., Battaglia, F, Hallett, M., et al. (1999). Dissociation of the pathways mediating ipsilateral and contralateral motor-evoked potentials in human hand and arm muscles. *Journal of Physiology, 518,* 895–906.

Zijdewind, I., & Kernell, D. (2001). Bilateral interactions during contractions of intrinsic hand muscles. *Journal of Neurophysiology, 85,* 1907–1913.

Zülch, K. J., & Müller, N. (1969). Associated movements in man. In P. J. Vinken & D. W. Bruyn (Eds.), *Handbook of clinical neurology* (Vol. 30, pp. 404–426). Amsterdam: Elsevier.

CHAPTER 18

Co-Occurrence of Motor Disorders with Other Childhood Disorders

DEBORAH DEWEY
SUSAN G. CRAWFORD
BRENDA N. WILSON
BONNIE J. KAPLAN

Health professionals who study children with developmental problems, and those who educate and treat them, tend to speak of *diagnostic categories*. Researchers and clinicians have attempted to classify childhood developmental disorders into discrete diagnostic categories such as those found in the fourth edition of the *Diagnostic and Statistical Manual of Mental Disorders* (DSM-IV; American Psychiatric Association, 1994) or the 10th edition of the *International Classification of Diseases* (ICD-10; World Health Organization, 1992). In many cases, however, children with these disabilities do not display just one discrete disorder but several disorders. For example, children with reading disabilities often have attention-deficit/hyperactivity disorder (ADHD), and children with ADHD frequently meet criteria for developmental coordination disorder (DCD). When this occurs, the term *comorbidity* has been used to refer to the fact that the child meets diagnostic criteria for more than one disorder.

Comorbid is a term that has been borrowed from medicine. Its original meaning indicated the presence of at least two diseases. An individual with diabetes and asthma, for instance, is said to be comorbid for these two diseases. In contrast, an individual reporting frequent urination and thirstiness is not said to be comorbid for these two conditions because they are symptoms; their co-occurrence suggests morbidity for a single disease, diabetes. When the term *comorbidity* was transferred to the mental health world, one element was missing that prevented its accurate application: the precise distinction between symptom and disease (or disorder). For instance, when a child has difficulties with learning, mood, behavior, and printing/writing, the child could be viewed as displaying a learning disability, ADHD, and/or DCD. The co-occurrence of these apparently disparate symptoms causes problems in both diagnosis and treatment. In addition, it raises questions about the etiology and mutual interdependence of various developmental disorders (Gilger, Pennington, & DeFries, 1992).

In this chapter, we begin with a discussion of some of the terminology that has been associated with the concept of comorbidity. We then address the issue of the extent of overlap of developmental disorders among children who display disorders in motor function. Because of our own research focus, we pay special attention to research involving children with DCD. We then examine research that has investigated the co-occurrence of motor problems with other developmental disorders in children with low birth weight and neurofibromatosis. This is followed by a discussion of neuroanatomical evidence that may account for the extensive overlap that is seen among developmental disorders. Finally, we present a new conceptual framework, which may assist researchers and educators to better understand the high rate of overlap among these various conditions.

THE EXTENT OF OVERLAP OF DEVELOPMENTAL PROBLEMS

Angold, Costello, and Erkanli (1999) provide an excellent overview of terms that are helpful when talking about comorbidity of common child and adolescent psychiatric disorders. It is important to note that when talking about childhood developmental problems such as DCD, ADHD, and learning disabilities we are referring to *disorders*, not diseases. Diseases are well-defined clinical entities whose etiologies are known, whereas disorders are behavioral and psychological syndromes that deviate from some standard of normality (Angold, 1988). As a result, the co-occurrence of several disorders may be due to a problem in the classification system rather than an association between underlying diseases (Angold et al., 1999). This does not mean, however, that there is no point in studying overlap of developmental disorders. Indeed, the investigation of these comorbidities may assist in correcting and validating the present classification systems.

One problem with the term *comorbidity* is that it can refer to a "multitude of different temporal relationships amongst disorders" (Angold et al., 1999, p. 59). Studies of children with developmental disorders have typically investigated the co-occurrence of disorders over a relatively short time span (Dewey, Kaplan, Crawford, & Wilson, 2002; Kaplan, Wilson, Dewey, & Crawford, 1998). For example, studies may investigate whether children with ADHD also display DCD and/or learning disabilities at the same time. However, when considering comorbidity, it is also important to investigate lifetime rates of disorders, as children with developmental disorders may display different types of disorders over their lifespan. Studies of children with DCD have reported that many of these children outgrow their motor problems at adolescence (Visser, Geuze, & Kalverboer, 1998). Other studies have reported that motor problems in children are associated with affective and anxiety disorders in adolescence (Ahonen, 1990; Gillberg & Gillberg, 1989; Safer, Shaffer, O'Conner, & Stokman, 1986). We do not know, however, if only the individuals who continue to display motor deficits are at risk for psychiatric problems in adolescence. Thus, knowing more about evolution of a developmental disorder would allow us to develop a better understanding of the course of the disorder over the individual's lifetime.

CO-OCCURRENCE OF MOTOR AND COGNITIVE IMPAIRMENTS

Motor problems in children may be due to medical and neurological conditions such as mild cerebral palsy, early-stage muscular dystrophy, congenital hypothyroidism, brain injury, and visual impairment (Barnett, Kooistra, & Henderson, 1998; Denckla & Roeltgen, 1992; Fox & Lent, 1996). In the case of DCD, which is estimated to occur in 5–8% of school-age children (American Psychiatric Association, 1994; Gubbay, 1975; Henderson & Hall, 1982), there is no identifiable neurological or medical cause. Children with DCD are distinguished from their typically developing peers by a pervasive slowness in the easy acquisition of everyday motor skills. As a result, their motor performance is significantly impaired so that daily activities at school (e.g., handwriting, participation in sports, and social interaction) and at home (e.g., self-care activities) are adversely affected.

Although DCD may occur in isolation, many children with this disorder display additional problems, including learning disabilities, speech/language deficits, and attention deficits (Cantell, Smyth, & Ahonen, 1994; Dewey et al., 2002; Dewey & Wall, 1997; Dewey, Wilson, Crawford, & Kaplan, 2000; Gordon & McKinlay, 1980; Kadesjo & Gillberg, 1998; Kaplan et al., 1998; Losse, et al., 1991; Roussounis, Gaussen, & Stratton, 1987; Snow, Blondis, & Brady, 1988). Children with DCD have also been noted to have deficits in visual perception, kinesthetic perception, and memory (Dewey, Crawford, Kaplan, & Wilson, 2003; Dwyer & McKenzie, 1994; Piek & Coleman-Carman, 1995; Rösblad, 2001; Smyth & Glencross, 1986; Wilson & McKenzie, 1998).

Learning and Language Difficulties

The co-occurrence of motor impairments and learning difficulties has been examined by a number of investigators. Gubbay (1975) reported that 50% of children with problems in motor coordination also had difficulties with academics. Drillien and Drummond (1983) found that 32% of children with motor problems had moderate problems in school and 32% had severe problems, whereas van Dellen, Vaessen and Schoemaker (1990) reported that a third of their sample of clumsy children ($n = 31$) had repeated a grade compared to one child in the comparison group. Kaplan and colleagues (1998) found that 56% of their sample of children with DCD had reading problems. Dewey and colleagues (2000) reported that 33% of their sample of children with DCD displayed reading problems and an additional 36% had reading problems and ADHD.

Studies that have examined movement deficits in children with dyslexia and learning problems have reported high rates of motor difficulties in these populations (Fawcett & Nicolson, 1995; Gottesman, Hankin, Levinson, & Beck, 1984; Nicolson & Fawcett, 1994; Silver, 1992; Sugden & Wann, 1987). Investigators have found that like children with DCD, children with dyslexia and learning problems have difficulties with continuous tapping tasks (Geuze & Kalverboer, 1994; Wolff, Michel, Ovrut, & Drake, 1990). Dewey and Wall (1997) noted that children with language impairments displayed significant difficulties with motor tasks. Further, deficits in the production of familiar hand postures have been reported in children with specific language impairments (Hill, Bishop, & Nimmo-Smith, 1998). Powell and Bishop (1992) investigated whether children with specific language impairment might be particularly impaired on motor skills that involved rapidly changing movements. In fact, what they found was that these children were impaired on all 19 measures of motor function included in their test battery, not just those that reflected slow processing rates. Thus, among children with learning/language impairments there appears to be a high prevalence of motor problems. It is important, however, to keep in mind that not all children with learning/language impairments (i.e., reading disability, math disability, spelling disability, and specific language impairment) have poor motor coordination. Conversely, not all children with poor motor coordination have learning/language problems.

Visual–Perceptual Motor Deficits

As Chapter 13 (Wilson, this volume) provides a detailed discussion of the visual–perceptual deficits found in children with DCD, we discuss them only briefly here. Visual–perceptual deficits have been found to be more common in children with DCD than in typically developing children. In a series of studies, Hulme and colleagues (Hulme & Lord, 1986; Hulme, Smart, & Moran, 1982; Hulme, Smart, Moran, & McKinlay, 1984; Hulme & Snowling, 1992) assessed the visual–perceptual skills of children with DCD on tasks such as discrimination of shape, area, slope, pattern, line length, and size constancy. Results indicated that the children with DCD were less proficient than typically developing children on these tests. Henderson, Barnett, and Henderson (1994) also found that children with DCD performed poorly on tests of visual–perceptual discrimination.

Investigations that have examined the visual–motor skills of children with DCD have found that these children perform more poorly than do comparison children (Dewey & Kaplan, 1994; Parush, Yochman, Cohen, & Gershon, 1998). Even when the motor component is removed from tests of visual perception, children with DCD have been found to be less proficient (Parush et al., 1998). Wilson and McKenzie (1998) showed that children with DCD were inferior to comparison children on almost all measures of information processing and the greatest deficits were found in the area of visuospatial processing. Furthermore, these deficits were found to be more pronounced for visual–perceptual tasks that demanded a motor response; however, impairments were still found on visual–perceptual tasks without motor responses. Thus, visual–perceptual abilities appear to be a specific area of deficiency in children with DCD (Wilson & McKenzie, 1998).

Memory Deficits

Visual memory deficits have also been reported in children with DCD. In a study by Dwyer and Mackenzie (1994), children with DCD and comparison children were asked to reproduce geometric patterns immediately or after a 15-second delay. No difference was found between groups in terms of their ability to reproduce the pattern immediately; however, the children with DCD were much less accurate after the time delay. In a related study, Skorji and McKenzie (1997) examined children's ability to reproduce a sequence of simple movements immediately after presentation and after a 15-second time delay. Consistent with the previous study, there were no differences in performance between children with DCD and comparison children immediately after presentation, but children with DCD were significantly more affected by the time delay. Henderson and colleagues (1994) found, however, that children with DCD were impaired in their ability to reproduce geometric patterns even when no time delay was introduced. Dewey and colleagues (2003) examined general memory functioning in children with DCD, children "suspect" for DCD, and typically developing children using the Wide Range Assessment of Memory and Learning (WRAML; Sheslow & Adams, 1990). Results indicated that on the General Memory Index of the WRAML, children with DCD obtained significantly lower scores than the "suspect" children and the typically developing children. Examination of children's performance on the individual subtests of the WRAML indicated that the children with DCD had difficulty on tests that assessed immediate recall of verbal and nonverbal information such as numbers, letters, pictures, and visual sequences. They also performed more poorly on subtests that assessed their ability to learn and retain verbal information (i.e., Verbal Learning) and their ability to learn and remember the association between a specific sound and symbol (i.e., Sound–Symbol). Interestingly, the children with DCD did not differ from the other two groups in their ability to immediately reproduce designs from memory (i.e., Design Memory) or in their ability to learn and remember the location of nonrepresentational pictures on a board (i.e., Picture Memory). When we examined the children's ability to retain information after a 10–15-minute delay, both children with DCD and the children "suspect" for DCD showed deficits on Story Memory and Sound Symbol; however, no impairments were noted on Picture Memory. The findings of the foregoing studies suggest that children with DCD evidence impairment in memory; however, this impairment does not appear to be confined to visual memory but includes impairments in verbal memory.

Attention Deficits

Chapter 14 (Piek & Pitcher, this volume) provides a detailed review of the literature on the co-occurrence of attention problems and motor problems in children with DCD; therefore, we provide only a brief overview here. The most extensive work on this issue has been done by Gillberg and colleagues who have proposed their own term to differentiate this subgroup: *deficits in attention, motor control, and perception* (DAMP; Gillberg & Rasmussen, 1982; Gillberg, Rasmussen, Carlstrom, Svenson, & Waldenstrom, 1982; Hellgren, Gillberg, & Gillberg, 1994; Kadesjo & Gillberg, 1998). Kadesjo and Gillberg (1998) reported that there was a considerable overlap between ADHD and DCD, with about half of each diagnostic group also meeting the criteria for the other diagnosis. Other investigators have also reported that as many as half of all children with ADHD fit the diagnosis for DCD (Barkley, DuPaul, & McMurray, 1990; Denckla & Rudel, 1978; Fox & Lent, 1996; Kaplan, Crawford, Wilson, & Dewey, 2000; Kaplan et al., 1998; Piek, Pitcher, & Hay, 1999; Szatmari, Offord, & Boyle, 1989).

Nonverbal Learning Disabilities

Because of the high rate of co-occurrence of motor problems with learning difficulties, Rourke's (1995) description of children with the syndrome of nonverbal learning disabilities (NLD) is of particular interest. He describes children with NLD as exhibiting bilateral psychomotor coordination deficiencies, difficulty with complex movement skills, deficits in visual–spatial–organizational abilities and tactile perception. All these difficulties have been associated with DCD. In addition, children with NLD also display problems in reading comprehension, mathematics, speech and language, concept formation, problem solving, and attention to and memory of tactile and visual stimuli. Similar deficits have been reported in children identified with DCD.

Socioemotional Problems

More recent studies have begun to investigate the overlap among DCD, ADHD, learning disabilities, and behavioral and emotional problems (Dewey et al., 2002; Kaplan, Dewey, Crawford, & Wilson, 2001). Kaplan and colleagues (2001) reported that 50% of their sample of 179 children met criteria for the diagnosis of at least two of the following disorders: reading disability (RD), ADHD, DCD, oppositional defiant disorder (OPD), conduct disorder (CD), depression, and anxiety. Dewey and colleagues (2002) found that children with movement problems were at risk for social and peer relationship problems and were more likely to report somatic symptoms such as general aches and pains, headaches, and tiredness. Longitudinal outcome studies have reported that children with DCD are more immature, socially isolated, and passive than are comparison children (Ahonen, 1990; Cantell, 1998; Cantell et al., 1994). In addition, somatic symptoms were more common in the children with DCD (Cantell, 1998). Studies that have followed children with DCD and ADHD (i.e., DAMP) report that these children are at risk for a number of psychiatric and personality disorders. Hellgren, Gillberg, Bagenholm, and Gillberg (1994) found that more than half of the adolescents with DAMP had psychiatric or personality disorders compared to only one-tenth of the control group. The psychiatric symptoms displayed by these adolescents ranged from affective and anxiety disorders to personality disorders, including social negativism and withdrawal. Follow-up of these individuals at 22 years of age revealed that 58% of the ADHD/DCD group had a poor outcome and that antisocial personality disorder, alcohol abuse, criminal offending, reading disorders, and low educational level were overrepresented in this group (see Ahonen, Kooistra, Viholainen, & Cantell, Chapter 12, this volume, for a more detailed discussion of the socioemotional difficulties of children with DCD).

The foregoing research indicates that DCD is associated with other disorders of development. Furthermore, children with DCD are at risk for developing a number of behavioral and emotional problems in adolescence and adulthood, which may have a significant influence on their long-term psychosocial functioning.

CO-OCCURRENCE OF MOTOR AND COGNITIVE IMPAIRMENTS IN OTHER DEVELOPMENTAL PROBLEMS

The previous section focused on the co-occurrence of DCD and problems in learning, attention, behavior, and socioemotional functioning. As noted in other chapters in this book, children with conditions such as cerebral palsy, muscular dystrophy, Tourette syndrome, head injury, and autism spectrum disorders display motor and visual motor difficulties, as well as neurocognitive impairments. Thus, in many developmental disorders, motor and neurocognitive impairments often co-occur. In the following section, we briefly discuss the motor, visual motor, and associated neurocognitive problems that have been found in children with two other conditions that are not reviewed elsewhere in this book, very low birth weight (VLBW) and neurofibromatosis type 1 (NF1).

Very Low Birth Weight

Most children born with VLBW (birth weight < 1,500 grams) and extreme low birth weight (ELBW; birth weight < 1,000 grams) display IQ scores within the normal range of intelligence (Hack et al., 1992; Victorian Infant Collaborative Study Group, 1991; Whitfield, Grunau, & Holsti, 1997). These children, however, frequently lag behind their normal birth weight (NBW; birth weight > 2,500 grams) peers in terms of their development of many neurocognitive abilities. Among these children, an increased prevalence of problems has been reported in areas such as language comprehension, memory, motor, and visual–motor abilities (Dewey, Crawford, Creighton, & Sauve, 1999; Gorga, Stern, Ross, & Nagler, 1991; Grunau, Whitfield, & Davis, 2003; Hack et al., 1992; Hack, Taylor, Klein, Schatschneider, & Mercuri-Minich, 1994; Keller, Ayub, Saigal, & Bar-Or, 1998; Klein, Hack, & Breslau, 1989; Rickards et al., 1993; Saigal, Rosenbaum, Szatmari, & Campbell, 1991; Whitfield et al., 1997). Children with VLBW have also been found to do less well in school and to use more special resources than children with NBW (Hack et al., 1992; Saigal et al., 1991; Whitfield et al., 1997).

Examination of the research literature on the neurocognitive problems associated with children with VLBW and ELBW without neurosensory deficits shows that difficulties in motor and perceptual abilities have been consistently reported (Dewey et al, 1999; Grunau et al. , 2003; Hack et al., 1992; Herrgard, Luoma, Tuppurainen, Karjalainen, & Martikainen, 1993; Hunt, Cooper, & Tooley, 1988; Jongmans, Mercuri, Dubowitz, & Henderson, 1998; Klein et al., 1989; Marlow, Roberts, & Cooke, 1989; Rickards et al., 1993; Saigal et al., 1991; Vohr & Gracia Coll, 1985). Studies of preterm children at *preschool* have reported that visuospatial and motor problems were the most frequent neurodevelopmental abnormalities found (25–30% of the children) (Herrgard et al., 1993; Mutch, Leyland, & McGee, 1993) with lower birth weights associated with more significant motor impairment (Mutch et al., 1993). Keller and colleagues (1998) compared the neuromotor abilities of children with ELBW, VLBW, and NBW. Consistent with Mutch's findings, they found that the children with ELBW displayed poorer coordination, poorer strength, and slower reaction times.

Studies examining the motor outcomes of children with VLBW free of major sensorineural impairments at *school age* have reported that a significant number of preterm children continue to display problems in visual–motor abilities and motor coordination (i.e., 30–40%), as well as difficulties in cognition, language, and behavior (Dewey et al., 1999; Hack et al., 1992; Jongmans, Demetre, Dubowitz, & Henderson, 1996; Keller et al., 1998; Marlow et al., 1989; Pharoah, Stevenson, Cooke, & Stevenson, 1994; Rickards et al., 1993; Roth et al., 1994; Saigal et al., 1991; Whitfield et al., 1997). Jongmans and colleagues (1996) assessed 165 preterm children who were 6 years of age. They found that 36% of these children had motor coordination problems, 13% had reading problems, and 10% had both motor and reading problems.

Marlow and colleagues (1989) reported that the performance of children with VLBW on motor tests at 6 years of age was the best predictor of school problems at 8 years. Rickards and colleagues (1993) and Hack and colleagues (1992) found that children with VLBW without major neurological abnormality had significantly poorer scores on visual motor and fine motor measures, as well as measures of intelligence, expressive language, memory function, and hyperactivity than did children with NBW. In contrast, Saigal and colleagues (1991) found that children with ELBW who were considered normal neurologically were comparable to controls on measures of intelligence, language, and academic achievement but fared significantly less well in motor performance. Whitfield and colleagues (1997) reported that children with ELBW performed significantly poorer on fine motor, gross motor, and visual–motor tests compared to full-term controls. Keller and colleagues (1998) noted that the neuromotor performance of children with ELBW was poorer than children with VLBW and NBW. Studies that have followed children with VLBW and ELBW into adolescence and adulthood report that they continue to display significant motor difficulties (Losse et al., 1991; Powls, Botting, Cooke, & Marlow, 1995; Whitfield et al., 1997). The foregoing findings indicate that many children and adolescents with VLBW and ELBW continue to display impairments in motor, visual–motor, and perceptual abilities as they mature and that these impairments could be particular areas of vulnerability for children with VLBW and ELBW (Keller et al., 1998; Whitfield et al., 1997).

Neurofibromatosis

NF1 is one of the most common genetic disorders with a prevalence of approximately 1 in 4,000 individuals. It is characterized by abnormal cell growth and tissue differentiation that can affect multiple organ systems including the central and peripheral nervous systems. Research has indicated that NF1 is associated with a broad range of relatively nonspecific cognitive impairments including lowered IQ (i.e., IQs in the high 80s to low 90s), learning disabilities, language impairments, executive function deficits, and poor motor and visuospatial skills (Ozonoff, 1999).

Studies that have investigated the motor skills of children with NF1 have reported a variety of abnormalities in gross and fine motor function. Children with NF1 have been found to have significantly more difficulty with balance and gait on neurological examination (Chapman, Waber, Bassett, Urion, & Korf, 1996; Eldridge et al., 1989; Hofman, Harris, Bryan, & Denckla, 1994). North and colleagues (1994) reported that approximately one-quarter of their sample displayed mild motor impairments on the Test of Motor Impairment (Stott, Moyes, & Henderson, 1984), a standardized measure of fine and gross motor function, and another half of the participants had moderate to severe motor coordination difficulties. Zoller, Rembeck, and Backman (1997) found that adults with NF1 had slowed performance on a finger-tapping task, a measure of fine motor speed, whereas Moore, Slopis, Schomer, Jackson, and Levy (1996) reported that children with NF1 did not display deficits on finger tapping; however, on a measure of fine motor coordination (i.e., Grooved Pegboard) the performance of these children was approximately one standard deviation lower than the published norms. Ferner, Hughes, and Weinman (1996) reported that NF1 patients had significantly slower mean reaction times on a simple motor task. Parental reports of the motor skills of children with NF1 are consistent with the above findings (Dilts et al.,

1996). In summary, these studies indicate that deficits in fine and gross motor ability are a common feature of NF1 and may be aspects of the phenotype of this disorder.

Deficits in visual–motor and visual–spatial–perceptual skills have also been reported in individuals with NF1. Eliason (1986) found that most of his sample of children with NF1 (20 out of 23) had visual–perceptual impairments. Stine and Adams (1989) reported that the performance of individuals with NF1 on visual–perceptual tests and tests of visual–motor integration was two standard deviations below population norms and one and a half standard deviations below the participants' own IQ scores, suggesting that visual–perceptual deficits may be a primary feature of this disorder. A number of recent studies have also documented impairments in visual–spatial–perceptual skills in individuals with NF1 (Bawden et al., 1996; Dilts et al., 1996; Hofman et al., 1994; Moore et al., 1996; Zoller et al., 1997). Some studies, however, have not found this pattern. North and colleagues (1994) reported that children with NF1 did not display significant impairments on a test of visual–motor integration relative to a normative sample or to their own overall intellectual ability.

In summary, the research literature suggests that NF1 is associated with impairments in visual–spatial–perceptual functioning. It should be noted, however, that the deficits in motor and visual–perceptual skills that are seen in children with NF1 are part of a broader spectrum of impairments (i.e., lowered intelligence, language, learning, and executive function) displayed by these individuals.

BRAIN–BEHAVIOR RELATIONSHIPS

The foregoing discussion suggests that there is a close relationship between impairments in motor development and impairments in other areas of cognition and behavior. Diamond (2000) stated that "motor development and cognitive development may be much more interrelated than has been previously appreciated. Indeed, they may be fundamentally intertwined" (p. 44). What then is the neural basis for this relationship?

Cerebellum and Frontal Lobe

Until very recently, the neocerebellum and the prefrontal cortex were not thought to be involved in the same functions. The cerebellum was thought to be critical primarily for motor skills, whereas the dorsolateral prefrontal cortex was considered critical for complex cognitive abilities (Diamond, 2000). Evidence from neuroimaging studies, however, suggests that there is a close relationship between these two brain regions. Coactivation of the contralateral neocerebellum and the dorsolateral prefrontal cortex has been found with the verbal fluency task (Schlosser et al., 1998), the verb generation task (Raichle et al., 1994) and the Wisconsin card sorting test, a classic test of prefrontal brain function (Berman et al., 1995). Coactivation of these two regions has also been reported with nonmotor, working-memory tasks (Awh et al., 1996; Desmond, Gabrieli, Wagner, Ginier, & Glover, 1997; deZubicaray et al., 1998). The foregoing functional neuroimaging studies have also found that on cognitive tasks, increased activation of the dorsolateral prefrontal cortex is associated with increased activation in the contralateral cerebellum and that both the cerebellum and the prefrontal cortex are most active when the task is novel or when conditions change.

Once the task becomes familiar and does not demand as much concentration, both cerebellar and prefrontal activation decrease. Similarly, for motor tasks, cerebellar neurons are most active during the early stages of learning (Flament, Ellermann, Ugurbil, & Ebmer, 1994; Van Mier, et al., 1994). Once the task has been practiced, cerebellar activation decreases. Thus, the aforementioned studies show that cognitive task activation of the dorsolateral prefrontal cortex and the neocerebellum are highly correlated and that both the cerebellum and the prefrontal cortex appear to be involved in the learning of new tasks.

Studies of patients with brain damage provide support for the close association between the neocerebellum and the dorsolateral prefrontal cortex. It has been noted that cerebellar patients often do poorly on tasks that are associated with prefrontal functions such as verbal fluency (Schmahmann & Sherman, 1998), verb generation (Fiez et al., 1996), planning (Schmahmann & Sherman, 1998), and working memory (Fiez et al., 1996; Schmahmann & Sherman, 1998).

Studies of children with developmental problems provide further support for the close relationship between motor and cognitive functioning. As noted in previous sections of this chapter, children with motor impairments frequently display ADHD, learning disabilities, and specific language disorder. Motor and visual–motor impairments are frequently reported in children with ADHD, learning disabilities, and language disorders and in children with VLBW, Tourette syndrome, NF1, and autism spectrum disorders. Finally, children with nonprogressive (i.e., cerebral palsy) and progressive motor disorders (i.e., Duchenne muscular dystrophy) also display cognitive deficits (see Blondis, Chapter 5, this volume).

Neuroimaging and behavioral studies provide support for the interrelationship between motor and cognitive impairments in these populations. Several neuroimaging studies have reported that children with ADHD have smaller cerebellums than do normal controls (Berquin et al., 1998; Castellanos, 1997; Castellanos et al., 1996; Mostofsky, Reiss, Lockhart, & Denckla, 1998) and that they have significant reductions in the size of the frontal cortex (Castellanos et al., 1996; Filipek et al., 1997). They have also reported that children with ADHD show unusual prefrontal activity (Amen, Paldi, & Thisted, 1993; Vaidya et al., 1998). Neuroimaging studies of individuals with dyslexia have also found abnormalities in the activation of the cerebellum associated with a sequence of finger movements (Nicolson et al., 1999). Investigations of the motor behavior of children with ADHD also suggest that their motor impairments are associated with cerebellar dysfunction (problems in balance, rapid alternating movements, and consistently producing movements of the correct distance or correct timing) (Diamond, 2000). Problems in timing precision on bimanual tasks, a cerebellar function (Ivry & Keele, 1989; Keele & Ivry, 1990), have also been reported in children with dyslexia (Wolff et al., 1990). Thus, children with cognitive impairments (e.g., ADHD and dyslexia) display concomitant motor problems that appear to be associated with cerebellar dysfunction.

Numerous studies of children with autistic spectrum disorder have found evidence of pathology in the cerebellum (Bailey et al., 1998; Courchesne, 1991, 1997; Gaffney, Tsai, Kuperman, & Minchin, 1987; Guerin et al., 1996). Children with autism spectrum disorders also display certain cognitive and behavioral deficits that suggest frontal lobe dysfunction (i.e., deficits in attention, set-shifting, cognitive planning, and problem solving) (Hughes, Russell, & Robbins, 1994; Pennington & Ozonoff, 1996; Rumsey & Hamburger, 1990; Townsend, Harris, & Courchesne, 1996). Recent neuropathological and neuroimaging studies have found evidence that provides neuro-anatomical support for the hypothesis that these individuals have frontal lobe damage. Carper and Courchesne (2000) found that the frontal lobe volume was increased in some patients with autism and that this increase correlated with the degree of cerebellar abnormality.

The aforementioned findings support the close link between cerebellar and frontal lobe functions and indicate that the cerebellum and the frontal cortex are parts of an interconnected neural system in which the dysfunction at one site can cause mal-development of other brain sites (Carper & Courchesne, 2000; Diamond, 2000). Investigators have shown that abnormal neural activity can affect the development of the cerebral cortex (Killackey, 1990; Quartz & Sejnowski, 1997); therefore, abnormal neural activity in the cerebellar projections to the frontal cortex could cause mal-development of the frontal lobes and any other brain region receiving this input (Carper & Courchesne, 2000; Diamond, 2000). Diamond (2000) suggests that another reason why abnormalities of the neocerebellum and the prefrontal cortex occur in the same disorders may be because both regions "have extended periods of maturation; insults too late in development to affect the maturation of other neural structures can have profound consequences for both prefrontal and cerebellar development" (p. 49). Thus, the coexistence of frontal and cerebellar abnormalities helps in explaining the co-occurrence of motor and cognitive impairments in children with various developmental disorders.

Basal Ganglia

Research has also suggested that the basal ganglia and specifically the caudate nucleus are important for movement control such as selecting the proper movement, the appropriate muscles to perform the movement, or the appropriate force to execute the movement (Groves, 1983; Stelmach & Worringham, 1988). It has also been shown that the caudate is a major output structure of dorsolateral prefrontal cortex (Selemon & Goldman-Rakic, 1988). Damage to the basal ganglia and caudate, as seen in Parkinson's disease and Huntington's chorea, results in significant problems in movement control (Albin, Young, & Penney, 1989; Halliday et al., 1998). Studies of children with ADHD have found size reductions and reduced left–right asymmetry in the caudate nucleus (Filipek et al., 1997; Hynd et al., 1993). Neuroimaging studies have also reported reduced activity in the caudate in children with ADHD during the performance of cognitive tasks relative to control children (Lou, Henriksen, Bruhn, Borner, & Nielsen, 1989; Teicher, Ito, Glod, & Barber, 1996; Vaidya et al., 1998). The caudate has also been implicated in Tourette syndrome. In a study of monozygotic twins concordant for tics, Hyde and colleagues (1995) found that the right caudate nucleus was significantly reduced in the more severely affected twin. Thus, the caudate nucleus appears to play an important role in both motor and cognitive functioning in some children with developmental disorders.

Right-Hemisphere Dysfunction

As noted previously, many children with developmental disorders display not only motor problems but also problems in visual–motor integration. In fact, problems in visual–motor integration and visual perception have been found to be areas of particular difficulty for children with DCD, VLBW, cerebral palsy (i.e., spastic diplegia), Tourette syndrome, and NF1. But what do we know about the neural basis for deficits in visual–motor integration? Studies of adult patients with brain damage suggest that both cerebral hemispheres contribute to visual–motor integration but that the right hemisphere may have a more important role given the greater frequency of visual–motor problems with right-hemisphere lesions (Damasio, 1985). Lesions of the parietal cortex, particularly when the injury is on the right, result in impaired visual perception and deficits in fine motor coordination associated with visual guidance (Andersen, 1987). Neuroimaging studies of preterm children with spastic diplegia have also reported that lesions in the parietal and/or occipital white matter are associated with visuospatial deficits (Goto, Ota, Iai, Sugita, & Tanabe, 1994). Finally, Rourke (1995) states that nonverbal learning disabilities, which are found in children with DCD and Asperger syndrome, have visuospatial deficits as a major feature, and are the result of lesions in the white matter of the right hemisphere. Thus, there is a large body of evidence that suggests that the nondominant (i.e., right) hemisphere, and particularly the parietal lobe, is involved in visuospatial processes that contribute to visual–motor integration. Visual–motor integration, however, also requires the exchange of information between the parietal region and the motor areas of the frontal cortex (Quintana & Fuster, 1993) with the subcortical areas providing an integrative function (Alexander, Delong, & Strick, 1986). As a result, deficits in visual–motor integration may arise from frontal and subcortical, as well as parietal, lobe lesions (Marshall et al., 1994).

Conclusion

The foregoing discussion emphasizes the close interconnections of the various brain regions that are involved in motor and cognitive functions. Because of these interconnections, abnormalities in one area of the brain such as the cerebellum may have a detrimental effect on the development of another region (i.e., frontal lobe). These bidirectional influences may result in the variety of "comorbidities" that are found in children with developmental disorders, with different combinations of disorders resulting depending on the parts of the neural system that are affected. Thus, damage to slightly different areas of the cerebellum, frontal lobe, parietal lobe, or the caudate might result in a very different pattern of cognitive and motor strengths and weaknesses.

ATYPICAL BRAIN DEVELOPMENT
AS A NEW CONCEPTUAL FRAMEWORK

The foregoing review suggests that there are several ways in which the term *comorbidity* is unsatisfactory. Surely the greatest problem is the fact that comorbidity of developmental disorders is the rule, not the exception. The scientific world has gone to great pains to prove what every clinician and educator already knows: It is an unusual child whose development is atypical in only one area. Thus children with reading disabilities often have ADHD, children with ADHD frequently meet criteria for some other psychiatric condition, and children with DCD and no other disability are found only rarely.

A second problem with our current conceptualization of comorbidity in relation to DCD and the other developmental disorders is that the etiology of these disorders is probably variable. There is research in support of both genetic and environmental factors contributing to the development of these problems. Indeed, it is not likely that one common factor alone will ever explain a significant majority of developmental cases in the population. In support of this variability is the fact that the neuroanatomy of developmental disorders also varies. The research to date indicates that one-to-one correspondence simply does not exist for developmental learning disabilities and specific regions of the brain.

Elsewhere, we have proposed a new conceptual framework for thinking about developmental disorders: atypical brain development (ABD) (Dewey et al., 2002; Gilger & Kaplan, 2001; Kaplan et al., 1998, 2001). The ABD concept is intended to resolve several problems—the growing awareness that developmental disabilities are typically nonspecific and heterogeneous and also the growing scientific literature showing that comorbidity of symptoms and syndromes is the rule rather than the exception. ABD does not itself represent a specific disorder or disease. It is a term that can be used to address the full range of developmental disorders that are found to be overlapping much of the time in any sample of children with these disorders.

According to an ABD conceptualization, the structural or activational anomalies in the brain of an individual with a developmental disability are probably numerous, though they may be more heavily focused in one region or another perhaps giving rise to a person's primary diagnosis. Therefore, the symptoms exhibited by people (e.g., motor, reading, math, spelling, attentional, or some combination) will depend on the relative amount of anomalous development in primary ability areas of the brain (e.g., supplementary motor areas or connections in, around, or to and from the parietal lobe) and which of the many other brain areas are also affected. Of course, there will be individuals with ABD who have anomalies in a very localized area, but such cases are probably in the minority.

If one accepts that the brain is responsible for all behavior, then individual differences in behavior are due to individual differences in brain development and activity, whether these individual differences are genetic or environmental in origin. Consequently, the idea of ABD has some similarities to an older, once-popular theory of etiology—namely, minimal brain dysfunction, or MBD (Clements & Peters, 1962; Rie & Rie, 1980). The concept of MBD is flawed, however, which is why its usefulness declined out over the years.

We think that the concept of ABD is superior to that of MBD for several reasons. First, *atypical* appropriately differs from the MBD concept of *dysfunction* or *damage* in that it can encompass phenomena such as children with superior intelligence, nonverbal disabilities, hyperlexia, and more (Gardner, 1982; Pennington, 1991; Rourke & Tsatsanis, 1996). Second, the term *brain* serves as a reminder that all learning and behavior are brain-based. Third, the term *development* accurately designates the fact that developmental disorders are probably the result of prenatal, and to a lesser extent early postnatal, brain growth and elaboration, including that which is due to genes and intrauterine environmental effects (Duane, 1999; Galaburda, Schrott, Sherman, Rosen, & Denenberg, 1996; Hynd, Semrud-Clikeman, & Lyytinen, 1991; Lyon & Chhabra, 1996; Pennington, 1991; Plante, 1991; Raff, 1996; Shapleske, Rossell, Woodruff, & David, 1999). Many extraordinary skills may also arise from the same developmental processes. In the ABD conceptualization, superlative skills represent natural biological potentials developed in conjunction with environmentally fostered elaborations (Gardner, 1982; Geary, 1996; West, 1999). Finally, ABD differs significantly from MBD because the latter was thought to be a unitary syndrome where a fairly specific collection of symptoms was required for diagnosis (Clements & Peters, 1962). In contrast, ABD is meant to serve as a unifying concept of etiology, the expression of which is variable within and across individuals. ABD does not itself represent a specific disorder or syndrome and ABD does not pertain to brain injury, trauma, or disease in the classic medical sense. Rather, ABD is a concept developed to describe the developmental variation of the brain. It is a practical concept that highlights the variable etiology of developmental problems, their variable neuroanatomical basis, and the enormous overlap of symptoms that we have incorrectly referred to as comorbidity.

ACKNOWLEDGMENTS

Grants from the Alberta Children's Hospital Foundation, the Alberta Mental Health Research Board, and the Canadian Institutes of Health Research supported the preparation of this chapter and some of the reported research.

REFERENCES

Ahonen, T. (1990). *Developmental coordination disorders in children: A developmental neuropsychological follow-up study* (Jyvaskyla Studies in Education, Psychology, and Social Research, 78). Jyvaskyla: University of Jyvaskyla.

Albin, R. L., Young, A. B., & Penney, J. (1989). The functional anatomy of basal ganglia disorders. *Trends in Neuroscience, 12,* 366–375.

Alexander, G. E., Delong, M. R., & Strick, P. L. (1986). Parallel organization of functionally segregated circuits linking basal ganglia and cortex. *Annual Review of Neuroscience, 9,* 357–381.

Amen, D. G., Paldi, F., & Thisted, R. A. (1993). Brain SPECT imaging. *Journal of American Academy of Child and Adolescent Psychiatry, 32,* 1080–1081.

American Psychiatric Association. (1994). *Diagnostic and statistical manual of mental disorders* (4th ed.). Washington, DC: Author.

Andersen, R. A. (1987). Inferior parietal lobule function in spatial perception and visuomotor integration. In F. Plum, V. B. Mountcastle, & S. R. Geiger (Eds.), *The handbook of physiology. Section 1: The nervous system, Vol. 5. Higher functions of the brain* (pp. 483–518). Bethesda, MD: American Physiological Society.

Angold, A. (1988). Childhood and adolescent depression I: Epidemiological and aetiological aspects. *British Journal of Psychiatry, 152,* 601–617.

Angold, A., Costello, E. J., & Erkanli, A. (1999). Comorbidity. *Journal of Child Psychology and Psychiatry, 40,* 57–87.

Awh, E., Jonides, J., Smith, E. E., Schumacher, E. H., Koeppe, R. A., & Kazt, S. (1996). Dissociation of storage and rehearsal in verbal working memory: Evidence from positron emission tomography. *Psychological Science, 7,* 25–31.

Bailey, A., Luthert, P., Dean, A., Harding, B., Janota, I., Montgomery, M., et al. (1998). A clinicopathological study of autism. *Brain, 121,* 889–905.

Barkley, R. A., DuPaul, G. J., & McMurray, M. B. (1990). A comprehensive evaluation of attention deficit hyperactivity disorder with and without hyperactivity. *Journal of Consulting and Clinical Psychology, 58*, 775–789.

Barnett, A. L., Kooistra, L., & Henderson, S. E. (1998). Editorial: "Clumsiness" as syndrome and symptom. *Human Movement Science, 17*, 435–447.

Bawden, H., Dooley, J., Buckley, D., Camfield, P., Gordon, K., Riding, M., et al. (1996). MRI and nonverbal cognitive deficits in children with neurofibromatosis 1 referred for learning disabilities are sex-specific. *American Journal of Medical Genetics, 67*, 127–132.

Berman, K. F., Ostrem, J. L., Randoulph, C., Gold, J., Goldberg, T. E., Coppola, R., et al. (1995). Physiological activation of a cortical network during performance of the Wisconsin Card Sorting Test: A positron emission tomography study. *Neuropsychologia, 33*, 1027–1046.

Berquin, P. C., Gidd, J. N., Jacobsen, L. K., Burger, S. D., Krain, A. L., Rapoport, J. L., et al. (1998). Cerebellum in attention-deficit hyperactivity disorder. A morphometric MRI study. *Neurology, 50*, 1087–1093.

Cantell, M. (1998). Developmental coordination disorder in adolescence: Perceptual–motor, academic and social outcomes of early motor delay. *LIKES-Research Report on Sport and Health, 112*.

Cantell, M. H., Smyth, M. M., & Ahonen, T. P. (1994). Clumsiness in adolescence: Educational, motor and social outcomes of motor delay detected at 5 years. *Adapted Physical Activity Quarterly, 11*, 115–129.

Carper, R. A., & Courchesne, E. (2000). Inverse correlation between frontal lobe and cerebellum sizes in children with autism. *Brain, 123*, 836–844.

Castellanos, F. X. (1997). Toward a pathophysiology of attention-deficit/hyperactivity disorder. *Clinical Pediatrics, 36*, 381–393.

Castellanos, F. X., Giedd, J. N., Marsh, W. L., Hamburger, S. D., Vaituzis, A. C., Dickstein, D. P., et al. (1996). Quantitative brain magnetic resonance imaging in attention-deficit hyperactivity disorder. *Archives of General Psychiatry, 53*, 607–616.

Chapman, C. A., Waber, D. P., Bassett, N., Urion, D. K., & Korf, B. R. (1996). Neurobehavioral profiles of children with neurofibromatosis I referred for learning disabilities and sex-specific. *American Journal of Medical Genetics, 67*, 127–132.

Clements, S. G., & Peters, J. E. (1962). Minimal brain dysfunctions in the school-age child. *Archives of General Psychiatry, 6*, 185–197.

Courchesne, E. (1991). Neuroanatomical imaging in autism. *Pediatrics, 87*, 781–790.

Courchesne, E. (1997). Brainstem, cerebellar and limbic neuroanatomical abnormalities in autism. *Current Opinions in Neurobiology, 7*, 269–278.

Damasio, A. R. (1985). Disorders of complex visual processing: Agnosias, achromatopsia, Balint's syndrome and related difficulties of orientation and construction. In M. M. Mesulam (Ed.), *Principles of behavioral neurology* (pp. 259–288). Philadelphia: Davis.

Denckla, M. B., & Roeltgen, D. P. (1992). Disorders of motor function and control. In I. Rapin & S. J. Segalowitz (Eds.), *Handbook of neuropsychology. Vol. 6: Child neuropsychology* (pp. 455–476). New York: Elsevier Science.

Denckla, M. B., & Rudel, R. G. (1978). Anomalies of motor development in hyperactive boys free of learning disabilities. *Annals of Neurology, 3*, 231–233.

Desmond, J. E., Gabrieli, J. D. E., Wagner, A. D., Ginier, B. I., & Glover, G. H. (1997). Lobular patterns of cerebellar activation in verbal working memory and finger tapping tasks as revealed by functional MRI. *Journal of Neuroscience, 17*, 9675–9685.

Dewey, D., Crawford, S. G., Creighton, D. E., & Sauve, R. S. (1999). Long-term neuropsychological outcomes in very low birth weight children free of sensorineural impairments. *Journal of Clinical and Experimental Neuropsychology, 21*, 851–65.

Dewey, D., Crawford, S., Kaplan, B., & Wilson, B. (2003). Memory abilities in children with developmental coordination disorder. *Journal of the International Neuropsychological Society, 9,* 210.

Dewey, D., & Kaplan, B. J. (1994). Subtyping of developmental motor deficits. *Developmental Neuropsychology, 10,* 265–284.

Dewey, D., Kaplan, B. J., Crawford, S. G., & Wilson, B. N. (2002). Developmental coordination disorder: Associated problems in attention, learning, and psychosocial adjustment. *Human Movement Science, 21,* 905–918.

Dewey, D., & Wall, K. (1997). Praxis and memory deficits in language impaired children. *Developmental Neuropsychology, 13,* 507–512.

Dewey, D., Wilson, B. N., Crawford, S. G., & Kaplan, B. J. (2000). Comorbidity of developmental coordination disorder with ADHD and reading disability. *Journal of the International Neuropsychological Society, 6,* 152.

deZubicaray, G. I., Williams, S. C., Wilson, S. J., Rose, S. E., Brammer, M. J., Bullmore, E., et al. (1998). Prefrontal cortex involvement in selective letter generation: A functional magnetic resonance imaging study. *Cortex, 34,* 389–401.

Diamond, A. (2000). Close interrelation of motor development and cognitive development and the cerebellum and prefrontal cortex. *Child Development, 71,* 44–56.

Dilts, C. V., Carey, J. C., Kircher, J. C., Hoffman, R. O., Creel, D., Ward, K., et al. (1996). Children and adolescents with neurofibromatosis 1: A behavioral phenotype. *Journal of Developmental and Behavioral Pediatrics, 17,* 229–39.

Drillien, C., & Drummond, M. (1983). *Clinics in developmental medicine, Vol. 86: Developmental screening and the child with special needs: A population study of 5000 children.* London: S.I.M.P. with Heinemann Medical.

Duane, D. D. (Ed.). (1999). *Reading and attention disorders: Neurobiological correlates.* Timonium, MD: York Press.

Dwyer, C., & McKenzie, B. E. (1994). Visual memory impairment in clumsy children. *Adapted Physical Activity Quarterly, 11,* 179–189.

Eldridge, R., Denckla, M. B., Bien, E., Myers, S., Kaiser-Kupfer, M. I., Pikus, A., et al. (1989). Neurofibromatosis type 1 (Recklinghausen's disease). Neurologic and cognitive assessment with sibling controls. *American Journal of Diseases of Children, 143,* 833–837.

Eliason, M. J. (1986). Neurofibromatosis: Implications for learning and behavior. *Developmental and Behavioral Pediatrics, 7,* 175–179.

Fawcett, A. J., & Nicolson, R. I. (1995). Persistent deficits in motor skill of children with dyslexia. *Journal of Motor Behavior, 27,* 235–240.

Ferner, R. E., Hughes, R. A. C., & Weinman, J. (1996). Intellectual impairments in neurofibromatosis 1. *Journal of Neurological Sciences, 138,* 125–133.

Fiez, J. A., Raife, E. A., Balota, D. A., Schwarz, J. P., Raichle, M. E., & Petersen, S. E. (1996). A positron emission tomography study of the short-term maintenance of verbal information. *Journal of Neuroscience, 16,* 808–22.

Filipek, P. A., Semrud-Clikeman, M., Steingard, R. J., Renshaw, P. F., Kennedy, D. N., & Biederman, J. (1997). Volumetric MRI analysis comparing subjects having attention-deficit hyperactivity disorder with normal controls. *Neurology, 48,* 589–601.

Flament, D., Ellermann, J., Ugurbil, K., & Ebmer, T. J. (1994). Functional magnetic resonance imaging (fMRI) of cerebellar activation while learning to correct for visuomotor errors. *Society for Neuroscience Abstracts, 20,* 20.

Fox, M. A., & Lent, B. (1996). Clumsy children: Primer on developmental coordination disorder. *Canadian Family Physician, 42,* 1965–1971.

Gaffney, G. R., Tsai, L. Y., Kuperman, S., & Minchin, S. (1987). Cerebellar structure in autism. *American Journal of Diseases in Children, 141,* 1330–1332.

Galaburda, A. M., Schrott, L. M., Sherman, G. F., Rosen, G., & Denenberg, V. H. (1996). Animal models of developmental dyslexia. In C. Chase, G. Rosen, & G. Sherman (Eds.), *De-*

velopmental dyslexia: Neural, cognitive and genetic mechanisms (pp. 3–14). Baltimore: York Press.

Gardner, H. (1982). Giftedness: Speculations from a biological perspective. In G. Feldman (Ed.), *New directions in child development: Approaches to giftedness and creativity* (pp. 47–60), San Francisco: Jossey-Bass.

Geary, D. (1996). Sexual selection and sex differences in mathematical ability. *Behavioral and Brain Sciences, 19,* 229–284.

Geuze, R. H., & Kalverboer, A. F. (1994). Tapping a rhythm: A problem of timing for children who are clumsy and dyslexic? *Adapted Physical Activity Quarterly, 11,* 203–213.

Gilger, J. W., & Kaplan, B. J. (2001). Atypical brain development: A conceptual framework for understanding developmental learning disabilities. *Developmental Neuropsychology, 20,* 465–481.

Gilger, J. W., Pennington, B. F., & DeFries, J. C. (1992). A twin study of the etiology of comorbidity: Attention-deficit hyperactivity disorder and dyslexia. *Journal of the American Academy of Child and Adolescent Psychiatry, 31,* 343–348.

Gillberg, C., & Rasmussen, P. (1982). Perceptual, motor and attentional deficits in six-year-old children: Background factors. *Acta Paediatrica Scandinavica, 71,* 121–129.

Gillberg, C., Rasmussen, P., Carlstrom, G., Svenson, B., & Waldenstrom, E. (1982). Perceptual, motor and attentional deficits in six-year-old children: Epidemiological aspects. *Journal of Child Psychology and Psychiatry, 23,* 131–134.

Gillberg, I. C., & Gillberg, C. (1989). Children with preschool minor neurodevelopmental disorders. IV: Behaviour and school achievement at age 13. *Developmental Medicine and Child Neurology, 31,* 3–13.

Gordon, N., & McKinlay, I. (1980). *Helping clumsy children.* New York: Churchill Livingstone.

Gorga, D., Stern, F. M., Ross, G., & Nagler, W. (1991). The neuromotor behavior of preterm and full-term children by three years of age: Quality of movement and variability. *Journal of Developmental and Behavior Pediatrics, 12,* 102–107.

Goto, M., Ota, R., Iai, M., Sugita, K., & Tanabe, Y. (1994). MRI changes and deficits of higher brain functions in preterm diplegia. *Acta Paediatrica, 83,* 506–511.

Gottesman, R. L., Hankin, D., Levinson, W., & Beck, P. (1984). Neurodevelopmental functioning of good and poor readers in urban schools. *Journal of Developmental and Behavioral Pediatrics, 5,* 109–115.

Groves, P. M. (1983). A theory of the functional organization of the neostriatum and the neostriatal control of voluntary movement. *Brain Research Reviews, 286,* 109–132.

Grunau, R. E., Whitfield, M. F., & Davis, C. (2003). Patterns of learning disabilities in children with extremely low birth weight and broadly average intelligence. *Archives of Pediatric and Adolescent Medicine, 156,* 615–620.

Gubbay, S. S. (1975). *The clumsy child.* London: Saunders.

Guerin, P., Lyon, G., Barthelemy, C., Sostak, E., Chevrollier, V., Garreau, B., et al. (1996). Neuropathological study of a case of autistic syndrome with severe mental retardation. *Developmental Medicine and Child Neurology, 38,* 203–211.

Hack, M., Breslau, N., Aram, D., Weissman, B., Klein, N., & Borawski-Clark, E. (1992). The effect of very low birth weight on neurocognitive abilities at school age. *Journal of Developmental and Behavioral Pediatrics, 13,* 412–420.

Hack, M., Taylor, H. G., Klein, N., Schatschneider, C., & Mercuri-Minich, N. (1994). School-age outcomes in children with birth weights under 750 g. *New England Journal of Medicine, 331,* 753–759.

Halliday, G. M., McRitchie, D. A., Macdonald, V., Double, K. L., Trent, R. J., & McCusker, E. (1998). Regional specificity of brain atrophy in Huntington's disease. *Experimental Neuropsychology, 154,* 663–672.

Hellgren, L., Gillberg, C., & Gillberg, I. C. (1994). Children with deficits in attention, motor control and perception (DAMP) almost grown up: The contribution of various background factors to outcome at the age of 16 years. *European Child and Adolescent Psychiatry, 3*, 1–15.

Hellgren, L., Gillberg, I. C., Bagenholm, A., & Gillberg, C. (1994). Children with deficits in attention, motor control and perception (DAMP) almost grown up: Psychiatric and personality disorders at age 16 years. *Journal of Child Psychology and Psychiatry, 35*, 1255–1271.

Henderson, S. E., Barnett, A., & Henderson, L. (1994). Visuospatial difficulties and clumsiness: On the interpretation of conjoined deficits. *Journal of Child Psychology and Psychiatry, 35*, 961–969.

Henderson, S. E., & Hall, D. (1982). Concomitants of clumsiness in young school children. *Developmental Medicine and Child Neurology, 24*, 448–460.

Herrgard, E., Luoma, L., Tuppurainen, K., Karjalainen, S., & Martikainen, A. (1993). Neurodevelopmental profile at five years of children born at < 32 weeks gestation. *Developmental Medicine and Child Neurology, 35*, 1083–1096.

Hill, E. L., Bishop, D. V. M., & Nimmo-Smith, I. (1998). Representational gestures in developmental coordination disorder and specific language impairment: Error-types and the reliability of ratings. *Human Movement Science, 17*, 655–678.

Hofman, K. J., Harris, E. L., Bryan, R. N., & Denckla, M. B. (1994). Neurofibromatosis type 1: The cognitive phenotype. *Journal of Pediatric, 124*(Suppl.), S1–S8.

Hughes, C., Russell, J., & Robbins, T. W. (1994). Evidence for executive dysfunction in autism. *Neuropsychologia, 32*, 477–492.

Hulme, C., & Lord, R. (1986). Clumsy children—A review of recent research. *Child: Care, Health and Development, 12*, 257–269.

Hulme, C., Smart, A., & Moran, G. (1982). Visual perceptual deficits in clumsy children. *Neuropsychologia, 20*, 475–481.

Hulme, C., Smart, A., Moran, G., & McKinlay, I. (1984). Visual kinaesthetic and cross-modal judgements of length by clumsy children: A comparison with young normal children. *Child: Care, Health and Development, 10*, 117–125.

Hulme, C., & Snowling, M. (1992). Deficits in output phonology: An explanation of reading failure? *Cognitive Neuropsychology, 9*, 47–72.

Hunt, J. V., & Cooper, B. A. B., Tooley, W. H. (1988). Very low birth weight infants at 8 and 11 years of age: Role of neonatal illness and family status. *Pediatrics, 82*, 596–603.

Hyde, T. M., Stacey, M. E., Coppola, R., Handel, S. F., Rickler, K. C, & Weinberger, D. R. (1995). Cerebral morphometric abnormalities in Tourette's syndrome: A quantitative MRI study of monozygotic twins. *Neurology, 45*, 1176–1182.

Hynd, G., Semrud-Clikeman, M., & Lyytinen, H. (1991). Brain imaging in learning disabilities. In J. Orbrzut & G. Hynd (Eds.), *Neuropsychological foundations of learning disabilities* (pp. 475–511). New York: Academic Press.

Hynd, G. W., Herm, K. L., Novey, E. S., Eliopulos, D., Marshall, R., Gonzalez, J. J., et al. (1993). Attention-deficit hyperactivity disorder and asymmetry of the caudate nucleus. *Journal of Child Neurology, 8*, 339–347.

Ivry, R. B., & Keele, S. W. (1989). Timing functions of the cerebellum. *Journal of Cognitive Neuroscience, 1*, 136–152.

Jongmans, M., Demetre, J. D., Dubowitz, L., & Henderson, S. E. (1996). How local is the impact of a specific learning difficulty on premature children's evaluation of their own competence? *Journal of Child Psychology and Psychiatry, 37*, 565–568.

Jongmans, M. J., Mercuri, E., Dubowitz, L. M. S., & Henderson, S. E. (1998). Perceptual–motor difficulties and their concomitants in six-year-old children born prematurely. *Human Movement Science, 17*, 629–654.

Kadesjo, B., & Gillberg, C. (1998). Attention deficits and clumsiness in Swedish 7-year-old children. *Developmental Medicine and Child Neurology, 40*, 796–804.

Kaplan, B. J., Crawford, S. G., Wilson, B. N., & Dewey, D. (2000). Does "pure" ADHD exist? *Journal of the International Neuropsychological Society, 6*, 153.

Kaplan, B. J., Dewey, D. M., Crawford, S. G., & Wilson, B. N. (2001). The term "comorbidity" is of questionable value in reference to developmental disorders: Data and theory. *Journal of Learning Disabilities, 34*, 555–565.

Kaplan, B. J., Wilson, B. N., Dewey, D. M., & Crawford, S. G. (1998). DCD may not be a discrete disorder. *Human Movement Science, 17*, 471–490.

Keele, S. W., & Ivry, R. (1990). Does the cerebellum provide a common computation for diverse tasks? A timing hypothesis. *Annals of the New York Academy of Sciences, 608*, 179–207.

Keller, H., Ayub, B. V., Saigal, S., & Bar-Or, O. (1998). Neuromotor ability in 5 to 7-year-old children with very low or extremely low birthweight. *Developmental Medicine and Child Neurology, 40*, 661–666.

Killackey, H. A. (1990). Neocortical expansion: An attempt toward relating phylogeny and ontogeny. *Journal of Cognitive Neuroscience, 2*, 1–17.

Klein, N. K., Hack, M., & Breslau, N. (1989). Children who were very low birth weight: Developmental and academic achievement at nine years of age. *Journal of Developmental and Behavioral Pediatrics, 10*, 32–37.

Losse, A., Henderson, S. A., Elliman, D., Hall, D., Knight, E., & Jongmans, M. (1991). Clumsiness in children: Do they grow out of it? A 10-year follow-up study. *Developmental Medicine and Child Neurology, 33*, 55–68.

Lou, H. C., Henriksen, L., Bruhn, P., Borner, H., & Nielsen, J. B. (1989). Striatal dysfunction in attention deficit and hyperkinetic disorder. *Archives of Neurology, 46*, 48–52.

Lyon, R. G., & Chhabra, V. (1996). The current state of science and the future of specific reading disability. *Mental Retardation and Developmental Disabilities Research Reviews, 2*, 2–9.

Marlow, N., Roberts, B. L., & Cooke, R. W. I. (1989). Motor skills in extremely low birth weight children at the age of 6 years. *Archives of Disease in Childhood, 64*, 839–847.

Marshall, R. S., Lazar, R. M., Binder, J. R., Desmond, D. W., Drucker, P. M., & Mohr, J. P. (1994). Intrahemispheric localization of drawing dysfunction. *Neuropsychologia, 32*, 493–502.

Moore, B. D., Slopis, J. M., Schomer, D., Jackson, E. F., & Levy, B. M. (1996). Neuropsychological significance of areas of high signal intensity on brain MRIs of children with neurofibromatosis. *Neurology, 46*, 1660–1668.

Mostofsky, S. H., Reiss, A. L., Lockhart, P., & Denckla, M. B. (1998). Evaluation of cerebellar size in attention-deficit hyperactivity disorder. *Journal of Child Neurology, 13*, 434–439.

Mutch, L., Leyland, A., & McGee, A. (1993). Patterns of neuropsychological function in a low-birthweight population. *Developmental Medicine and Child Neurology, 35*, 943–956.

Nicolson, R. I., & Fawcett, A. J. (1994). Comparison of deficits in cognitive and motor skills among children with dyslexia. *Annals of Dyslexia, 44*, 147–164.

Nicolson, R. I., Fawcett, A. J., Berry, E. L., Jenkins, I. H., Dean, P., & Brooks, D. J. (1999). Association of abnormal cerebellar activation with motor learning difficulties in dyslexic adults. *Lancet, 353*, 1662–1667.

North, K., Joy, P., Yuille, D., Cocks, N., Mobbs, E., Hutchins, P., et al. (1994). Specific learning disability in children with neurofibromatosis type 1: Significance of MRI abnormalities. *Neurology, 44*, 878–883.

Ozonoff, S. (1999). Cognitive impairment in neurofibromatosis type 1. *American Journal of Medical Genetics, 89*, 45–52.

Parush, S., Yochman, A., Cohen, D., & Gershon, E. (1998). Relation of visual perception and visual-motor integration for clumsy children. *Perceptual and Motor Skills, 86*, 291–295.

Pennington, B. F. (1991). *Diagnosing learning disorders: A neuropsychological framework.* New York: Guilford Press.

Pennington, B. F., & Ozonoff, S. (1996). Executive functions and developmental psychopathology. *Journal of Child Psychology and Psychiatry, 37,* 51–87.

Pharoah, P. O. D., Stevenson, C. J., Cooke, R. W. I., & Stevenson, R. C. (1994). Clinical and subclinical deficits at 8 years in a geographically defined cohort of low birthweight infants. *Archives of Disease in Childhood, 70,* 264–270.

Piek, J. P., & Coleman-Carman, R. (1995). Kinaesthetic sensitivity and motor performance of children with developmental co-ordination disorder. *Developmental Medicine and Child Neurology, 37,* 976–984.

Piek, J. P., Pitcher, T. M., & Hay, D. A. (1999). Motor coordination and kinaesthesis in boys with attention deficit-hyperactivity disorder. *Developmental Medicine and Child Neurology, 41,* 159–165.

Plante, E. (1991). MRI findings in the parents and siblings of specifically language-impaired boys. *Brain and Language, 41,* 67–80.

Powell, R. P., & Bishop, D. V. M. (1992). Clumsiness and perceptual problems in children with specific language impairment. *Developmental Medicine and Child Neurology, 34,* 755–765.

Powls, A., Botting, N., Cooke, R. W. I., & Marlow, N. (1995). Motor impairment in children 12 to 13 years old with a birthweight of less than 1250 g. *Archives of Disease in Childhood, 72,* F62–F66.

Quartz, S. R., & Sejnowski, T. J. (1997). The neural basis of cognitive development: A constructivist manifesto. *Behavioural Brain Science, 20,* 537–556.

Quintana, J., & Fuster, J. M. (1993). Spatial and temporal factors in the role of prefrontal and parietal cortex in visuomotor integration. *Cerebral Cortex, 3,* 122–132.

Raff, M. (1996). Neural development: Mysterious no more? *Science, 274,* 1063.

Raichle, M. E., Fiez, J. A., Videen, T. O., MacLeod, A. M., Pardo, J. V., Fox, P. T., et al. (1994). Practice-related changes in human brain functional anatomy during nonmotor learning. *Cerebral Cortex, 4,* 8–26.

Rickards, A. L., Kitchen, W. H., Doyle, L. W., Ford, G. W., Kelly, E. A., & Callanan, C. (1993). Cognitive, school performance and behavior in very low birth weight and normal birth weight children at 8 years of age: A longitudinal study. *Journal of Developmental and Behavioral Pediatrics, 14,* 363–368.

Rie, H., & Rie, E. (1980). *Handbook of minimal brain dysfunctions: A critical review.* New York: Wiley.

Rösblad, B. (2001). Visual perception in children with developmental coordination disorder. In S. A. Cermak & D. Larkin (Eds.), *Developmental coordination disorder* (pp. 104–116). Albany, NY: Delmar.

Roth, S. C., Baudin, J., Pezzani-Goldsmith, M., Townsend, J., Reynolds, E. O. R., & Stewart, A. L. (1994). Relation between neurodevelopmental status of very preterm infants at one and eight years. *Developmental Medicine and Child Neurology, 36,* 1049–1062.

Rourke, B., & Tsatsanis, K. D. (1996). Syndrome of nonverbal learning disabilities: Psycholinguistic assets and deficits. *Topics in Language Development, 16,* 30–44.

Rourke, B. P. (Ed.). (1995). *Syndrome of nonverbal learning disabilities: Neurodevelopmental manifestations.* New York: Guilford Press.

Roussounis, S. H., Gaussen, T. H., & Stratton, P. (1987). A 2-year follow-up study of children with motor coordination problems identified at school entry age. *Child: Care, Health and Development, 13,* 377–391.

Rumsey, J. M., & Hamburger, S. D. (1990). Neuropsychological divergence of high-level autism and severe dyslexia. *Journal of Autism and Developmental Disorders, 20,* 155–168.

Safer, S. Q., Shaffer, D., O'Conner, P. A., & Stokman, C. (1986). Hard thoughts on neurological soft signs. In M. Rutter (Ed.), *Developmental neuropsychiatry* (pp. 133–143). Edinburgh, Scotland: Churchill Livingstone.

Saigal, S., Rosenbaum, P., Szatmari, P., & Campbell, D. (1991). Learning disability and school problems in a regional cohort of extremely low birth weight (1000G) children: A comparison with term controls. *Journal of Developmental and Behavioral Pediatrics, 12,* 294–300.

Schlosser, R., Hutchinson, M., Joseffer, S., Rusinek, H., Saarimaki, A., Stevenson, J., et al. (1998). Functional magnetic resonance imaging of human brain activity in a verbal fluency task. *Journal of Neurology Neurosurgery, and Psychiatry, 64,* 492–498.

Schmahmann, J. D., & Sherman, J. C. (1998). The cerebellar cognitive affective syndrome. *Brain, 121,* 561–579.

Selemon, L. D., & Goldman-Rakic, P. S. (1988). Common cortical and subcortical targets of the dorsolateral prefrontal and posterior parietal cortices in the rhesus monkey: Evidence for a distributed neural network subserving spatially guided behavior. *Journal of Neuroscience, 8,* 4049–4068.

Shapleske, J., Rossell, S. L., Woodruff, P. W. R., & David, A. S. (1999). The planum temporale: A systematic, quantitative review of its structural, functional and clinical significance. *Brain Research Reviews, 29,* 26–49.

Sheslow, D., & Adams, W. (1990). *Wide Range Assessment of Memory and Learning.* Wilmington, DE: Jastak.

Silver, L. B. (Ed.). (1992). *The misunderstood child: A guide for parents of children with learning disabilities.* Blue Ridge Summit, PA: Tab Books.

Skorji, V., & McKenzie, B. E. (1997). How do children who are clumsy remember modelled movements? *Developmental Medicine and Child Neurology, 39,* 404–408.

Smyth, T. R., & Glencross, D. J. (1986). Information processing deficits in clumsy children. *Australian Journal of Psychology, 38,* 13–22.

Snow, J. H., Blondis, T., & Brady, L. (1988). Motor and sensory abilities with normal and academically at-risk children. *Archives of Clinical Neuropsychology, 3,* 227–238.

Stelmach, G. E., & Worringham, C. J. (1988). The preparation and production of isometric force in Parkinson's disease. *Neuropsychologia, 26,* 93–103.

Stine, S. B., & Adams, W. V. (1989). Learning problems in neurofibromatosis patients. *Clinical Orthopedics and Related Research, 245,* 43–48.

Stott, D. H., Moyes, F. A., & Henderson, S. E. (1984). *The Test of Motor Impairment—Henderson revision.* San Antonio, TX: Psychological Corp.

Sugden, D. A., & Wann, C. (1987). Kinaesthesis and motor impairment in children with moderate learning difficulties. *British Journal of Educational Psychology, 57,* 225–236.

Szatmari, P., Offord, D., & Boyle, M. (1989). Ontario Child Health Study: Prevalence of attention deficit disorder with hyperactivity. *Journal of Child Psychology and Psychiatry, 30,* 219–230.

Teicher, M. H., Ito, Y., Glod, C. A., & Barber, N. I. (1996). Objective measurement of hyperactivity and attentional problems in ADHD. *Journal of American Academy of Child and Adolescent Psychiatry, 35,* 334–342.

Townsend, J., Harris, N. S., & Courchesne, E. (1996). Visual attention abnormalities in autism: Delayed orienting to location. *Journal of the International Neuropsychological Society, 2,* 541–550.

Vaidya, C. J., Austin, G., Kirkorian, G., Ridlehuber, H. W., Desmond, J. E., Glover, G. H., et al. (1998). Selective effects of methylphenidate in attention deficit hyperactivity disorder: A functional magnetic resonance study. *Proceedings of the National Academy of Sciences USA, 95,* 14494–14499.

van Dellen, T., Vassen, W., & Schoemaker, M. (1990). Clumsiness: Definition and selection of subjects. In A. F. Kalverboer (Ed.), *Developmental biopsychology* (pp. 135–152). Ann Arbor: University of Michigan Press.

Van Mier, H., Petersen, S. E., Tempel, L. W., Perlmutter, J. S., Snyder, A. Z., & Raichle, M. E. (1994). Practice related changes in a continuous motor task measured by PET. *Society for Neuroscience Abstracts, 20,* 361.

Victorian Infant Collaborative Study Group. (1991). Eight-year outcome of infants with birthweight at 500 to 900 grams: Continuing regional study of 1979 and 1980 births. *Journal of Pediatrics, 118,* 761–767.

Visser, J., Geuze, R. H., & Kalverboer, A. F. (1998). The relationship between physical growth, the level of activity and the development of motor skills in adolescence: Differences between children with DCD and controls. *Human Movement Science, 17,* 573–608.

Vohr, B. R., & Gracia Coll, C. T. (1985). Neurodevelopmental and school performance of very low-birth-weight infants: A seven-year longitudinal study. *Pediatrics, 76,* 345–350.

West, T. G. (1999). The abilities of those with reading disabilities: Focusing on the talents of people with dyslexia. In D. D. Duane (Ed.), *Reading and attention disorders: Neurobiological correlates* (pp. 213–241). Baltimore: York Press.

Whitfield, M. F., Grunau, R. V., & Holsti, L. (1997). Extremely premature (800 g) schoolchildren: Multiple areas of hidden disability. *Archives of Diseases in Childhood, 77,* F85–F90.

Wilson, P. H., & McKenzie, B. E. (1998). Information processing deficits associated with developmental coordination disorder: A meta-analysis of research findings. *Journal of Child Psychology and Psychiatry, 39,* 829–840.

Wolff, P. H., Michel, G. F., Ovrut, M., & Drake, C. (1990). Rate and timing precision of motor coordination in developmental dyslexia. *Developmental Psychology, 26,* 349–359.

World Health Organization. (1992). *The ICD-10 classification of mental and behavioural disorders: Clinical descriptions and diagnostic guidelines.* Geneva, Switzerland: Author.

Zoller, M. E., Rembeck, B., & Backman, L. (1997). Neuropsychological deficits in adults with neurofibromatosis type 1. *Acta Neurolica Scandinavica, 95,* 225–232.

CHAPTER 19

Psychosocial Functions of Children and Adolescents with Movement Disorders

MOTOHIDE MIYAHARA
BRYANT J. CRATTY

This chapter discusses psychosocial functioning of children and adolescents with motor disorders, which involves the interplay of several sets of variables such as self-concept, coping patterns, and the availability of social support. We first explore the terms *motor disorders, disablement, impairment, disability*, and *handicap* within the frameworks proposed by the International Classification of Impairments, Disabilities, and Handicaps (ICIDH; World Health Organization, 1980) and the International Classification of Functioning and Disability (ICFD; World Health Organization, 2001). The protective mechanisms of self-concept, coping strategies, and social support associated with optimal psychosocial functioning are then examined. The chapter concludes with a discussion of the implications for interventions based on research evidence on self-esteem, coping skills, and social support.

WORLD HEALTH ORGANIZATION CLASSIFICATIONS

Before discussing how motor disorders can influence the social and emotional development of children, we delineate what we mean by the terms *motor disorders, disablement, impairment, disability*, and *handicap* using frameworks proposed by the ICIDH (World Health Organization, 1980) and the ICFD (World Health Organization, 2001). The ICIDH was developed to meet the change in health focus from disorders to the consequences of disorders. Childhood motor disorders are often congenital and chronic, persisting into adolescence and adulthood. Identifying and naming of motor disorders, however, fails to provide essential information about the long-term consequences of these problems, such as the level of care, service needs, disability benefits, and social integration. To systematically classify such consequences, the ICIDH and the ICFD use an umbrella term, *disablement*. The ICIDH refers to the process of disablement in a linearly progressive manner from impairment (body level) to disability (person level) to handicap (social level). The revised ICFD has replaced the term *disability* with *activity limitation* and *handicap* with *participation restriction*, thus recognizing the interaction between impairment, activity and participation from a multidimensional perspective.

Motor disorders are health conditions that may lead to disablement. This disablement can be due to physiological and/or psychosocial factors. Whether the etiology of motor disorders is organic, psychogenic, or a combination of both, a motor disorder is an intrinsic medical condition that occurs within the individual. An *impairment* refers to a loss of function, a *disability* indicates a lack of ability to perform an activity as a result of impairment, and a *handicap* denotes a social disadvantage caused by a discrepancy between the individual's performance and the expectation from the society (ICIDH; World Health Organization, 1980). Children experience motor disorders at the body level as skeletal and disfiguring impairments, at the personal level as personal care, locomotor, body disposition, and dexterity disabilities, or at the society level as physical independence, mobility, and social integration handicaps. Hence, the children's quality of life, their self-esteem, and their social integration cannot be directly associated with a specific movement disorder but, rather, with how the disorder is experienced by the children in the surrounding environment at the body, personal, and societal levels. In the following section, we explore self-perceptions of children with motor impairments and physical disabilities.

SELF-CONCEPT

In discussing children's views or perceptions of their motor impairments and physical disabilities, we face problems of terminology. Terms such as *self-concept, self-esteem*, and *self-image* are often loosely applied. For example, the distinction between *self-concept* and *self-esteem* is not always clear, and the two terms are often used interchangeably. However, some investigators (e.g., King, Shultz, Steel, Gilpin, & Cathers, 1993; Specht, King, & Francis, 1998) define self-concept as how people view themselves and self-esteem as how people value themselves. We use the definition of self-concept provided by Shavelson, Hubner, and Stanton (1976) in our discussion of children's self-perceptions of physical disability. According to this definition, self-perceptions are developed through the experience in and the interpretation of the individual condition. A child with a motor disorder experiences the motor disorder and interprets its consequences at body, personal, and social levels. For the purposes of this chapter, self-esteem is defined as an evaluation of information contained in the self-concept (Pope, McHale, & Craighead, 1988).

Researchers of self-concept and self-esteem have postulated either a unidimensional or a multidimensional model of the constructs and have developed assessment tools with structures that reflect these models. Examples of unidimensional scales include the Rosenberg Self-Esteem Scale (Rosenberg, 1965), the Coopersmith Behavior Rating Form (Coopersmith, 1967), and the Piers–Harris Self-Concept Scale for Children (Piers & Harris, 1969). These unidimensional scales rate self-concept or self-esteem as high or low. The developers of the scales presume that general self-concept or self-esteem is so dominant that it is difficult to differentiate it into specific domains (Harter, 1982, 1985; Marsh, 1997).

These unidimensional scales have been used with children and adolescents with various levels of physical disabilities. Cratty, Ikeda, Martin, Jennett, and Morris (1970) administered the Piers–Harris Self-Concept Scale for Children (Piers & Harris, 1969) to a group of children with coordination problems (N = 133) and a group of age- and gender-matched controls. They reported lower self-concepts in children with coordination problems. Shaw, Levine, and Belfer (1982) also used the Piers–Harris Self-Concept Scale for Children to investigate whether gross motor delay was associated with lower self-concept in boys with learning disabilities aged 8–11. Twelve children with gross motor delay were compared to 11 boys without the delay. Results revealed no group differences. Henderson, May, and Umney (1989) administered a modified version of the Piers–Harris Scale to children with motor difficulties and a matched control group. In the absence of a significant correlation between positive statement items (e.g., "I am a happy person") and negative items (e.g., "I am unpopular"), the researchers examined the group differences in the two types of items separately. There was a significant group difference only on the subtotal scores of negative statement items. Although the researchers concluded that motor difficulties were associated with lower self-esteem, our reanalysis of the total scores revealed no significant group difference. Of the previous studies, only Cratty and colleagues' (1970) study found that mild to moderate movement disorders were associated with lower self-concept. Therefore, findings of the past studies do not provide strong evidence for lower general (i.e., as measured by a unidimensional scale) self-concept in children with mild to moderate physical disabilities.

Studies have also investigated general self-concept in children with severe motor disorders. Teplin, Howard, and O'Connor (1981) used the Coopersmith Behavior Rating Form (Coopersmith, 1967) and compared a group of 15 children (7 males, 8 females) with cerebral palsy between 4 and 8 years of age to a group of control children matched for age, gender, ethnicity, IQ, and socioeconomic status. Results revealed no group differences. Harvey and Greenway (1984) administered the Piers–Harris Scale to children with physical disabilities, such as cerebral palsy and spina bifida, who were 9–11 years of age. Compared to control children, the children with physical disabilities exhibited lower self-concept. Arnold and Chapman (1992) administered the Rosenberg Self-Esteem Scale (Rosenberg, 1965) to adolescents with physical disabilities, including cerebral palsy and spina bifida, and found that the adolescents with physical disability were not significantly different on this measure of self-esteem compared to age-matched able-bodied controls. These findings suggest that even severe disorders, such as cerebral palsy and spina bifida, are not always associated with lower general self-concept. Thus, the evidence that motor disorders, whether mild, moderate, or severe, are associated with poorer self-concept on unidimensional measures is equivocal.

In their multidimensional model of self-concept, Shavelson and colleagues (1976) place the general self at the apex of a hierarchy of the physical, academic, and social domains. This domain-specific nature of self-concept has been demonstrated by subsequent factor-analytic studies. Among children 4–7 years of age, Harter and Pike (1984) found that self-concept was divisible into two factors: perceived competence and social acceptance. In children 8–12 years of age, Harter (1982) identified four factors, cognitive competence in school, social competence with peers, physical competence in sports, and general self-worth. Among fourth graders, Marsh and Hocevar (1985) failed to confirm Shavelson's single higher-order factor model with general self-concept at the peak of the hierarchy, but three higher-order factors (verbal, math, nonacademic) reflected lower component variables (physical abilities, physical appearance, peer relationships, parent relationships, reading ability, math ability, school). These studies support the multidimensionality of self-concept.

An example of the multidimensionality of self-concept in a real-world setting was once made clear to us when a parent described the effects of the mainstream placement of her daughter with spina bifida in a regular school. On one hand, the child felt good about herself while participating in the academic exercises in the classroom. In contrast, she reportedly suffered a psychic diminution of her physical self when faced with participation in both formal and informal activities on the playground. This case clearly illustrates that self-concept is indeed, multidimensional. Furthermore, it raises the following questions: "Is this child's general self-concept influenced by her uneven competence in the academic and physical domains?" and "Does the personal importance she places on each domain affect her general self-concept?"

Three studies (Losse et al., 1991; Schoemaker & Kalverboer, 1994; Skinner & Piek, 2001) that examined multiple domains of self-esteem among children and adolescents who were diagnosed as being "clumsy" or with developmental coordination disorder provide some clues that may assist in answering these questions. Losse and colleagues (1991) used the Perceived Competence Scale for Children (PCSC; Harter, 1982) to evaluate multiple domains of self-esteem among 16-year-olds who had been identified as being "clumsy" at the age of 10 years. Compared to IQ-matched controls, the clumsy adolescents exhibited poorer motor coordination and lower physical, social, and overall self-esteem (i.e., mean of all four domains). However, their cognitive and general self-esteem were similar to the controls. In the second study, Schoemaker and Kalverboer (1994) administered the Pictorial Scale for Perceived Competence and Social Acceptance for Young Children (PCSAS; Harter & Pike, 1984) to 18 clumsy children and an age- and gender-matched control group. The clumsy children scored significantly worse than did the control children on the physical competence and social acceptance subscales. The third study by Skinner and Piek (2001) used a revision of the PCSC (Harter, 1985) and examined the effect of poor motor coordination on psychosocial life in children and adolescents. The 8- to 10-year-old children with coordination disorder reported lower levels of competence on the scholastic, athletic, physical appearance, and global self-worth subscales. Among adolescents 12 to 14 years of age, lower levels of competence were found on the social acceptance, athletic competence, physical appearance, and global self-worth scales. The findings support the multidimensionality of self-concept and suggest that in some children general self-concept may be intact, though they may evidence poor self-concepts in specific domains.

Gender differences may add another dimension to the stigma of public visibility. Consistent with traditional gender stereotypes, girls tend to have lower physical self-esteem and higher social self-esteem than do boys from preadolescence to early adulthood (Marsh, 1989). If girls are more vulnerable than boys to the stigmatization of the body due to physical disabilities, their physical self-esteem may well be at increased risk. Several studies have examined gender differences in self-esteem among children and adolescents with physical disabilities.

Among children with mild to moderate movement problems, low self-concept was not as pronounced among the group of girls surveyed (Cratty et al., 1970). The investigators suggested that girls might not have predicated as much of their feelings about the self on physical skill performance as did the boys in this study. Around the same time, a study by Meissner, Thoreson, and Butler (1967) found that female adolescents with highly visible physical disabilities showed more negative self-concept than did the other groups, such as male adolescents with highly visible physical disabilities and female adolescents without highly visible physical disabilities.

Magill and Hurlbut (1986) compared male adolescents with cerebral palsy to counterparts without disabilities and female adolescents with cerebral palsy to counterparts without disabilities on the multidimensional Tennessee Self-Concept Scale (Fitts, 1965). Although no main effect was found for disability, there was a significant main effect for gender, and a significant interaction effect between disability and gender for physical self-esteem and social self-esteem. Female adolescents with cerebral palsy rated themselves lower than did the other groups. On physical self-esteem, although no difference existed between male adolescents with cerebral palsy and female adolescents without disabilities, female adolescents with cerebral palsy were significantly lower than the other groups. The female adolescents with cerebral palsy exhibited the same pattern on the social self-esteem as on physical self-esteem. More recently, Larkin and Parker (1997) investigated gender differences among adolescents with a history of motor learning difficulties. Although the female adolescents perceived some of their physical abilities (e.g., activity, endurance, and coordination) to be lower than those of the males with motor learning difficulties, no gender differences were revealed on their self-rating of appearance and global self-esteem.

In summary, female adolescents with physical disabilities seem to be more at risk of low physical self-esteem than male counterparts. Physical disability also appears to affect the global self-worth and social self-esteem of female adolescents if disabilities are severe or highly visible. It is likely that in addition to gender differences, age, severity of physical disabilities, and the cultural emphasis on physical ability and appearance together contribute to multidimensional self-esteem.

COPING PATTERNS AND COMPENSATION STRATEGIES

Crocker and Major (1989) have proposed three coping mechanisms that protect the self-esteem of individuals, including those who are targets of negative attitudes, stereotypes, and treatment, thus physically handicapped. One of the coping mechanisms involves devaluing the domain in which they find themselves at a disadvantage and instead valuing other areas of competence. For example, the child with spina bifida described earlier in this chapter may make light of physical activities, and regard her academic achievements as more important. This could result in her maintaining her overall self-esteem. The second coping mechanism is concerned with the selection of a reference group. An athlete with a physical disability may not compare him- or herself with able-bodied athletes but with athletes with the same disability. A third mechanism used by individuals with disabilities to protect self-esteem is to discount the negatives attitudes directed toward the stigmatized group to which they belong. In such a case, the individual does not take the prejudices personally.

Recent studies have begun to investigate whether individuals with motor impairments use these coping mechanisms to protect self-esteem. Appleton and colleagues (1994) examined the devaluing and reference group hypotheses in 79 young adolescents with spina bifida and the same number of age- and gender-matched controls. They administered the Self-Perception Profile for Learning Disabled Students and its accompanying importance scale (Renick & Harter, 1988) and asked the spina bifida group whether they used people with physical disabilities or without for comparison on each of the domains. The spina bifida group rated themselves as less competent than the control group on the academic, athletic, and social domains, but there was no group difference on other areas of competence and on global self-worth. All domains were rated as equally important by both groups. There was a greater gap between the perceived competence scales and importance scales for the spina bifida group than for the control group on the academic, athletic, social competence, and physical appearance domains. It is noteworthy that the majority of youngsters with spina bifida compared themselves to able-bodied peers. Thus, neither the devaluing hypothesis nor the reference group hypothesis were supported. Appleton and colleagues suggested that young people with spina bifida might employ compensatory strategies that were not measured in this study and emphasized a need for qualitative studies of coping strategies within the spina bifida population.

The devaluing hypothesis and the reference group hypothesis were also tested by Specht and colleagues (1998) in their study on the self-esteem and coping strategies of 19 adolescents with spina bifida or cerebral palsy aged 13–18 years. The Self-Perception Profile for Adolescents (Harter, 1988) was used to measure multidimensional self-concept. The importance of the domains was assessed by the Importance Rating Scale for Adolescents (Harter, 1988). Although general self-concept was not lower than the standardization norms, social acceptance, athletic competence, and job competence were rated significantly lower by the adolescents with spina bifida or cerebral palsy. The participants also devalued the domains of social acceptance, athletic competence, romantic appeal, and job competence. Therefore, it was concluded that these adolescents were using a selective devaluing strategy (i.e., a strategy of specifically devaluing domains in which they performed poorly) to protect their general self-esteem.

To test the reference group hypothesis and the stigmatized group hypothesis, Specht and colleagues (1998) examined the spontaneous use of reference group (with or without disabilities) and the causal attributions of negative social events in adolescents with physical disabilities. Results indicated that most participants used able-bodied people as their reference group, and only a few (4 out of 19) considered their physical disabilities the prevalent cause of negative social events. Specht and colleagues concluded that these results provided support for the devaluing hypothesis.

The devaluing hypothesis was further examined in children with developmental coordination disorder (DCD) by Piek, Dworcan, Barrett, and Coleman (2000). Thirty-six children with DCD were compared to 36 children without DCD matched for age, gender, and verbal IQ. The Self Perception Profile for Children (Harter, 1985) was used to assess general self-worth, domain-specific self-concept (i.e., scholastic competence, social acceptance, athletic competence, physical appearance, and behavioral conduct) and the importance of each domain. The only significant group difference in self-concept was found on athletic competence and no group differences were noted on any of the importance domains. The lack of group difference in global self-worth suggests that children with DCD do not devalue the athletic domain to maintain their global self-worth.

In summary, the findings of the foregoing studies suggest that individuals with physical disabilities do not always use the strategies proposed by Crocker and Major (1989) to maintain their self-esteem. The devaluing hypothesis was supported neither by Appleton and colleagues (1994) nor by Piek and colleagues (2000). Although Specht and colleagues' (1998) study suggests that adolescents with physical disabilities used a selective devaluing strategy, no control group was sampled from the same population base. Coupled with the small sample size, this finding by Specht and colleagues is not entirely convincing. The reference group hypothesis was also not supported by both Appleton and colleagues and Specht and colleagues. Finally, to the best of our knowledge, no study has examined whether people with physical disabilities protect their self-esteem by not taking negative social attitudes personally. Thus, research that examines this specific mechanism of protecting self-esteem is needed.

Interestingly, a lack of group difference in global self-worth has been consistently reported in studies that have examined self-esteem in children with physical disabilities (e.g., Arnold & Chapman, 1992; Teplin et al., 1981). The maintenance of global self-worth despite low perceived athletic competence was also observed in children and adolescents with DCD (Cantell, Smyth, & Ahonen, 1994; Maeland, 1994; van Rossum & Vermeer, 1990) and those with spina bifida or acquired spinal cord injuries (Antle, 2000). How do young individuals with motor disorders maintain general self-esteem, by comparing themselves to those without motor disorders, and without devaluing the physical domain?

The coping strategies used by individuals with physical disabilities may be elusive, and questionnaire surveys may not detect them due to the inherent biases associated with social desirability. For example, it is generally acceptable to consider all academic, physical, and social domains as important. Even if some individuals regard athletic skills as unimportant, they may still state that athletic skills are important on the questionnaire. There is also a risk of self-deceptive positivity. High self-esteem is important to many, so they may respond to questions that assess self-esteem in a positive manner. Llewellyn and Chung (1997) raise the question as to whether it is possible and useful to measure the self-concept of young people with physical disabilities. It is true that the survey method enables us to obtain information about a large number of people, but actual microbehaviors employed for the compensation of motor impairment may not be detectable in quantitative studies using questionnaires. Appleton and colleagues (1994) suggested employing a qualitative research approach, including case studies and naturalistic observation.

Several published reports contain clinical observations of compensatory behaviors, purportedly reflecting social maladjustment, among motorically challenged youngsters. For example, Brooks (1992) listed quitting, avoiding, cheating, clowning and regressing, controlling, being aggressive and bullying, being passive–aggressive, denying, rationalizing, and being impulsive as compensatory behaviors. These behaviors appeared to be ways of avoiding confrontations, which might reveal deficient physical skills, as well strategies that called attention to nonphysical aspects of the self, which may be deemed to be more intact than the physical self (Cratty, 1994). Other compensatory social behaviors that may be used by children with physical disabilities are (1) avoiding games with peers entirely—strategies include habitually offering to help the teacher during recesses, or staying home from school with a feigned illness during days in which some fitness test is given at the school; (2) disguising the problems with "pretend" play strategies—they may follow the ball in a soccer game but take care not to go too close so that they avoid the attention of children on the other side, or they might also stand in line to take their turns at some game, like playing hand ball against a wall, but when it is their turn to participate quickly assume a position at the end of the line without risking competition; (3) being overly aggressive during times designated for outdoor recreational activities—boys who chase others, rather than play in games, are suspect in this respect; and (4) participating in forms of play typical of less mature youngsters—a boy of 6 or 7 who prefers sandbox play, often with an equally maladroit friend rather than participating in more complex and threatening team games, is an example of this type of avoidance strategy. These clinically observed examples of compensatory patterns are not easily detected by using the questionnaire survey method.

Although psychosocial variables need to be predetermined and limited in number in the questionnaire survey method, the case-study method provides insights into the process of how a wide range of variables change over time (Yin, 2003). In the clinical and educational settings, we can easily follow targeted cases for a period of time in order to investigate the effect of age on psychosocial functions. In contrast, questionnaire surveys require a large sample for sufficient statistical power, and therefore, cross-sectional studies are often the method of choice to minimize the cost for time, labor, and continuity. The disadvantage of cross-sectional studies lies in the validity of age-related changes; developmental changes are inferred from different cohorts which mask individual variation.

Longitudinal multiple case studies of children with physical disabilities are a useful way of examining developmental influences on psychosocial life. Minde (1972) and Minde, Hackett, Killou, and Silver (1978) conducted a longitudinal case study that followed 34 children with cerebral palsy from school entry to early adolescence using bi-annual formal psychiatric interviews. Over this period, not only were the researchers able to identify personal stress events (e.g., parents' divorce) that influenced the psychosocial well-being of the children and families, but they were also able to examine general developmental issues. For instance, upon their entry into a segregated school, the children experienced a temporary depressive period after realizing their own differences from their peers without disabilities. As the children grew up, both children and parents became aware of the permanence of the physical disabilities, personal and occupational identities of the children, and the fact that parents withdrew from direct child care.

Among young people with Duchenne muscular dystrophy, developmental influences on psychosocial life are of particular importance as individuals with this disorder face deteriorating physical functions and death during adolescence or early adulthood. Suzuki (1995) conducted a multiple case study to examine the process of coping with the disease and fear of death by conducting weekly interviews with five young people with Duchenne muscular dystrophy who were between 16 and 27 years of age for periods ranging from 1 year and 5 months to 2 years. In-depth interviews revealed individual coping strategies: (1) some seemed to distance themselves from the disease by rationalizing or being angry at it; (2) others expressed anxiety, fear, and depression.

One individual seemed to accept the disease, stating that it was natural for him to have the disease and not necessarily unfair as in the case of acquired disabilities by violence. This person was the only one that spoke of death directly. He was still afraid of death but ready for it. He wanted to die in a right way. "Quality of life does not depend on the length of life, but how life is lived," he stated. Others referred to death by talking about related issues, such as gender differences in lifespan, AIDS, and the hardship of living with Duchenne muscular dystrophy.

Compared to questionnaire studies, longitudinal multiple case studies of children with physical disabilities provide information on psychosocial issues that are unique to specific disorders. Hence, more research which uses this approach in the investigation of self-concept and coping strategies in children with physical disabilities is warranted.

As noted previously, the questionnaire survey method is vulnerable to respondent bias. On the other hand, the case-study method and the naturalistic observation method are subject to observer bias. Trying to detect compensatory strategies in children with movement disorders, we may well interpret their behaviors in such a way that portrays stories suitable to explain the compensation phenomena. There is also a problem of generalizability from circumstantial samples. It may not be possible to generalize a specific compensatory strategy from the observed cases to other individuals. Keeping the limitations of both quantitative and qualitative methods in mind, researchers need to further examine the coping mechanism of children with physical disabilities to better identify the factors that are associated with positive outcomes across the various dimensions of self-concept (i.e., athletic, academic, social, and physical appearance).

SOCIAL SUPPORT

Caring and helping are essential ingredients for successful development of youth. Children and adolescents with physical disabilities may have particular needs for social support to manage activities of daily living, social stigma, and discrimination. Social support is defined as an exchange of resources from providers to recipients, which is intended to enhance the well-being of the recipient (Shumaker & Brownell, 1984). Social support can be categorized into emotional support, esteem support, belonging support, network support, appraisal support, tangible support, instrumental support, and informational support (Wilcox & Vernberg, 1985). Cohen and MacKay (1984) present a stress-buffering hypothesis which assumes that the detrimental effects of psychological stress can be lessened or eliminated if one has a strong support system. In the face of stigmatization and discrimination, young people with physical disabilities and their family members may reduce the impact of negative social attitudes by using various types of social support (e.g., emotional support, esteem support, belonging support, and network support). If a youngster with physical disability needs personal assistance to perform some activities of daily living, the youngster and the family members may appreciate instrumental and tangible support from the other family members and caregivers. Informational support may assist people in obtaining advocacy information and in learning how to assert their rights and effectively fight against discrimination. At times, parents may be uncertain about the nature of disability and anxious about its developmental course. They may be reassured by informational support from community agencies and support groups. Thus, social support could help young people with physical disabilities and their families to cope with challenges they face. In this section, we begin with a critical review of questionnaire survey studies that have investigated social support in young people with chronic physical disabilities. Then we turn our attention to interview studies conducted with youngsters with progressive physical disabilities.

Three recent questionnaire studies have examined the relationship between social support and self-esteem in young people with physical disabilities. Antle (2000) administered the Social Support Scales (Harter, 1985; Neemann & Harter, 1986) and the Self-Perception Scales (Harter, 1988; Renick & Harter, 1988) to a total of 85 children and adolescents aged 8–18 years with spina bifida or acquired spinal cord injuries. Significant correlations were revealed between perceived social support from close friends and parents and global self-worth. In a regression model, which was used to predict global self-worth from gender, age, diagnosis, and social support from parents, social support from parents was the strongest predictor ($R^2 = .12$). Piek and colleagues (2000) also used the Harter's Self-Perception Scales (Harter, 1985), and compared 36 children with DCD to the same number of control children. There was no group difference on the perceived social support measures. Although social support was significantly correlated with global self-worth in the control group, the correlation was not significant in the children with DCD. Skinner and Piek (2001) further studied the perception of social support among children and adolescents with DCD and this time found that young people with DCD felt less socially supported than did the matched controls. Instrumental support was significantly correlated with global self-worth in adolescents with DCD and adolescents in the control group. Thus, Antle's and Skinner and Piek's studies provide support for the stress-buffering hypothesis (Cohen & MacKay, 1984).

What are the practical implications of their findings? Because perceived support from parents contributed most significantly to the maintenance of general self-esteem, Antle (2000) proposed that social workers should facilitate parents' supportive roles for their children with spina bifida or acquired spinal cord injuries into the late adolescence. How about children and adolescents with developmental coordination disorder? Although Piek and colleagues (2000) and Skinner and Piek (2001) found no significant correlation between global self-esteem and social support among children with DCD, Skinner and Piek did obtained a significant correlation between instrumental support and global self-worth among adolescents with the disorder. Because social support is not associated with global self-esteem in childhood but in adolescence, support from significant others may play an increasingly important role in individuals with DCD as it persists into adolescence. However, this hypothesis needs to be examined in a longitudinal study.

Of the various functions of social support mentioned earlier, some categories overlap (e.g., emotional support and belonging support); however, a distinction has been made between emotional and instrumental support in the studies of children and family with physical disabilities. Emotional support is the love and care perceived by recipients. Instrumental support is the provision of materials and services that contribute to the execution of tasks that may not be otherwise accomplished or may be more difficult to accomplish. The sources of social support can be informal, such as friends and family members, or formal, such as the department of disability support service in a residing city. The studies that examined the network types of mothers of children

TABLE 19.1. Summary of Group Comparison Studies Employing Unidimensional and Multidimensional Measures of Self-Esteem in Children and Adolescents with Movement Disorders

Authors (year)	Measures	Age (yr)	Movement disorders (MD)	N MD group	N Control group	Findings
			Unidimensional measures			
			Moderate physical disabilities			
Cratty et al. (1970)	PHSCSC	5–12	Perceptual-motor deficiencies	133	133	Control > MD
Shaw et al. (1982)	PHSCSC	8–12	Gross motor delay	12	11	No group difference
Henderson et al. (1989)	PHSCSC	7–11	Movement difficulties	18	18	Control > MD in negative statements; no group difference in positive statements
			Severe physical disabilities			
Teplin et al. (1981)	CBRF	4–8	CP	15	15	No group difference
Harvey & Greenway (1984)	PHSCSC	7–15	CP, spina bifida, etc	33	18	Control > MD
Arnold & Chapman (1992)	RSES	15–17	CP, spina bifida, etc	15	35	No group difference
			Multidimensional measures			
			Moderate physical disabilities			
Losse et al. (1991)	PCSC	16	Clumsy	17	17	Control > MD in physical, social domains
Schoemaker & Kalverboer (1994)	PCSAS	6–9	Clumsy	18	18	Control > MD in physical, social domains, extroversion
Skinner & Piek (2001)	SPPC	8–10	DCD	58	58	Control > MD in scholastic competence, athletic competence, physical appearance, global self-worth
	SPPA	12–14		51	51	Control > MD in social acceptance, athletic competence, physical appearance, global self-worth

Note. MD, movement disorders; DCD, developmental coordination disorder; CP, cerebral palsy; PHSC, Piers–Harris Self-Concept Scale for Children; CBRF, Coopersmith Behavior Rating Form; RSES, Rosenberg Self-Esteem Scale; PCSC, Perceived Competence Scale for Children; PCSAS, Pictorial Scale for Perceived Competence and Social Acceptance for Young Children; SPPC, Self-Perception Profile for Children; SPPS, Self-Perception Profile for Adolescents.

with disabilities have found that these mothers took advantage of both formal and informal support networks (Findler, 2000; Kitagawa, Nanakida, & Imashioya, 1995; Seybold, Fritz, & Macphee, 1991).

Progressive neuromuscular disorders, such as Duchenne muscular dystrophy, have a distinct prognosis: death during adolescence or early adulthood. Because of such a devastating consequence, young people with the disorders and their families may encounter unique psychosocial issues and may require specific social support. Both informational and emotional support seems particularly important for the parents when receiving the diagnosis as they want to obtain specific information and feel understood (Green & Murton, 1996). Informational support needs to be individualized because parents without higher education tend to receive inadequate information (Green & Murton, 1996). Emotional support should be available at hospitals and the muscular dystrophy associations because parental anxiety and depression could have an impact not only on themselves but also on their children's behaviors (Thompson, Zeman, Fanurik, & Sirotkin-Roses, 1992). Although family adjustment to muscular dystrophies is an ongoing complex individual process, many families experience similar emotions and feelings (Miller, 1990). Because *frankness* and *empathy* are highly valued by parents (Green & Murton, 1996), staff at hospitals and muscular dystrophy associations may need special communication and counseling training to provide sufficient informational and emotional support.

In summary, social support is beneficial for the children and adolescents with physical disabilities and their family members. Social workers may be able to facilitate family support (Antle, 2000), and schoolteachers could encourage peer support. To receive social support from significant others, it is useful for recipients to have good social skills. The next section discusses intervention programs that use social skills training and the cognitive-behavioral techniques.

IMPLICATIONS FOR INTERVENTION

Public concerns about children's self-esteem have been consciously addressed since the 1980s, and books and programs promoting positive self-esteem have proliferated. In such a social climate, it is taken for granted that the enhancement of self-esteem in children and adolescents with disabilities is necessary and important because they have been perceived as being at risk of low self-esteem. In an attempt to improve the self-esteem of children with disabilities, Pope and colleagues (1988) developed a treatment program in response to a request from a regular school. Like many other programs of this kind, it employs a cognitive-behavioral approach. The components of their program consist of problem solving, self-talk in controlling feelings and behaviors, attribution retraining, goal setting, social skills training, communication skills, and modifying standards for physical attractiveness and performance. Although the program is fairly comprehensive, no empirical data have demonstrated the effectiveness of the program for the children with disabilities.

Few studies have examined the efficacy of self-esteem programs for children with physical disabilities; however, two are reported in the literature (King, Specht, Warr-Leeper, Redekop, & Risebrough, 1997; Todis, Irvin, Singer, & Yovanoff, 1993). Todis and colleagues (1993) developed a parent intervention program that attempted to foster self-esteem in children with physical disabilities. Stress management, behavior management, assertive training, and advocacy skills were taught in six weekly classes. The themes of the classes were derived from interviews with personally and professionally successful adults who had grown up with physical disabilities. The themes included independence through self-determination and responsibility, leisure activities, peer interaction, assertiveness, coping with difficult situations such as teasing and discrimination, and advocacy skills for parents and children. Qualitative assessment of the program outcome showed that parents increased their awareness of how their parenting practices could influence their children's self-esteem. The Self-Esteem Parent Program Questionnaire, developed by the researchers to assess parents' perceptions of children's performance in choice and responsibility, leisure activities, peer interaction, assertiveness, coping, parent advocacy, and self-advocacy was administered prior to and after the parent intervention program. The comparison of the pre- and post-intervention questionnaire scores indicated an improvement in assertive behavior, coping, and advocacy skills of children and parents after the intervention. This intervention study, however, only involved parents. No direct measure of the children's self-esteem was obtained. Thus, whether this intervention resulted in improved self-esteem in the children is open to question.

King and colleagues (1997) conducted a 10-week social skills training program with 11 withdrawn unpopular children with cerebral palsy or spina bifida. The program taught the children social skills, such as initiating interactions with peers, verbal and nonverbal communication, conversation skills, interpersonal problem solving, and coping with difficult others. Results indicated that the training significantly enhanced the children's perception of social acceptance measured by the Self Perception Profile for Children (Harter, 1985). However, the enhancement was not sustained 24 weeks after the end of the training. In addition, no significant improvement was observed on the global self-worth subscale, or on the scales for classmate support and close friend support at the end of the training. Although the index of loneliness did not improve significantly by the end of the training, a significant improvement emerged 24 weeks after the training was over. Thus, support for the effectiveness of this social skills training program is rather weak and limited to temporary improvement of the children's perception of social acceptance and a delayed reduction of loneliness.

In light of a dearth of intervention studies that involved children with physical disabilities, we discuss a meta-analysis study of social skills training for students with emotional or behavioral disorders (Magee, Kavale, Mathur, Rutherford, & Forness, 1999). This study found that social skills training was not very effective if training was conducted in small group settings. Rather, the results of this meta-analysis suggested that social skills training is more effective if the training is integrated into the school, playground, and home settings. Therefore, it is possible that children with physical disabilities may benefit more from social skills training conducted in real-life situations.

CONCLUSIONS

In conclusion, the empirical evidence provides little support for the notion that low general self-concept or self-esteem is found among young people with physical disabilities. Rather, it appears that children with disabilities tend to evidence low self-concept in specific domains that appear to be related to their disability, such as athletic competence, physical appearance, and social acceptance. Coping mechanisms to protect global self-esteem in the presence of poor physical self-esteem were examined; however, the research evidence provided by questionnaire studies to support these mechanisms is negligible. It is possible that the coping strategies used by individuals with physical disabilities are temporary and situation-specific tactics, which may not be detected by gross questionnaire surveys. Evidence is emerging on the buffering effect of social support for children with motor impairments and their families. However, more research is needed into this. Finally, intervention programs including stress coping, assertiveness training, and support networking may be beneficial to enhance the quality of psychosocial life in children with motor impairments and their families; however, research that focuses on the types of programs that are most effective is needed.

REFERENCES

Antle, B. J. (2000). Seeking strengths in young people with physical disabilities: Learning from the self-perceptions of children and young adults. *Dissertation Abstract International, 60*(10-A), 3795.

Appleton, P. L., Minchom, P. E., Ellis, N. C., Elliott, C. E., Böll, V., & Jones, P. (1994). The self-concept of young people with spina bifida: A population-based study. *Developmental Medicine and Child Neurology, 36*, 198–215.

Arnold, P., & Chapman, M. (1992). Self-esteem, aspirations and expectations of adolescents with physical disability. *Developmental Medicine and Child Neurology, 34*, 97–102.

Brooks, R. B. (1992). Self-esteem during the school years: Its normal development and hazardous decline. *Pediatric Clinics of North America, 39*, 537–550.

Cantell, M. H., Smyth, M. M., & Ahonen, T. P. (1994). Clumsiness in adolescence: educational, motor, and social outcomes of motor delay detected at 5 years. *Adapted Physical Activity Quarterly, 11*, 115–129.

Cohen, S., & McKay, G. (1984). Social support, stress and the buffering hypothesis: A theoretical analysis. In A. Baum, S. E. Taylor, & J. E. Singer (Eds.), *Handbook of psychology and health* (Vol. 4, pp. 253–267). Hillsdale, NJ: Erlbaum.

Coopersmith, S. (1967). *The antecedents of self-esteem.* San Francisco: Freeman.

Cratty, B. J. (1994). *Clumsy child syndromes: Descriptions, evaluation and remediation.* Chur, Switzerland: Harwood.

Cratty, B. J., Ikeda, N., Martin, M. M., Jennett, C., & Morris, M. (1970). *Movement activities, motor ability and the education of children.* Springfield, IL: Thomas.

Crocker, J., & Major, B. (1989). Social stigma and self-esteem: The self-protective properties of stigma. *Psychological Review, 96*, 608–630.

Findler, L. S. (2000). The role of grandparents in the social support system of mothers of children with a physical disability. *Families in Society: Journal of Contemporary Human Services, 81*, 370–381.

Fitts, W. H. (1965). *Tennessee Self Concept Scale manual.* Nashville, TN: Counselor Recordings and Tests.

Green, J. M., & Murton, F. E. (1996). Diagnosis of Duchenne muscular dystrophy: Parents' experiences and satisfaction. *Child: Care, Health and Development, 22*, 113–128.

Harter, S. (1982). The Perceived Competence Scale for Children. *Child Development, 53*, 87–97.

Harter, S. (1985). *Manual for the Self Perception Profile for Children: Revision of the Perceived Competence Scale for Children.* Denver, CO: University of Denver Press.

Harter, S. (1988). *Manual for the Self-Perception for Adolescents.* Denver, CO: University of Denver Press.

Harter, S., & Pike, R. (1984). The pictorial scale of Perceived Competence and Social Acceptance for Young Children. *Child Development, 55*, 1969–1982.

Harvey, D. H., & Greenway, A. P. (1984). The self-concept of physically handicapped children and their non-handicapped siblings: An empirical investigation. *Journal of Child Psychology and Psychiatry and Allied Disciplines, 25*, 273–284.

Henderson, S. E., May, D. S., & Umney, M. (1989). An exploratory study of goal-setting behaviours, self-concept and locus of control in children with movement difficulties. *European Journal of Special Needs Education, 4*, 1–15.

King, G. A., Shultz, I. Z., Steele, K., Gilpin, M., & Cathers, T. (1993). Self-evaluation and self-concept of adolescents with physical disabilities. *American Journal of Occupational Therapy, 47*, 132–140.

King, G. A., Specht, J. A., Warr-Leeper, G., Redekop, W. K., & Risebrough, N. (1997). Social skills training for withdrawn unpopular children with physical disabilities. *Rehabilitation Psychology, 42*, 47–60.

Kitagawa, N., Nanakida, A., & Imashioya, H. (1995). Effects of social support on mothers of children with disabilities. *Japanese Journal of Special Education, 33*, 35–44.

Larkin, D., & Parker, H. E. (1997). Gender differences in physical self-descriptions of adolescents with a history of motor learning difficulties. *Australian Educational and Developmental Psychologist, 14*, 63–71.

Llewellyn, A., & Chung, M. C. (1997). The self-esteem of children with physical disabilities: Problems and dilemmas of research. *Journal of Developmental and Physical Disabilities, 9*, 265–275.

Losse, A., Henderson, S., Elliman, D., Hall, D., Knight, E., & Jongmans, M. (1991). Clumsiness in children-do they grow out of it? A 10-year follow-up study. *Developmental Medicine and Child Neurology, 33*, 55–68.

Maeland, A. F. (1994). Self-esteem in children with motor coordination problems (clumsy children). *Handwriting Review*, 128–133.

Magee, Q. M., Kavale, K. A., Mathur, S. R., Rutherford, R. B. Jr., & Forness, S. R. (1999). A meta-analysis of social skill interventions for students with emotional or behavioral disorders. *Journal of Emotional and Behavioral Disorders, 7*, 54–64.

Magill, J., & Hurlbut, N. (1986). The self-esteem of adolescents it cerebral palsy. *American Journal of Occupational Therapy, 40*, 402–407.

Marsh, H. W. (1997). The measurement of physical self-concept: A construct validation approach. In K. R. Fox (Ed.), *The physical self: From motivation to well-being*. Champaign, IL: Human Kinetics.

Marsh, H. W. (1989). Age and sex effects in multiple dimensions of self-concept: Preadolescence to early adulthood. *Journal of Educational Psychology, 81*, 417–430.

Marsh, H. W., & Hocevar, D. (1985). The application of confirmatory factor analysis to the study of self-concept: First and higher order factor structures and their invariance across age groups. *Psychological Bulletin, 97*, 562–582.

Meissner, A. L., Thoreson, R. W., & Butler, A. J. (1967). Relation of self-concept to impact and obviousness of disability among male and female adolescents. *Perceptual and Motor Skills, 24*, 1099–1105.

Miller, R. M. (1990). Family response to Duchenne muscular dystrophy. *Loss, Grief and Care, 4*, 31–42.

Minde, K. K. (1978). Coping styles of 34 adolescents with cerebral palsy. *American Journal of Psychiatry, 135*, 1344–1349.

Minde, K. K., Hackett, J. D., Killou, D., & Silver, S. (1972). How they grow up: 41 physically handicapped children and their families. *American Journal of Psychiatry, 128*, 1554–1560.

Neemann, J., & Harter, S. (1986). *Manual for the self-perception profile for college students*. Denver, CO: University of Denver.

Piek, J. P., Dworcan, M., Barrett, N. C., & Coleman, R. (2000). Determinants of self-worth in children with and without developmental coordination disorder. *International Journal of Disability, Development and Education, 47,* 259–272.

Piers, E., & Harris, D. (1969). *The Piers–Harris Children's Self-Concept Scale.* Nashville, TN: Counselor Recordings and Tests.

Pope, A. W., McHale, S. M., & Craighead, W. E. (1988). *Self-esteem enhancement with children and adolescents.* Oxford, UK: Pergamon.

Renick, M. J., & Harter, S. (1988). *Manual for the Self-Perception Profile for Learning Disabled Students.* Denver, CO: University of Denver Press.

Rosenberg, M. (1965). *Society and the adolescent self-image.* Princeton, NJ: Princeton University Press.

Schoemaker, M. M., & Kalverboer, A. F. (1994). Social and affective problems of children who are clumsy: How early do they begin? *Adapted Physical Activity Quarterly, 11,* 130–140.

Seybold, J., Fritz, J., & MacPhee, D. (1991). Relation of social support to the self-perceptions of mothers with delayed children. *Journal of Community Psychology, 19,* 29–36.

Shavelson, R. J., Hubner, J. J., & Stanton, G. C. (1976). Validation of construct interpretations. *Review of Educational Research, 46,* 407–441.

Shaw, L., Levine, M. D., & Belfer, M. (1982). Developmental double jeopardy: a study of clumsiness and self-esteem in children with learning problems. *Developmental and Behavioral Pediatrics, 3,* 191–196.

Shumaker, S. A., & Brownell, A. (1984). Toward a theory of social support: Closing conceptual gaps. *Journal of Social Issues, 40,* 11–36.

Skinner, R. A., & Piek, J. P. (2001). Psychosocial implications of poor motor coordination in children and adolescents. *Human Movement Science, 20,* 73–94.

Specht, J. A., King, G. A., & Francis, P. V. (1998). A preliminary study of strategies for maintaining self-esteem in adolescents with physical disabilities. *Canadian Journal of Rehabilitation, 11,* 109–116.

Suzuki, K. (1995). Psychological world of parents with Duchenne muscular dystrophy: Attitude toward the illness and death. *Japanese Journal of Child and Adolescent Psychiatry, 36,* 271–284.

Teplin, S. W., Howard, J. A., & O'Connor, M. J. (1981). Self-concept of young children with cerebral palsy. *Developmental Medicine and Child Neurology, 23,* 730–738.

Thompson, R. J., Zeman, J. L., Fanurik, D., & Sirotkin-Roses, M. (1992). The role of parents stress and coping and family functioning in parent and child adjustment to Duchenne muscular dystrophy. *Journal of Clinical Psychology, 48,* 11–19.

Todis, B., Irvin, L. K., Singer, G. H. S., & Yovanoff, P. (1993). The self-esteem parent program: quantitative and qualitative evaluation of a cognitive-behavioral intervention. In G. H. S. Singer & L. E. Powers (Eds.), *Families, disability, and empowerment: Active coping skills and strategies for family interventions* (pp. 203–229). Baltimore: Brookes.

van Rossum, J. H. V., & Vermeer, A. (1990). Perceived competence: A validation study in the field of motoric remedial teaching. *International Journal of Disability, Development and Education, 37,* 71–81.

Wilcox, B. L., & Vernberg, E. M. (1985). Conceptual and theoretical dilemmas facing social support research. In I. G. Sarason & B. R. Sarason (Eds.), *Social support: Theory, research and application* (pp. 3–20). Boston: Martinus Nijhoff.

World Health Oganization. (1980). *International classification of impairments, disabilities, and handicaps.* Geneva: Author.

World Health Oganization. (2001). *ICIDH-2: International classification of functioning, disability and health.* Geneva: Author.

Yin, R. K. (2003). *Case study research: Design and methods* (3rd ed.). Thousand Oaks, CA: Sage.

CHAPTER 20

Implications of Movement Difficulties for Social Interaction, Physical Activity, Play, and Sports

DAWNE LARKIN
JANET SUMMERS

Children with mild motor impairments and motor learning difficulties encounter many challenges in their day-to-day living. In this chapter we explore the implications that emerge from limitations in the coordination and control of movement and we focus on issues that can arise for children who have these problems. Although some children have additional learning difficulties in specific cognitive domains or more pervasive behavioral difficulties, we do not address how these complexities complicate their motor learning, rather, we focus on how a movement problem might constrain development in the social and physical domains. We discuss the impact of movement difficulties on social development, daily activity, physical activity, play, and sports. We also address some ways to modulate motor behavior and provide the child with culturally appropriate motor skills so that he or she can participate in a physically active life and overcome some of the social and physical limitations that occur with movement difficulties.

Movement difficulties are sometimes referred to as "hidden" motor deficits because they remain unrecognized and the associated complications are attributed to problems with behavior and attention. These "hidden" motor deficits encompass a range of terms (Cermak, Gubbay, & Larkin, 2002; Peters, Barnett, & Henderson, 2001) such as developmental coordination disorder (DCD; American Psychiatric Association, 1994), dyspraxia, and motor learning difficulties. The motor difficulties can be found in a range of conditions such as attention-deficit/hyperactivity disorder (ADHD), autism, cerebral palsy, head injuries, hemiplegia, hypotonia, academic learning disabilities, and syndromes such as *cri du chat* and Praeder–Willi. Whether the child has DCD or dyspraxia alone or with a co-occurring condition, the motor difficulties can be socially and psychologically debilitating if they are not recognized, understood, and addressed. Evidence is accruing that the long-term implications can be negative (see Cantell & Kooistra, 2002, for review; see also Fitzpatrick & Watkinson, 2003; Kirby & Drew, 1999) and failure to address the motor problems can limit independent development.

Why do movement deficits affect the lifestyle of children? Movement, so often taken for granted, is essential for our interactions with our social and physical environment. The interplay between action, perception, and cognition is manifest as we search and monitor our environments, explore spatial concepts, solve motor problems, express our ideas, and relate to people. Movement contributes to our efficiency in the perceptual and cognitive domains. Efficient movement allows us to do more with less effort, and, as a result, energy remains for additional activities. For example, the smooth coordination of the eye, head, and trunk provides the basis for easy manipulation (Bertenthal & von Hofsten, 1998) and the subsequent exploration of objects. By contrast, self-regulated exploration requires more energy and is made harder by impaired coordination and labored locomotion. Overall, the developmental pathways available to the child are limited by these motor difficulties.

Motor development has increasing influence on general development during the early years (Anderson et al., 2001; Hadders-Algra, 2000; Sporns & Edelman, 1993; Thelen, 1995, 2000; Touwen, 1998). Consequently, motor impairment is predicted not only to have negative influences on motor development but also to have more pervasive effects across development. The constraints on development may manifest at the morphological, social, emotional, and cognitive levels of observation. These constraints can lead to negative events and may contribute to overall, or specific, differences in the developmental pathway of the child.

Predictions about the implications of motor difficulties for general development vary by theoretical perspective. Unlike the perspectives that are biased toward nature or nurture, the framework that drives our thinking focuses on the interactive effects between the organism and the environment (Gottlieb, 1998; Newell, 1986; Thelen, 1995, 2000). This framework accommodates a number of issues that have intrigued and frustrated researchers and clinicians who work with children with motor learning difficulties or DCD. For example, from an interactive framework we would predict the heterogeneity of the population, the increased incidence of learning difficulties, the increased incidence of behavioral problems, and the negative social implications. Such a framework allows one to explore a number of questions, such as the following: (1) How early are the motor difficulties likely to impinge on the developmental pathway? (2) What initially does a parent perceive that causes concern? (3) Is it that the infant fails to achieve "motor milestones" when expected or are the infant's actions perceived and interpreted differently? (4) What are the social and behavioral implications of motor learning difficulties in the playground and do these associated difficulties contribute to overall attitudes to others and to school in general? Research to date tells us little about the influence of movement difficulties on these interactions.

MOTOR DIFFICULTIES AND SOCIAL INTERACTION

During infancy and childhood, movement provides a pathway to both social and motor development. The development of action is, in part, contingent upon interactions between the infant and parent or caregiver. This relationship is interdependent and reciprocating depending on the motor response of the infant as well as that of the parent (Trevarthen & Burford, 1993). If an infant with mild motor impairment is unable to move appropriately, social interaction can be compromised, consequently limiting social as well as motor development.

Studies of infant motor development help us to understand some of the difficulties to which infants with motor difficulties might be exposed. Danis, Bourdais, and Ruel (2000) demonstrate the importance of social interaction in early motor learning. They report that during the development of prehension, maternal behaviors are influenced by, and in turn influence, infants' behavior. There was reciprocation between motor and social learning. As the infants' responses toward toys changed from gross motor activity to grasping and manipulating, the mothers' behaviors changed from presenting the toy out of reach, then within reach, and then no activity on the toy, as the infant became more competent. What are the implications of motor constraints on this type of interactive communication? What happens if there is a limited response from the infant to the mother's stimulation? Does the mother stimulate even more or lose interest? Social interactions can influence the developmental pathway of the child with motor difficulties in a number of ways. Infants need an environment that blends social interaction with motor activity. Regular physical play during infancy and early childhood can contribute to more optimal social and physical development. Of particular importance is parental knowledge of the contribution of movement to the overall development of the child. Without this understanding, the infant with motor impairment can be deprived of the support necessary for optimal development.

As the social context changes with age, motor impairments and motor learning problems are likely to have different effects on social skill development of the child with motor difficulties. One of the more distressing aspects of motor impairment is the rejection by peers during primary school (Barbour, 1996; Smyth & Anderson, 2000; Summers & Larkin, 2002; Symes, 1972). What is it about the child with movement difficulties that makes him or her the object of other children's rejection? The rejection can occur because the child does not have the skills to participate in the play and "spoils" the game (discussed in more detail later), or it could be influenced by implicit recognition of the child's motor problem. Movement is a means of personal expression. Ramsden (1992) says, " For every individual, the complex and unceasing interplay of movement qualities forms a pattern which is one of the most telling expressions of a person's individuality" (p. 222). She says that we vary the intensity and combinations of movement elements to express ourselves through our actions. Thus, the nonverbal communication of children who have difficulties with control and coordination of movement might appear more constrained or unusual when compared with typical children. This could further contribute to (1) rejection by peers; (2) the use of derogatory terms to describe their movement and behavior; and (3) the consequent social isolation. On the flipside, if a child with motor difficulties has an inability to read movement, that is a difficulty with movement perception, as opposed to difficulty with static perception; such a deficit might have implications for both social–emotional learning, reading of facial expressions, and more general motor learning.

The social context also modulates motor development (Cintas, 1995; Hopkins & Westra, 1989) such that parents' limited knowledge and biases can contribute to an enriched or deprived motor experience. Sprinkle and Hammond (1997) report case studies of children with motor difficulties whose parents did not encourage involvement in physical activity and sport. In one case the parents feared that the child would have an accident; in the other it was a dislike for the competitive sport environment. Often parents do not understand the contribution of physical activity to the normal growth and development of the musculoskeletal and the cardiorespiratory systems, nor do they realize that movement deprivation might further compromise the development of their child whose motor skills are already lagging.

Although there is limited documentation of the influence of impaired movement on the development of the social relationship between the infant and caregiver, parents of children with DCD report concerns about the social interaction with other family members (Chia, 1997; Gibson, 1996; Schoemaker & Kalverboer, 1994; Summers & Larkin, 2002; Taylor, 1990). The negative interactions occur with mothers, fathers, siblings, grandparents, and other relatives who do not understand the motor problem. These negative social interactions revolve around issues of motor performance such as slowness in dressing, untidiness, and messy mealtime behavior, discussed later. Parents report avoiding grandparents who are intolerant of the child's eating behaviors and limiting social interaction with critical relatives. Thus, it is not surprising that parents of adolescents with movement difficulties report higher stress levels when asked about family functioning and family health than do parents of matched controls (Larkin & Parker, 1999).

The early social–emotional experiences of children with DCD appear to carry over into adolescence (Cantell & Kooistra, 2002; Losse et al., 1991) and into later life. Research by Fitzpatrick and Watkinson (2003) showed that many adults reporting movement difficulties have negative memories from their childhood. They experienced failure in sport and physical education and subsequently were humiliated and embarrassed by their very public performances and the reactions of others to their behavior. While some adults with movement difficulties learn to deal with their movement limitations and lowered movement confidence, others remain alienated and still carry the social scars from their experiences during childhood and adolescence (Fitzpatrick & Watkinson, 2003; Larkin & Parker, 1999).

Do the social implications of motor difficulties differ for females and males? There are a few lines of evidence that support differences in attitudes and expectations of girls and boys in the movement domain. These differences may affect the recognition and social support received by girls and boys with motor impairment. Perhaps gender expectations about motor performance contribute to different reactions to motor impairment in boys and girls. The limited evidence does show that observations and judgments of movement performance are not always well matched for either girls or boys. Research with infants demonstrates that differences in perceptions of motor performance start during the first year of life. In a study of 11-month-old males and females crawling on a slope, mothers underestimated the motor performance of infant girls and overestimated the motor performance of infant boys (Mondschein, Adolph, & Tamis-LeMonda, 2000).

Our own research has reinforced that recognition of the motor performance levels of boys and girls is often inaccurate when based on movement observation. In our study involving teachers' observations of over 2,000 primary schoolchildren, only 2.3% of the children were identified with motor difficulties (Revie & Larkin, 1993a) despite population studies in this country (Larkin & Rose, 1999) and in Sweden (Kadesjö & Gillberg, 1999), suggesting that the incidence of motor difficulties may be over 10%. More boys were identified but with less accuracy than girls, with the girls scoring very poorly in comparison to the boys on a movement assessment battery (Arnheim & Sinclair, 1979). Girls were only identified by teachers if they had quite severe motor difficulties. Differences in the play behavior of boys and girls, discussed later, might contribute further to different expectations in the movement domain.

Although the nonverbal communications manifest through the inefficient movement of children with DCD are implicitly acknowledged and evaluated by families and peers, explicitly the motor problems often remain unrecognized. This is probably one of the reasons these children are labeled as "lazy" and parents, relatives, and peers do not understand their neuromotor difficulties. Many professionals who deal with young children still fail to recognize the condition (Fox & Lent, 1996; Revie & Larkin, 1993a). Consequently, neither the parents nor the children receive needed social support (Dyspraxia Foundation, 1998; Stephenson, McKay, & Chesson 1991; Stephenson & McKay, 1989) that could modulate the negative influences on the social development of these children and adolescents.

In summary, motor difficulties are likely to have an impact on social development and social interactions in a negative way. In turn, the reciprocal interactions between motor and social development can create an environment that contributes to avoidance of motor activities and further limits motor development. Recognition of the motor difficulty accompanied by social support might change the developmental pathway sufficiently to eliminate some of the long-term problems associated with motor impairments (Cantell, Smyth, & Ahonen, 1994; Fitzpatrick & Watkinson, 2003; Losse et al., 1991).

MOTOR DIFFICULTIES AND DAILY LIVING

One of the criteria for DCD according to the fourth edition of *Diagnostic and Statistical Manual of Mental Disorders* (DSM-IV; American Psychiatric Association, 1994) is difficulty with activities of daily living (ADL) requiring motor coordination. Because many daily activities involve coordination and control of movement, it is not surprising that children with DCD have difficulty getting dressed and organized for school. To get off to school, these children are more likely to need help with grooming, packing their bag, and preparing their lunch. In a study that compared Australian and Canadian 6- and 8-year-old children with DCD to matched controls, parents reported that children with DCD require more time and supervision to dress in the morning. To avoid frustration for the family and the child, parents reported using various strategies such as getting the child up earlier and laying out his or her clothes, assisting with dressing, and constant prompts to stay on track. Parents selected suitable clothing, typically t-shirts and velcro-closing shoes, to make dressing easier (Summers, Larkin, & Dewey, 2001a, 2001b). These findings are similar to those reported in Scotland (Chesson, McKay, & Stephenson, 1990) where two-thirds of the parents of children with motor learning difficulties reported difficulties with ADL. Children were slow at tasks and family routines were influenced by the child's difficulties. Morning routines, mealtimes, and homework were sources of stress to mothers.

The motor profiles of children with DCD differ, with some children experiencing more difficulty with gross motor skills than fine motor skills, while others have difficulty in both areas (Summers et al., 2001a, 2001b). Children with fine motor difficulties were likely to experience more problems with ADL that relied on manipulative skills. At home these include meal-related tasks such as using knives and forks, household chores such as stacking dishes or tidying drawers, and grooming. At school, these children experienced particular difficulty with motor skills such as drawing and writing, which contributed to slower schoolwork. When children had general problems with coordination and control, some aspects of grooming and personal hygiene became a problem both at home and at school. In addition, many of these children had difficulties with simple activities that require locomotion, such as moving around in the classroom and from classroom to classroom.

The difficulties in performing essential daily activities interfered with family dynamics and the daily routine at home and at school. Nevertheless, individual difficulties in performing ADL varied quite markedly depending on the child, the child's motor profile, and the attitude of the major caregiver. Although most parents reported many similar difficulties when their children performed daily tasks, parents used different strategies to deal with the issues. Examples with dressing illustrate these differences. Most parents reported the time it took their child to dress. However, some parents focused on the slow but arduous process of teaching their child independent dressing skills; other parents resorted to dressing the child or allowing the child to sleep in his or her clothing in order to deal with the time constraints of the morning routine (Summers et al., 2001a, 2001b). Overall, parents reported the need for more structure in the daily routine to overcome some of these motor difficulties and the frustrations that arise with daily activities (Summers et al., 2001a, 2001b).

MOTOR DIFFICULTIES AND PHYSICAL ACTIVITY

Childhood is a time when physical play and physical activity predominate (Eaton, McKeen, & Campbell, 2001). It is a time when fundamental motor skills including running, jumping, hopping, and skipping are developed and refined. During this period, children with DCD, dyspraxia, and mild cerebral palsy manifest a number of problems with motor coordination and control (see Williams, 2002, for a review). Children with ADHD, autism, and Down syndrome are also likely to demonstrate some of these movement difficulties, as are some children with acquired brain damage resulting from accidents or diseases. A major concern is that motor learning difficulties or movement impairments increase the probability that children will withdraw from physical activity. Physical health is at real risk for adolescents and adults who drop out or withdraw from physical activity in the first years of school and who have very low participation levels. Relative inactivity in children with motor learning difficulties seems to interfere with normal development of fitness, including aerobic and motor fitness, strength, and anaerobic power (O'Beirne, Larkin, & Cable, 1994; Raynor, 2001). Body mass index and endomorphy are higher in some of these children (Larkin, Hoare, & Kerr, 1989). Those children with increased body weight and decreased activity are more likely to become obese with all the attendant health risks. In turn, lower fitness levels lead to greater difficulty in performing motor skills efficiently, and this has implications for perceptions of movement competence and movement confidence. In addition, children with low levels of physical activity and low fitness levels are more likely to report that they are lonely (Page, Frey, Talbert, & Falk, 1992).

In this section of the chapter, we focus on the implications of motor learning difficulties on motor skill performance and physical fitness. Although the evidence that crawling skills develop later in children who have motor learning difficulty is equivocal (Hoare, 1991; Stephenson, McKay, & Chesson, 1990), other locomotor skills including walking (Hoare, 1991; Taylor 1990), cycling (Taylor, 1990), and hopping are achieved later than average. When children with DCD do acquire these skills, the quality of the performance is generally inefficient so that even if they spend similar amounts of time compared to their peers in skill mastery (Smyth & Anderson, 2000), they are more likely to automate "bad habits."

We draw on some common motor skills to identify the movement difficulties frequently limiting the production of efficient skills. Many of these difficulties can be eliminated with appropriate task teaching, specific feedback, and persistence. The task-specific approach to teaching motor skills to children with DCD involves intensive teaching of culturally appropriate fundamental motor skills that are precursors to more complex playground and sport skills. Teaching generally occurs individually or in small groups with a high pupil-to-teacher ratio. Technique and quality of movement are emphasized and timely feedback focuses on task efficiency by providing knowledge of performance to the learner. The child is explicitly taught strategies of how to deal with the dynamic spatial and temporal demands of the environment. Teaching and reteaching with feedback, social support through the learning process, and motivation by reinforcing small gains eventually result in a more competent performance of the task (Larkin & Parker, 2002). The focus is on attaining a movement pattern that looks good, is efficient, and can be adapted to different contexts. Research to date provides good support for the use of the task-specific approach with children with DCD (Pless & Carlsson, 2000; Revie & Larkin, 1993b).

FUNDAMENTAL MOTOR SKILLS

Fundamental motor skills such as running, jumping, hitting, kicking, and catching are essential skills for casual play and competitive sports. Difficulties with or failure to achieve these motor skills precludes a child from many culturally based activities and exposes him or her to peer ridicule and rejection.

Running

Generally children with motor learning problems do learn to run; however, without teaching, they are unlikely to develop an efficient technique. As a consequence, running is difficult and the energy required is increased. Aspects of performance that regularly contribute to the inefficient technique include (1) an unstable head that moves from side to side or up and down; (2) a trunk that rotates excessively and arms that swing across the body rather than in the direction of the run; (3) excessive flexion at the hips; (4) limited leg drive; and (5) flat foot landing (Larkin & Hoare, 1991; Larkin & Parker, 2002). Running practice without teaching tends to reinforce these inefficient techniques so that they become "habits" and are increasingly difficult to change.

An inefficient running technique can result in reduced involvement in physical activity for a few reasons. The first is that the movement requires a lot of energy and is hard to do. If maintaining balance is an issue, then the resulting falls can be painful and reduce movement confidence. Another reason is that the inefficient technique and falls elicit peer ridicule, and sometimes parent and teacher ridicule. Peers will clearly articulate to the child, "You run funny." This decreases the likelihood of inclusion in play activities and also influences the child's perceptions of movement competence.

Because running is such a basic skill, it is helpful to the child to improve the technique of his or her running style. This can be done with task-specific teaching provided by a competent coach or physical educator. It involves analysis of the technique, and elimination of established inefficient movement patterns, with regular movement-based feedback to establish a more efficient technique (Larkin & Parker, 2002). Changing and developing the technique require patience and perseverance. The benefits to children are that they eventually come to run more efficiently and they no longer are teased about their inefficient running performance. They are able to participate in running as a fitness activity and some children begin to enjoy running and to participate successfully in cross-country running.

Hitting

Hitting skills are necessary for a range of games, from T-ball and golf, where the ball is stationary, to tennis, baseball, field hockey, cricket, and ice hockey, where a moving object (i.e., ball or puck) is hit, often on the run. Basic hitting skills are difficult for children with coordination problems, yet T-ball is a game that children often want to play because their friends or peer-group value it. When it comes to learning to hit, positioning and technique contribute to the inefficient performance (Larkin & Hoare, 1991). Children learning to hit a ball often have some of the difficulties experienced by children with motor learning problems; however, they overcome them rapidly with good teaching. Children with motor learning difficulties maintain inefficient practices for longer despite coaching and feedback. They can have difficulty achieving a consistent and efficient grip on the hitting implement. They regularly have problems with the initial positioning of their body in relation to the ball. They may stand too close or too far away, making it difficult to hit the ball. They generally position themselves front on, instead of side on to the ball and the direction of the hit. This positioning prevents them from developing the rotational forces to apply to the ball. When they know all the elements of the technique they can still have difficulty with timing so that the movement looks disjointed. Some children with movement problems do not overcome the timing problem and are probably better directed to less complex motor skills where multisegmental timing is not so crucial. Others achieve an acceptable level of performance after a period of coaching and perseverance on the part of the motivated child and teacher. Achieving competence in these skills opens the door to lifetime social activities such as golf and tennis.

One issue that continues to haunt us, as we attempt to understand the implications of motor deficits for the control and coordination of movement skills, is that we have yet to identify the different factors that can perturb motor learning and motor control. Understanding this will help us to deal better with the problems that arise. We can then assist children to develop skills that draw on their best resources. Identifying subtypes of movement problems (see Dewey, 2002, for a review) contributes to our understanding of the relative strengths and weaknesses that children with movement difficulties bring to the learning environment. For example, there are children who appear to have better dynamic balance than static balance. Motor learning of specific tasks might vary if the underlying problem was one of balance rather than motor coordination. If the motor problem arose from problems with both balance and coordination, then that would mean more severe motor learning difficulties with a wider range of physical activities. When we consider some of the underlying motor deficits manifest (e.g., slower reaction time, slower movement time, and increased co-contraction) by children with DCD (Raynor, 2001; Williams, 2002), it is not surprising that they have such difficulty achieving these fundamental motor skills.

PHYSICAL FITNESS

There now is sufficient research available to suggest that children with motor learning difficulties, DCD, or dyspraxia have lower fitness levels when contrasted with control groups with no motor impairment. While Gubbay (1975) suggested that " 'the clumsy child' is to be regarded as one ... whose physical strength, sensation, and coordination are virtually normal by the standards of routine conventional neurological assessment" (p. 39), data comparing these children to normative samples indicate that their lower levels of strength and power could limit their ability to efficiently carry out a number of physical activities.

Our data indicate that they have lower levels of anaerobic power and they tire more readily (O'Beirne et al., 1994). These children who were 7, 8, and 9 years of age produced significantly lower levels of work than did their better coordinated peers on the Wingate Anaerobic test (Bar-Or, 1983, 1987) which involves a 30-second all-out trial on a bicycle ergometer. We particularly chose this task as the bicycle constrains their movement and subsequently controls for some of the coordination difficulties that are inherent to the children's condition. Despite this attempt to control for their coordination difficulties, they had significantly lower peak and mean power output, but their mean heart rate was similar to that of the control group, suggesting that they were working as hard. Of particular interest were the results from the fatigue index that provided an estimate of local muscular fatigue. Fatigue decreased with age in the control group, but it increased with age in the group with coordination difficulties.

To further reduce the confounding of coordination in the measurement of strength and power, Raynor (2001) used simple tasks, knee flexion, and knee extension under isometric and isokinetic conditions to look at differences between a group of boys with DCD and a control group. She found that boys with DCD produced significantly lower levels of flexor and extensor force in comparison to the control group. Raynor suggested that the increased levels of muscular coactivation found with the DCD group could contribute to their lower strength and power.

Aerobic fitness also appears to be lower in children with DCD. Again, the measurement of this aspect of fitness is confounded by coordination difficulties and lower limb power, so we must be cautious about interpretation of the tests. With this in mind, children with DCD and other movement difficulties consistently show low levels of aerobic fitness on tests including the 800 meter run, the 1.6 kilometer run, and the multistage shuttle run (see Hands & Larkin, 2002, for review). Among the factors that contribute to the lower levels of fitness, apparent among children with DCD is their lower level of vigorous activity (Bouffard, Watkinson, Thompson, Causgrove Dunn,

& Romanow, 1996; Kuiper, Reynders, & Rispens, 1997; Rarick & McKee, 1949), as well as their tendency to play less active games (Cratty, Ikeda, Martin, Jennet, & Morris, 1970; Smyth & Anderson, 2000). This withdrawal or avoidance of vigorous physical activity could further contribute to differences in their motor developmental pathway as it is during middle childhood that children are particularly active (Eaton et al., 2001) and there is a remarkable increase in anaerobic power as a function of physical activity. Withdrawal from physical activity could also compromise the development of the neuromuscular system, the cardiorespiratory system, and the musculoskeletal system.

Bouffard and colleagues (1996) propose an activity deficit hypothesis for children with movement difficulties. That is, they withdraw from movement and the subsequent low level of activity results in low levels of physical fitness. The activity deficit hypothesis overlaps with the hypoactivity hypothesis, which proposes that the system deteriorates as a function of disuse (Bar-Or, 1983). Both propositions have far-reaching implications for this group in that both motor learning and performance will suffer a related downward spiral. In addition, the healthy lifestyle that is associated with the active life will be compromised. We need research to explore whether children with DCD, who withdraw from physical activity, are more likely to be overweight and more susceptible to cardiovascular disease and other lifestyle diseases as they age.

IMPLICATIONS FOR PHYSICAL PLAY AND LEISURE

Action and interaction are important aspects of play. In the early years, a child's play is often directed toward parents (Trevarthen & Aitken, 2001). In the preschool years, it becomes more directed toward peers. Once a child reaches school, play is an important part of social interaction with peers and the social rejection discussed earlier interferes with involvement in play and games. Because boys and girls have different styles of play (Barbour, 1996, 1999; Cratty et al., 1970), and boys' play involves more physically aggressive activities, the possibility arises that boys with motor learning difficulties are at greater risk of rejection in the social play setting than are girls with similar movement problems. In an American study, Barbour (1996) reported that boys tend to play in the playground with boys who have similar motor skill levels, while girls interact with a more heterogeneous grouping. In a British study of playground behavior, Smyth and Anderson (2000) found that girls with DCD were less likely to be involved in informal team games than were girls without DCD, and when they were involved in these games they were more likely to be less active. Although the boys with DCD played less football, they were quite similar to boys in the control group in the time that they spent in informal team games, such as tag and hide and seek.

It is clear that children with motor learning difficulties have different strategies for coping with their difficulties. As Smyth and Anderson (2000) note, their participation is more variable than that of their age-matched peers. One coping strategy used by children with movement difficulties is to play with younger children (Rarick & McKee, 1949). Another way to cope with movement difficulties is to spend less time in situations that require physical play. For example, children with movement difficulties are less likely to spend time on playground equipment such as swings and bars (Barbour, 1999; Bouffard et al., 1996). Boys with DCD are more likely to be observed in the playground with a book (Smyth & Anderson, 2000). They are also more likely to be involved in fantasy play (Cratty et al., 1970; Smyth & Anderson, 2000). Children with low levels of motor skill spend less time in playgrounds than do their coordinated peers (Rarick & McKee, 1949), and in the playground they are more likely to spend time just watching a game (Smyth & Anderson, 2000). They are also less likely to play with a large group (Barbour, 1999; Rarick & McKee, 1949; Smyth & Anderson, 2000) and more likely to play with one or two children or remain on their own (Bouffard et al., 1996; Smyth & Anderson, 2000).

A study that followed children from a movement program into adolescence (Larkin & Parker, 1999) showed that their involvement in physical recreation differed from that of an age- and gender-matched normative sample. There was a significant difference in the number of recreational activities between the group that had motor learning difficulties with a median score of 4 and the control group with a median score of 7. In contrast, the group with a history of motor learning difficulties was involved in significantly more sedentary hobbies than were the control group. Thus, the adolescents who had difficulties with motor learning were less involved in physical recreation; however, they compensated by being involved in less active recreational pursuits.

The research to date indicates that children with motor difficulties generally participate in play that is less active and in keeping with their limited motor abilities. If our aim is to provide them with a healthy lifestyle, it is important to direct them to recreational activities that help to maintain an optimal level of physical fitness and health. For young children, playgrounds with a variety of equipment and materials appear to facilitate more varied opportunities for play (Barbour, 1999). Children with motor difficulties are more likely to be drawn to the "sedentary society" and replace active games with sedentary recreational activities. Encouraging active play through well-planned school and community facilities will benefit these children socially and emotionally if good coaching is matched with appropriate social support. The environment needs to provide opportunities for continued participation, and these activities need to be fun.

IMPLICATIONS FOR PARTICIPATION IN SPORTS

The difficulties encountered in the sporting domain vary with cultural demands and the demands of the sport. Generally, involvement in team sports increases in importance through the mid-primary school years when children are more active (Eaton et al., 2001). This is a time when children play in groups, and sport contributes to the social status of boys (Chase & Dummer, 1992). Unfortunately, fundamental motor skills, such as running, throwing, hitting, and catching, are inefficient in children with DCD. Therefore, they often lack the basic skills for participation in sports. Even when they are coached to perform the skills with good technique, they often lack speed. When we add the complexity of the open environment where a player has to deal with a moving ball and moving offenders and defenders, it is not surprising that the children with motor difficulties are less likely to participate. Boys with movement difficulties are less likely to play games such as football (Cratty et al., 1970; Smyth & Anderson, 2001). Cratty and colleagues (1970) found that 63% of boys with movement difficulties ($n = 105$) reported that they played football in comparison to 88% of their age-matched group without movement difficulties. In their playground observation study, Smyth and Anderson (2001) found that boys with DCD were more likely to participate in playground football in grade 2 than in higher grades, but in the higher grades, the boys with DCD played significantly less football than did their peers.

We studied the activity patterns of adolescents who had a history of motor learning difficulties (Larkin & Parker, 1999). During elementary school, these children were exposed to a movement enrichment program in a socially supportive environment. In response to a question that probed for their favorite physical activity, the adolescents with motor difficulties had a higher incidence of bicycle riding, swimming, and hitting sports, whereas the matched adolescent control group preferred team games, including basketball, football, and netball. The combined motor, cognitive, and spatial demands of these sports are generally too complex for children with motor impairments. However, some of the 86 adolescents with motor difficulties identified team games as their favorite physical activity (basketball = 9, netball = 2, football = 7). Not surprisingly, adolescents with motor impairments also were more likely to report that they had no favorite physical activity ($n = 10$) compared to adolescents in the control group ($n = 2$).

Apart from the physical difficulty of participation in sport, psychosocial difficulties also provide further barriers to participation. When it comes to team sports, children with motor difficulties are the last to be chosen (Short & Crawford, 1984). They report low levels of social support from classmates and best friends (Rose, Larkin, & Berger, 1994). Their confidence to participate is eroded by interactions with their peers (Symes, 1972). Their self-perceptions of competence in sport are lower (Larkin & Parker, 1997), and they are more likely to perceive themselves as less competent in the athletic domain (Rose, Larkin, & Berger, 1997). Their motivation for challenging physical activities is likely to be lower (Rose, Larkin, & Berger, 1998) and competitive team sports would certainly be challenging for them. Because fun is a major reason for participation in sport, it is easy to see why children with motor difficulties would avoid involvement in many sports.

Even in less complex and less competitive sports, children with DCD find it difficult to participate without additional coaching and social support. In countries such as Australia, where children start swimming classes early and many children can swim by 6 years of age, children with motor learning difficulties become conspicuous because they are unable to keep up with the levels achieved by their peers. Whereas 5- to 6-year-olds regularly learn freestyle (Parker & Blanksby, 1997), children with motor impairments are much older as they require many more lessons to achieve competent levels of skill. Because this is a culturally appropriate achievement for children, the failure to achieve at a socially acceptable age contributes further to the anxiety of both the child and the parent. Parents of children with movement difficulties ask swimming teachers to focus on the aspects of a child's swimming necessary to pass levels already passed by the child's peer group. Typical problems that the children encounter include fear of putting the face in the water and fear of floating on their back. They generally have a very inefficient freestyle and backstroke kick that originates from the knee rather than the hip. Although this is acceptable with younger children, it is viewed differently in older children, setting them apart from their peers and exposing them to teasing by peers. In instances in which they do not have good trunk stability it becomes extremely difficult for the child to control the many degrees of freedom necessary to produce an efficient and coordinated stroke. Coordinating the efficient kick with the efficient arm stroking and the breathing is extremely complex and thus very difficult for these children. Whereas most children are taught swimming in small groups, children with motor problems need one-on-one attention so that the teacher can provide specific coaching and feedback. It takes them many times longer to learn a stroke competently even with competent teaching.

Children with coordination difficulties, after persistent task-specific instruction, are generally able to handle sports such as swimming and bicycling, where the movement demands are relatively repetitive and the environmental demands are not changing or are relatively predictable. However, some children are highly motivated and manage to participate in more complex sports. For those children who are diagnosed with more obvious motor impairments such as cerebral palsy, there are social structures in place so that they can participate in sports that cater for their disability. Children with intellectual disabilities, where there is also a high incidence of motor impairment, also have associations that provide for physical leisure and sport. By contrast, children with DCD, dyspraxia, and motor learning problems are excluded from these special groups and also marginalized in mainstream groups. While some of the children with coordination difficulties have no desire to participate in sport, some want to participate in the socially acceptable sports. Further, some of these children are successful in participating, particularly if the coach and parents are supportive and the motivational climate focuses on participation rather than winning.

Because there is the possibility of psychosocial harm when children attempt to participate in sport, it is important that parents and professionals provide a supportive environment and, where possible, direct the child toward activities that draw on the child's best resources. When a child wants to participate in a sport even though he or she clearly lacks the basic skills, three approaches can be worked on sequentially or in parallel: (1) the child needs extra coaching in the basic skills, the rules, and strategies; (2) the team chosen needs to have a coach who is patient and helpful with children with motor learning difficulties; and (3) the parent needs to listen carefully to the child so that if the child needs to terminate involvement in a sport, the parent is supportive. Such approaches can avoid the trauma of social rejection and teasing, and the embarrassment of a public show of movement incompetence.

We generally direct children with movement difficulties toward lifetime sports, such as swimming, cycling, sailing, 10-pin bowling, and golf. We advise parents to ensure that the children have professional coaching when they take up the sport to enhance the chances of successful participation and to avoid the development of inefficient movement patterns. If by adolescence they have competence in just one skill (e.g., swimming or bicycling) and can perform that activity with relative ease and confidence, they have a socially acceptable way of coping with the expectation of peers as well as a lifetime physical activity.

SUMMARY AND CONCLUSION

Motor difficulties constrain the developmental pathways available to children. The motor difficulties can limit social interactions, participation in ADL at home and at school, and participation in culturally based physical activities. The child with motor difficulties has less efficient movement and has to work harder to achieve motor skills. Subsequent withdrawal from an active life will compromise development of the musculoskeletal and cardiorespiratory systems and lead to low levels of fitness. In turn, this can increase the risk of health-related problems. However, the developmental pathway can be facilitated by the early identification of motor problems, educating parents and professionals on the need for social support, and providing the child with a movement enrichment program and skill specific interventions. Although limited research is available, most children are able to achieve sufficient levels of skill to enjoy participating in some physical activities. The learning of physical skills, such as swimming, cycling, and sailing, opens a pathway to lifetime social participation and long-term physical health.

As we consider the long-term implications of mild motor deficits (see Figure 20.1), we need to consider the interplay of positive and negative assets that the child has (e.g., strong cognitive skills, a sense of humor, motivation, an ability to play, and supportive or nonsupportive parents and teachers). Some children with motor difficulties live in an environment that increases their ability to deal with their limited resources; others live in situations in which the deficit is exacerbated by life's circumstances. Cultural expectations that vary for girls and boys may lead to different implications based on gender. Thus, cultural and life chances can lead to different developmental pathways such that a motor deficit can have very different implications for social development, involvement in physical activity, play, and sport. Public policy and educational strategies are needed to ensure that these children have access to physical activity in socially supportive environments that facilitate movement skill development and enjoyment.

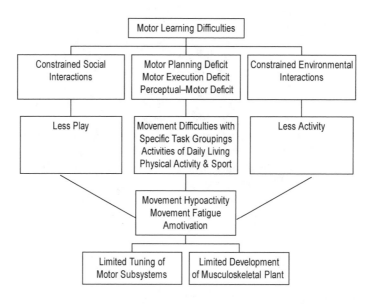

FIGURE 20.1. Ongoing implications of mild motor learning deficits.

ACKNOWLEDGEMENTS

While writing this chapter Janet Summers was diagnosed with a glioblastoma multiforme brain tumor. Sadly, she passed away in September 2003. Janet held an appointment as a Lecturer in the School of Occupational Therapy, Curtin University of Technology, Perth, Australia. She was in the final stages of completing her PhD thesis in the School of Human Movement and Exercise Science, The University of Western Australia, Perth, Australia. Her research focused on the performance of activities of daily living in children with developmental coordination disorder, an area of investigation that had received very little attention in the research literature. She will be sorely missed by her colleagues and the many students whose lives she touched.

REFERENCES

American Psychiatric Association. (1994). *Diagnostic and statistical manual of mental disorders* (4th ed.). Washington, DC: Author.

Anderson, D. I., Campos, J. J., Anderson, D. E., Thomas, T. D., Witherington, D.C., Uchiyama, I., et al. (2001). The flip side of perception-action coupling: Locomotor experience and the ontogeny of visual-postural coupling. *Human Movement Science, 20,* 461–487.

Arnheim, D., & Sinclair, W. A. (1979). *The clumsy child: A program of motor therapy* (2nd ed.). St. Louis, MO: Mosby.

Barbour, A. C. (1996). Physical competence and peer relations in 2nd-graders qualitative case studies of recess play. *Journal of Research in Childhood Education, 11,* 35–46.

Barbour, A. C. (1999). The impact of playground design on the play behaviors of children with differing levels of physical competence. *Early Childhood Research Quarterly, 14,* 75–98.

Bar-Or, O. (1983). *Pediatric sports medicine for the practitioner.* New York: Springer Verlag.

Bar-Or, O. (1987). Pathophysiological factors which limit the exercise capacity of the sick child. *Sports Science, 4,* 381–394.

Bertenthal, B., & Von Hofsten, C. (1998). Eye, head and trunk control: The foundation of manual development. *Neuroscience and Biobehavioral Reviews, 22,* 515–520.

Bouffard, M., Watkinson, E. J., Thompson, L. P., Causgrove Dunn, J. L., & Romanow, S. K. E. (1996). A test of the activity deficit hypothesis with children with movement difficulties. *Adapted Physical Activity Quarterly, 13,* 61–73.

Cantell, M., & Kooistra, L. (2002). Long-term outcomes of developmental coordination disorder. In S. A. Cermak & D. Larkin (Eds.), *Developmental coordination disorder* (pp. 23–38). Albany, NY: Delmar Thomson Learning.

Cantell, M., Smyth, M. M., & Ahonen, T. P. (1994). Clumsiness in adolescence: Educational, motor and social outcomes of motor delay detected at 5 years. *Adapted Physical Activity Quarterly, 11,* 129–155.

Cermak, S. A., Gubbay, S. S., & Larkin, D. (2002). What is developmental coordination disorder? In S. A. Cermak & D. Larkin (Eds.), *Developmental coordination disorder* (pp. 2–22). Albany, NY: Delmar Thomson Learning.

Chase, M. A., & Dummer, G. M. (1992). The role of sports as a social status determinant for children. *Research Quarterly for Exercise and Sport, 63,* 418–424.

Chesson, R., McKay, C., & Stephenson, E. (1990). Motor/learning difficulties and the family. *Child: Care, Health and Development, 16,* 123–138.

Chia, S. H. (1997). The child, his family, and dyspraxia. *Professional Care of Mother and Child, 7*(4), 105–107.

Cintas, H. L. (1995). Cross-cultural similarities and differences in development and the impact of parental expectations on motor behavior. *Pediatric Physical Therapy, 7,* 103–111.

Cratty, B. J., Ikeda, N., Martin, M. M., Jennet, C., & Morris, M. (1970). *Movement activities,* motor ability and the education of children (pp. 45–85). Springfield, IL: Charles C. Thomas.

Danis, A., Bourdais, C., & Ruel, J. (2000). The co-construction of joint action between mothers and 2–4-month-old infants: The mother's role. *Infant and Child Development, 9,* 181–198.

Dewey, D. (2002). Subtypes of developmental coordination disorder. In S. A. Cermak & D. Larkin (Eds.), *Developmental coordination disorder* (pp. 40–53). Albany, NY: Delmar Thomson Learning.

Dyspraxia Foundation. (1998). *Member's questionnaire—June 1997 awareness and diagnosis.* [Online]. Available from http://www.emmbrook.demon.co.uk/dysprax/report.html.

Eaton, W. O., McKeen, N. A., & Campbell, D. W. (2001). The waxing and waning of movement: Implications for psychological development. *Developmental Review, 21,* 205–223.

Fitzpatrick, D., & Watkinson, J. (2003). The lived experience of physical awkwardness: Adults' retrospective views. *Adapted Physical Activity Quarterly, 20,* 279–297.

Fox, A. M., & Lent, B. (1996). Clumsy children primer on developmental coordination disorder. *Canadian Family Physician, 42,* 1965–1971.

Gibson, R. C. (1996). The effects of dyspraxia on family relationships. *British Journal of Therapy and Rehabilitation, 3,* 101–105.

Gottlieb, G. (1998). Normally occurring environmental and behavioral influences on gene activity: From central dogma to probabilistic epigenesis. *Psychological Review, 105,* 792–802.

Gubbay, S. S. (1975). *The clumsy child: A study in developmental apraxic and agnosic ataxia.* London: Saunders.

Hadders-Algra, M. (2000). The neuronal group selection theory: A framework to explain variation in normal motor development. *Developmental Medicine and Child Neurology, 42,* 566–572.

Hands, B., & Larkin, D. (2002). Physical fitness and developmental coordination disorder. In S. A. Cermak & D. Larkin (Eds.), *Developmental coordination disorder* (pp. 172–184). Albany, NY: Delmar Thomson Learning.

Hoare, D. (1991). *Classification of movement dysfunctions in children: Descriptive and statistical approaches.* Unpublished doctoral thesis, University of Western Australia, Nedlands, Western Australia, Australia.

Hopkins, B., & Westra, T. (1989). Maternal expectations of their infants' development: Some cultural differences. *Developmental Medicine and Child Neurology, 32,* 384–390.

Kadesjö, B., & Gillberg, C. (1999). Developmental coordination disorder in Swedish 7-year-old children. *Journal of the American Academy of Child and Adolescent Psychiatry, 38,* 820–828.

Kirby, A., & Drew, S. (1999, October). *Is DCD a diagnosis that we should be using for adults? Is clumsiness the issue in adults and adolescents?* Paper presented at the 4th biennial workshop on children with developmental coordination disorder, "From Research to Diagnostics and Intervention," Groningen, The Netherlands.

Kuiper, D., Reynders, K., & Rispens, P. (1997, May). *Leisure time physical activity in children with movement difficulties: A pilot study.* Paper presented at the 11th International Symposium for Adapted Physical Activity, Quebec.

Larkin, D., & Hoare, D. (1991). *Out of step: coordinating kids' movement.* Nedlands, Australia: Active Life Foundation.

Larkin, D., Hoare, D., & Kerr, G. (1989, August). *Structure/function interactions: A concern for the poorly coordinated.* Poster presentation at the 7th IFAPA International Symposium, Berlin.

Larkin, D., & Parker, H. E. (1997). Gender differences in physical self-descriptions of adolescents with a history of motor learning difficulties. *Australian Educational and Developmental Psychologist, 14,* 63–71.

Larkin, D., & Parker, H. E. (1999). Physical activity profiles of adolescents who experienced motor learning difficulties. In D. Drouin, C. Lepine, & C. Simard (Eds.), *Proceedings of the 11th International Symposium for Adapted Physical Activity* (pp. 175–181). Quebec, Canada.

Larkin, D., & Parker, H. E. (2002). Task-specific intervention for children with developmental coordination disorder: A systems view. In S. A. Cermak & D. Larkin (Eds.), *Developmental coordination disorder* (pp. 234–247). Albany, NY: Delmar Thomson Learning.

Larkin, D., & Rose, B. (1999, October). *Use of the McCarron Assessment of Neuromuscular Development for DCD identification.* Paper presented at the 4th biennial workshop on children with a developmental coordination disorder, Groningen, The Netherlands.

Losse, A., Henderson, S. E., Elliman, D., Hall, D., Knight, E., & Jongmans, M. (1991). Clumsiness in children—Do they grow out of it? A 10-year follow-up study. *Developmental Medicine and Child Neurology, 33,* 55–68.

Mondschein, E. R., Adolph, K. E., & Tamis-Le Monda, C. S. (2000). Gender bias in mothers' expectations about infant crawling. *Journal of Experimental Child Psychology, 77,* 304–316.

Newell, K. M. (1986). Constraints on the development of coordination. In M. G. Wade & H. T. A. Whiting (Eds.), *Motor development in children: Aspects of coordination and control* (pp. 341–360). The Hague, The Netherlands: Nijhoff.

O'Beirne, C., Larkin, D., & Cable, T. (1994). Coordination problems and anaerobic performance in children. *Adapted Physical Activity Quarterly, 11,* 141–149.

Page, R. M., Frey, J., Talbert, R., & Falk, C. (1992). Children's feelings of loneliness and social dissatisfaction: Relationship to measures of physical fitness and activity. *Journal of Teaching Physical Education, 11,* 211–219.

Parker, H. E., & Blanksby, B. A. (1997). Starting age and aquatic skill learning in young children: Mastery of prerequisite water confidence and basic aquatic locomotion skills. *Australian Journal of Science and Medicine in Sport, 29*(3), 83–87.

Peters, J. M., Barnett, A. L., & Henderson, S. E. (2001). Clumsiness, dyspraxia and developmental coordination disorder: How do health and educational professional in the UK define the terms? *Child: Care, Health and Development, 27,* 399–412.

Pless, M., & Carlsson, M. (2000). Effects of motor skill intervention on developmental coordination disorder: A meta-analysis. *Adapted Physical Activity Quarterly, 17,* 381–401.

Ramsden, P. (1992). The Action Profile[r] system of movement assessment for self development. In H. Payne (Ed.), *Dance movement therapy: theory and practice* (pp. 218–241). London: Routledge.

Rarick, G. L., & McKee, R. (1949). A study of twenty third-grade children exhibiting extreme levels of achievement on tests of motor proficiency. *Research Quarterly, 20,* 142–152.

Raynor, A. (2001). Strength, power, and coactivation in children with developmental coordination disorder. *Developmental Medicine and Child Neurology, 43,* 676–684.

Revie, G., & Larkin, D. (1993a). Looking at movement: Problems with teacher identification of poorly coordinated children. *ACHPER National Journal, 40,* 4–9.

Revie, G., & Larkin, D. (1993b). Task specific intervention with children reduces movement problems. *Adapted Physical Activity Quarterly, 10,* 29–41.

Rose, B., Larkin., D. & Berger, B. G. (1994). Perceptions of social support in children of low, moderate, and high coordination. *ACHPER Healthy Lifestyles Journal, 41*(4), 18–21.

Rose, B., Larkin, D., & Berger, B. (1997). Coordination and gender influences on the perceived competence of children. *Adapted Physical Activity Quarterly, 14,* 210–221.

Rose, B., Larkin, D., & Berger, B. (1998). The importance of motor coordination for children's motivational orientations in sport. *Adapted Physical Activity Quarterly, 15,* 316–327.

Schoemaker, M. M., & Kalverboer, A. F. (1994). Social and affective problems of children who are clumsy: How early do they begin? *Adapted Physical Activity Quarterly, 11,* 130–140.

Short, H., & Crawford, J. (1984). Last to be chosen the awkward child. *Pivot, 2*, 32–36.

Smyth, M. M., & Anderson, H. I. (2000). Coping with clumsiness in the school playground: Social and physical play in children with coordination impairments. *British Journal of Developmental Psychology, 18*, 389–413.

Smyth, M. M., & Anderson, H. I. (2001). Football participation in the primary school playground: The role of coordination impairments. *British Journal of Developmental Psychology, 19*, 369–379.

Sporns, O., & Edelman, G. M. (1993). Solving Bernstein's problem: A proposal for the development of coordinated movement by selection. *Child Development, 64*, 960–981.

Sprinkle, J., & Hammond, J. (1997). Family, health, and developmental background of children with developmental coordination disorder. *Australian Educational and Developmental Psychologist, 14*(1), 55–62.

Stephenson, E., & McKay, C. (1989). A support group for parents of children with motor-learning difficulties. *British Journal of Occupational Therapy, 52*(5), 181–183.

Stephenson, E., McKay, C., & Chesson, R. (1990). An investigative study of early developmental factors in children with motor/learning difficulties. *British Journal of Occupational Therapy, 53*(1), 4–6.

Stephenson, E., McKay, C., & Chesson, R. (1991). The identification and treatment of motor/learning difficulties: Parent's perceptions and the role of the therapist. *Child: Care, Health and Development, 17*, 91–113.

Summers, J., & Larkin, D. (2002, June). *Social relationships of children with developmental coordination disorder.* Paper presented at the World Federation of Occupational Therapy Conference, Sweden.

Summers, J., Larkin, D., & Dewey, D. (2001a). *Engagement in and performance of activities of daily living by 6 & 8 year old children in Australia and Canada.* Paper presented at the 21st annual meeting of the Australian Occupational Therapy Association, Brisbane, Australia.

Summers, J., Larkin, D., & Dewey, D. (2001b). *Performance of activities of daily living by 6 and 8 year old children with developmental coordination disorder.* Paper presented at the Paediatric Occupational Therapy Conference, Sydney, Australia.

Symes, K. (1972). Clumsiness and the sociometric status of intellectually gifted boys. *Bulletin of Physical Education, 9*, 35–40.

Taylor, M. J. (1990). Marker variables for early identification of physically awkward children. In G. Doll-Tepper, C. Dahms, B. Doll, & H. von Selzam (Eds.), *Adapted physical activity* (pp. 379–386). Berlin: Springer-Verlag.

Thelen, E. (1995). Motor development: A new synthesis. *American Psychologist, 50*(2), 79–95.

Thelen, E. (2000). Motor development as foundation and future of developmental psychology. *International Journal of Behavioral Development, 24*, 385–397.

Touwen, B. C. L. (1998). The brain and development of function. *Developmental Review, 18*, 504–526.

Trevarthen, C., & Aitken, K. J. (2001). Infant intersubjectivity: Research theory and clinical implications. *Journal of Child Psychology and Psychiatry, 42*, 2–48.

Trevarthen, C., & Burford, B. (1993). The central role of parents: How they can give power to a motor impaired child's acting, experiencing and sharing. *European Journal of Special Needs Education, 10*, 138–148.

Williams, H. G. (2002). Motor control in children with developmental coordination disorder. In S. A. Cermak & D. Larkin (Eds.), *Developmental coordination disorder* (pp. 117–137). Albany, NY: Delmar Thomson Learning.

CHAPTER 21

Approaches to the Management of Children with Motor Problems

HELENE J. POLATAJKO
SYLVIA RODGER
AMEET DHILLON
FARRAH HIRJI

Development occurs at a rapid pace during childhood. For many children this follows a well-documented sequence at a predictable pace. However, some children have developmental disorders, or experience a disease or injury in early childhood that impedes the normal course of development, often resulting in lifelong deficits. All systems of human function are susceptible to disease or disorder, including the motor system. According to Sugden and Keogh (1990), motor problems in children can range from complete paralysis of movement to movements that are abrupt or uncoordinated. When a child's motor system is affected, a number of important lifelong problems can occur. Thus, it is imperative that these problems are addressed. Parents of children with motor problems frequently seek the advice of professionals in the management of these problems with the hope of mitigating against their effects, as much as possible, or eliminating the problems altogether.

The professional literature provides a broad range of approaches, each intended to maximize the developmental potential of children with motor problems. The available approaches address a variety of motor problems, come from a variety of theoretical perspectives, and have variable impact on the motor performance of children. In this chapter, the contemporary approaches being used by professionals in the treatment of children's motor problems are reviewed with a particular focus on the empirical evidence that supports their use. The purpose of this chapter is to provide an overview of the approaches that appear in the literature rather than an exhaustive review of all available approaches, thus the discussion is limited to major current approaches. The intention is to provide the reader with an overview of the literature from an evidence-based perspective so that informed decisions can be made about best practices in the treatment of motor problems in children.

A large number of childhood conditions have motor sequelae. In some cases, these are primary (e.g., cerebral palsy [CP] and developmental coordination disorder [DCD]); in others, they are secondary (e.g., intellectual disabilities, attention-deficit/ hyperactivity disorder [ADHD], and autism spectrum disorders [ASD]). In most cases, management is focused on the primary sequelae of a condition; hence the treatment literature is similarly focused. Earlier in this volume, the major childhood conditions that have motor sequelae were discussed. The literature reveals six conditions with primary developmental motor disorders to be the most prevalent, specifically CP, DCD, spina bifida, muscular dystrophy, acquired brain injury (including pediatric stroke), and Tourette syndrome (TS). The focus of this chapter is on the rehabilitation or remediation of the motor-based performance problems of children with these disorders. As these disorders have been discussed in detail in previous chapters, only the treatment approaches are described here. The approaches to be discussed are those identified in the literature as particularly relevant to these populations. The chapter provides an overview of the relevant treatment approaches and a summary of the evidence regarding the efficacy and efficiency of the approaches.

THE IDENTIFICATION AND CLASSIFICATION OF APPROACHES

To determine which treatment approaches are being used with children with primary motor problems, a comprehensive literature review of journal articles from 1982 to 2002 was conducted using four computerized literature-indexing databases: CINAHL, EMBASE, MEDLINE, and PsycINFO; in addition, pediatric textbooks were scanned and the Internet was searched. Any articles describing treatment for children with CP, DCD, spina bifida, muscular dystrophy, acquired brain injury (ABI; including pediatric stroke), or TS were considered. For each developmental motor disorder explored, the generic key words used to search the databases were *treatment* and *children*. For DCD, *developmental coordination disorder, DCD,* and *clumsy child syndrome* were used, for CP, *cerebral palsy,* and *CP* were used, and for TS, the only key words used were *Tourette syndrome.* For spina bifida and muscular dystrophy the key words used were *spina bifida or muscular dystrophy,* and for ABI the key words were *traumatic brain injury* and *stroke.* Articles were eliminated if they provided information solely on pharmacological or surgical management of these disorders. In some cases, articles reported results of treatment involving a combination of treatment approaches, such as surgical management and exercise (e.g., Bach & McKeon, 1991). A total of 106 journal articles were obtained that had some focus on treatment for these six developmental motor disorders.

An overview of these articles revealed that approaches to the treatment of the motor problems of these six populations of children take a variety of forms. They range from medical/curative approaches to educational/functional approaches. Some of them are very specific, often tailored to specific conditions such as the use of botoxilin (Suputtitada, 2000; Yablon, 2001) or hyperbaric oxygen treatment (Bischof, 2001; Collet et al., 2001) for children with CP, or specific electric stimulation of muscle groups by physical therapists (Sommerfelt, Markestad, Berg, & Saetesdal, 2001; Wright & Granat, 2000) for children with CP and muscular dystrophy. Others are quite generic, often intended to address motor problems in general, such as pediatric physical therapy (Eigsti, Aretz, & Shannon, 1990; Mulligan, Climo, Hansen, & Mauga, 2000) or functional physical therapy (Ketelaar, Vermeer, 't Hart, van Petegem-van Beek, & Helders, 2001). Some treatments are relatively obscure, while others enjoy broad use. This latter group, referred to here as the major treatment approaches addressing the motor problems of children with CP, DCD, spina bifida, muscular dystrophy, ABI, and TS, includes cognitive approaches, conductive education, and compensatory approaches; exercise, medical, pharmacological, and neurodevelopmental treatment; sensory integration; and surgical approaches.

Each treatment approach is distinct from the others, each resting on distinct theoretical underpinning. However, a number of the approaches are derived from similar theoretical roots and can be broadly classified as *process-focused* or *performance-focused*. The *process-focused* approaches are those that emphasize the role of the components of motor performance, typically from a developmental, hierarchical perspective. These approaches frequently focus on "fixing" the underlying dysfunctional motor components or "curing" the disorder. In contrast, the *performance-focused* approaches focus on skill acquisition and environmental or task adaptation, frequently emphasizing the role of learning and task or environmental modification in motor-based performance. In this chapter, these two classifications are used to group the major treatment approaches addressing the motor problems of children with CP, DCD, spina bifida, muscular dystrophy, ABI, and TS. The major treatment approaches have been classified as follows: (1) process-focused approaches, which include neurodevelopmental treatment and sensory integration; and (2) performance-focused approaches, which include cognitive approaches (e.g., cognitive orientation for daily occupational performance), conductive education, compensatory approaches (e.g., adaptive or specialized equipment, devices, and orthotics), and exercise (focused on muscle strengthening).

Each of these approaches is briefly described and then discussed in terms of the evidence for effectiveness. While the literature contained a number of medical, including pharmacological and surgical, approaches, these were considered beyond the scope of this chapter and are not discussed here.

THE MAJOR TREATMENT APPROACHES

As indicated previously, the treatment of motor problems in children is frequently discussed from a conditions perspective. Table 21.1 summarizes the treatment approaches used for children with CP, DCD, spina bifida, muscular dystrophy, ABI (including pediatric stroke), and TS. As can be seen, articles were found for all six conditions, but none were found for pediatric stroke. While there is a large literature on the treatment of stroke in adults, this literature is not necessarily relevant for the treatment of children. Hence, pediatric stroke is not discussed any further in this chapter. The studies located within the ABI category therefore refer primarily to traumatic injury. In viewing Table 21.1, it should be noted that within any one study more than one treatment approach may have been used. Studies often contrasted two types of treatment such as SI and perceptual motor in DCD, or cognitive and pharmacological

TABLE 21.1. Number of Papers Found by Type of Treatment Approach and Motor Disorder

Motor disorder	Treatment approach						
	Process		Performance				
	NDT	SI	Cognitive	CE	Compensatory	Exercise	Other
ABI	1	1	4		1		5
CP	14	1		7	6	3	6
DCD		4	8				7
MD					3	7	
SB	2	1	1	1	8		
TS			10				8
Totals	17	7	23	8	18	10	25

Note. ABI, acquired brain injury; CP, cerebral palsy; DCD, developmental coordination disorder; MD, muscular dystrophy; SB, spina bifida; TS, Tourette syndrome; NDT, neurodevelopmental treatment; SI, sensory integration; CE, conductive education.

interventions in TS. It is noteworthy that the category "other" includes interventions that (1) were not clearly specified in the study but listed under the professional disciplines involved, such as physiotherapy or occupational therapy; (2) referred to the use of eclectic management encompassing several approaches; or (3) encompassed pharmacological management or techniques, surgical interventions, or additional interventions such as ambulatory therapy. In addition, the category "other" refers to approaches that appear in the literature only as comparison treatments rather than the focus of the enquiry (e.g., perceptual–motor and direct skill training[1]).

Of particular interest in Table 21.1 is the observation that while in a few cases treatment approaches appear to be condition-specific, in most cases treatments are used for several conditions (i.e., they appear to be condition-neutral). For example, physical exercise seems to be relatively condition-specific as it appears only in the treatment literature for children with CP and muscular dystrophy, while SI appears to be condition-neutral as it is described as a treatment for most of the six primary conditions (ABI, CP, DCD, spina bifida). Furthermore, some conditions appear to be treated in an almost unitary way, while others are treated in a variety of ways. For example, children with TS appear primarily to be treated with cognitive approaches, whereas children with ABI, CP, and spina bifida appear to be treated with numerous approaches.

Process-Focused Approaches

As noted earlier, *process-focused* approaches emphasize the role of the components of motor performance and tend to focus on "fixing" the underlying dysfunctional motor components or "curing" the disorder.

---

[1]Perceptual–motor or direct skill treatment only appeared in this literature search as comparators, even though they are recognized and prominent in the treatment literature for other disability groups (e.g., learning disabilities). Therefore, these approaches are not discussed in this chapter.

Neurodevelopmental Treatment

Dr. Karel Bobath, a medical practitioner and his wife, a physiotherapist, began developing neurodevelopmental treatment (NDT) approximately 40 years ago (Stanton, 1997). Since then, NDT has continued to evolve, influenced by research and new knowledge from neurophysiology, movement sciences, and other theoretical frameworks, particularly motor control, motor learning (Bly, 1991; Miles-Breslin, 1996; Whiteside, 1997), and biomechanical approaches. Within NDT, movement disorders are seen as a dysfunction of the normal postural control mechanism. The three main components of the normal postural control mechanism are normal postural tone, reciprocal innervation, and variation of movement (Mayston, 2000, 2001). NDT is a widely used form of treatment for motor disorders and disturbances of posture and movement in children and adults. In particular, it is widely used by physical and occupational therapists (DeGangi, Hurley, & Linscheid, 1983).

NDT is a "hands-on" approach, which involves three primary treatment techniques: inhibition, facilitation, and specific sensory stimulation. These techniques are used to prepare the child's postural and motor systems before and during goal-directed activity. While working with the child, the therapist is sensitive to the child's own activity and uses key points of control to grade and gradually withdraw his or her hands, allowing the child to take over the movement. Key points of control are where the therapist places his or her hands to effect changes in patterns of posture and movement in other parts of the body. During treatment the therapist is continually assessing and reevaluating the effects of the techniques used and adjusting his or her handling accordingly.

The aim of NDT is to modify the abnormal patterns of posture and movement and to facilitate more normal patterns of movement, preparing and enabling the child to engage in goal-directed functional activities. Treatment involves preparation, practice, and repetition of normal postures and movements within the context of functional tasks.

NDT focuses on encouraging typical developmental movement patterns in children with motor disorders to reduce abnormal patterns that may be exhibited (Fetters & Kluzik, 1996). The NDT approach emphasizes early intervention, as it attempts to prevent abnormal movement patterns from arising (Stanton, 1997). Each child's ability to move is seen to be dependent on righting reactions that keep the head in line with the trunk and the rest of the body, and equilibrium reactions that enable children to maintain their balance when their center of gravity is displaced (Hedges, 1988). NDT attempts to evoke these righting and equilibrium reactions to facilitate normal posture, balance, and movement in children with motor disorders.

The treatment process involves preparation for the task and repetition of the sensory motor components of a task. These are followed by practice in the context of a functional task and then integration and carryover in the everyday context (e.g., at home) (Mayston, 2001). Preparation involves processes of tone education/activation/modification, mobilization, active muscle lengthening, achieving postural alignment, and practice of specific components of movement/transitions. For example, a child with hypotonia may need more active trunk control in sitting with alignment of his head on trunk to assist oral efficiency for eating and drinking, or to enable more successful eye–hand coordination. Sensory techniques such as light touch and weight shift may be used to achieve postural alignment, combined with compression to achieve increased postural/trunk muscle activity against a stable base of support at the pelvis. Preparation is followed by engaging the child in a functional or goal-directed activity (e.g., eating) and play activities using hand function.

Inhibition techniques are also used in preparation to achieve tone reduction to enable increased range and variation of movement, or to smooth out fluctuating tone to enable midrange control. For example, a child with increased tone and restricted movements at the shoulder may be limited in his ability to reach forward to engage in hand–mouth exploration and manipulation. Techniques of elongation with traction may be used to lengthen trunk, scapular, and humeral muscles to achieve postural and joint alignment. This may be followed by the therapist guiding the child into a shoulder-weight-bearing position (e.g., over a therapy roll), in preparation for a hand or hand–mouth play activity. Facilitation occurs when the therapist uses her hands to physically guide the child's movement. Facilitation assists movements initiated by the child and aims to help the child experience more normal movement (e.g., using light touch to guide reaching). Specific sensory stimulation techniques are used in preparation and to assist inhibition and facilitation. Sensory techniques use tactile, proprioceptive, and vestibular input and include light touch, compression (light, intermittent, sustained deep), tapping and sweeping, placing and holding, traction, weight bearing, and weight shifting (Boehme, 1988).

This approach does not advocate that parents learn specific NDT techniques to carry over at home (e.g., as an exercise program). Through the dynamic interaction between the child and therapist in therapy sessions, therapists learn about the child's responses and which techniques are most effective. The therapist then aims to show parents different ways of positioning and handling their child during daily routines, such as dressing, eating and drinking, and playtime, to help reinforce the use of more normal postures and more normal patterns of movement. In NDT, the use of positioning with equipment, including splints, is seen as an adjunct to therapy and important to the overall management of the child's condition and ability to participate in their everyday life and community.

Sensory Integrative Therapy

Sensory integrative therapy (SI) evolved from the work of Dr. A. J. Ayres, an occupational therapist, working in the 1960s and 1970s with children with learning disabilities. She noted that these children appeared to have difficulty organizing sensory input and devised a therapy to help children do that. SI has its roots in developmental theory and is based on the premise that children must organize sensory information in the brain in order to make an adaptive motor response (Parham & Mailloux, 1998). An adaptive response results if children are successful in meeting challenges within their environment. SI therapy proposes that inadequate sensory processing leads to maladaptive motor responses. SI problems may present as difficulty responding to touch, problems in concentration, and/or difficulty with movement sensations such as swinging (Haerle, 1992).

SI dysfunction refers to an inability to use sensation effectively to make appropriate adaptive responses (Chu, 1989). It may involve one or more sensory systems and affect responses at a postural and/or a conceptual level. SI dysfunction can lead to delayed motor development and affect a child's ability to interpret sensations and use them to form meaningful concepts, which are necessary for learning and motor planning (Chu, 1989).

If children are unable to adapt adequately to the demands of their environment and have a poor sensory processing system, SI therapy may be used (Hinojosa, Kramer, & Pratt, 1998). The central principle in SI therapy is the provision of planned and controlled sensory input to elicit an adaptive response, thereby enhancing the organization of brain mechanisms (Chu, 1989). The primary aim of SI is to enhance the ability of the nervous system to effectively use sensory information for functional activities (Parham & Mailloux, 1998).

SI theory postulates that treatment should be applied on an individual basis to ensure a child-centered approach, which also fosters the development of rapport between the child and the clinician. SI may also be provided in a small group setting. The child is given choices as to the sensory and movement activities he or she performs, while the clinician provides some structure to the treatment session. The SI environment typically consists of a large therapy room or gymnasium, with a wide assortment of specialized equipment such as suspended equipment, ramps, and equipment and materials that evoke tactile, proprioceptive, and vestibular responses (Parham & Mailloux, 1998). The room is also equipped with mats and large pillows to ensure the child's safety during vestibular activities such as swinging and spinning. The child is viewed as an active participant in treatment and is encouraged to perform activities that challenge his or her sensory processing abilities. Activities include constant motion stimulation such as swinging in a hammock or standing on a balance board, and performing multiple activities simultaneously such as sitting on a T stool while catching a ball with two hands (Parham & Mailloux, 1998).

Performance-Focused Approaches

In contrast to the process-focused approaches, the performance-focused approaches emphasize adaptive learning, performance outcomes, and skill development and acquisition.

Conductive Education

The conductive education approach was developed by Andras Peto. It is based on learning theory and is primarily used for children with motor disorders who do not have associated cognitive impairments. Peto viewed motor disorders as learning difficulties that do not require medical treatment but, rather, a teaching program to facilitate all areas of child development (Stanton, 1997).

The primary goal of conductive education is to encourage the developmental process that may be delayed in children with motor disorders so that the children can gain independence in daily activities (Hedges, 1988). The basic premise of conductive education is to teach a child how to learn. Conductive education discourages the use of adaptive and mobility aids but emphasizes the importance of a "normal" environment. The child is an active participant in conductive education and his or her motivation and determination are central aspects to the success of this treatment approach (Stanton, 1997).

According to Hedges (1988), there are four basic elements of conductive education: the conductor, the group, the program, and rhythmical intention. The conductor may have an educational background as a teacher, nurse, physiotherapist, or occupational therapist; however, the essential quality is that he or she is trained in conductive education. The conductor is responsible for guiding and teaching children and providing a positive and nurturing learning environment. There is typically more than one conductor for each group of children. Groups consist of up to 20 children who are matched according to age and general abilities (Hedges, 1988). Group work is an essential aspect of conductive education, as children are motivated to keep up with their peers and are provided with support from the group based on individual accomplishments (Stanton, 1997).

In essence this approach relies on the child's own active participation, problem-solving abilities, and initiative rather than on the physical handling and the skill of the therapist (Robinson, McCarthy, & Little, 1989). All motor problems are viewed as difficulties in learning and the aim is to stimulate the developmental motor process through education. The catalyst in this approach is a specially trained conductor who has a key role in educating, motivating, and involving children in all their daily activities. Children are organized into small groups with similar abilities and are facilitated to learn the movements and skills necessary for daily living activities.

The conductor structures the child's schoolday to provide opportunities to practice normal movement patterns in functional activities (Chu, 1989). All the movement patterns demonstrated by the conductor are based on the basic motor patterns typical of normal motor development. The conductor makes use of a specific learning method called rhythmical intention by which children verbalize their intention of movement. Movement is carried out rhythmically while counting from 1 to 5 or dynamically to illustrate the direction of movement. Through verbal regulation and rhythmical intention, a child is taught to continuously initiate and complete movement patterns as part of functional tasks. Task analysis is used to break functional tasks into their component parts and subsequently to teach the child the motor plan or sequence for that functional task (Hedges, 1988). Rhythmic intention incorporates vocalization of the action while the child performs the movement. The theory behind "rhythmic intention" is that speech and active motion reinforce each other (Hedges, 1988). The conductive education program consists of tasks that are part of activities of daily living such as walking, dressing, and clapping (Stanton, 1997), which are broken down into individual steps to facilitate independent movement (Hedges, 1988). The aim is to enable children to develop their own patterns of functional movements and to be able to transfer that learning into tasks throughout the day.

Cognitive Approaches

These approaches employ a range of behavioral reinforcement and learning techniques that enable children to consistently exhibit appropriate motor responses. Cognitive-behavioral techniques require the therapist to provide praise or positive reinforcement of approximations, as well as achievement of the desired response or motor skill. This reinforcement helps children to subsequently initiate their own movements (Manella

& Varni, 1981). Cognitive-behavioral techniques such as rewarding behavior that is incompatible with tics, substitution of more socially acceptable rituals, habit reversal, and use of competing responses are frequently used concurrently with pharmacological intervention for children with TS to modify or eliminate tics (Carr, 1995; Dodick & Adler, 1992; Parker, 1985; O'Quinn & Thompson, 1980; Robertson, 2000; Tolchard, 1995).

Recently, there have been a number of investigations of the use of cognitive approaches with children with DCD. One such approach, cognitive orientation to daily occupational performance (CO-OP), was developed for children identified with DCD (Polatajko, Mandich, Missuina, et al., 2001). CO-OP has its origins in learning theory as it views DCD as a motor learning difficulty rather than a neurodevelopmental problem (Polatajko, Mandich, Miller, & Macnab, 2001). It aims to assist children to discover the specific cognitive strategies necessary to enhance their ability to perform the everyday tasks of childhood that they want to, or are expected to, perform (Polatajko & Mandich, 2004).

The CO-OP approach is client-centered. It uses global and domain-specific strategies as well as guided discovery of strategies to enable the child to achieve his or her self-selected goals. It is typically administered by an occupational therapist and involves active participation by both the child and caregivers. Parents are encouraged to observe as many sessions as possible to assist their children in generalizing their learning. Each child chooses individual goals, which increases motivation and transfer of learning (Polatajko & Mandich, 2004).

A key feature of CO-OP is *dynamic performance analysis* (DPA), which attempts to determine when a child encounters difficulty in performing an activity (Polatajko & Mandich, 2004). This leads to the identification of performance breakdowns that have an impact on skill acquisition. Once these breakdowns are identified by the therapist, a global strategy known as *Goal-Plan-Do-Check* is taught to the child as a framework for solving motor-based peformance problems. The child is then guided to discover *domain-specific strategies* to enable occupational performance (Polatajko & Mandich, 2004). CO-OP can be used with any number of motor-based, child-chosen occupations such as catching a ball, biking, handwriting, and using cutlery.

Compensatory Approach

The compensatory approach focuses on supporting a person's ability to function to enhance his or her well-being. Within this approach the successful completion of the activity or occupation is the primary goal to enable independent functioning. Compensatory approaches are widely used by physical and occupational therapists, orthotists, and prosthetists (Foster, 1996). This approach encompasses a number of specific interventions such as the use of specialized equipment (e.g., wheelchairs, standers, walkers, braces, and crutches), adaptive devices (e.g., modified computer keyboards), and orthopedic rehabilitation (e.g., use of orthotics and casting) to promote motor development and skill acquisition and to increase or maintain independent function (Eigsti et al., 1990). Adaptive equipment, assistive devices, or orthotics are prescribed for children to maintain or increase functional independence (Eigsti et al., 1990). The goals are to minimize secondary musculoskeletal deformities and to make children as functionally independent as possible.

Skeletal disorders resulting from spina bifida, CP, muscular dystrophy, and ABI often restrict joint range of motion and decrease muscle strength. Orthopedic rehabilitation includes the use of splints that provide functional positioning, maintain passive stretching to elongate soft tissues or muscles, and correct deformities. This approach applies principles of biomechanical intervention to provide appropriate feedback to the body for correction of these musculoskeletal abnormalities (Foster, 1996).

Another intervention that has been used to increase upper and lower extremity support in children with motor disorders is casting (Cottalorda, Gautheron, Metton, Charmet, & Chavrier, 2000; Portela, 1990). Inhibitive casting is most often used with children with CP. Casts are used as a treatment approach to maintain joints in a functional position, thus decreasing muscle tone and promoting mobility (Law et al., 1997).

Exercise Therapy

This approach is primarily used with children and adolescents with muscular dystrophy for strength training of weak muscle groups. During exercise, therapy resistance is provided through the use of weights and manual resistance provided by the therapist to a particular muscle or muscle group that is functionally useful but weak. Electrical stimulation of specific muscles or muscle groups may also be used to counter the deterioration in muscle activity and enhance muscle strength. Exercise therapy builds muscle strength and affects muscle fiber histopathology. Weak muscles are strengthened through a range of isometric, concentric, and eccentric exercises. For children with CP, resistive exercise has been used to increase lower limb muscle strength and enhance mobility (Haney, 1998).

In contrast to specific stimulation of muscle groups and use of graded resistance for strengthening, there is literature describing the use of general physical activity and exercise with children with motor disorders to reduce stress, evoke calming and relaxation, enhance emotional well-being, and improve performance in various sporting activities. Chapter 20 (Larkin & Summers, this volume) provides a more in-depth discussion of this literature. Children with TS may also benefit from exercise as they reportedly experience fewer tics when involved in physical activity (Haerle, 1992). Physical exercise is also used to provide a calming effect on children who seek out increased stimulation. Exercise is a treatment modality that is used in conjunction with other approaches to assist with enhancing relaxation and well-being, as well as stress management for children with motor disorders (Haerle, 1992).

CHARACTERIZING THE LITERATURE
IN TERMS OF LEVELS OF EVIDENCE

As indicated previously, a review of the literature for children with CP, DCD, spina bifida, muscular dystrophy, ABI, and TS yielded 106 papers describing treatment. These papers varied greatly in quality and the level of evidence provided. Thus, it was decided to characterize the literature before critically appraising it for the level of evidence provided. The categories used were those identified by Bailey (1997): *descriptive, research*, or *opinion*. A paper was classified as *descriptive* if the investigator described objective observations of the characteristics of the sample but did not manipulate any variables, impose any control, or randomize subjects to attain a result. Types of descriptive studies included were correlational, surveys, case studies, and observational studies. Papers were classified as *research* if they reported on research with some attempt at implementing control and manipulation of variables. Randomized controlled trials, repeated measures designs, pretest–posttest design or single systems designs were included. Papers were classified as *opinion* papers if the author expressed a subjective viewpoint on an issue based on experience, without reporting on a study; the author subjectively reported or reflected on his or her analysis of a particular intervention strategy without manipulating any conditions. Literature reviews were classified according to the type of studies reviewed in the article. For example, if the majority of studies were *descriptive* in nature, the literature review was placed in the descriptive category. If the review addressed research studies in which there was some sort of randomization and a control group and strict inclusion criteria were applied for studies, it was classified as a systematic review (e.g., Brown & Burns, 2001) and included as a *research* study. Meta-analyses characterized by statistical manipulation of the data were also classified as *research* studies (e.g., Pless & Carlsson, 2000). Table 21.2 depicts the classification of the 106 papers found. Specific research studies included in the systematic review and meta-analysis were excluded from further review to avoid double counting of studies.

The vast majority of the treatment papers in the literature, irrespective of the type of disorder, were *descriptive* ($N = 50$), or *opinion* papers ($N = 26$) (see Table 21.2). Only 30 of the 106 papers identified reported experimental *research* on actual treatment studies for children with motor disorders. The most frequently researched developmental motor conditions were CP and muscular dystrophy. For the conditions ABI and TS, no research studies were found, with the articles in these two areas being predominantly descriptive or opinion based.

TABLE 21.2. Study Type by Motor Disorder

Motor disorder	Study type		
	Opinion	Descriptive	Research
ABI	2	6	0
CP	10	16	10
DCD	2	11	5
MD	0	2	14
SB	5	4	1
TS	7	11	0
Totals	26	50	30

Note. ABI, acquired brain injury; CP, cerebral palsy; DCD, developmental coordination disorder; MD, muscular dystrophy; SB, spina bifida; TS, Tourette syndrome.

To determine the evidence for best practices, the 30 research studies were examined for the levels of evidence they yielded. The "Hierarchy of Levels of Evidence for Evidence-Based Practice" described by Moore, McQuay, and Gray, cited in Holm (2000), was used. In this hierarchy, *Level I* evidence, which is the highest level of evidence, is described as "at least one systematic review of multiple well-designed randomized controlled trials" (Holm, 2000, p. 576). Meta-analytic studies or systematic reviews provide strong evidence and have rigorous methodological procedures including well-defined study criteria for inclusion and use of studies that have randomized controlled clinical trials. These studies use statistical analysis to evaluate the data from multiple studies. *Level II* evidence includes studies that involve at least one randomized control trial that is an acceptable size. *Level III* encompasses experimental studies in which the subject sample has not been randomized, such as time-series, matched case-controlled studies, cohort, and single group pretest–posttest designs. *Level IV* includes evidence from well-designed nonexperimental studies in which the sample has been selected from more than one center or research group. *Level V* provides the lowest level of evidence and includes opinion papers written by respected authorities based on clinical evidence, descriptive studies, and reports of expert committees (Holm, 2000).

Table 21.3 displays the levels of evidence found in the treatment literature. As can be seen only 19 of the 30 research studies provided Level I, II, or III evidence. The remaining 11 studies provided Level IV or V evidence. Level IV and V studies were not included in any further discussion, as the focus of this chapter is on experimental research. Taken as a whole, Table 21.3 demonstrates that this literature has very few Level I studies. Indeed there were only two: a systematic review by Brown and Burns (2001) on NDT for children with CP and the meta-analysis by Pless and Carlsson (2000) on interventions for children with DCD. Furthermore, there were few Level II studies; there were three randomized clinical trials (RCTs): one RCT investigating CO-OP for children with DCD (Miller, Polatajko, Missiuna, Mandich, & Macnab, 2001); one investigating strength training for children with muscular dystrophy (Lindeman et

TABLE 21.3. Levels of Evidence in the Studies of Treatment Approaches

| Levels of evidence[a] | Treatment approach | | | | | | |
| | Process | | Performance | | | | |
	NDT	SI	Cognitive	CE	Compensatory	Exercise	Other
I[b]	1 CP	1 DCD					
II		1 DCD	1 CP			1 MD	
III	2 CP	1 DCD	2 DCD	1 CP	1 SB	5 MD 2 CP	
Totals	3	2	2	3	1	8	0

Note. NDT, neurodevelopmental treatment; SI, sensory integration; CE, conductive education.
[a] Levels IV and V do not appear here because they were judged to be inadequate for determining best practice.
[b] None of the studies included in the systematic reviews are included in this table, to prevent double counting.

al., 1995); and one investigating NDT for children with CP (Reddihough, King, Coleman, & Catanese, 1998). The majority of studies (*N* = 15) provided Level III evidence, covering all six treatment approaches. There were no studies providing evidence within Levels I–III for TS or ABI.

DETERMINING BEST PRACTICES

The treatment approaches are next discussed in terms of the research evidence available to support their use with these developmental motor disorders. Table 21.4 provides a detailed description of the 19 research studies that provide Level I, II, or III evidence.

Process-Focused Approaches

The Evidence: Neurodevelopmental Treatment

Three research studies addressed NDT for children with CP (see Table 21.4). There was one Level I study, the systematic review of NDT by Brown and Burns (2001). Brown and Burns included 17 studies from a list of 147 relevant citations on the use of NDT with high-risk infants and children with CP. These studies were assessed for concealment of treatment allocation and the quality of the RCT using the Quality Assessment of Randomised Clinical Trials (QARCT) Scale developed by Jadad and colleagues (1996). This scale, similar to the criteria used in this chapter, assesses the quality of a study based on methodological rigor and assessment of the level of evidence using Sackett's Levels of Evidence (LEO; Sackett, 1989). These guidelines rate levels of evidence of treatment efficacy ranging from descriptive case studies to RCTs, and hence reflect the levels of methodological sophistication of study designs used. The systematic review process used by Brown and Burns was detailed clearly and high levels of agreement were reported between the two independent reviewers for each stage of their review process. Level of agreement for stage two using kappa was .932 and for assignment of levels of evidence according to Sackett's criteria was 0.678. Results were reported separately for children with CP and high-risk infants. Eleven of the 17 studies researched NDT treatment for children with CP. Brown and Burns concluded that the findings were equivocal, with six studies reporting benefits and four reporting no benefit. One study reported inconclusive results due to the concurrent use of two interventions (NDT and posterior rhizotomy). Brown and Burns concluded that there was insufficient evidence to reach a clear decision regarding the efficacy of NDT for children with CP.

The two remaining studies revealed Level III evidence. One study using a one-group pre–posttest design (Adams, Chandler, & Schuhmann, 2000) demonstrated improvement in gait velocity and stride length as a result of NDT in 40 children with CP. Fetters and Kluzik (1996) using a two-group repeated measures design found no significant treatment effect as a result of NDT, or practice, on reaching skills in eight children. As each group received some therapy, no conclusions could be drawn about the effect of no therapy.

TABLE 21.4. Detailed Description of Level I, II, and III Studies

Treatment approach	Authors (year)	Purpose	Study design	N	Results
		Process approaches			
NDT: CP—Level I					
NDT	Brown & Burns (2001)	To determine the effects of NDT in pediatrics, including CP	Systematic review	17 studies; 11 CP (6 high-risk infants)	Effect inconclusive for CP: 6 studies showed benefits, 4 no benefits, 1 unclear.
NDT: CP—Level III					
NDT	Adams, Chandler, & Schuhmann (2000)	To evaluate gait improvement	One group, pre–posttest design	40	Improvement in gait velocity and stride length.
NDT	Fetters & Kluzik (1996)	To evaluate the effectiveness of NDT, vs. practice on reaching	Two-group, repeated-measures, crossover design; pre–posttest design	5 NDT then practice; 3 the reverse	No significant effect on the dependent variables after 5 days of either NDT or practice.
SI: DCD—Level I					
SI and other motor skill intervention	Pless & Carlsson (2000)	To determine if there is sufficient evidence for the use of specific skills, SI, and general ability approach	Meta-analysis	13 studies	The specific skills approach was the most effective, with SI being the least effective.
SI: DCD—Level III					
SI and other	Davidson & Williams (2000)	To determine if SI and perceptual motor treatment is effective	Pre–posttest single-group study	37	After a 10-week block of SI and perceptual–motor and at 12-month follow-up, statistically significant improvements were found for fine motor skill and visual–motor integration.

474

Performance approaches

	Reference	Purpose	Design	Sample	Results
Cognitive: DCD—Level II					
CO-OP vs. CTA	Miller, Polatajko, Missiuna, Mandich, & Macnab (2001)	To determine the effectiveness of CO-OP relative the contemporary approach (CTA)	Two-group RCT	10 CO-OP, 10 CTA	CO-OP group performed significantly better in skill acquisition and some measures of transfer.
Cognitive: DCD—Level III					
CO-OP	Polatajko, Mandich, Miller, & Macnab (2001)	2 series of single-case design studies:			
		Series One examining the effectiveness of CO-OP on skill acquisition and transfer;	Series One: 1 single-case design study with 9 replications	Series One: 10	Significant improvement in skill acquisition and some measures of transfer.
		Series Two examining the effectiveness of CO-OP on skill acquisition, only	Series Two: 1 single-case design study with 3 replications	Series Two: 4	Significant improvement in skill acquisition.
CE: CP—Level II					
CE vs. NDT	Reddihough, King, Coleman, & Catanese (1998)	Examine the relative effects of CE and NDT for under 3-year-olds	Two-group RCT, pre–posttest	34 CE, 34 NDT	No significant differences between groups.
CE): CP—Level III					
CE vs. EI	Catenese, Coleman, King, & Reddihough (1995)	Examine the relative effects of CE and EI for school-age children with CP	Two-group, pre–posttest design	17 CE, 17 EI	CE group had significantly more gains in motor and parent coping, both groups had cognitive gains with EI having the higher gains.

(continued)

TABLE 21.4. (continued)

Treatment approach	Authors (year)	Purpose	Study design	N	Results
Compensatory: Spina bifida—Level III					
Orthopedic brace treatment	Muller & Nordwall (1994)	Evaluate effectiveness of the Boston brace for halting the progression of scoliosis	One-group, repeated-measures design	21	Significant finding that progression of scoliosis can be treated with a Boston-type brace if the curvature is less than 45°.
Exercise: CP—Level III					
Exercise	Damiano & Abel (1998)	To determine if strength training produces lower limb functional outcomes	One-group, pre–posttest design	11	Significant improvements in strength with significant increases in gait velocity.
Exercise	Schindl, Forstner, Kern, & Hesse (2000)	To determine if treadmill training improves gait/ambulation	One-group, pre–posttest design	10	General improvement in motor functions including walking in 8 out of 10 children.
Exercise: MD—Level II					
Exercise vs. no exercise	Lindeman et al. (1995)	To determine the effects of strength training on lower limb muscles on MD and MD neuropathy (MDN) cases	Two-group RCT, strength training vs. no training	MD: 15 exercise, 15 control; MDN: 14 exercise, 14 control	MD group: showed no effect. MDN: showed moderate effect in strength and function.
Exercise: MD—Level III					
Exercise (electrical stimulation and ankle exercise)	Belanger & Gilles (1990)	Compare the contractile and functional properties of exercised and non exercised muscle	Two-group nonrandomized sample selection; random assignment, repeated-measures design	3 exercise 3 control	No effect, no improvement in muscle strength due to lack of compliance.

476

Exercise and surgical procedure on the lower extremity	Bach & McKeon (1991)	Evaluate results of a single surgical intervention followed by exercise on lower extremity contractures and ambulation	One group with subjects as own control, nonrandomized sample selection, repeated-measures design	13	Significant finding that surgical intervention followed by exercise can stabilize and prolong ambulation.
Exercise	Milner-Brown & Miller (1988b)	To examine the efficacy of weight training of elbow flexors and knee extensors for strengthening	One group, contrasting exercised and nonexercised contralateral muscle groups, pre–posttest design	12	Significant finding, high-resistance weight training increases muscle strength when disease progression is minimal.
Exercise and electrical stimulation	Milner-Brown & Miller (1988a)	Measure the effects of electric stimulation and weight training of the knee extensors and ankle dorsiflexors	One group, contrasting exercised and nonexercised contralateral muscle groups, pre–posttest design	10	Significant finding of increased muscle strength of markedly weak muscles when using weights and electric stimulation of the knee; no effect on ankle.
Exercise	Tollback et al. (1999)	Evaluate effects of a high resistance weight training of the knee extensors on muscle strength	One group, contrasting exercised and nonexercised contralateral muscle groups, pre–posttest design	9	Significant finding of strength gain in knee extensors during high-resistance training.

Note. NDT, neurodevelopmental treatment; SI, sensory integration; CF, conductive education; CO-OP, cognitive orientation to daily occupationl performance; EI, early intervention; CP, cerebral palsy; DCD, developmental coordination disorder; MD, muscular dystrophy; RCT, randomized controlled trial.

On the basis of these three research studies, no firm conclusions can be drawn about the efficacy of NDT as an intervention over other interventions. While children with CP in the Adams and colleagues (2000) studies demonstrated improvements with NDT, the lack of a control group receiving no treatment makes it impossible to determine whether the intervention itself or other factors resulted in these changes.

The Evidence: Sensory Integration

Only two research studies were found investigating the use of SI; both investigated its use with children with DCD (see Table 21.4). First, Pless and Carlsson (2000) conducted a meta-analysis to determine the relative benefits of SI, specific skills training, and the general ability approach for children with DCD. Their meta-analysis of 13 research studies demonstrated that the specific skills approach was the most effective approach for children with DCD, with SI being the least effective approach. This Level I study provides the strongest evidence for clinicians with regard to the best treatment among these three approaches (SI, specific skills, and general ability). SI was not supported as an effective intervention for children with DCD. The other study by Davidson and Williams (2000) provides Level III evidence regarding the efficacy of SI. In this study of 37 children with DCD, it was found that a combination of SI and perceptual–motor treatment resulted in significant improvements in visual–motor and fine motor skills in children after a 10-week block of therapy. This study used a pretest–posttest single-group design. The limitations of the study include the lack of a control group and the mix of SI and perceptual–motor treatment, making it impossible to extract the relative benefit of SI versus perceptual–motor activities, or no treatment.

In summary, on the basis of a stringent meta-analysis revealing Level I evidence, SI is the least effective approach to use for children with DCD. While SI was also used with children with ABI, CP, and spina bifida, the lack of empirical studies makes it impossible to draw any conclusions about its effectiveness with these other conditions.

Performance-Focused Approaches

The Evidence: Conductive Education

Two empirical studies were located that addressed conductive education for children with CP. One study by Reddihough and colleagues (1998) was an RCT that examined the relative effects of conductive education ($N = 34$) versus NDT ($N = 34$) for children under 3 years of age. This study used a relatively large sample and provides Level II evidence that there were no significant differences in outcome between the two groups. The second study by Catanese, Coleman, King, and Reddihough (1995) involved 34 children, 17 receiving conductive education and 17 receiving early intervention services. Catanese and colleagues used a two-group pre–posttest design. The conductive education group made significantly more gains in motor skills and parental coping, while the early-intervention group had higher gains in cognitive skills. This limited research evidence is insufficient to reach any conclusions regarding the relative effect of CE as compared to NDT or early intervention in improving the motor outcomes for young children with CP.

The Evidence: Cognitive Approaches

While cognitive approaches were commonly reported with children with ABI, DCD, and TS, the only cognitive approach to have been extensively investigated is CO-OP. Two research studies (Miller, Missiuna, Macnab, Malloy-Miller, & Polatajko, 2001; Polatajko, Mandich, Missiuna, et al., 2001) have investigated the effectiveness of CO-OP for children with DCD. Polatajko et al. reported on two series of studies of CO-OP with DCD providing Level III evidence. In the first series, one single case design study with pre- and posttest measures and nine replications were reported. This provided evidence for the effectiveness of CO-OP in promoting skills acquisition and transfer in children 7–12 years with DCD. The second series reported involved one single-case design study with three replications. This study demonstrated the effectiveness of the treatment with a new therapist and resulted in significant improvements in motor skill acquisition. The Level II study by Miller, Missiuna and colleagues (2001) involved a two-group RCT with 20 children. Ten children received 10 individual sessions of CO-OP and 10 received 10 individual sessions of contemporary occupational therapy treatment (CTA). The CO-OP group performed significantly better in skill acquisition and some measures of transfer. The children receiving CO-OP reported higher levels of satisfaction and performance with goals as measured by the Canadian Occupational Performance Measure (COPM). The findings of this series of studies suggests that CO-OP shows promise as an effective intervention for promoting skill acquisition and transfer in children 7–12 years with DCD.

The Evidence: Compensatory Approaches

Compensatory approaches have been widely used for children with CP, muscular dystrophy, and spina bifida (see Table 21.1). Orthopedic intervention was most frequently discussed to correct the spinal deformities or limited mobility due to deformities in the lower extremities. Only one study using compensatory approaches was found that could be categorized within the top three levels of evidence. This study by Muller and Nordwall (1994) investigated the use of orthopedic braces with 21 children with spina bifida to halt the progress of scoliosis. The Boston Brace was found to be effective in treating progressive scoliosis if the curvature was less than 45 degrees when the brace was fitted. It is impossible to make any global conclusions about the use of compensatory approaches as most of these studies were descriptive and covered a wide range of varied treatment approaches from bracing and orthopedic rehabilitation to the use of orthotics and casting.

The Evidence: Exercise Therapy

Therapeutic use of exercise was the most researched treatment approach, involving 8 of the 19 research studies. Exercise was used for management of some of the motor sequelae experienced by children with CP and muscular dystrophy. In terms of its use in CP, the two studies reviewed provided Level III evidence of its efficacy. Both studies addressed lower limb outcomes in terms of lower limb functioning (Damiano & Abel, 1998) and gait or ambulation (Schindl, Forstner, Kern, & Hesse, 2000) in children with CP. They both used single-group pre–posttest designs with small numbers of subjects ($n = 10$, $n = 11$). In both studies, children benefited from strength or treadmill training resulting in ambulation (Schindl et al., 2000) or increases in strength and gait velocity (Damiano & Abel, 1998). These studies lacked a control or comparison (no treatment or alternate treatment) group and therefore there was no subject randomization. This reduces the strength of the findings.

Specific exercise training was the most commonly used intervention for children and adolescents with muscular dystrophy with six research studies providing Level II or Level III evidence of treatment efficacy. The other treatment approach used with muscular dystrophy was the compensatory approach; however, none of these studies were empirical. The Level II study by Lindeman and colleagues (1995) was an RCT that investigated strength training versus no training for adolescents and young adults with muscular dystrophy and muscular dystrophy neuropathy (MDN). This study used reasonable numbers, with 30 subjects with muscular dystrophy and 28 subjects with MDN, randomly assigned to treatment and no treatment. While the muscular dystrophy group showed no effect of treatment, the MDN group demonstrated a moderate treatment effect in relation to strength and function. In terms of the Level III studies, two studies involved electrical stimulation and exercise (Belanger & Gilles, 1990; Milner-Brown & Miller, 1988a). While the Milner-Brown and Miller (1988a) study demonstrated significant findings of increased muscle strength when using weights and electrical stimulation of the muscles of the knee, no effect was found for the muscles of the ankle. This study used a one-group pre–posttest design with 10 subjects with no control group. In the Belanger and Gilles (1990) study, two groups (control and experimental) were used with random assignment of subjects to groups increasing the strength of the design. However, this study had only six subjects, three allocated to each group. No treatment effect was found, with compliance with training being problematic.

The study by Bach and McKeon (1991) used both surgical management and a physiotherapy exercise program with 13 subjects. Significant improvements in stability and ambulation were found as a result of this combined approach. There was no control group and a convenience sample was used. Both Milner-Brown and Miller (1988b) and Tollback and colleagues (1999) investigated the efficacy of weight training on knee extensors, with Milner-Brown and Miller also looking at elbow flexors. These studies had small numbers ($n = 9$, $n = 12$). Both studies demonstrated significant improvements in strength as a result of high-resistance weight training. However, they both lacked control groups, which detracted from the strength of the findings. The lack of randomization also increased the probability of the results occurring due to chance or biased sample selection.

In summary, all the one-group studies for muscular dystrophy demonstrated significant findings; however, neither of the two group studies that involve more scientific control (Belanger & Gilles, 1990) and the RCT (Lindeman et al., 1995) demonstrated any significant effects of exercise for individuals with muscular dystrophy.

SUMMARY AND CONCLUSIONS

The results of this literature review indicate that there are six main treatment approaches that are typically used in the treatment of children with primary motor problems. The results also suggest that similar treatment approaches are used in the management of children with CP, spina bifida, and ABI, namely NDT, SI, conductive education, exercise, cognitive, compensatory, and other. Children with muscular dystrophy tend to be treated using exercise and compensatory approaches, while children with TS tend to be treated using cognitive and other (often pharmacological) treatments. Children with DCD appear to be treated with SI, cognitive, and other approaches (such as perceptual–motor). The majority of the treatment literature is descriptive or opinion based in nature with only a few papers providing empirical evidence regarding the effectiveness of these treatment approaches.

One of the most commonly used treatment approaches for motor disorders in children is NDT. Although this approach is widely used in the clinical realm by both occupational therapists and physiotherapists, there is relatively little published research on its efficacy. The research articles exploring NDT reported no significant effects of increasing the intensity of NDT, and no significant improvement in reaching after 5 days of NDT (Fetters & Kluzik, 1996; Law et al., 1997). The descriptive literature focusing on the efficacy of NDT also provided no concrete evidence as several studies demonstrated no significant effects of NDT when applied to children with CP (DeGangi et al., 1983; Lilly & Powell, 1990). Therefore, there is a need for more valid and reliable empirical studies examining the usefulness of NDT for children with motor disorders.

Another treatment approach that is used by occupational therapists in treating motor disorders including CP and DCD is SI. According to a meta-analysis conducted by Pless and Carlsson (2000), the least effective treatment approach for the motor disorders seen in children with DCD was SI. Additional literature on the efficacy of SI was mostly of the opinion type (Chu, 1989) and therefore fails to lend any empirical support for the use of SI in the clinical environment.

The search for research studies of cognitive treatment approaches for children with motor disorders did not yield a large amount of literature, except in the area of DCD. The CO-OP approach has recently received increasing attention with regard to its success in improving these children's performance in daily tasks. The research article by Polatajko, Mandich, Missiuna, and colleagues (2001) detailed the studies that have been performed to validate CO-OP as a new and effective treatment approach for this disorder. Additional descriptive literature (Polatajko, Mandich, Missiuna, et al., 2001; Mandich, Polatajko, Macnab, & Miller, 2001; Mandich, Polatajko, Missiuna, & Miller, 2001) has provided more information on CO-OP and its application for children with DCD. A pilot RCT supports the Level III reports of the effectiveness of this approach.

In reference to conductive education, the majority of conductive education articles were opinion papers, although two research studies were found providing inconclusive evidence regarding the efficacy of this approach for children with CP. Given the intensive nature of this intervention and the expense required in training as a conductor, further empirical support is required before the use of this approach can be justified.

The compensatory studies covered a broad range of treatment interventions. The use of specialized equipment was typically combined with another treatment approach, making it difficult to draw any conclusions about the relative benefits of treatment components within this approach. There are limited empirical data on the use of compensatory approaches.

Exercise as a treatment modality for children with motor disorders has not received an overwhelming amount of attention. However, there are some research articles that provided some support for its use for children with CP and muscular dystrophy. Both treadmill training and general strength training produced general improvements in motor functioning and strength (Haney, 1998; Schindl et al., 2000). Further research is required to demonstrate the utility of this treatment modality.

Intervention for motor disorders in children remains controversial, as there is no proven best practice approach for any specific disorder. The results from this review challenge clinical practice due to the small number of empirical studies on interventions for children with developmental motor disorders. In those research studies identified, there was often a lack of rigorous experimental design leading to poor support for the use of NDT for children with CP, SI for children with DCD or conductive education for children with CP, and only mixed support for muscle strengthening exercise for children with CP or muscular dystrophy. There is a developing body of research to support the use of CO-OP as a cognitive intervention for children with DCD. Only one empirical study as an example of compensatory approaches was located and that was in relation to the use of orthopedic braces to prevent ongoing progression of scoliosis in children with spina bifida. The wide range of techniques used within the compensatory approach makes generalization of findings impossible. In conclusion, there is insufficient quality research to date to demonstrate conclusively best practices; however, some are more promising than others.

IMPLICATIONS FOR RESEARCHERS

The findings of this literature review indicate a great need for an increase in scientifically rigorous research studies that explore treatment approaches for children with developmental motor disorders. More rigorous empirical evidence is needed supporting the use or disuse of many of the treatment approaches that are widely employed by clinicians.

While many clinicians appear to use eclectic approaches for management of children with a range of developmental motor disorders, and some authors encourage therapeutic eclecticism (Chu, 1989), from a research perspective, it is impossible to determine the efficacy of combined approaches that, for example, incorporate components of SI and perceptual–motor. In addition, the results of treatment vary according to each individual, as there is no "typical child" with movement problems. The heterogeneous nature of these developmental motor disorders makes studying treatment outcome difficult. Therefore, there is a need for research studies that clearly indicate the nature of the treatment approach under investigation, that describe the duration and intensity of treatment, that clearly outline the subject characteristics and the inclusion and exclusion criteria for subject selection, and that use the most rigorous designs for studying treatment efficacy. RCTs remain the gold standard for efficacy studies. If treatment *A* is to be compared with treatment *B*, it is critical that each treatment is described as clearly as possible and that a "pure" form of the treatment under investigation is provided. There is also a need for prospective, longitudinal repeated measures designs that enable the researcher to determine the effect of the intervention over time.

IMPLICATIONS FOR CLINICIANS

Treatment for motor disorders is an area of significance for both families of children with movement problems and for clinicians. Children with motor disorders experience difficulty performing many activities that are central to engaging in the occupations of childhood. Depending on the type and severity of the disorder, children with movement problems may also experience secondary attentional, behavioral, and psychosocial difficulties that can further confound the treatment of the disorder (see Dewey, Crawford, Wilson, & Kaplan, Chapter 18, this volume). Throughout the literature the importance of parent/caregiver involvement in the management of conditions such as CP, TS, and DCD is emphasized. It is imperative that treatment encompasses a family-centered approach to ensure generalizability of skills learned from the treatment facility to the home and school environment.

It is difficult for clinicians to make confident decisions about which treatment approach to use when there is insufficient research evidence for treatment of various childhood motor disorders. As a result, clinicians must rely on their clinical experience and judgment, along with the individual client and family needs, to determine the best approach. As a clinician, it is essential that the treatment approach used is appropriate for the client. If a variety of approaches are combined in an effort to be holistic in treating children with motor disorders, it is important that clinicians clearly understand the theoretical underpinnings of each approach and its relative compatibility or lack of compatibility. This chapter has offered a classification of treatment approaches as either process-focused or performance-focused, as one way of differentiating the treatment approaches presented. Clinicians must also be mindful of the setting in which they provide services, the philosophy and experiences of other team members, and the expectations and requirements of their employers, as these external factors will have an impact on the type of treatment approach used. The present climate of consumer empowerment and economic restraint also means that clinicians must remain current in terms of the best evidence available regarding the efficacy of various treatment approaches in order to justify their treatment decisions to consumers and funding bodies alike.

REFERENCES

Adams, M. A., Chandler, L. S., Schuhmann, K. (2000). Gait changes in children with cerebral palsy following a neurodevelopmental treatment course. *Pediatric Physical Therapy, 12,* 114–120.

Bach, K., & McKeon, J. (1991). Orthopedic surgery and rehabilitation for the prolongation of brace-free ambulation of patients with Duchenne muscular dystrophy. *American Journal of Physical Medicine and Rehabilitation, 70,* 323–330.

Bailey, D. M. (1997). *Research for the health professional: A practical guide* (3rd ed.). Philadelphia: Davis.

Belanger, A., & Gilles, N. (1990). Compliance to and effects of a home strengthening exercise program for adult dystrophic patients: a pilot study. *Physiotherapy Canada, 43,* 24–30.

Bischof, F. M. (2001). An evidence-based review of hyperbaric oxygen for children with cerebral palsy. *South African Journal of Physiotherapy, 57,* 21–22.

Bly, L. (1991). A historical and current view of the basis of NDT. *Pediatric Physical Therapy, 3,* 131–135.

Boehme, R. (1988). *Improving upper body control: An approach to assessment and treatment of tonal dysfunction.* Tucson, AZ: Therapy Skill Builders.

Brown, G. T., & Burns, S. A. (2001). The efficacy of neurodevelopmental treatment in paediatrics: A systematic review. *British Journal of Occupational Therapy, 64,* 235–244.

Carr, J. E. (1995). Competing responses for the treatment of Tourette syndrome and tic disorders. *Behaviour Research and Therapy, 33,* 455–456.

Catanese, A. A., Coleman, G. J., King, J.A., & Reddihough, D. S. (1995). Evaluation of an early childhood programme based on principles of conductive education: The Yoralla project. *Journal of Paediatrics and Child Health, 31,* 418–422.

Chu, S. (1989). The application of contemporary treatment approaches in occupational therapy for children with cerebral palsy. *British Journal of Occupational Therapy, 52,* 343–348.

Collet, J. P., Vanasse, M., Marois, P., Amar, M., Goldberg, J., Lambert, J., et al. (2001). Hyperbaric oxygen for children with cerebral palsy: A randomized multicentre trial. *Lancet, 357,* 582–586.

Cottalorda, J., Gautheron, V., Metton, G., Charmet, E., & Chavrier, Y. (2000). Toe-walking in children younger than six years with cerebral palsy. *Journal of Bone and Joint Surgery, 82,* 541–544.

Damiano, D. L., & Abel, M. F. (1998). Functional outcomes of strength training in spastic cerebral palsy. *Archives of Physical Medicine and Rehabilitation, 79,* 119–126.

Davidson, T., & Williams, B. (2000). Occupational therapy for children with developmental co-ordination disorder: A study of the effectiveness of a combined sensory integration and perceptual-motor intervention. *British Journal of Occupational Therapy, 63,* 495–499.

De Gangi, G. A., Hurley, L., & Linscheid, T. R. (1983). Toward a methodology of the short-term effects of neurodevelopmental treatment. *American Journal of Occupational Therapy, 37,* 479–484.

Dodick, D., & Adler, C. H. (1992). Tourette's syndrome. Current approaches to recognition and management. *Postgraduate Medicine, 92,* 299–307.

Eigsti, H., Aretz, M., & Shannon, L. (1990). Pediatric physical therapy in a rehabilitation setting. *Pediatrician, 17,* 267–77.

Fetters, L., & Kluzik, J. (1996). The effect on Tourette syndrome of neurodevelopmental treatment versus practice on the reaching of children with spastic cerebral palsy. *Physical Therapy, 76,* 346–357.

Foster, M. (1996). Theoretical frameworks. In A. Turner, M. Foster, & S. E. Johnson (Eds.), *Occupational therapy for physical dysfunction. Principles, skills and practice* (pp. 27–59). New York: Churchill Livingstone.

Haerle, J. (Ed.). (1992). *Children with Tourette syndrome: A parents' guide.* Rockville, MD: Woodbine House.

Haney, N. B. (1998). Muscle strengthening in children with cerebral palsy. *Physical and Occupational Therapy in Pediatrics, 18,* 149–157.

Hedges, K. (1988). The Bobath and conductive education approaches to cerebral palsy treatment-management and education models. *New Zealand Journal of Physiotherapy, 16,* 6–12.

Hinojosa, J., Kramer, P., & Pratt P. (1998). Foundations of practice: developmental principles, theories, and frames of reference. In J. Case-Smith, A. Allen, & P. Pratt (Eds.), *Occupational therapy for children* (pp. 25–45). St. Louis, MO: Mosby.

Holm, M. B. (2000). The 2000 Eleanor Clarke Slagle Lecture: Our mandate for the new millennium: Evidence-based practice. *American Journal of Occupational Therapy, 54,* 575–585.

Jadad, A. R., Moore, R. A., Carroll, D., Jenkinson, C., Reynolds, J. M., Gavaghan, D. J., et al. (1996). Assessing the quality of reports of randomised clinical trials: Is blinding necessary? *Controlled Clinical Trials, 17,* 1–12.

Ketelaar, M., Vermeer, A., 't Hart, H., van Petegem-van Beek, E., & Helders, P. J. M. (2001). Effects of a functional therapy program on motor abilities of children with cerebral palsy. *Physical Therapy, 81*, 1534–1545.

Law, M., Russell, D., Pollack, N., Rosenbaum, P., Walter, S., & King, G. (1997). A comparison of intensive neurodevelopmental therapy plus casting and a regular occupational therapy program for children with cerebral palsy. *Developmental Medicine and Child Neurology, 39*, 664–670.

Lilly, L. A., & Powell, N. J. (1990). Measuring the effects of neurodevelopmental treatment on the daily living skills of 2 children with cerebral palsy. *American Journal of Occupational Therapy, 44*, 139–145.

Lindeman, E., Leffers, P., Spaans, F., Drukker, J., Reulen, J., & Kerckhoffs, M., et al. (1995). Strength training in patients with myotonic dystrophy and hereditary motor and sensory neuropathy: a randomized clinical trial. *Archives of Physical Medicine and Rehabilitation, 76*, 612–619.

Mandich, A. D., Polatajko, H. J., Macnab, J. J., & Miller, L. T. (2001). Treatment of children with Developmental Coordination Disorder: What is the evidence? *Physical and Occupational Therapy in Pediatrics, 20*, 51–68.

Mandich, A. D., Polatajko, H. J., Missiuna C., & Miller, L. T. (2001). Cognitive strategies and motor performance in children with developmental coordination disorder. *Physical and Occupational Therapy in Pediatrics, 20*, 125–143.

Manella, E., & Varni, J. (1981). Behavior therapy in a gait-training program for a child with myelomeningocele. *Physical Therapy, 61*, 1284–1287.

Mayston, M. J. (2000). Compensating for CNS dysfunction. *Physiotherapy, 86*, 612.

Mayston, M. J. (2001, Spring). The Bobath concept today. *Synapse*, pp. 32–34.

Miles-Breslin, D. M. (1996). Motor learning theory and the neurodevelopmental treatment approach: A comparative analysis. *Occupational Therapy in Health Care, 10*, 25–40.

Miller, L., Missiuna, C., Macnab, J., Malloy-Miller T., & Polatajko, H. (2001). Clinical description of children with developmental coordination disorder. *Canadian Journal of Occupational Therapy, 68*, 5–15.

Miller, L. T., Polatajko, H. J., Missiuna, C., Mandich, A. D. & Macnab, J. J. (2001). A pilot trial of a cognitive treatment for children with developmental coordination disorder. *Human Movement Science, 20*, 183–210.

Milner-Brown, H. S., & Miller, R. G. (1988a). Muscle strengthening through electric stimulation combined with low-resistance weights in patients with neuromuscular disorders. *Archives of Physical Medicine and Rehabilitation, 69*, 14–19.

Milner-Brown, H. S., & Miller, R. G. (1988b). Muscle strengthening through high-resistance weight training in patients with neuromuscular disorders. *Archives of Physical Medicine and Rehabilitation, 69*, 14–18.

Muller, E. B., & Nordwall, A. (1994). Brace treatment of scoliosis in children with myelomeningocele. *Spine, 19*, 151–155.

Mulligan, H., Climo, K., Hanson, C., & Mauga, P. (2000). Physiotherapy treatment intensity for a child with cerebral palsy: A single case study. *New Zealand Journal of Physiotherapy, 28*, 6–12.

O'Quinn, A. N., & Thompson, R. J. (1980). Tourette's syndrome: An expanded view. *Pediatrics, 66*, 420–423.

Parham, C., & Mailloux, Z. (1998). Sensory Integration. In J. Case-Smith, A. Allen, & P. Pratt (Eds.), *Occupational therapy for children* (pp. 307–352). St. Louis, MO: Mosby.

Parker, K. (1985). Helping school age children cope with Tourette Syndrome. *Journal of School Health, 55*, 30–32.

Pless, M., & Carlsson, M. (2000). Effects of motor skill intervention on developmental coordination disorder: A meta-analysis. *Adapted Physical Activity Quarterly, 17*, 381–401.

Polatajko, H., & Mandich, A. (2004). *Enabling occupation in children: The Cognitive Orientation to Daily Occupational Performance (CO-OP) approach.* Ottowa: CAOT Publications.

Polatajko, H., Mandich, A., Miller, L., & Macnab, J. (2001). Cognitive orientation to daily occupational performance (CO-OP): Part II—The evidence. *Physical and Occupational Therapy in Pediatrics, 20,* 83–106.

Polatajko, H., Mandich, A., Missiuna, C., Miller, L., Macnab, J., Malloy-Miller, T., et al. (2001). Cognitive orientation to daily occupational performance (CO-OP): Part III—The protocol in brief. *Physical and Occupational Therapy in Pediatrics, 20,* 107–123.

Portela, A. L. (1990). Lower extremity casting in the treatment of cerebral palsy. *Physical and Occupational Therapy in Pediatrics, 10,* 121–132.

Reddihough, D. S., King, J., Coleman, G., & Catanese, T. (1998). Efficacy of programmes based on conductive education for young children with cerebral palsy. *Developmental Medicine and Child Neurology, 40,* 763–770.

Robertson, M. M. (2000). Invited review: Tourette syndrome, associated conditions and the complexities of treatment. *Brain, 123,* 426–462.

Robinson, R. O., McCarthy, O. T., & Little, T. M. (1989). Conductive education at the Peto Institute, Budapest. *British Medical Journal, 299,* 1145–1149.

Sackett, D. L. (1989). Rules of evidence and clinical recommendations on the use of antithrombotic agents. *Chest, 95*(2, Suppl.), 2S–4S.

Schindl, M. R., Forstner, C., Kern, H., & Hesse, S. (2000). Treadmill training with partial body weight support in nonambulatory patients with cerebral palsy. *Archives of Physical Medicine and Rehabilitation, 81,* 301–306.

Sommerfelt, K., Markestad, T., Berg, K., & Saetesdal, I. (2001). Therapeutic electrical stimulation in cerebral palsy: A randomized controlled cross-over trial. *Developmental Medicine and Child Neurology, 43,* 609–613.

Stanton, M. (1997). *Cerebral palsy handbook: A practical guide for parents and carers.* London: Vermillion.

Sugden, D. A., & Keogh, J. F. (1990). *Problems in movement skill development.* Columbia: University of South Carolina Press.

Suputtitada, A. (2000). Managing spasticity in pediatric cerebral palsy using a very low does of Botulunum toxin type A. *American Journal of Physical Medicine and Rehabilitation, 79,* 320–326.

Tollback, A., Eriksson, S., Wredenberg, R., Jenner, G., Vargas, R., Borg, K., et al. (1999). Effects of high resistance training in patients with myotonic dystrophy. *Scandinavian Journal of Rehabilitative Medicine, 31,* 9–16.

Tolchard, B. (1995). Treatment of Gilles de la Tourette Syndrome using behavioural psychotherapy: A single case example. *Journal of Psychiatric and Mental Health Nursing, 2,* 233–236.

Whiteside, A. (1997, September–October). Clinical goals and application of NDT facilitation. *NDTA Network,* pp. 1–14.

Wright, P. A., & Granat, M. H. (2000). Therapeutic effects of functional electrical stimulation of the upper limb of eight children with cerebral palsy. *Developmental Medicine and Child Neurology, 42,* 724–727.

Yablon, S. A. (2001). Botulinum neurotoxin intramuscular chemodenervation: Role in the management of spastic hypertonia and related motor disorders. *Physical Medicine and Rehabilitation Clinics of North America, 12,* 833–874.

Index